T0293723

Fc Receptors and their Antibodies: Role in Disease and Immunotherapy

Fc Receptors and their Antibodies: Role in Disease and Immunotherapy

Editor: Remy Nelson

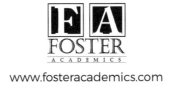

www.fosteracademics.com

www.fosteracademics.com

Cataloging-in-Publication Data

Fc receptors and their antibodies : role in disease and immunotherapy / edited by Remy Nelson.
    p. cm.
Includes bibliographical references and index.
ISBN 978-1-64646-603-0
1. Fc receptors. 2. Immunoglobulins. 3. Immune response. 4. Immunotherapy.
5. Immune response--Regulation. I. Nelson, Remy.
QR185.8.F33 F373 2023
616.079--dc23

© Foster Academics, 2023

Foster Academics,
118-35 Queens Blvd., Suite 400,
Forest Hills, NY 11375, USA

ISBN 978-1-64646-603-0 (Hardback)

This book contains information obtained from authentic and highly regarded sources. Copyright for all individual chapters remain with the respective authors as indicated. All chapters are published with permission under the Creative Commons Attribution License or equivalent. A wide variety of references are listed. Permission and sources are indicated; for detailed attributions, please refer to the permissions page and list of contributors. Reasonable efforts have been made to publish reliable data and information, but the authors, editors and publisher cannot assume any responsibility for the validity of all materials or the consequences of their use.

Trademark Notice: Registered trademark of products or corporate names are used only for explanation and identification without intent to infringe.

Contents

Preface

Fc receptor is a protein which is present on the surface of cells such as macrophages, B lymphocytes, mast cells, neutrophils, basophils and human platelets. Fc receptors allow the cells to connect with antibodies which are attached to the microbe's surface, and help the cells in identifying and eliminating the pathogens. Antibodies (Ab) protect against infectious agents by binding to pathogens and preventing their entry into target cells. They also facilitate the recruitment of Fc-receptor bearing cells that can eliminate pathogens or infected cells by mediating phagocytosis or cytotoxic activity known as Fc-mediated functions. Antibodies can be classified as neutralizing (nAb) antibodies and non-neutralizing (non-nAb) antibodies. Neutralizing (nAb) antibodies can mediate both functions and non-neutralizing (non-nAb) antibodies are limited to Fc-mediated functions. Non-nAb plays an important role in providing protection against a variety of viral infections, including smallpox, sindbis, yellow fever, ebola, and influenza. It also provides protection from non-viral infections such as tuberculosis and malaria. This book provides comprehensive insights on Fc receptors and their antibodies, as well as their role in disease and immunotherapy. It will serve as a reference to a broad spectrum of readers.

All of the data presented henceforth, was collaborated in the wake of recent advancements in the field. The aim of this book is to present the diversified developments from across the globe in a comprehensible manner. The opinions expressed in each chapter belong solely to the contributing authors. Their interpretations of the topics are the integral part of this book, which I have carefully compiled for a better understanding of the readers.

At the end, I would like to thank all those who dedicated their time and efforts for the successful completion of this book. I also wish to convey my gratitude towards my friends and family who supported me at every step.

Editor

Induction of Fc-Mediated Effector Functions Against a Stabilized Inner Domain of HIV-1 gp120 Designed to Selectively Harbor the A32 Epitope Region

Maria L. Visciano[†], Neelakshi Gohain[†], Rebekah Sherburn, Chiara Orlandi, Robin Flinko, Amir Dashti, George K. Lewis, William D. Tolbert and Marzena Pazgier[*‡]

Division of Vaccine Research of Institute of Human Virology, University of Maryland School of Medicine, Baltimore, MD, United States

*Correspondence:
Marzena Pazgier
marzena.pazgier@usuhs.edu

[†] *These authors have contributed equally to this work*

[‡] **Present Address:**
Marzena Pazgier, Infectious Disease Division of Department of Medicine of Uniformed Services of University of the Health Sciences, Bethesda, MD, United States

Recent clinical trials and studies using nonhuman primates (NHPs) suggest that antibody-mediated protection against HIV-1 will require α-HIV envelope humoral immunity beyond direct neutralization to include Fc-receptor (FcR) mediated effector functions such as antibody-dependent cellular cytotoxicity (ADCC). There is also strong evidence indicating that the most potent ADCC response in humans is directed toward transitional non-neutralizing epitopes associated with the gp41-interactive face of gp120, particularly those within the first and second constant (C1–C2) region (A32-like epitopes). These epitopes were shown to be major targets of ADCC responses during natural infection and have been implicated in vaccine-induced protective immunity. Here we describe the immunogenicity of ID2, an immunogen consisting of the inner domain of the clade A/E 93TH057 HIV-1 gp120 expressed independently of the outer domain (OD) and stabilized in the CD4-bound conformation to harbor conformational A32 region epitopes within a minimal structural unit of HIV-1 Env. ID2 induced A32-specific antibody responses in BALB/c mice when injected alone or in the presence of the adjuvants Alum or GLA-SE. Low α-ID2 titers were detected in mice immunized with ID2 alone whereas robust responses were observed with ID2 plus adjuvant, with the greatest ID2 and A32-specific titers observed in the GLA-SE group. Only sera from groups immunized in the presence of GLA-SE were capable of mediating significant ADCC using NKr cells sensitized with recombinant BaL gp120 as targets and human PBMCs as effectors. A neutralization response to a tier 2 virus was not observed. Altogether, our studies demonstrate that ID2 is highly immunogenic and elicits A32-specific ADCC responses in an animal host. The ID2 immunogen has significant translational value as it can be used in challenge studies to evaluate the role of non-neutralizing antibodies directed at the A32 subregion in HIV-1 protection.

Keywords: HIV envelope, ID (Inner domain) immunogen, ADCC (Antibody dependent cellular cytotoxicity), A32 epitope, Fc-mediated effector function

INTRODUCTION

The design of immunogens which induce broadly protective antibody responses against human immunodeficiency virus type 1 (HIV-1) is a major goal of HIV-1 vaccine development. This goal is formidable as HIV-1 evades immune surveillance via a number of escape mechanisms (1–3). Over the last few years neutralizing humoral responses have been observed to overcome some of these obstacles and provide protection in a subpopulation of chronically infected individuals (1, 4–9). Despite the significant progress in identification and characterization of broadly neutralizing antibodies (bnAbs) there are still multiple, challenging obstacles in the design of a successful candidate immunogen which, when coupled with appropriate immunization strategies, can induce effective neutralizing responses *in vivo* (10). These challenges are primarily linked to the unusual structural features associated bnAbs; such as the long complementary determining region 3 (CDR H3) and the high level of somatic mutation of the variable (V) domain. The frequency of B cells for these unusual antibodies is very low and the time required for their full development from progenitors is remarkably long (11), making them very complex candidates for vaccine design.

By contrast, less is known about mechanisms of vaccine induced humoral responses that act solely through Fc-mediated effector functions, including antibody-dependent cell-mediated cytotoxicity (ADCC). Epitopes involved solely in Fc-mediated processes are usually exposed late during viral entry and are thus targeted by antibodies that lack direct neutralizing activity. One group of these potent ADCC targets constitute the CD4-inducible (CD4i) epitopes within the gp120 molecule, referred to as Cluster A epitopes (12–16). These epitopes become exposed on the target cell surface during viral entry after envelope trimers engage the host CD4 receptor and they persist on newly infected cell surfaces for extended periods of time (17–20), reviewed in (21–23). They are also expressed at the surface of infected cells, but only in cell populations that retain some levels of the CD4 receptor which is required for triggering envelope trimers on budding virions (15, 16, 23). We recently isolated and characterized, at the molecular level, the complexes of CD4-triggered gp120 with a number of monoclonal antibodies (mAbs) known to be capable of potent Fc-receptor mediated function from memory B cells of HIV-1 infected individuals that recognize the A32-like epitope within the Cluster A epitope region (14, 24, 25). Based on these studies, we mapped the A32 epitope into the highly conserved constant regions 1 and 2 (C1–C2) of the gp120 inner domain in the CD4-bound conformation. We also found that A32-like antibodies differ significantly from those involved in neutralization as they mostly possess moderate length CDR H3 loops and low degrees of V affinity maturation and therefore bypass the frequently observed somatic hypermutation hurdle in eliciting a protective antibody response (12, 26, 27). The high sequence conservation of the A32 epitope among different HIV isolates indicates the possibility that ADCC responses specific for this epitope region may be cross-reactive and multiple strains would therefore undergo limited immune escape. Indeed, the recent vaccination strategy tested in the RV144 vaccine trial

partially confirmed these predictions. A32-like responses were induced with the RV144 vaccine and ADCC responses directed to the A32 epitope region were implicated in its protective effect (28). In the absence of IgA responses, ADCC correlated with a reduced infection risk (29, 30) with a very narrow array of antibody specificities involved in the protective effect. RV144 ADCC specificities included the linear epitopes in the V2 loop region (31) and the CD4-inducible conformational epitopes within the A32 region (32, 33), confirmed by blocking the plasma ADCC activity with the A32 Fab (32). Furthermore, most ADCC mAbs (19 of 23) isolated from vaccine recipients targeted multiple related but distinct conformational epitopes in the A32 region (31, 32). These antibodies displayed low levels of V_H chain somatic mutation (0.5–1.5%) and mediated cross-clade ADCC activity; clade B and CRF01 AE, as well as clade C, which was not represented in the vaccine (32); a canarypox ALVAC prime with the E.92TH023 gp120 membrane anchored insert and an AIDSVAX B/E gp120 boost.

Here we describe the immunogenicity of a gp120 sub domain immunogen, referred to as ID2, designed by our group to stimulate humoral responses involving solely FcR-effector mechanisms designed to elicit an ADCC response in the absence of a neutralizing response (34). ID2 consists of the inner domain (ID) of the clade A/E HIV-1 gp120 93TH057 isolate and was made to confer the minimal structural unit of gp120 stably presenting the non-neutralizing epitopes in the A32 region without any other known epitopes present (34). When injected into BALB/c mice, ID2 was able to elicit cross-clade A32-like antibody responses with ADCC activities against $gp120_{BaL}$ coated cells.

MATERIALS AND METHODS

ID2 Immunogen Expression and Purification

A HEK 293 cell line stably expressing the ID2 immunogen was generated using the plasmid previously used for transient protein production, as in (34). Freestyle 293 medium (Gibco) from cells grown for 6–7 days (8% CO2 at 37°C in shaker flasks rotating at 145 rpm) after inoculation (1 × 10⁶ cells/ml) was collected and passed through a 0.45 μm filter. ID2 was purified from the media using an N5-i5 IgG affinity column, which was made by coupling N5-i5 IgG to protein A resin using the Pierce protein A IgG plus orientation kit (Thermo Fisher Sci.). Media was passed over the column after equilibration in phosphate buffered saline (PBS) pH 7.2. The column was washed with 5–10 column volumes of PBS pH 7.2 and ID2 protein eluted with 0.1 M glycine pH 3.0. Elution fractions were concentrated and dialyzed against PBS pH 7.2 prior to use in animal studies.

Immunization and Blood Collections

BALB/c mice were purchased from The Jackson Laboratory and housed in the animal facility managed by BIOQUAL's, Inc., Rockville, MD. The mice were cared for in accordance with the Association for the Assessment and Accreditation of Laboratory Animal Care International (AAALAC) standards and all procedures involving animals were approved by the University

Committee on Use and Care of Animals (UCUCA) of BIOQUAL, Inc. 6–8 weeks old BALB/c mice (male and female, 6 animals per group) were immunized at week 0, 2, 4, and 8 via IP injections of 20 μg of ID2 protein in different adjuvants. The control group received ID2 immunogen in PBS and two adjuvants were also trialed; ID2 immunogen in Alum (2% aluminum hydroxide wet gel suspension, InvivoGen, Catalog # vac-alu-250), and ID2 immunogen in GLA-SE adjuvant (stable oil-in water emulsion containing TLR-4 agonist developed by Infectious Disease Research Institute, Catalog # IDRI-GLA-SE, known also under the name EM082). Serum samples were collected prior to immunization and 2 weeks after each immunization according to the scheme shown in **Figure 1**.

Detection of Serum Immunoglobulin Specific for ID2

The presence and titers of total IgG, IgG1, IgG2a, IgG2b or IgG2c, IgG3, IgA, and IgM antibodies, specific for ID2 recombinant protein in sera of immunized mice were determined by an Enzyme Linked Immunosorbent Assay (ELISA) using a 100-μL-per-well volume format. Blocking Buffer (Tris-buffered saline (TBS; 10 mM Tris and 100 mM NaCl; pH 8.0) with 5% no fat dry milk and 0.1% Nonidet P-40) was used as blocking solution and as diluting solution for sera and detecting Abs. TBS-T buffer (TBS with 0.1% Tween-20) was used as washing solution. ELISAs were performed as follows: ID2 recombinant protein (0.5 μg/ml) was adsorbed onto ELISA plates (Immunoblot 2HB Thermo, Milford, MA) overnight at 4°C. The plates were washed three times and incubated with 100 μl blocking buffer per well for 2 h at room temperature. Serially diluted sera, beginning at 1:100, were then added and allowed to react with the coated antigen for 2 h at 37°C. Sera was removed, the plates washed, and alkaline phosphatase-conjugated goat anti-mouse IgG (Sigma cat#A3562), IgG1, IgG2a, IgG2b, IgG2c, and IgG3 (SouthernBiotech cat# 1071-04, 1081-04, 1091-04, 1078-04, 1103-04, respectively), IgA and IgM antibodies (SouthernBiotech cat #1040-04 and 1021-04, respectively) diluted 1:1000 in blocking buffer, were added followed by incubation for 1 h at 37°C. After removal of unbound antibody and washing, the Blue Phos Microwell Phosphatase Substrate System (KPL 50–88-00) was used as a substrate to quantitate bound antibody. After 15 min incubation at room temperature, the reaction was stopped using APstop Solution (KPL 50-89-00) and the optical density was read on a microplate reader (SpectraMax Paradigm Multi-Mode Detection Platform Molecular Devices) at 620 nm. The anti-ID2 antibody half-max binding serum titer was calculated using a Microsoft Excel iteration formula.

Competition ELISAs

To determine if the immunization with ID2 immunogen had induced Cluster A like serum Abs, sera from the terminal bleed were tested for their ability to compete with Cluster A mAbs (A32, N5-i5) for the binding to ID2 in an ELISA setting. Plates were coated o/n at 4°C with 0.5 μg/ml of ID2. Ten-fold serial dilutions of immune sera and pre-immunization sera were mixed 1:1 with biotinylated human CD4i anti-envelope mAb at a concentration correspondent to the half max binding

concentrations for each tested mAb; 0.66 μg/mL of A32 and 0.2 μg/ml of N5-i5. The mixtures were then added to previously washed and blocked plates. As a control, a 10-fold dilution of unbiotinylated CD4i mAbs A32 and N5-i5, starting at 10 μg/mL, were tested in the same assay. Sera and Abs were prepared as 2x solutions. After 2 h incubation at r.t. assay wells were washed and incubated with avidin-AP (Invitrogen 1:1,000 dilution) and then with the Blue Phos Microwell Phosphatase Substrate System. Biotinylated-mAb binding was determined by measuring absorbance at 620 nm. Competition percentage was calculated using GraphPad Prism as follows: 0% inhibition was defined as the mean OD value of the lowest serial dilution of the pre-immunization sera ($1:10^6$) while 100% inhibition was defined as the mean OD value of the highest concentration tested for unbiotinylated mAbs A32 and N5-i5 (10 μg/ml).

Sera Reactivity With Denatured ID2 Protein

To assess if immunization with ID2 recombinant protein elicited serum antibodies recognizing conformational epitopes on ID2, pooled sera collected 2 weeks after the last immunization were incubated in solution o/n at 4°C with 1 μg/mL of denatured ID2. ID2 recombinant protein denaturation was performed as previously described in Moore et al. (35), with little modification. Briefly ID2 protein (final concentration 200 μg/ml) was mixed with 10 mM DTT, 0.1% SDS (Sigma-Aldrich), 0.1% FBS (GIBCO-Termo Fisher Scientific), and incubated at 70°C for 10 min. After incubation, the denatured protein was diluted 1:10 in TBS and stored at −20°C until used. The mixtures of denatured protein and pooled sera were then added to a plate coated with ID2. Pooled sera from each group were used as a control. Goat anti-mouse IgG Alkaline Phosphatase conjugated was used as secondary Ab. Plates were read at 620 nM after addition of Blue Phos Microwell Phosphatase Substrate System as previously described.

Antibody-Dependent Cell-Mediated Cytotoxicity (ADCC)

The ADCC activity of immunoglobulins present in mouse sera collected at week 10 were tested with the optimized rapid fluorometric antibody-dependent cellular cytotoxicity (RFADCC) assay (36). Briefly, EGFP-CEM-NKr-CCR5SNAP cells sensitized with recombinant BaL gp120 were used as targets and human PBMCs were utilized as effectors. Sera were serially diluted three-fold starting at 1:100 through 1:1,968,300 together with control mAbs (N5-i5-positive and Synagis-negative controls). After 2 h of incubation the samples were fixed and collected (at approximately 20,000 events per sample) on a Fortessa Special Order instrument (BD Biosciences) and analyzed using FlowJo software (Tree Star, Ashland, OR). ADCC activity (shown as % cytotoxicity) was defined as the percentage of EGFP-CEM-NKr-CCR5-SNAP target cells that lost GFP staining but retained the CCR5-SNAP tag staining. The results represent the average of the samples tested in triplicate and normalized to the N5-i5 positive control. Max lysis was defined as the maximum percent lysis at any sera concentration. Ec_{50} was determined using a GraphPad prism formula of Log(agonist) vs. Normalized response for a variable slope.

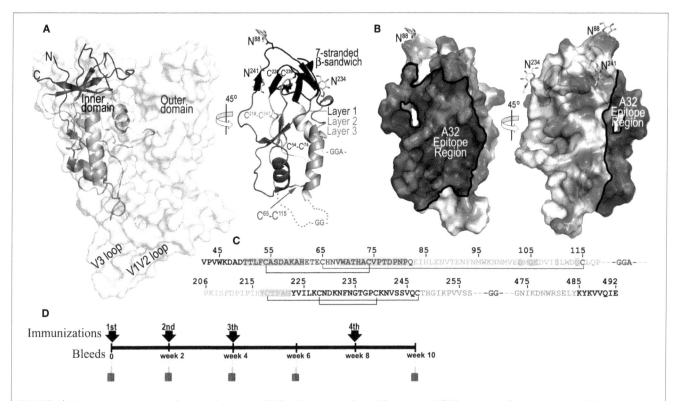

FIGURE 1 | ID2 immunogen design and immunization scheme. **(A)** Putative and crystallographic structure of ID2 immunogen. Putative structure of ID2 is shown overlaid over the structure of full length gp120 from the CD4-triggered BG505 SOSIP trimer (PDB code:1U1F) and a 45° rotation shows the crystal structure of ID2 immunogen from the ID2-Fab A32 complex structure (PDB code:4YC2). "Layered" architecture of gp120 inner domain is shown with the 7-stranded β-sandwich colored black, layer 1 in blue, layer 2 in cyan, layer 3 in light orange. The C^{65}-C^{115} disulfide bond introduced to stabilize ID2 in the CD4-bound conformation and GGA(GG)-linkers are shown in red. Sugars at positions 88, 234, and 241 are shown as sticks. The region of ID2 disordered in the ID2-Fab A32 complex are show as broken lines. **(B)** The A32 epitope region in the context of ID2 immunogen. The gp120 residues involved in binding of A32 and A32-like antibodies N5-i5, 2.2c, N60-i3, JR4 are highlighted in black over the ID2 molecule. The molecular surface is displayed over the ID2 molecule and the electrostatic potential is shown as red for negative, blue for positive, and white for apolar. **(C)** Primary sequence of the ID2 construct (from gp120 sequence of clade A/E 93TH057 isolate) with disulfide bonds and –GG—linkers shown. Residues forming the A32 epitope region are highlighted in gray. **(D)** Schematic of immunization protocol.

Neutralization Assay

Mouse sera collected 2 weeks after the 4th immunization and pre-immune sera, were tested in a TZM-bl assay for the presence of neutralizing antibodies. Briefly, 3-fold serial dilution (starting from 1/100 dilution) of sera were mixed with JR-FL pseudo-virus (TCID of 45000 Relative Luminescence Unit) and incubated at 37°C in 5% CO_2 atmosphere for 60 min at room temperature. TZM-bl cells (10,000/well in complete RPMI with 11 μg/mL DEAE-Dextran) were then added to the sera-pseudo virus mix and plates were incubated for 48 h at 37°C in 5% CO_2 atmosphere. One hundred and Fifty Microliter of supernatant were removed and 100 μL/well of BrightGlo was then added to each well and after a 2 min incubation to allow complete cell lysis, 100μL from each well was transferred to 96 well black plates. Plates were read with a luminometer using the Promega BrightGlo program. Percent neutralization was determined by calculating the difference in average relative luminescence units (RLU) between virus control (no serum/antibody) and test wells (cells + serum or antibody sample + virus), dividing this result by the difference in average RLU between virus control (cell + virus) and cell only wells, and multiplying by 100.

Statistical Analysis

Differences in responses between ID2 alone, ID2+Alum, and ID2+GLA-SE were analyzed using a Two-way ANOVA with Bonferroni post-test comparing every sample to every other sample. All statistical analysis was carried out using GraphPad Prism (Version 5 for Windows, San Diego, CA, USA). ****represents statistical significance of $P < 0.0001$, ***$P < 0.001$, **$P < 0.01$, and *$P < 0.05$. Blue stars represent the difference between ID2 alone and ID2 + Alum, red stars represent differences between ID2 alone and ID2 + GLA-SE and purple stars represent differences between ID2 + Alum and ID2 + GLA-SE.

RESULTS

ID2 as an Immunogen Candidate Selectively and Stably Presents the A32 Region

ID2 was designed to stably present the conformational CD4-inducable epitopes of the A32 region within a minimal structural unit of gp120 without any other known (neutralizing or non-neutralizing) epitopes present (34). The design of ID2 was guided by detailed analysis of the epitope structures of A32 and several A32-like antibodies (14, 24, 25) that involve the Env antigen binding residues exclusively within the gp120 inner domain of the constant regions 1 and 2 (C1–C2). Through several steps of structure-guided design we obtained a construct consisting of only 154 residues of the gp120 inner domain which is stabilized in the CD4-bound conformation by the addition of a C_{65}-C_{115} disulfide bond (**Figures 1A–C**). In the ID2 construct the outer domain, variable loops and receptor binding sites were removed to form a minimal structural unit which engrafts only the A32 epitope region. **Figures 1A,B** show the putative and crystallographic structure of ID2, determined previously in a complex with the Fab of the A32 antibody. ID2 constitutes only one third of the full length gp120 molecule with the A32 epitope region mapping to almost half of the ID2 surface. In addition, a significant area of the ID2 face which does not harbor the A32 epitope is masked by N-glycosylation (asparagines at positions 88, 234, and 241) most likely rendering this part of molecule immunologically silent (**Figures 1B,C**). We showed previously that ID2 is folded to fully preserve the conformation of the inner domain as seen in the context of CD4-triggered gp120 and stably presents the functional A32 epitopes within the C1–C2 region and thus constitutes a novel immunogen candidate for selective induction of A32-like responses (34).

To evaluate if ID2 indeed is capable of selective induction of humoral response to the desired A32 region we performed immunogenicity studies using the recombinant preparation of ID2 obtained by mammalian cell culture (to preserve wild-type glycosylation) and BALB/c mice as an animal host. Purified ID2 protein, 20 µg per injection, was used to immunize groups of mice (6 animals per group) in the absence of adjuvant (in PBS) and with two adjuvant choices; Alum (2% aluminum hydroxide wet gel suspension) and GLA-SE (a stable oil-in water emulsion containing TLR-4 agonist adjuvant developed by Infectious Disease Research Institute). Immunizations were done according to the immunization scheme shown in **Figure 1D** with three immunizations in 2-week intervals and a fourth at week 8. Sera was collected 2 weeks after each immunization and analyzed individually for each mouse.

Immunization With Recombinant ID2 Protein Induced Specific Anti-ID2 Responses in BALB/c Mice

Sera collected 2 weeks after each immunization were tested in a sandwich ELISA to assess the presence of specific anti-ID2 serum antibodies. As shown in **Figures 2A–D**, immunization with ID2 with and without adjuvant elicited an anti-ID2 humoral immune response in all immunized mice, although with significant differences among the 3 immunization groups. Some mice immunized with ID2 without adjuvant developed a weak anti-ID2 specific humoral immune response with a half max binding titers above 1:500, but only after the 4th immunization (**Figure 2E**). In contrast, titers and kinetics of the humoral immune response was quite different in mice immunized with ID2 delivered alongside Alum or GLA-SE adjuvants. In both groups the immunization induced a detectable specific humoral immune response after the 1st immunization, however, only mice injected with ID2+Alum had higher levels of specific IgG compared to ID2 injected alone (**Figure 2A**). After 2 and 3 injections, both adjuvants induced significant levels of ID2-specific IgG above mice injected with ID2 alone (**Figures 2B,C**) and following the final injection, specific IgG levels were significantly higher in the GLA-SE adjuvant group compared to the Alum group (**Figure 2D**). For mice immunized in GLA-SE, all sera showed an enhancement in the anti-ID2 specific antibody immune response from 1 to 2 logs after each immunization with half-max binding titers ranging from 1:3,400 to 1:36,000 after the 4th immunization (**Figures 2D,E**). Altogether, these results clearly indicate that recombinant protein ID2 is immunogenic and that such immunogenicity can be improved by administrating the recombinant protein in combination with an adjuvant. As for the adjuvant, our data clearly suggested that mice immunized with ID2 in GLA-SE produced higher titers of anti-ID2 serum antibodies.

Immunization With ID2 Immunogen Induces an Antibody Response Specific for the Conformational Epitopes Within the A32 Region

By design ID2 consists of two faces; a face that harbors the conformational epitopes of the A32 region and a face that is exposed by the removal of the OD which does not have any known epitope targets. Although the epitopes within the newly exposed face are not known, this face might harbor epitopes that are rendered immunodominant by their exposure. To assess if the antibody response induced by ID2 is indeed specific for the desired A32 epitope region we tested sera collected after the final immunization in a competition ELISA with mAb A32 and the A32-like antibody N5-i5 (14). Our assay format was designed to detect if serum antibodies inhibited the binding of mAb A32 or N5-i5 to the recombinant ID2 protein immobilized on microplates. As shown in **Figures 3A,B**, the immune sera of mice immunized with ID2 alone were not able to inhibit the binding of the tested mAbs to the coated ID2 protein. In contrast, mice immunized either with ID2 in Alum or in GLA-SE elicited antibodies capable of blocking A32 (**Figure 3A**) and N5-i5 (**Figure 3B**) at a significantly higher level than sera from mice injected with ID2 alone. Sera from mice immunized with the GLA-SE adjuvant inhibited the binding of over 80% of both N5-i5 and A32, significantly higher than mice injected in the presence of Alum. These data indicate that immunization with ID2 leads to elicitation of a serum antibody response specific for Env targets that overlap with epitopes recognized by the A32 region antibodies A32 and N5-i5 with the adjuvant GLA-SE eliciting the most robust humoral responses.

Next, we asked if the elicited antibody responses were directed toward conformational or linear epitopes within the ID2 immunogen. Pooled sera collected after the final immunization were incubated in solution with denatured ID2 (dID2) protein

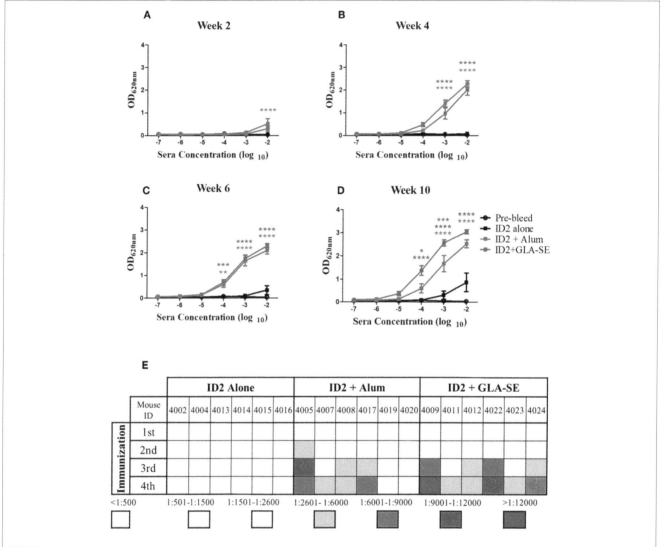

FIGURE 2 | Kinetics and titers of anti-ID2 immune response in immunized mice. Sera collected 2 weeks after each immunization were tested in ELISA for the presence of anti-ID2 specific immune responses (total αID2 IgG). Each sample was assayed in duplicate, displayed is the Mean ± SEM of the 6 mice in each group for **(A)** Week 2, **(B)** Week 4, **(C)** Week 6, and **(D)** Week 10. **(E)** The half-max binding for each individual mouse, identified with a unique number, at each time point following an immunization (1–4) was calculated. $n = 6$ mice for each group. **** represents statistical significance of $P < 0.0001$, ***$P < 0.001$, **$P < 0.01$, and *$P < 0.05$. Blue stars represent the difference between ID2 alone and ID2 + Alum, red stars represent differences between ID2 alone and ID2 + GLA-SE and purple stars represent differences between ID2 + Alum and ID2 + GLA-SE.

and then probed in ELISAs with non-denatured ID2 immunogen coated on microplates. As shown in **Figure 3C**, after being adsorbed with denatured ID2 in solution, sera of all 3 immunization groups were still able to bind the non-denatured ID2. The residual sera of mice immunized with ID2 + GLA-SE adjuvant showed higher levels of binding to conformationally intact ID2 than mice injected with ID2 alone and GLA-SE led to significantly higher levels than alum. This indicates that immunization with ID2 protein alone or in combination with adjuvants leads to elicitation of sera antibodies that recognize and bind conformational ID2 epitopes with a higher titer of conformational antibodies present in sera of mice immunized with the GLA-SE adjuvant.

Sera of Mice Immunized With ID2 in GLA-SE Mediates ADCC

The ID2 immunogen was designed to harbor A32 or A32-like epitopes involved in potent ADCC responses against target cells during the earliest stage of viral entry i.e., at the interaction of gp120 of the Env trimer with the host cell receptor CD4 (14, 21–23, 37) and HIV infected/budding cells which retain CD4 at the target cell surface. Antibodies recognizing the A32 region epitopes were shown to lack conventional neutralizing activities [(12–16, 38), reviewed in (21–23)]. To test if ID2 elicited antibodies capable of ADCC against CD4 inducible (CD4i) targets of a cross clade gp120 we characterized the terminal sera of immunized mice with the optimized RFADCC assay

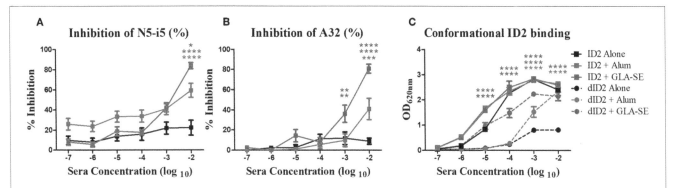

FIGURE 3 | Epitope and conformational specificity of serum antibodies elicited in immunized mice. Sera collected 2 weeks after the final immunization (week 10) were tested for their ability to compete with Cluster A biotinylated mAbs for the binding to ID2 recombinant protein in ELISA. Plates were coated with 0.5 μg/mL of ID2 and serum was incubated with **(A)** A32 and **(B)** N5-i5 (right panel) at half max binding concentrations. Each sample was assayed in duplicate before calculation of % inhibition from the average. **(C)** To assess if immunization with ID2 alone or in combination with adjuvants induced serum antibodies recognizing conformational or linear epitopes different dilutions of pooled sera collected 2 weeks after the last immunization (week 10) were mixed o/n at 4°C with a fixed concentration of denatured ID2. Sera were then reacted in ELISA on ID2 coated plates. Anti-mouse IgG alkaline phosphatase conjugated was used to detect the binding of serum antibodies. **** represents statistical significance of $P < 0.0001$, ***$P < 0.001$, **$P < 0.01$ and *$P < 0.05$. Blue stars represent the difference between ID2 alone and ID2 + Alum, red stars represent differences between ID2 alone and ID2 + GLA-SE and purple stars represent differences between ID2 + Alum and ID2 + GLA-SE.

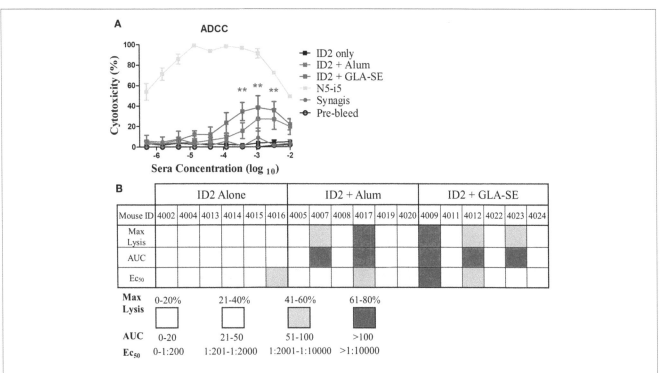

FIGURE 4 | ADCC in sera from mice immunized with ID2 with and without adjuvant. **(A)** Pre-immune sera and sera collected after the last immunization were tested in Rapid Fluorescence ADCC assay against EGFP-CEM-NKr-CCR5SNAP cells sensitized with recombinant BaL gp120 to assess their ability to mediate cytotoxicity. Results are reported as % Cytotoxicity, in relation to maximal cytotoxicity by N5-i5. All samples were analyzed in triplicate before calculating the % cytotoxicity from the mean. No statistical difference existed between ID2+Alum and ID2+GLA-SE at any sera concentration, determined using a Two-way ANOVA test with Bonferroni post-test. **(B)** The maximum lysis (%), Area under the curve (AUC) and Ec_{50} for each individual mouse, identified with a unique number, at each time point following the final immunization was calculated. Max lysis was defined as the maximum percent lysis at any sera concentration. Area under the curve (AUC) was calculated using an Excel formula. Ec_{50} was determined using a GraphPad prism formula of Log(agonist) vs. Normalized response for a variable slope. $N = 6$ for each group. ** represents statistical significance of $P < 0.01$. Red stars represent differences between ID2 alone and ID2 + GLA-SE.

(36) using NKr cells sensitized with recombinant BaL gp120. As shown in **Figure 4A**, sera from mice immunized with ID2 in the absence of adjuvant showed no ADCC activity, with cytotoxicity readings comparable to the negative control Synagis and the pre-bleed samples. Sera analyzed from mice immunized with ID2 + Alum were capable of modest but not significant ADCC

above ID2 alone samples with peaks of cytotoxicity for sera dilutions of 10^2-10^4. In contrast, sera from mice injected with ID2 + GLA-SE elicited significant ADCC when compared to ID2 alone (**Figures 4A,B**).

ID2 was designed specifically to contain no known neutralizing epitope targets (34) in order to closely mimic the response observed in the RV144 vaccine trial in which ADCC in the absence of neutralization was associated with protection (28). To test if the ID2 immunized sera contained any neutralizing antibodies we performed a standard neutralization TZM-bl assay against the Tier 2 clade B virus JRFL. This virus was selected to represent a biologically relevant strain for demonstrating neutralization. The recent publication by Montefiori et al. (39) concludes that tier 2 viruses represent the Env conformation of most circulating viruses and are therefore the most appropriate for determining neutralization potential of antibodies. Using sera collected after the last immunization and mAbs A32 and P7 as respective negative and positive controls, we were able to determine that none of the tested sera was able to robustly neutralize the JRFL virus (**Figure 5**).

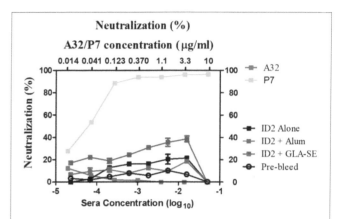

FIGURE 5 | Neutralization in sera from mice immunized with ID2 with and without adjuvant. Sera were tested in a TZM-bl assay for the presence of neutralizing activities against clade B Tier 2 JRFL pseudo-virus. Sera from Pre-bleed (Hollow circle), ID2 Alone (Black square), ID2 + Alum (Blue square), and ID2 + GLA-SE (Red square) were diluted and assayed for their ability to neutralize a clade B Tier 2 JR pseudo-virus (Bottom X axis). These samples were run alongside diluted A32 antibody (orange square) for a negative control and P7 antibody (green square) as a positive control, beginning at 10 μg/ml (Top X axis).

Mice Immunized With ID2 in GLA-SE Show a Larger Diversity of Anti-ID2 Ig Subclasses

In addition to showing that ADCC in the absence of robust neutralization was adequate for protection against HIV, the RV144 trial also highlighted the importance of the type of antibody repertoire raised. A strong IgG response in the absence of IgA conferred the best protection (28). We therefore aimed to determine the antibody repertoire triggered in response to ID2 in the presence and absence of adjuvants. We tested sera collected after the last immunization (week 10) for the presence of anti-ID2 specific IgG1, IgG2a, IgG2b, IgG2c, IgG3, IgA, and IgM (**Figures 6A–G**). As expected, the IgG1 subclass was detected in all immunization groups albeit with different titers. Mice immunized with ID2 alone had very low half-max binding titers, ranging between 1:341 and 1:2,344 (**Figure 6H**). The addition of Alum increased the level of ID2-specific IgG1 with half-max binding titers ranging from 1:7,597 to 1:66,337 in these sera. The half-max binding titers were similar for mice immunized in the presence of GLA-SE, ranging between 1:16,678 and 1:72,864. In contrast, significant differences existed in titers of IgG2a and 2b subclasses between the Alum and GLA-SE adjuvant groups. Mice immunized in the presence of Alum generated a very low titer for both IgG2a and 2b, with half max binding titers for both below 1:500 in all but two mice, while the addition of GLA-SE resulted in half max binding titers for IgG2a ranging between 1:1,833 and 1:20,585 and for IgG2b between 1:572 and 1:3,139 (**Figures 5B,C,H**). Low levels of anti-ID2 specific IgG2c, IgG3, IgA, and IgM responses were detected only in sera of mice immunized in presence of GLA-SE adjuvant (**Figures 6D–G**). Combined, these data indicate that immunizations with GLA-SE adjuvant induce a larger diversity of anti-ID2 IgG subclasses as compared to Alum.

DISCUSSION

Antibodies capable of effective Fc-mediated effector functions, including ADCC, have recently received increasing interest as important components of a vaccine induced humoral response. Although the enthusiasm for this type of antibody function was mostly evoked by the RV144 trial, the evidence also exists from vaccination strategies with Env immunogens in non-human primates (NHP) that link FcR effector functions of antibodies with post-infection control of viremia and/or blocking HIV-1 acquisition, often in the absence of neutralization (40–45), reviewed in (27).

Correlate analyses of the infection risk in the RV144 trial have indicated two gp120 epitope regions; the conformational C1-C2 and the linear V2 loop epitopes, as the major players involved in the Fc-mediated protective response (21, 22, 46). Although only the ADCC response of antibodies directed at the crown of the V2 loop region directly correlated with a lower risk of infection (29–31) the non-neutralizing C1-C2-specific A32-like antibodies synergized with the weakly-neutralizing V2 antibodies (33) to deliver ADCC against neutralization resistant tier 2 isolates. The synergistic crosstalk between antibodies directed at these two epitopes was recognized to be an important component of the protective effect of the RV144 vaccine trial suggesting that C1-C2- and V2-specifc antibodies may act in tandem in a polyfunctional antibody profile to deliver a broad and potent Fc-effector response (33).

Similarly, antibodies specific for Cluster A epitope region (including the A32 subregion) and the co-receptor binding site correlated with sterilizing heterologous protection against SHIV162p3 in NHPs immunized with the conformationally constrained gp120 immunogen, full-length single chain (FLSC) (41, 47). As with the RV144 trial, no correlation

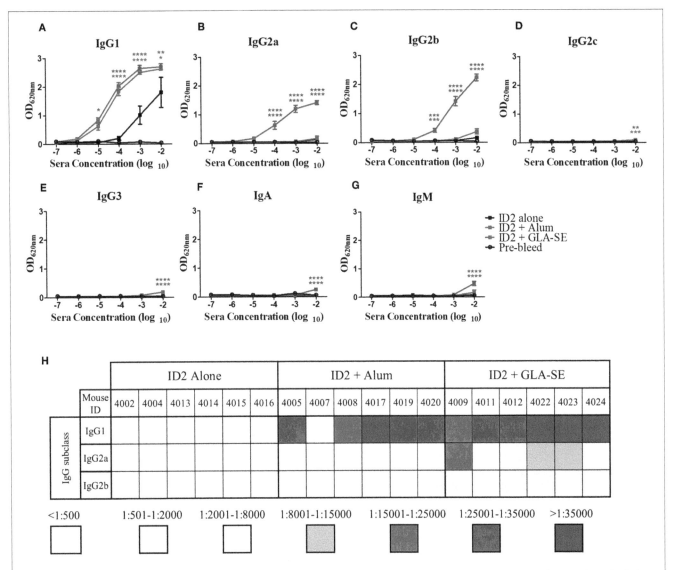

FIGURE 6 | Evaluation of IgG subclasses, IgA and IgM elicited in immunized mice. 10-fold dilutions of pre-immunized (pre-bleed, Black circle) and immunized mice sera collected after last immunization (week 10), were evaluated in ELISA to assess the IgG subtypes; **(A)** IgG1, **(B)** IgG2a, **(C)** IgG2b, **(D)** IgG2c, **(E)** IgG3, as well as **(F)** IgA, and **(G)** IgM induced with no adjuvant (Black square), with Alum (Blue square), or with GLA-SE (Red square). **(H)** The half-max binding for each individual mouse sera sample, identified by an individual number, for the terminal bleed was calculated and displayed for IgG1, IgG2a, and IgG2b. $n = 6$ mice for each group. **** represents statistical significance of $P < 0.0001$, ***$P < 0.001$, **$P < 0.01$, and *$P < 0.05$. Blue stars represent the difference between ID2 alone and ID2 + Alum, red stars represent differences between ID2 alone and ID2 + GLA-SE and purple stars represent differences between ID2 + Alum and ID2 + GLA-SE.

between neutralizing activity and protection was observed in these studies pointing again at a role for Fc-mediated effector function in protection against SHIV-1 transmission. In both the RV144 and FLSC trials described above the C1–C2 specific antibodies acted in tandem with antibodies directed at other Env epitopes to contribute to the vaccine efficacy through Fc effector mechanisms. The question remains open if antibodies directed at these non-neutralizing epitope targets could alone afford protection or if they act only as a component of a polyclonal response with antibodies targeting other epitopes. This question has not been addressed, mostly due to the lack of an appropriate immunogen

which could selectively bear only this conformational epitope target.

In this study, we investigated the immunogenicity and ability to induce an effective cross-clade ADCC response of a new immunogen candidate ID2, developed previously in our laboratory, as a minimal structural unit of HIV Env stably presenting the non-neutralizing epitopes within the A32 region (C1–C2 epitopes). ID2 consists of the inner domain construct stabilized in CD4-bound conformation by C_{65}-C_{115} disulfide bond preserving the A32 region epitopes in the context of CD4-triggered full length gp120, derived from a clade A/E strain, without the complication of any other known neutralizing epitopes. We immunized BALB/c mice intraperitoneally (IP) with 4 doses of ID2 (20 μg /dose) over a period of 8 weeks with three immunizations with 2 weeks intervals and one final immunization delivered 4 weeks later to assess the induction of a memory antibody response. ID2 was administered either alone or with an adjuvant: Alum or GLA-SE. The resulting immune sera were evaluated for the presence of anti-ID2 antibodies (total IgG, IgG subclasses, IgA, and IgM) as well as for their capacity to bind to conformational A32 region epitopes and compete for the binding with mAbs specific for those epitopes. Immune sera were also tested in our RFADCC assay for their ability to mediate ADCC with CEM-NKr-CCR5 target cells sensitized with recombinant gp120 from the Clade B HIV-1$_{BaL}$ isolate and to neutralize a Tier 2 strain of HIV-1. Our results showed that immunization with ID2 alone elicited no or very low anti-ID2 serum antibodies and those elicited were only after the 4th immunization, whereas mice in the groups immunized with ID2 in adjuvants showed robust anti-ID2 responses. Of the two adjuvants, mice immunized with ID2 in GLA-SE exhibited higher anti-ID2 titers at the end of study (week 10) as compared with the Alum group. Interestingly, both groups showed comparable titers after the 3rd immunization, but while in the GLA-SE group the 4th immunization boosted the immune response significantly above the alum group, mice in the Alum group presented a comparable titer to week 6. These data indicate that administration of ID2 in combination with GLA-SE induces enhanced and easily boosted responses to the target antigen. This agrees with the data regarding GLA-SE as an adjuvant, which was designed to promote strong and long lasting T_H1 responses to protein vaccine antigens (48, 49). Quality analyses of the immune responses elicited by ID2 with adjuvants indicated that antibodies elicited by ID2 with GLA-SE were directed more toward conformational epitopes within the A32 region as shown by the ability of these sera to inhibit the binding of mAb A32 and the A32-like mAb N5-i5 to ID2 and by the residual binding of sera previously incubated with a denatured/linear ID2. Differences were also detected in terms of the IgG isotypes of the elicited antibodies. Mice immunized with ID2 in Alum produced mostly IgG1 antibodies, whereas the immunization with ID2 in GLA-SE induced a broader range and a higher titer of IgG isotypes IgG1, IgG2a, and IgG2b, together with low but detectable IgG3 in addition to IgA and IgM. This difference in antibody isotypes between the two adjuvant groups likely explains the significant higher titers of total IgG in the GLA-SE adjuvant group over the alum group following the final immunization.

ADCC was only significantly increased over the negative control in sera isolated from the GLA-SE adjuvant group, indicating that high titers of ID2-specific mouse IgG1, IgG2a, and IgG2b in addition to small amounts of other isotypes are required for effective RFADCC. In addition to generating more diverse isotypes of ID2 specific antibodies, immunizing with GLA-SE also led to the generation of more specific antibodies – as indicated by significantly higher percent competition for both A32 and N5-i5 antibodies. Interestingly, some sera displayed high ADCC yet low levels of ID2-specific IgG and an absence of class switching from IgG1. One example of this is sample 4,007; when looking at the individual data for the competition

ELISA, 4,007 sera inhibits the binding of A32 by 39.7% at the highest sera concentration and N5-i5 by 45%, an average amount for A32 and below average for N5-i5 when compared to other mice in the Alum group. One possibility for a more potent ADCC response is that antibodies to different epitopes were raised in this particular mouse. While the design of ID2 prevents the elicitation of classical C11-like antibodies, some antibodies may be specific for C11-like epitopes which would not have been identified by the competition ELISAs carried out. One known examples of an antibody which could be raised to this area of ID2 is JR4 (24). As previously reported, the RFADCC assay (36) uses antigen sensitized NKr cells and human PBMCs, in which mostly monocyte activity (through their FcγRIIA receptors) is measured. Although interactions between mouse immunoglobulins and human FcγRs are largely understudied there are reports indicating that human FcγRIIA binds mouse IgG1, 2a, and 2b, but not mouse IgG3 (50). All together this suggests that the presence of IgG1 and IgG2a in immunized mouse sera is sufficient to stimulate human PBMCs to mediate the killing of cross-clade antigen sensitized NKr cells.

In conclusion, these results indicate that ID2 can be highly immunogenic, especially when administered together with GLA-SE as an adjuvant, and that the elicited immune response can mediate ADCC in a RFADCC assay using human PBMCs as effector cells. None of the immune sera showed robust neutralization activity against the tier 2 JRFL virus indicating that ID2 as an immunogen induces mostly a humoral immune response against the desired non-neutralizing epitopes within the A32 region. ID2 in combination with GLA-SE was successfully utilized to demonstrate that Fc-effector mechanisms in the absence of strong neutralizing antibodies could be directed toward the A32 subregion which has the potential for HIV-1 protection and ID2 could therefore be utilized for future studies in a NHP challenge study.

AUTHOR CONTRIBUTIONS

MV, NG, WT, and MP designed, performed research, and analyzed the data. AD, CO, RF, and GL carried out assays and analyzed the ADCC data. RS analyzed the data. MV, RS, and MP wrote the paper. All authors read the manuscript and provided comments or revisions.

ACKNOWLEDGMENTS

We thank our IHV colleagues for outstanding support of the studies leading to the ideas presented above. This work was supported by NIH Grants: NIAID R01 AI116274 to MP, R01AI129769 to MP and Andres Finzi and NIAID P01 AI120756 to Georgia Tomaras.

REFERENCES

1. Kwong PD, Doyle ML, Casper DJ, Cicala C, Leavitt SA, Majeed S, et al. HIV-1 evades antibody-mediated neutralization through conformational masking of receptor-binding sites. *Nature.* (2002) 420:678–82. doi: 10.1038/nature01188

2. Phogat S, Wyatt RT, Hedestam GBK. Inhibition of HIV-1 entry by antibodies: potential viral and cellular targets. *J Intern Med.* (2007) 262:26–43. doi: 10.1111/j.1365-2796.2007.01820.x

3. Schief WR, Ban Y-EA, Stamatatos L. Challenges for structure-based HIV vaccine design. *Curr Opin HIV AIDS.* (2009) 4:431. doi: 10.1097/COH.0b013e32832e6184

4. Agarwal A, Hioe CE, Swetnam J, Zolla-Pazner S, Cardozo T. Quantitative assessment of masking of neutralization epitopes in HIV-1. *Vaccine.* (2011) 29:6736–41. doi: 10.1016/j.vaccine.2010.12.052

5. Correia BE, Ban Y-EA, Holmes MA, Xu H, Ellingson K, Kraft Z, et al. Computational design of epitope-scaffolds allows induction of antibodies specific for a poorly immunogenic HIV vaccine epitope. *Structure.* (2010) 18:1116–26. doi: 10.1016/j.str.2010.06.010

6. Joyce JG, Krauss IJ, Song HC, Opalka DW, Grimm KM, Nahas DD, et al. An oligosaccharide-based HIV-1 2G12 mimotope vaccine induces carbohydrate-specific antibodies that fail to neutralize HIV-1 virions. *Proc Natl Acad Sci USA.* (2008) 105:15684–9. doi: 10.1073/pnas.0807837105

7. Klasse PJ, Sanders RW, Cerutti A, Moore JP. How can HIV-type-1-env immunogenicity be improved to facilitate antibody-based vaccine development? *AIDS Res Hum Retroviruses.* (2012) 28:1–15. doi: 10.1089/aid.2011.0053

8. Krachmarov CP, Honnen WJ, Kayman SC, Gorny MK, Zolla-Pazner S, Pinter A. Factors determining the breadth and potency of neutralization by V3-specific human monoclonal antibodies derived from subjects infected with clade A or clade B strains of human immunodeficiency virus type 1. *J Virol.* (2006) 80:7127–35. doi: 10.1128/JVI.02619-05

9. Wei X, Decker JM, Wang S, Hui H, Kappes JC, Wu X, et al. Antibody neutralization and escape by HIV-1. *Nature.* (2003) 422:307–12. doi: 10.1038/nature01470

10. Burton DR, Weiss RA. A boost for HIV vaccine design. *Science.* (2010) 329:770–3. doi: 10.1126/science.1194693

11. Briney BS, Willis JR, Jr, Crowe JE Jr. Human peripheral blood antibodies with long HCDR3s are established primarily at original recombination using a limited subset of germline genes. *PLOS ONE.* (2012) 7:e36750. doi: 10.1371/journal.pone.0036750

12. Acharya P, Tolbert WD, Gohain N, Wu X, Yu L, Liu T, et al. Structural definition of an antibody-dependent cellular cytotoxicity response implicated in reduced risk for HIV-1 infection. *J Virol.* (2014) 88:12895–906. doi: 10.1128/JVI.02194-14

13. Ferrari G, Pollara J, Kozink D, Harms T, Drinker M, Freel S, et al. An HIV-1 gp120 envelope human monoclonal antibody that recognizes a C1 conformational epitope mediates potent antibody-dependent cellular cytotoxicity (ADCC) activity and defines a common ADCC epitope in human HIV-1 serum. *J Virol.* (2011) 85:7029–36. doi: 10.1128/JVI.00171-11

14. Guan Y, Pazgier M, Sajadi MM, Kamin-Lewis R, Al-Darmarki S, Flinko R, et al. Diverse specificity and effector function among human antibodies to HIV-1 envelope glycoprotein epitopes exposed by CD4 binding. *Proc Natl Acad Sci USA.* (2013) 110:E69–78. doi: 10.1073/pnas.1217609110

15. Veillette M, Désormeaux A, Medjahed H, Gharsallah N-E, Coutu M, Baalwa J, et al. Interaction with cellular CD4 exposes HIV-1 envelope epitopes targeted by antibody-dependent cell-mediated cytotoxicity. *J Virol.* (2014) 88:2633–44. doi: 10.1128/JVI.03230-13

16. Veillette M, Coutu M, Richard J, Batraville L-A, Dagher O, Bernard N, et al. The HIV-1 gp120 CD4-bound conformation is preferentially targeted by antibody-dependent cellular cytotoxicity-mediating antibodies in sera from HIV-1-infected individuals. *J Virol.* (2015) 89:545–51. doi: 10.1128/JVI.02868-14

17. Finnegan CM, Berg W, Lewis GK, DeVico AL. Antigenic properties of the human immunodeficiency virus envelope during cell-cell fusion. *J Virol.* (2001) 75:11096–105. doi: 10.1128/JVI.75.22.11096-11105.2001

18. Finnegan CM, Berg W, Lewis GK, DeVico AL. Antigenic properties of the human immunodeficiency virus transmembrane glycoprotein during cell-cell fusion. *J Virol.* (2002) 76:12123–34. doi: 10.1128/JVI.76.23.12123-12134.2002

19. Mengistu M, Ray K, Lewis GK, DeVico AL. Antigenic properties of the human immunodeficiency virus envelope glycoprotein Gp120 on virions bound to target cells. *PLoS Pathog.* (2015) 11:e1004772. doi: 10.1371/journal.ppat.1004772

20. Ray K, Mengistu M, Lewis GK, Lakowicz JR, DeVico AL. Antigenic properties of the HIV envelope on virions in solution. *J Virol.* (2014) 88:1795–808. doi: 10.1128/JVI.03048-13

21. Lewis GK, Guan Y, Kamin-Lewis R, Sajadi M, Pazgier M, DeVico AL. Epitope target structures of fc-mediated effector function during HIV-1 acquisition. *Curr Opin HIV AIDS.* (2014) 9:263–70. doi: 10.1097/COH.0000000000000055

22. Pollara J, Bonsignori M, Moody MA, Pazgier M, Haynes BF, Ferrari G. Epitope specificity of human immunodeficiency virus-1 antibody dependent cellular cytotoxicity [ADCC] responses. *Curr HIV Res.* (2013) 11:378–87. doi: 10.2174/1570162X113116660059

23. Veillette M, Richard J, Pazgier M, Lewis GK, Parsons MS, Finzi A. Role of HIV-1 Envelope Glycoproteins conformation and accessory proteins on ADCC responses. *Curr HIV Res.* (2016) 14:9–23. doi: 10.2174/1570162X13666150827093449

24. Gohain N, Tolbert WD, Acharya P, Yu L, Liu T, Zhao P, et al. Cocrystal structures of antibody N60-i3 and antibody JR4 in complex with gp120 define more cluster A epitopes involved in effective antibody-dependent effector function against HIV-1. *J Virol.* (2015) 89:8840–54. doi: 10.1128/JVI.01232-15

25. Tolbert WD, Gohain N, Alsahafi N, Van V, Orlandi C, Ding S, et al. Targeting the late stage of HIV-1 entry for antibody-dependent cellular cytotoxicity: structural basis for env epitopes in the C11 region. *Structure.* (2017) 25:1719–31.e4. doi: 10.1016/j.str.2017.09.009

26. Lewis GK, Pazgier M, Evans DT, Ferrari G, Bournazos S, Parsons MS, et al. Beyond viral neutralization. *AIDS Res Hum Retroviruses.* (2017) 33:760–4. doi: 10.1089/aid.2016.0299

27. Lewis GK, Pazgier M, DeVico AL. Survivors remorse: antibody-mediated protection against HIV-1. *Immunol Rev.* (2017b) 275:271–84. doi: 10.1111/imr.12510

28. Rerks-Ngarm S, Pitisuttithum P, Nitayaphan S, Kaewkungwal J, Chiu J, Paris R, et al. Vaccination with ALVAC and AIDSVAX to Prevent HIV-1 Infection in Thailand. *N Engl J Med.* (2009) 361:2209–20. doi: 10.1056/NEJMoa0908492

29. Chung AW, Ghebremichael M, Robinson H, Brown E, Choi I, Lane S, et al. Polyfunctional Fc-effector profiles mediated by IgG subclass selection distinguish RV144 and VAX003 vaccines. *Sci Transl Med.* (2014) 6:228ra38. doi: 10.1126/scitranslmed.3007736

30. Yates NL, Liao H-X, Fong Y, deCamp A, Vandergrift NA, Williams WT, et al. Vaccine-induced env V1–V2 IgG3 correlates with lower HIV-1 infection risk and declines soon after vaccination. *Sci Transl Med.* (2014) 6:228ra39. doi: 10.1126/scitranslmed.3007730

31. Haynes BF, Gilbert PB, McElrath MJ, Zolla-Pazner S, Tomaras GD, Alam SM, et al. Immune-Correlates analysis of an HIV-1 vaccine efficacy trial. *N Engl J Med.* (2012) 366:1275–86. doi: 10.1056/NEJMoa1113425

32. Bonsignori M, Pollara J, Moody MA, Alpert MD, Chen X, Hwang K-K, et al. Antibody-dependent cellular cytotoxicity-mediating antibodies from an hiv-1 vaccine efficacy trial target multiple epitopes and preferentially use the VH1 gene family. *J Virol.* (2012) 86:11521–32. doi: 10.1128/JVI.01023-12

33. Pollara J, Bonsignori M, Moody MA, Liu P, Alam SM, Hwang K-K, et al. HIV-1 vaccine-induced C1 and V2 Env-specific antibodies synergize for increased antiviral activities. *J Virol.* (2014) 88:7715–26. doi: 10.1128/JVI.00156-14

34. Tolbert WD, Gohain N, Veillette M, Chapleau J-P, Orlandi C, Visciano ML, et al. Paring down HIV Env: design and crystal structure of a stabilized inner domain of HIV-1 gp120 displaying a major ADCC target of the A32 region. *Structure.* (2016) 24:697–709. doi: 10.1016/j.str.2016.03.005

35. Moore JP, Ho DD. Antibodies to discontinuous or conformationally sensitive epitopes on the gp120 glycoprotein of human immunodeficiency virus type 1 are highly prevalent in sera of infected humans. *J Virol.* (1993) 67:863–75.

36. Orlandi C, Flinko R, Lewis GK. A new cell line for high throughput HIV-specific antibody-dependent cellular cytotoxicity (ADCC) and cell-to-cell virus transmission studies. *J Immunol Methods.* (2016) 433:51–8. doi: 10.1016/j.jim.2016.03.002

37. Kramski M, Stratov I, Kent SJ. The role of HIV-specific antibody-dependent cellular cytotoxicity in HIV prevention and the influence of the HIV-1 Vpu protein. *AIDS.* (2015) 29:137–44. doi: 10.1097/QAD.0000000000000523

38. Ding S, Veillette M, Coutu M, Prévost J, Scharf L, Bjorkman PJ, et al. A highly conserved residue of the HIV-1 gp120 inner domain is important for antibody-dependent cellular cytotoxicity responses mediated by anti-cluster A antibodies. *J Virol.* (2016) 90:2127–34. doi: 10.1128/JVI.02779-15

39. Montefiori DC, Roederer M, Morris L, Seaman MS. Neutralization tiers of HIV-1. *Curr Opin HIV AIDS.* (2018) 13:128. doi: 10.1097/COH.0000000000000442

40. DeVico A, Fouts T, Lewis GK, Gallo RC, Godfrey K, Charurat M, et al. Antibodies to CD4-induced sites in HIV gp120 correlate with the control of SHIV challenge in macaques vaccinated with subunit immunogens. *Proc Natl Acad Sci USA.* (2007) 104:17477–82. doi: 10.1073/pnas.0707399104

41. Fouts TR, Bagley K, Prado IJ, Bobb KL, Schwartz JA, Xu R, et al. Balance of cellular and humoral immunity determines the level of protection by HIV vaccines in rhesus macaque models of HIV infection. *Proc Natl Acad Sci USA.* (2015) 112:E992–9. doi: 10.1073/pnas.1423669112

42. Gómez-Román VR, Florese RH, Patterson LJ, Peng B, Venzon D, Aldrich K, et al. A simplified method for the rapid fluorometric assessment of antibody-dependent cell-mediated cytotoxicity. *J Immunol Methods.* (2006) 308:53–67. doi: 10.1016/j.jim.2005.09.018

43. Gómez-Román VR, Florese RH, Peng B, Montefiori DC, Kalyanaraman VS, Venzon D, et al. An adenovirus-based HIV subtype B prime/boost vaccine regimen elicits antibodies mediating broad antibody-dependent cellular cytotoxicity against non-subtype B HIV strains. *J Acquir Immune Defic Syndr.* (2006) 43:270–7. doi: 10.1097/01.qai.0000230318.40170.60

44. Malkevitch NV, Patterson LJ, Aldrich MK, Wu Y, Venzon D, Florese RH, et al. Durable protection of rhesus macaques immunized with a replicating adenovirus-SIV multigene prime/protein boost vaccine regimen against a second SIVmac251 rectal challenge: role of SIV-specific CD8+ T cell responses. *Virology.* (2006) 353:83–98. doi: 10.1016/j.virol.2006.05.012

45. Smith AJ, Wietgrefe SW, Shang L, Reilly CS, Southern PJ, Perkey KE, et al. Live SIV vaccine correlate of protection: immune complex-inhibitory Fc receptor interactions that reduce target cell availability. *J Immunol.* (2014) 193:3126–33. doi: 10.4049/jimmunol.1400822

46. Lewis GK. Qualitative and quantitative variables that affect the potency of Fc- mediated effector function *in vitro* and *in vivo*: considerations for passive immunization using non-neutralizing antibodies. *Curr HIV Res.* (2013) 11:354–64. doi: 10.2174/1570162X113116660060

47. Fouts TR, Tuskan R, Godfrey K, Reitz M, Hone D, Lewis GK, et al. Expression and characterization of a single-chain polypeptide analogue of the human immunodeficiency virus type 1 gp120-CD4 receptor complex. *J Virol.* (2000) 74:11427. doi: 10.1128/JVI.74.24.11427-11436.2000

48. Carter D, Fox CB, Day TA, Guderian JA, Liang H, Rolf T, et al. A structure-function approach to optimizing TLR4 ligands for human vaccines. *Clin Transl Immunol.* (2016) 5:e108. doi: 10.1038/cti.2016.63

49. Desbien AL, Cauwelaert ND, Reed SJ, Bailor HR, Liang H, Carter D, et al. IL-18 and subcapsular lymph node macrophages are essential for enhanced B cell responses with TLR4 agonist adjuvants. *J Immunol.* (2016) 197:4351–9. doi: 10.4049/jimmunol.1600993

50. Bruhns P. Properties of mouse and human IgG receptors and their contribution to disease models. *Blood.* (2012) 119:5640–9. doi: 10.1182/blood-2012-01-380121

2

The Complex Association of FcγRIIb with Autoimmune Susceptibility

J. Sjef Verbeek*, Sachiko Hirose and Hiroyuki Nishimura

Department of Biomedical Engineering, Toin University of Yokohama, Yokohama, Japan

*Correspondence:
J. Sjef Verbeek
j.s.verbeek@toin.ac.jp

FcγRIIb is the only inhibitory Fc receptor and controls many aspects of immune and inflammatory responses. The observation 19 years ago that $Fc\gamma RIIb^{-/-}$ mice generated by gene targeting in 129 derived ES cells developed severe lupus like disease when backcrossed more than 7 generations into C57BL/6 background initiated extensive research on the functional understanding of this strong autoimmune phenotype. The genomic region in the distal part of Chr1 both in human and mice in which the $Fc\gamma R$ gene cluster is located shows a high level of complexity in relation to the susceptibility to SLE. Specific haplotypes of closely linked genes including the $Fc\gamma RIIb$ and $Slamf$ genes are associated with increased susceptibility to SLE both in mice and human. Using forward and reverse genetic approaches including in human GWAS and in mice congenic strains, KO mice (germline and cell type specific, on different genetic background), knockin mice, overexpressing transgenic mice combined with immunological models such as adoptive transfer of B cells from Ig transgenic mice the involved genes and the causal mutations and their associated functional alterations were analyzed. In this review the results of this 19 years extensive research are discussed with a focus on (genetically modified) mouse models.

Keywords: SLE, systemic lupus erythematosus, autoimmue disease, mouse model, Fcgamma receptor IIB, reverse genetics

INTRODUCTION

Antibodies (Ab) form immune complexes (IC) with their cognate antigen (Ag). IgG-ICs are potent activators of the immune system via cross-linking of receptors for the Fc part of IgG, FcγR, mainly expressed on the surface of cells of the innate immune system.

FcγRs belong to the Ig supergene family of leukocyte FcR and are transmembrane glycoproteins containing a ligand-binding α subunit with two or three extracellular Ig-like domains, a transmembrane and a cytoplasmic domain. In mice, the high-affinity FcγRI, binding monomeric IgG, and the low-affinity receptors for complexed IgG, FcγRIII, and FcγRIV are activating receptors. The α subunits of the activating receptors form a multi-subunit complex with a dimer of the common γ-chain (FcRγ) (1, 2) with an immunoreceptor tyrosine-based activation motif (ITAM). Cross-linking activating FcRs by IC initiates signal transduction via recruitment and subsequent activation of intracellular tyrosine kinases (3), switching on a large variety of effector mechanisms activating inflammatory cascades.

In humans, there are four activating FCGRs. The high-affinity FCGR1 (CD64) and the low-affinity FCGR3A (CD16A) are associated with the common γ chain whereas the low-affinity FCGR2A (CD32A), containing an ITAM in its cytoplasmic domain, and the low-affinity FCGR3B (CD16B), with a glycosylphosphatidylinositol (GPI) anchor, are single-chain receptors. All human

FCGR genes are clustered at the distal end of Chr1, a region associated with susceptibility to autoimmune diseases such as Systemic Lupus Erythematosus (SLE) (4). In mice the FcγRII, -III, and -IV genes are clustered at the distal end of Chr1, a region orthologous with SLE associated genomic intervals on human Chr1 and associated also with susceptibility to autoimmune disease (Lupus-like disease). *FcγRI* is located on Chr3 due to a translocation during evolution after mouse and human had diverged.

In both humans and mice, the activating FcγRs are counterbalanced by one inhibitory single-chain low-affinity receptor FcγRIIb (FCGR2B or CD32B) with an inhibitory motif named immunoreceptor tyrosine-based inhibition motif (ITIM) within its cytoplasmic domain. In addition, co-engagement of FcγRIIb and the ITAM containing B-cell receptor (BCR) on B cells forms an important negative feedback mechanism to control antibody production. This regulatory mechanism of cellular activation by the ITAM-ITIM motif pair, observed originally with FcγR, has been described for many other receptors in the immune system e.g., T cell receptors and B cell receptors (5, 6). This review focuses on the important but still puzzling immune regulatory role of the inhibitory FcγRIIb and the complex association of its impaired function with autoimmunity as studied extensively in mice.

GENERAL CHARACTERISTICS OF FcγRIIb

Isoforms

In humans and mice, there are two membrane-bound isoforms of FcγRIIb identified: FcγRIIb1 and b2 (7) resulting from alternative splicing. The cytoplasmic domain is encoded by three exons whose 5′ exon encodes a 47 amino acid motif that prevents coated pit localization, which inhibits FcγRIIb mediated endocytosis of soluble immune complexes. This exon is present in the mRNA that encodes the b1 isoform, the only isoform expressed on B cells, but absent in the mRNA that encodes the b2 isoform (8, 9) expressed on most innate immune cells. The ITIM dependent inhibition of cell activation is the same for both isoforms. Therefore, the name FcγRIIb is used in this review without making a distinction between the b1 and the b2 isoform.

Expression

In mice FcγRIIb is expressed on all innate immune cells and is the only FcγR expressed on B cells, including pre-, pro-, and mature B cells, memory B cells, plasma cells (10, 11) and B1 cells (12). Unlike many other B cell surface receptors, expression of FcgRIIb is not downregulated during plasma cell differentiation (10). FcγRIIb expression is modulated on different B cell subsets (11) and increases when the B cells become activated (11, 13). T cells do not intrinsically express FcγRs (14). However, it has been reported that expression of FcγRIIb but not any other FcγR, is upregulated in memory CD8$^+$ T cells after *Listeria monocytogenes* infection and tempers the function of these cells *in vivo* (15). Guilliams et al. showed that according to the microarray expression values extracted from public data sets the mRNA expression of FcγRIIb in mice is from high to low as follows: Inflammatory macrophages (Mφ), Ly6C^{hi}

classical monocyte, inflammatory monocyte-derived dendritic cell (moDC), lung CD11b$^+$ conventional or classical DC (cDC), Ly6C^{lo} patrolling monocyte, alveolar Mφ, follicular B cell, GC B cell, skin-draining lymph node CD11b$^+$ cDC, spleen CD8$^+$XCR1$^+$ cDC, spleen plasmacytoid DC (pDC), spleen CD11b$^+$ cDC, neutrophils, spleen Mφ, and NK cells (16). The overall FcγRIIb expression pattern is similar in mouse and human. In mouse cDCs the relatively low expression of FcγRIIb is higher than that of any activating FcγR.

FcγRIIb expression, relative to that of activating FcγRs, is tightly regulated. In mice, C5a rapidly down-regulates FcγRIIb on alveolar Mφ and upregulates FcγRIII on these cells (17, 18). IL-4 downregulates FcγRIIb expression on mouse activated B cells (13, 19). IFNγ increases FcγRIIb expression on B cells (19) and increases the expression of activating FcγR on myeloid effector cells in mice. In humans the Th2 cytokines IL-4, IL-10, and TGF-β increase FCGR2B expression and decrease activating FCGR expression on myeloid cells (20–22) whereas IFNγ decreases FCGR2B expression on these cells and increases activating FCGR expression (23).

FcγRIIb is also expressed on non-hematopoietic cells. Its expression is induced on FDC upon antigen stimulation (24). It has been calculated that almost 70% of total mouse body FcγRIIb is expressed on liver sinusoidal endothelial cells (LSEC) (25, 26). On mouse glomerular mesangial cells, TNFα/IL-1β upregulates FcγRIIb expression whereas IFNγ downregulates FcγRIIb expression and upregulates the activating FcγR (27).

Cellular Function

Co-aggregation of the inhibiting ITIM containing FcγRIIb with activating ITAM containing FcRs results in the recruitment of the inositol polyphosphate-5-phosphatase SHIP1 that counteracts the signals mediated by activating FcRs (3, 28). Therefore, FcγRIIb has a strong regulatory role in all the processes in which activating FcγR are involved. The ratio between activating and inhibiting signals determines the outcome of the cellular response to IgG-ICs. This ratio depends mainly on the following factors: (a) the relative affinities of the different antibody isotypes involved for the different FcγR, (b) the level of opsonization, and (c) the relative expression level of inhibitory and activating FcγR, which is partially determined by the cytokine milieu. The binding of FcγRIIb for IgG-IC is strongest for IgG1 and weakest for IgG2a. So, FcγRIIb expression has the highest impact on IgG1-IC. In addition, FcγRIIb can inhibit complement-mediated inflammation when co-engaged with Dectin-1 by galactosylated IgG1-ICs (29) indicating that its immune-modulatory function in the efferent response is not restricted to the regulation of activating FcγRs.

In B cells co-crosslinking of the BCR and FcγRIIb results in the inhibition of activation, proliferation, Ag internalization and Ab secretion (30–32). Moreover, *in vitro* studies have shown that FcγRIIb on B cells can induce apoptosis upon clustering (10, 12, 28, 33, 34).

FcγRIIb can also function as an endocytic receptor of small ICs. The endocytic properties of FcγRIIb depend on the presence of a di-leucine motif in the intracellular domain (8) and are independent of the ITIM.

Role in Different Tissues and Cell Types
Myeloid Effector Cells

In the efferent phase, FcγRIIb sets a threshold for the activation by IgG-IC of myeloid effector cells, e.g., monocytes, Mφs, and neutrophils. Crosslinking of activating FcγR by IgG-ICs induces effector mechanisms of these cells e.g., soluble IC clearance, antibody-dependent cell-mediated cytotoxicity (ADCC), antibody-dependent cellular phagocytosis (ADCP), the release of inflammatory mediators, degranulation, superoxide production, enhancement of Ag presentation, and cell maturation and proliferation. This includes also the regulation of high-affinity IgE receptor-mediated mast cell activation (35).

Lupus-prone (NZBxNZW)F1 mice deficient for the FcR γ chain, lacking functional activating FcγR, do not develop IC-mediated severe glomerulonephritis (GN), despite high autoantibody titers (36). This suggests that FcγR play a dominant role in the efferent phase of Ab-driven diseases including lupus-like disease and therefore FcγRIIb might have a strong protective role in such a disease. In addition, FcγRIIb might also inhibit an ongoing auto-Ab response by suppressing the activating FcγR dependent, IgG-IC-triggered release of inflammatory mediators and other immune regulatory molecules by myeloid effector cells.

Dendritic Cells

DCs are central regulators of immunity determining whether tolerance is induced, or an effective adaptive immune response is generated, bridging innate and adaptive immunity (37–39). DCs have the unique capacity to take up exogenous Ag via a variety of mechanisms and surface molecules, including FcγR, and subsequently process and present the Ag-derived peptides in their MHC molecules to prime naïve T cells. Three main subsets of DCs can be recognized, cDC, moDC and pDC. Their ontogeny and functions have been reviewed extensively (40, 41).

A series of observations suggest that FcγR on cDCs and moDCs can play a role in priming and regulation of adaptive immunity (16). Ag-specific IgG enhances Ab responses to soluble protein Ag via activating FcγRs, probably by increasing Ag presentation by dendritic cells to Th cells (42). Many laboratories have shown that soluble IgG-ICs strongly enhance cross-presentation by using either *in vitro* assays (43–45), or *in vivo* assays with *in vitro* loaded DCs from WT and FcγR KO mice (46–50). Signaling through the activating FcγRs results in lysosomal targeting of the Ag and importantly activation and maturation of the DCs (44), required for their migration to the lymph node and their presentation of Ag-derived peptides in MHC class I to CD8[+] T cells (49, 51). In mouse bone marrow-derived DCs (BMDCs), activating FcγRs modulate the expression of many genes, associated with T cell response induction, upon crosslinking by IgG-ICs. This is strongly regulated by FcγRIIb, setting a threshold for DC activation and maturation (52). *FcγRIIb*[−/−] mice showed an increased upregulation of costimulatory molecules, resulting in an enhanced capacity to generate antigen-specific T cell responses upon injection of IgG-ICs (52–54). However, *in vivo*, in mice, the role of FcγR in the presentation of soluble IgG-IC derived Ag is redundant (55, 56).

In mice, cDCs consist of two main subsets, type 1 cDC or cDC1 and Type 2 cDC or cDC2 (41). *In vivo* IgG-IC improve strongly cross-presentation of the cDC2 but not the cDC1 DCs. Only cDC2 mediated cross-presentation is FcγR dependent (57). Moreover, FcγRs are dispensable for the *in vivo* uptake of IgG-IC by cDC1 and cDC2 (56, 57). The *in vivo* cross-presentation of IgG-IC derived Ag by cDC1 is completely and by cDC2 partially dependent on C1q (56).

Because it has been shown that treatment with FCGR2B blocking antibodies results in spontaneous maturation of human DCs (58) it has been hypothesized that FCGR2B does not only regulate DC activation but also actively prevents unwanted spontaneous DC maturation by small amounts of circulating IC present in serum under non-inflammatory steady-state conditions (2).

IgG-ICs endocytosed by activating FcγR on DCs ends up in a degradative Lamp-1 positive compartment where it is slowly degraded into peptides (59). In contrast, antigen, endocytosed in the periphery via FcγRIIb on DCs, enters preferentially in a non-degradative Lamp-1 negative intracellular vesicular compartment, that recycles to the cell surface to transfer the native antigen via interaction with the BCR to B cells in the lymphoid organs. This indicates that DCs, migrating into extrafollicular areas (60) and the splenic marginal zones (MZ) (61), are not only important for the production of B cell activating components but also for the delivery of Ag to the BCR (62).

The question is whether in an autoimmune disease self-antigen containing IgG-IC can trigger DCs to promote autoreactive immune responses by presenting autoantigens or to release B and T cell activating cytokines and other stimulating factors breaking tolerance and whether FcγRIIb on DCs negatively regulates these processes. That is any way at a stage of the disease that some autoantibodies are already produced.

pDCs produce type I IFN in response to viral nucleic acids sensed through TLR7 and TLR9 (63, 64). Their main function is to control tolerance in the steady state (65, 66). Mouse pDCs express exclusively FcγRIIb (67). Conflicting results have been published regarding FcγRIIb facilitated T cell priming by mouse pDCs (56, 67, 68). *In vitro* uptake of IgG-ICs by mouse pDC is FcγRIIb dependent but does not promote Ag presentation to T cells (67), similarly to what has been shown with FcγRIIb mediated IC uptake in cDCs (62). In contrast, it has been reported that subcutaneous (s.c.) injection of *in vitro* IgG1-IC loaded pDCs induces strong Ag-specific CD4[+] and CD8[+] T cell responses although with lower efficiency than cDCs. The IgG1-IC-loaded pDC mainly promoted a Th2/tolerogenic environment *in vivo* (68). Human pDCs express besides low levels of FCGR2B, the activating FCGR2A and FCGR3B (16) and show FCGR2A dependent IgG enhanced Ag presentation to T cells (69). SLE patients have circulating ICs, containing small nuclear RNA and anti-small nuclear RNA IgG. pDCs can acquire such IC via FCGR mediated uptake resulting in stimulation of TLR7 and 8 and production of IFNα (70), a cytokine that is believed to play a central role in SLE pathogenesis (71). However, this requires FCGR2A and not FCGR2B (72). Therefore, it is unlikely that such a pathogenic process plays a role in lupus-like disease in mice.

B Cells and FDC

Primary B cells, developed and selected in the bone marrow, are recruited into GCs within the spleen and lymph nodes to undergo affinity maturation by Somatic Hypermutation (SHM). Three main mechanisms maintain self-tolerance in the primary B cell repertoire: central clonal deletion, receptor editing, clonal anergy induction (73). The first two effectively remove autoreactive B cells from the system. Clonal anergy occurs when self-reactive B cells interact with a self-Ag with relatively low avidity. The result is that BCR signaling is desensitized because of chronic exposure to self-antigens (74, 75) and differentiation into plasma cells is suppressed (76) resulting in the maintenance of anergic B cells with the potential to produce auto-Abs which can be recruited into GC (77). Anergic B cells can get T help if their BCR cross-reacts with foreign Ag but because of impaired BCR signaling FAS-mediated apoptosis is induced. However, extensive cross-linking by a foreign antigen can overcome the attenuated BCR signaling in anergic B cells inhibiting apoptosis (74). Autoreactive primary B cells can escape negative selection because of "clonal ignorance" when self-reactive B cells cannot encounter their self-Ag because it is hidden inside the cell. Development, responsiveness, and lifespan of ignorant cells is normal (76, 78, 79). The lack of T cell help after Ag contact induces apoptosis in ignorant self-reactive B cells in the periphery. However, it is striking that many auto-Abs are directed against intracellular Ags such as DNA. Therefore, it has been suggested that ignorant self-reactive B cells might be important for the development of SLE (77). So, the GC has to deal with three types of potential autoreactive B cells: anergic and ignorant, both recruited, and newly generated by somatic hypermutation in the GC reaction. Several mechanisms are in place in the GC to avoid the development of auto-Ab producing plasma cells. A very high concentration of self-Ag in the GC either overrules the binding of the BCR to foreign Ag presented by the FDC and apoptosis is induced, because of the lack of additional signals provided by the FDC (80), or/and blocks presentation of foreign Ag to follicular helper T cells (T_{FH}), whose survival signals are required. Alternatively, self-reactive B cells can be maintained temporarily until their self-reactivity is abrogated by somatic hypermutation (SHM) (81). Ignorant self-reactive primary B cells, activated by cross-reactive foreign Ag, can enter the GC to get T_{FH} help (82) and subsequently, receptor editing by SHM can destroy self-recognition and improve specificity for foreign antigen. However, this appears not sufficient to prevent that autoreactive B cells escape negative selection in the GC and enter the AFC (antibody-forming cell) pathway. More downstream tolerance checkpoints are required.

In the GC Ag is presented to B cells on the cell surface of FDC, mainly in the form of CR1/2 bound C3d-coated ICs. FcγRIIb is expressed on both the GC B cell and the FDC. Although FcγRIIb is upregulated on FDC in GC compared to non-GC FDC, its expression is relatively low compared to CR2 expression. Therefore, it is unlikely that FcγRIIb plays a role in the capture and presentation of Ag early on in the GC response

(83). It is unclear how a GC B cell becomes activated, because binding of its BCR to the Ag, within the FDC bound ICs, will also crosslink FcγRIIb on that B cell. It has been suggested that FcγRIIb expression on FDC competes with FcγRIIb expression on GC B cells by binding most of the Fc domains in the ICs (84). The outcome of co-engagement of BCR and FcγRIIb by ICs bound to FDC in GC might be dependent on the balance between concurrent activating and inhibiting signals, leading to stimulatory, inhibitory, or apoptotic responses (33, 85, 86). FcγRIIb might set a threshold for B-cell activation, that enables the selection of B cells with a BCR with sufficiently high affinity, to become activated. B cells with BCRs that have lost their affinity for the presented Ag during the process of affinity maturation by SHM will get only signals via crosslinking of FcγRIIb, which could result in induction of apoptosis as has been demonstrated *in vitro* (28, 33, 87, 88). In conclusion, the inhibitory FcγRIIb would be an important checkpoint for the deletion of potentially autoreactive B cells in the GC.

An additional apoptosis inducing mechanism in the bone marrow might also contribute to the control of autoreactive B cells (10). Long-lived plasma cells persist in the bone marrow. To provide room to newly generated plasma cells that migrate to the bone marrow after a new infection has occurred, a restricted number of plasma cells in the bone marrow has to be eliminated. Based on observations *in vitro* and *in vivo* in mice it has been hypothesized that plasma cells (which intrinsically lack BCR expression) are killed by apoptosis, induced by cross-linking of FcγRIIb highly expressed on these cells (10).

Non-immune Cells

On LSEC FcγRIIb might function as an endocytic scavenger receptor removing small IgG-IC from circulation to prevent systemic IC triggered inflammation (25). FcγRIIb on renal mesangial cells might protect against IgG-IC induced inflammation in the kidney (89). Both mechanisms might protect against the pathogenesis of IC-driven autoimmune diseases such as glomerulonephritis in SLE in the efferent phase. Because of the lack of an endothelial cell-specific Cre expressing strain that is not transcriptionally active during early hematopoiesis, required to generate endothelium-specific FcγRIIb deficient mice, the specific role of FcγRIIb on LSEC should be studied by applying transplantation of bone marrow from WT mice into lethally irradiated *FcγRIIb* KO mice.

FORWARD GENETICS: ASSOCIATION OF AUTOIMMUNITY AND FcγRIIb POLYMORPHISM

In Mice

The association between autoimmunity and *FcγRIIb* polymorphism is extensively studied in NZW and NZB inbred stains. NZB mice show limited autoimmunity (90) while NZW mice are not autoimmune although their B cells have intrinsic defects sufficient to break tolerance to nuclear antigens (91, 92). However, the (NZBxNZW)F1 offspring of an accidental cross between NZW and NZB mice (93) showed a severe lupus-like

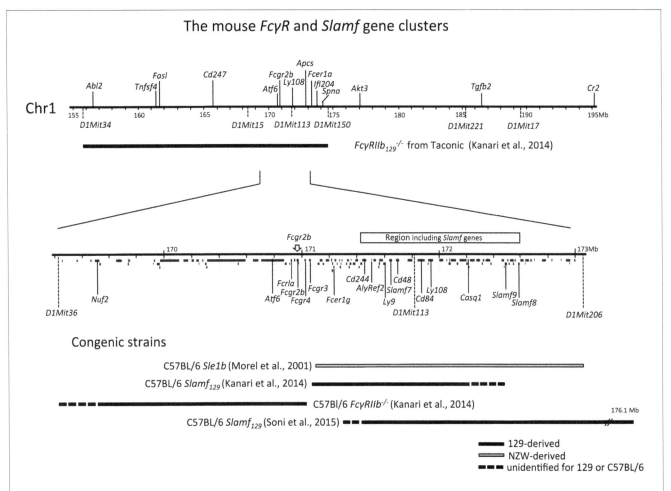

FIGURE 1 | Physical map of the sub-telomeric region of mouse chromosome 1. The upper horizontal line represents a 40 Mb genomic region including the 129 derived *FcγRIIb* flanking region present in the original *FyRIIB*$_{129}^{-/-}$ mouse, backcrossed more than 7 generations into C57BL/6 background. This *FcγRIIb* flanking region spans at a minimum the distance between the microsatellite markers *D1Mit34* and *D1Mit150* [horizontal black bar; (98)]. The lower horizontal line represents a magnification of the 3.8 Mb subregion located between microsatellite markers *D1Mit36* and *D1Mit206* showing a detailed map of the *FcγR* and *Slam* family gene clusters within this region. In addition, below the line, the location of all other coding genes in this region is shown according to the NCBI database. At the bottom, the congenic fragments present in the different *FcγRIIb*$^{-/-}$ and *Slamf*$_{129}$ C57BL/6 congenic strains, described in the text, are depicted as horizontal bars.

phenotype characterized by a gender-bias, expansion of activated B and CD4$^+$ T cells, splenomegaly, elevated serum ANA and IC-mediated GN causing renal failure and premature death at 10–12 months of age (94). By backcrossing (NZBxNZW)F1xNZW followed by brother-sister mating the NZM2410 recombinant inbred strain with a homozygous genome was generated (95–97). In this mouse four SLE susceptibility loci, *Sle1-4*, have been identified on different chromosomes. *Sle1* is located on the telomeric region of Chr1 syntenic to human 1q23 that has shown strong linkage to SLE susceptibility in all human studies. The *FcγR* gene cluster maps in this region (**Figure 1**) and is from NZW origin in NZM2410 mice. From the NZM2410 strain, C57BL/6 strains have been developed congenic for a single SLE susceptibility locus. The presence of *Sle1* appeared to be sufficient to break tolerance in C57BL/6 mice and to drive the production of high titers of anti-chromatin ANAs with a selective Ab reactivity to H2A/H2B/DNA sub-nucleosomes (99, 100).

Importantly, this step appears to be necessary for the induction of disease (100) making *Sle1* a key locus in the initiation of SLE. Transplantation of hematopoietic stem cells from C57BL/6 *Sle1* congenic mice into C57BL/6 recipient mice showed that *Sle1* causes independent B and T cell-intrinsic effects on the B cell response (101, 102).

Three *FcγRIIb* haplotypes [numbered I-III according to Jiang et al. (103), **Table 1**] have been recognized in inbred strains of mice and wild mice with variation in the promoter region and intron 3 (**Table 1**). Haplotype I with 2 deletions in the promoter region and one in intron 3 is found in autoimmune-prone strains and most wild mice and is associated with decreased expression of FcγRIIb on Mφ, activated B cells and GC B cells (11, 103–105). By using C7BL/6 congenic strains with the NZW (106) and NZB (107) allelic variants of *FcγRIIb* the effect of the deletions in haplotype I and II on B cell expression was studied. When immunized with KLH, FcγRIIb expression on splenic non-GC B

TABLE 1 | Allelic variants of mouse *FcγRIIb* gene and their association with impaired expression and autoimmune disease susceptibility.

Haplotype	Mouse strain	Genetic variation	Phenotype
I	NZB, BXSB, MRL, NOD, Wild mice 129	13 bp 5′ deletion in promoter 3 bp 3′ deletion in promoter 4 bp 5′ deletion in intron 3	Decreased expression on Mφ and activated and GC B cells. Autoimmune-prone (except 129)
II	NZW, SWR, SJL	4 bp 5′ deletion in intron 3 24 b 3′ deletion in intron 3	Decreased expression on GC B cells. Potential to accelerate autoimmunity
III	C57BL/6, BALB/c, DBA	No deletions	Not autoimmune

cells was high and similar in C7BL/6 and C57BL/6 *FcγRIIb~NZB~* congenic mice. In contrast, the expression on activated GC B cells was markedly down-regulated in C57BL/6 congenic *FcγRIIb~NZB~* mice and up-regulated in control C57BL/6 mice, in comparison with the expression levels on non-GC B cells. The downregulation of FcγRIIb expression on activated GC B cells was associated with an increase of IgG anti-KLH Ab titers. C57BL/6 *FcgRIIb~NZB~* congenic mice also showed lower FcγRIIb expression on Mφ compared with WT C57BL/6 mice (107). In a C57BL/6 knockin (KI) mouse model of the 5′ region of the haplotype I *FcγRIIb* gene (*FcγRIIb~NZB~*), FcγRIIb failed to be upregulated on activated and GC B cells resulting in enhanced early GC responses and low auto-Ab production without kidney disease as discussed later in more detail (11).

As mentioned earlier, *in vitro* cross-linking of FcγRIIb on B cells from C57BL/6 mice can induce apoptosis. However, plasma cells from autoimmune-prone NZB or MRL mice could not be killed *in vitro* by FcγRIIb cross-linking because of too little expression of the receptor (10). This might partially explain why these autoimmune-prone mice have larger numbers of plasma cells and might contribute to the autoimmune phenotype of these mice.

Similarly, to the *FcγRIIb~NZB~* allele, the *FcγRIIb~NZW~* allele in the C57BL/6 *Sle1* congenic strain did not upregulate its expression on GC B cells and plasma cells, as did the C57BL/6 allele, when immunized with SRBCs. However, in the absence of its *Sle1* flanking regions, *FcγRIIb~NZW~* did not induce an autoimmune phenotype but was associated with an increased number of class-switched plasma cells (108). This might indicate that the decreased expression of the *FcγRIIb~NZW~* allele is not sufficient for the development of autoreactive B cells but can result in the increase of the number of autoreactive B cells, induced by other lupus-susceptibility loci, by enhancing the production of class-switched plasma cells. This suggests that the *FcγRIIb~NZB~* (haplotype I) allele has a stronger impact on susceptibility to autoimmunity than the *FcγRIIb~NZW~* (haplotype II) allele (**Figure 2**). However, in one study comparing the phenotypes of C57BL/6 strains congenic for different intervals of the *Nba2* locus, a region on Chr1 of NZB mice corresponding to

the *Sle1~NZW~* locus, *FcγRIIb~NZB~* was identified as an autoimmune susceptibility gene (114), in another it was not (115). *Sle1* can be divided in four non-overlapping sub-loci: *Sle1a*, *-b*, *-c*, and *-d*. *Sle1b* is far the most potent autoimmune susceptibility locus causing almost the same phenotype as the whole *Sle1* locus: gender-biased spontaneous loss of immune tolerance to chromatin, the production of high titers of IgG auto-Abs with a penetrance of 90% at 9 months of age and increase of total IgM and B7-2 expression on B cells (116). This suggests that *Sle1b* mainly affects B cells. The genomic location of *Sle1b* was determined by phenotypic analysis (e.g., ANA production) of a series of C57BL/6 congenic strains carrying truncated *Sle1* intervals. C57BL/6 congenic mice with an NZW derived genomic fragment, containing the *FcγR* cluster, did not develop ANA whereas C57BL/6 mice, containing an adjacent 900 kb congenic NZW fragment expressing 24 genes including seven members of the highly polymorphic signaling lymphocytic activation molecules (*Slam*) cluster, did. This positions the *FcγR* cluster just outside the *Sle1b* locus (117) and confirms previous observations that *FcγRIIb* is located in between the *Sle1a* and *Sle1b* loci (113) (**Figure 1**). Together these data suggest that in C57BL/6 *Sle1* congenic mice the *FcγRIIb~NZW~* allele is not required for the development of an autoimmune phenotype, whereas the adjacent *Slam* cluster is. Because of these puzzling results, the questions remain why FcγRIIb is upregulated on GC B cells in non-autoimmune inbred strains such as C57BL/6 and BALB/c and why this is impaired in autoimmune-prone mouse strains and how does that contribute to the autoimmune phenotype of these mice.

Slam family (*Slamf*) member genes encode cell surface glycoproteins with extracellular binding domains that mediate stimulatory and/or inhibitory signaling via associations with members of the Slam-associated protein (SAP) family of signaling adaptors during cell-cell interactions between many hematopoietic cell types (118–120). They are the only genes within the *Sle1b* interval with obvious immunological functions (117). Most Slamf members act as self-ligand and are expressed on many lymphoid and myeloid cell subsets, platelets, and hematopoietic stem and progenitor cells. Slamf plays a role in the interaction of CD4⁺ T cells with cognate B cells, recruitment and retention of T cells within the emerging GCs (121–123), long-lasting T cell:B-cell contact, optimal T_FH function, T cell activation (124, 125), stabilization of B–T cell conjugates and sustaining effective delivery of T cell help required for GC formation (126, 127).

The *Slamf* genes show extensive polymorphisms (117) but only two haplotypes of the *Slamf* locus have been identified in laboratory mouse strains. Haplotype 1 is represented by C57BL/6 and related strains and haplotype 2 by all autoimmune-prone mouse strains, as well as many non-autoimmune mouse strains including BALB/c and 129. The polymorphism in *Slamf* member *Ly108* affects the expression of two alternatively spliced isoforms, Ly108-1 and, Ly108-2, which differ exclusively in their cytoplasmic region (117). Ly108-1 is dominantly expressed in T and B lymphocytes of mice with haplotype 2, whereas Ly108-2 is dominantly expressed in T and B cells of mice with haplotype 1. Modulation of the BCR signaling by Ly108-1 results in the impaired negative selection of B cells (128). Overexpression of

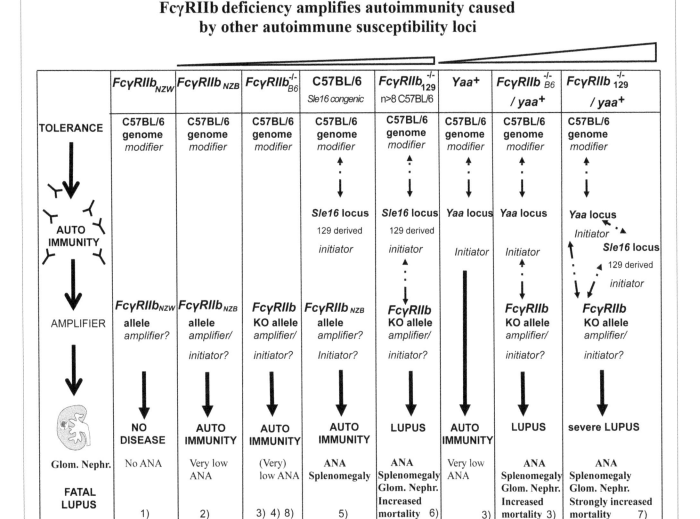

FIGURE 2 | Epistasis between the *FcγRIIb* KO alleles and the *Sle16 (Slam129)* and *Yaa* autoimmune susceptibility loci resulting in lupus-like disease in C57BL/6 mice. Epistatic interactions are indicated as dotted arrows. The FcγRIIb flanking *Sle16* genomic region contains the autoimmunity associated *Slamf129* haplotype 2 gene cluster (see **Figure 1**). (1) Rahman et al. (108); (2) Espéli et al. (11); (3) Boross et al. (109); (4) Li et al. (110); (5) Bygrave et al. (111); (6) Bolland and Ravetch (112); (7) Bolland et al. (113); (8) Kanari et al. (98). The increasing severity of autoimmune disease in the different mouse models is depicted on top.

both C57BL/6 derived non-autoimmune Ly108 and CD84 Slamf members was required to restore tolerance in autoimmune-prone C57BL/6 *Sle1* congenic mice (129), indicating that polymorphism in both *Slamf* genes contributes to the autoimmune phenotype of C57BL/6 *Sle1* congenic mice.

In the NZM2410 model four NZW-derived SLE suppressor loci have been identified (130). The presence of such suppressor loci might explain why NZW and also129 and BALB/c mice do not develop autoimmune disease, although they carry the type 2 *Slamf* haplotype.

In Humans

The reported copy number variation (CNV) in human *FCGR* genes does not involve *FCGR2B* (131–134). A series of single nucleotide polymorphisms (SNPs) have been reported to be located both in the promoter and the encoding region of

the human *FCGR2B* gene (135). Two SNPs are located in the promoter region at nucleotide positions−386 and −120 (−386G>C; *rs3219018* and −120A>T; *rs34701572*) (136) resulting in four haplotypes:−386G−120T (named *FCGR2B.1*), −386C−120T (*FCGR2B.2*),−386G−120A (*FCGR2B.3*), and −386C−120A (*FCGR2B.4*). The rare *FCGR2B.4* haplotype increased the transcription of *FCGR2B in vitro* and resulted in increased FCGR2B expression on EBV transformed B cells and primary B cells (137) and myeloid cells (138), compared to the more frequent *FCGR2B.1* haplotype. However, independently, others have shown that homozygosity of the −386C genotype decreases the transcription and surface expression of FCGR2B in peripheral B cells compared to the −386G homozygote genotype (139). Up till now, there is no explanation for these contradictory results.

In the transmembrane encoding fifth exon a non-synonymous C to T transition was identified, *rs1050501*, resulting in the substitution of isoleucine with threonine at position 232 (140), excluding the receptor from lipid rafts. This prevents interaction of FCGR2B with ITAM containing receptors such as the activating FCGR and the BCR (141, 142). Mφs from individuals homozygous for *FCGR2B^T232* showed a stronger phagocytic capacity of IgG-IC while the B cells of these individuals showed reduced FCGR2B-mediated inhibition of BCR-triggered proliferation (142).

GWAS analyses have shown an association between *rs1050501* and SLE (140, 143–147). Three meta-analyses confirmed these associations (147–149). The *FCGR2B^T232* homozygosity is associated with an odds ratio of 1.73, one of the strongest associations in SLE (147). Association of *rs1050501* with Rheumatoid Arthritis (RA) has been reported for a Taiwanese cohort (150).

The frequency of homozygosity of the *FCGR2B^T232* allele is only 1% in Caucasians and in contrast 5–11% in African and South-East Asian populations (151). This might be one of the explanations for the ethnic differences in SLE susceptibility. Malaria is endemic in Africa and South-East Asia. An association was found between decreased susceptibility for severe malaria and homozygosity for the *FCGR2B^T232* allele (135). So, increased protection against malaria by down-regulation of FCGR2B expression goes along with increased risk to develop SLE.

A significant but weak association has been observed between *SLAMF* and susceptibility to SLE. The weakness of the association might be explained by the limited size of the cohorts studied (152). An association study of UK and Canadian families with SLE has revealed multiple polymorphisms in several *SLAMF* genes (153). However, the strongest association with a non-synonymous SNP could not be replicated in independent Japanese and European cohorts of SLE patients (154, 155). Instead, another SNP was significantly associated with the susceptibility to SLE in another Japanese cohort (156). One large-scale case-control association study showed an association of two SNPs with increased susceptibility to RA, in two independent Japanese cohorts (155). In conclusion, these observations indicate that also in human's polymorphisms of *SLAMF* contribute to the susceptibility to autoimmune disease.

Overall, a model emerges from both studies with C57BL/6 *Sle* congenic mouse strains and human SLE (157), in which disease susceptibility arises through the co-expression of multiple genetic variants that have weak individual effects (152, 158). According to the "threshold liability" model, the severity of the autoimmune phenotype increases with the increasing number of autoimmunity associated allelic variants of autoimmune susceptibility genes in the genome. However, epistatic interactions might result in a more complex non-additive inheritance of the autoimmune phenotype (**Figure 2**). According to this "multiplicative model" the interactions of all susceptibility and suppressor alleles in the genome determine the susceptibility for autoimmune diseases of an individual (159). Importantly this means that the contribution of an individual gene to the autoimmune phenotype can vary depending on the presence of other susceptibility and suppressor genes

in the genome (the genomic context). This might explain the puzzling and contradictory results with the $Fc\gamma RIIb_{NZW}$ and $Fc\gamma RIIB_{NZB}$ haplotypes. To uncover the polygenic effects associated with a complex disease such as SLE not a single gene association approach but gene set analysis (GSA) is required (160). However, a reverse genetic approach might offer the opportunity to reconstruct an autoimmune phenotype by modifying a combination of a limited number of candidate genes in a well-defined genetic background.

REVERSE GENETICS

So far three $Fc\gamma RIIb$ KO mouse models have been published. The first published KO was generated by gene targeting in 129 derived ES cells (161) and subsequently backcrossed into the C57BL/6 background, here called $Fc\gamma RIIb_{129}^{-/-}$ mouse. This mouse on a not well-defined mixed genetic background was during 15 years (between 1996 and 2011) the only $Fc\gamma RIIb$ KO model available and has been extensively used resulting in an overwhelming amount of literature concerning the role of FcγRIIb in immune tolerance. Subsequently, independently, in two different laboratories $Fc\gamma RIIb$ KO mice were generated by gene targeting in C57BL/6 derived ES cells, here called $Fc\gamma RIIb_{B6}^{-/-}$ mice (109, 110). The published data regarding ANA titers of one of these mouse strains are inconsistent (162, 163) as are the autoimmune phenotypes of both C57BL/6 strains (109, 110). Moreover, it is still under debate to what extent the autoimmune phenotypes of the $Fc\gamma RIIb_{B6}^{-/-}$ mice differ from the autoimmune phenotype of the $Fc\gamma RIIb_{129}^{-/-}$ mice. Therefore, we discuss in chronological order these different models.

The $Fc\gamma RIIb$ KO Mouse on Mixed 129/C57BL/6 Background

The $Fc\gamma RIIb_{129}^{-/-}$ mouse develops elevated immunoglobulin levels in response to both T cell-dependent and T cell-independent Ags (161), have more plasma cells (10), and show an enhanced passive cutaneous anaphylaxis compared to WT controls (161). They develop arthritis (164) and Good pasture's syndrome-like disease (165) upon immunization with bovine collagen type II and type IV, respectively when backcrossed into the non-permissive ($H-2^b$ haplotype) C57BL/6 background. When backcrossed more than 7 generations into C57BL/6, but not BALB/c background, the $Fc\gamma RIIb_{129}^{-/-}$ mice started to develop spontaneously with high penetrance lupus-like disease. This autoimmune disease is characterized by gender bias, splenomegaly, increase of the proportion of different subsets of activated lymphocytes with age, high titers of ANA, IC-mediated GN and vasculitis in different organs resulting in proteinuria and premature death (112) very similar to the phenotype of the NZM2410 mouse we discussed earlier. This is surprising because, as we have seen, genetic studies revealed that lupus susceptibility is a multigenic phenotype. Monogenic autoimmune diseases are rare (158). However, the strong autoimmune phenotype of the $Fc\gamma RIIb_{129}^{-/-}$ mouse cannot be attributed exclusively to the deletion of the *FcgRIIb* alleles. This mouse has been generated by gene targeting in 129 derived ES cells and subsequently backcrossed into C57BL/6 background. Such a mouse is, even after 10–12 generations, not fully C57BL/6 but congenic for the 129 derived flanking regions of the targeted allele, containing still hundreds of genes of 129 origin (**Figure 1**). The 129 genome contains more than 1,000 non-synonymous mutations compared to the C57BL/6 genome (166). This is only one part of the problem. Epistasis between 129 derived loci and the C57BL/6 genome also occurs. It has been shown that mice without targeted alleles but congenic for the 129 derived distal-region of Chr1 (*Sle16*), a lupus-associated region including the autoimmune-prone haplotype 2 of the *Slamf* genes and the haplotype I of the *FcγRIIb* gene, develop a similar autoimmune phenotype as C57BL/6 *Sle1* congenic mice (111). That might explain why several mouse strains generated by targeting genes in the proximity of the *Slamf* locus in 129 derived ES cells, and backcrossed into C57BL/6 background, develop autoimmunity.

Strikingly, the $FcγRIIb_{129}^{-/-}$ mouse backcrossed more than seven generations into C57BL/6 background develops ANA with similar selective reactivity to H2A/H2B/DNA sub-nucleosomes as C57BL/6 *Sle1* congenic mice, however, with earlier onset, stronger penetrance, and higher titers. Irradiated $Rag^{-/-}$ C57BL/6 or $IgH^{-/-}$ C57BL/6 mice adoptively transferred with bone marrow from $FcγRIIb_{129}^{-/-}$ mice backcrossed more than seven generations into C57BL/6 background developed anti-chromatin antibodies and proteinuria, indicating that the disease is fully transferable, dependent on B cells. Myeloid $FcγRIIb^{-/-}$ cells are not required (112). This is in keeping with experiments, mentioned earlier, that show that the autoimmune phenotype of C57BL/6 *Sle1* congenic mice is completely reconstituted in C57BL/6 irradiated mice that received bone marrow from C57BL/6 *Sle1* congenic mice but not by the reciprocal reconstitution. This demonstrates that *Sle1* is functionally expressed in B cells (101) although impaired FcγRIIb expression seems to play a minor role in that model (113, 117). Taken together these data all point in the same direction: the strong lupus-like phenotype of the $FcγRIIb_{129}^{-/-}$ mice backcrossed more than seven generations into C57BL/6 background is caused by epistatic interaction between the $Slamf_{129}$ locus, the C57BL/6 genome, and $FcγRIIb^{-/-}$ (**Figure 2**), similar to the epistatic interactions between $FcγRIIb_{NZB}$ (haplotype I), $Slamf_{NZB}$ (haplotype 2) and the C57BL/6 genome in C57BL/6 *Nba2* congenic mice (114). As a consequence, the $FcγRIIb_{129}^{-/-}$ mouse suffers from the confounding effect that the $FcγRIIb_{129}$KO alleles are closely linked to the $Slamf_{129}$ locus associated with autoimmunity. This means that in most experimental conditions, no distinction can be made between $FcγRIIb^{-/-}$ and $Slamf_{129}$ mediated effects in these mice.

Ig gene analysis of ANA suggests that ANA develop in GCs (167–172). Therefore, analysis of the loss of tolerance in $FcγRIIb_{129}^{-/-}$ mice focused on GC (173). The role of FcγRIIb as an immune tolerance checkpoint has been studied in a transgenic mouse model in which the variable heavy chain (V_H) *3H9H-56R*, derived from a dsDNA specific hybridoma, or its variant *56RV_H*, with higher affinity binding to dsDNA, were inserted in the *Igh* locus (*IgM^a* allele) (174). Receptor editing, based on the use of specific light chains that abrogates the

dsDNA binding, is the main mechanism to maintain tolerance in these mice (175–177). The Ab selection process was compared between WT C57BL/6 and $FcγRIIb_{129}^{-/-}$ mice carrying the V_H transgenes (178). C57BL/6 mice expressing the high-affinity *56R* allele (B6.56R) developed low but significant anti-DNA titers, indicating that tolerance was broken, whereas C57BL/6 mice with the low-affinity *3H9* allele (B6.3H9) did not. Tolerance was also maintained in $FcγRIIb_{129}^{-/-}$ mice carrying the low-affinity *3H9* allele ($FcγRIIb_{129}^{-/-}$.3H9). The development of IgM-positive autoreactive B cells was similar in $FcγRIIb_{129}^{-/-}$ mice carrying the high-affinity *56R* allele ($FcγRIIb_{129}^{-/-}$.56R) and B6.56R mice. Moreover, $FcγRIIb_{129}^{-/-}$.3H9 mice and $FcγRIIb_{129}^{-/-}$.56R mice did not show differences in the populations of activated and GC B cells or T cells compared to B6.3H9 and B6.56R control mice. However, $FcγRIIb_{129}^{-/-}$.56R mice developed higher IgG anti-DNA titers compared to B6.56R mice. Taking together these observations suggest that the function of FcγRIIb in B6.56R mice is limiting the production of serum IgG anti-dsDNA. Analysis of hybridomas derived from these different mouse strains showed that a much higher percentage of hybridomas from $FcγRIIb_{129}^{-/-}$.56R mice secreted IgG antibodies compared to the hybridomas from B6.56R mice. Moreover, $FcγRIIb_{129}^{-/-}$.56R mice had a higher percentage of splenocytes with a plasma cell phenotype compared to B6.56R mice. The cross of the $FcγRIIb_{129}^{-/-}$ mice with autoimmune B cell receptor transgenic mice most likely bypasses the involvement of $Slamf_{129}$ (which is mainly responsible for the spontaneous development of autoreactive B cells in a C57BL/6 $Slamf_{129}$ congenic strain, as we will see later). So, in this case, the phenotype of the $FcγRIIb_{129}^{-/-}$.56R mouse can be completely attributed to the absence of FcγRIIb. From these results, it was concluded that the main function of FcγRIIb in the GC reaction is to control, as one of the latest checkpoints, the development of autoreactive IgG-secreting plasma cells and that most likely FcγRIIb deficiency modifies autoimmunity rather than initiates loss of tolerance (178). This was confirmed independently, in an experimental model with two V_H chain knockin strains, HKI65 and HKIR, with specificity for the hapten arsonate and a weak and strong specificity for DNA respectively (179). No indications for a role of FcγRIIb in primary or GC tolerance checkpoints were found. Only an increased number of plasma cells was detected in mice that received C57BL/6 HKIR/$FcγRIIb_{129}^{-/-}$ B cells. FcγRIIb seems to prevent autoimmunity by suppressing the production of autoreactive IgG from B cells that escaped negative selection in GC and enter the AFC pathway (179). This is also in agreement with observations in C57BL/6 $FcγRIIb_{NZW}$ congenic mice mentioned earlier (108). However, more recently it has been shown that the number of spontaneous (Spt) GC B cells is increased in 6–7 months old $FcγRIIb^{-/-}$ mice on a pure C57BL/6 background, suggesting that FcγRIIb deficiency dysregulates the Spt-GC B cell response [(163); **Table 3**] as will be discussed later.

The view that FcγRIIb acts as a suppressor of autoimmunity caused by other loci is supported by the observed synergism between $FcγRIIb^{-/-}$ and several autoimmune susceptibility loci. Just like the *Sle1* locus (100), $FcγRIIb^{-/-}$ interacts synergistically with the autoimmune susceptibility *Yaa* locus from BXSB autoimmune-prone mice, containing the *Tlr7* gene translocated from the X chromosome to the Y chromosome, resulting in strong acceleration of lupus-like disease in $Yaa^+Fc\gamma RIIb_{129}^{-/-}$ male mice (113) (**Figure 2**). MRL/*Fas^{lpr/lpr}* mice develop lupus-like disease whereas C57BL/6 *Fas^{lpr/lpr}* mice do not, likely due to suppressor activity of the C57BL/6 genome. However, C57BL/6 *Fas^{lpr/lpr}* $Fc\gamma RIIb_{129}^{-/-}$ mice develop systemic autoimmune disease (180). This is consistent with the presence of the haplotype I allelic variant of *Fc\gamma RIIb* in MRL mice with an impaired expression on B cell subsets. Mice deficient for both, deoxyribonuclease 1 like 3 (DNASE1L3) and FcγRIIb exhibit at the age of 10 weeks an IgG anti-dsDNA production higher than in 9 months old (NZBxNZW)F1 mice (181). The presence of either the *Yaa* locus or homozygosity for the *Fas^{lpr}* or *Dnase1l3* KO alleles is most likely sufficient to break tolerance. However, FcγRIIb prevents strong autoimmunity by suppressing the production of autoreactive IgG from B cells that have escaped negative selection and enter the AFC pathway. Because $Fc\gamma RIIb_{129}^{-/-}$ mice were used in the crosses mentioned a role for Slamf$_{129}$ cannot be excluded in these models as indicated by the much milder phenotype of the $Yaa^+ Fc\gamma RIIb_{B6}^{-/-}$ mouse on pure C57BL/6 background discussed later (109) compared to the severe lupus phenotype of the $Yaa^+Fc\gamma RIIb_{129}^{-/-}$ mouse (**Figure 2**). Nevertheless, these observations underscore the crucial role of FcγRIIb in the protection against the development of spontaneous autoimmunity determined by other autoimmune susceptibility loci.

Because of allelic exclusion, Ig transgenic mice do not have a normal B cell repertoire. Therefore, the development of self-reactive GC B cells and plasma cells was studied in $Fc\gamma RIIb_{129}^{-/-}$ mice by large scale Ig cloning from single isolated B cells to determine how loss of FcγRIIb influences the frequency at which autoreactive ANA-expressing B cells participate in GC reactions and develop in plasma cells under physiological conditions (173). In comparison with WT controls the following was observed in $Fc\gamma RIIb_{129}^{-/-}$ mice: (a) No skewing of *Ig* gene repertoire but enrichment for IgGs with highly positively charged IgH CDR3s which is associated with antibody autoreactivity; (b) lower numbers of somatic mutation; (c) increased numbers of polyreactive IgG$^+$ GC B cells and bone marrow plasma cells and (d) enrichment of nucleosome-reactive GC B cells and plasma cells. The overall frequency of ANAs was high in GC B cells but not in plasma cells. These results demonstrate that in $Fc\gamma RIIb_{129}^{-/-}$ mice IgG autoantibodies including ANAs are expressed by GC B cells and that somatic mutations contribute to the generation of high-affinity IgG antibodies suggesting that the $Fc\gamma RIIb^{-/-}$/Slamf$_{129}$ combination plays an important role in the regulation of autoreactive IgG$^+$ B cells which develop from non-self-reactive or low-self-reactive precursors by affinity maturation (173). It would be of great interest to repeat this analysis in $Fc\gamma RIIb_{B6}^{-/-}$ mice on pure C57BL6 background and C57BL/6 Slamf$_{129}$ congenic mice to define the individual contribution of the Slamf$_{129}$ locus and the $Fc\gamma RIIb$ KO alleles in the loss of immune tolerance in the C57BL/6 background.

Interestingly the frequency of high-affinity autoreactive IgG$^+$ plasma cells was relatively low, given the high frequency of autoreactive IgG$^+$ GC B cells. This can be explained by the existence of a tolerance checkpoint before GC B cells differentiate into spleen or bone marrow plasma cells, downstream of FcγRIIb and Slamf (173).

Complementation of the mutant phenotype of an organism by expression of a transduced WT gene is considered as the ultimate proof that the mutated gene is the cause of the phenotype. Irradiated autoimmune-prone BXSB, NZM2410, and $Fc\gamma RIIb_{129}^{-/-}$ mice transplanted with autologous bone marrow transduced with a viral vector expressing FcγRIIb showed reduced autoantibody levels and as a consequence much milder disease symptoms compared to mice that received autologous bone marrow transduced with an empty vector (182). These results were confirmed by using a transgenic mouse with a stable 2-fold B cell-specific overexpression of FcγRIIb (183). These mice hardly developed a lupus-like disease when backcrossed into autoimmune-prone MRL/*Fas^{lpr/lpr}* background. The underlying mechanism of these strong effects of overexpression of FcγRIIb is not known. These experiments mainly demonstrate that overexpression of FcγRIIb on B cells inactivates these cells resulting in a strong decrease in autoantibody production. Although they confirm a role of FcγRIIb in autoimmune disease they don't answer the intriguing question whether FcγRIIb deficiency is a modifier of autoimmunity rather than a primary initiator of the loss of tolerance.

FcγRIIb KO on a Pure C57BL/6 Background

To avoid the confounding effect of 129 derived flanking sequences (*Sle16*), independently, in two different laboratories $Fc\gamma RIIb^{-/-}$ mice were generated by gene targeting in C57BL/6 ES cells. To distinguish between these two models, one is called here $^{Le}Fc\gamma RIIb_{B6}^{-/-}$ (109) and the other $^{NY}Fc\gamma RIIb_{B6}^{-/-}$ (110). $^{Le}Fc\gamma RIIb_{B6}^{-/-}$ mice exhibit a hyperactive phenotype in the effector phase, although somewhat milder than $Fc\gamma RIIb_{129}^{-/-}$ mice, suggesting a contribution of *Sle16* to the phenotype of the $Fc\gamma RIIb_{129}^{-/-}$ mouse in the effector phase (109). Both KO mice develop very mild lupus-like disease (**Table 2**). Total IgG ANA was not significantly increased in 10 months old female $^{Le}Fc\gamma RIIb_{B6}^{-/-}$ mice compared to C57BL/6 mice although serum of 5% of these mice showed some total IgG anti-dsDNA and anti-ssDNA antibody titers just above (C57BL/6) baseline. In contrast, in 40% of 10 months old $^{NY}Fc\gamma RIIb_{B6}^{-/-}$ mice total IgG anti-nuclear Abs was significantly increased compared to C57BL/6 mice (110). But only five percent of $^{NY}Fc\gamma RIIb_{B6}^{-/-}$ mice showed premature death whereas mortality was not increased in $^{Le}Fc\gamma RIIb_{B6}^{-/-}$ mice although proteinuria and kidney pathology were significantly higher in these mice compared to C57BL/6 mice. The kidney phenotype in the absence of detectable ANA in $^{Le}Fc\gamma RIIb_{B6}^{-/-}$ mice points to a protective role of FcγRIIb in the kidney, in the efferent phase, as has also been shown in a model

TABLE 2 | Disease phenotypes of $Fc\gamma RIIb_{B6}^{-/-}$, C57BL/6 $Fc\gamma RIIB_{129}^{-/-}$ $Slamf_{B6}$ congenic, C57BL/6 $Slamf_{129}$ congenic and the original $Fc\gamma RIIb_{129}^{-/-}$ mice compared to WT C57BL/6 control mice at the age of 6–8 months.

Mouse Phenotype	$^{Le}Fc\gamma RIIb_{B6}^{-/-}$ [c]	C57BL6 $Fc\gamma RIIb_{129}^{-/-}$ $Slamf_{B6}$ Congenic[a]	$^{NY}Fc\gamma RIIb_{B6}^{-/-}$ [b,d]	C57BL/6 $Slamf_{129}$ Congenic[a,b]	$Fc\gamma RIIb_{129}^{-/-}$ [a,b,c,d]
Increased IgM	n.d.	−[a]	n.d.	−[a]	+[a]
Increased IgG[a]	n.d.	+ (♀)[a]	n.d.	−[a]	+ (♀ ♂)[a]
α-DNA	+ (♀) Total IgG Incidence 5%[c]	+ (♀) IgG2c[a]	++ (♀) IgG2c[b] Total IgG[d]	+++ IgG2c/2b[b] (♀) IgG2c[a]	++++++ (♀) IgG2c[a,b] IgG2b[b] Total IgG[a,d]
α-histone	− (♀) Total IgG[c]	n.d.	++ (♀) IgG2c[b]	+++ IgG2c/2b[b]	++++++ IgG2c/2b[b] Total IgG[c]
α-nuclear	+ (♀) Total IgG[c]	+ (♀) IgG2c[a]	++ (♀) IgG2c[b] Total IgG Incidence 40%[d]	+++ IgG2c[a,b] IgG2b[b]	++++++ (♀) IgG2c[a,b] IgG2b[b] Total IgG[a,d]
Kidney pathology	+ (♀)[c]	+ (♀)[a]	++[b]	−[a,b]	+++++[a,b,c]
IgG-IC deposition in glomeruli	+ (♀)[c]	+ (♀)[a]	++ (♀)[b]	+ (♀)[b] − (♀)[a]	++++ (♀ ♂)[a,b,c]
C3 deposition	+[c]	n.d.	−[b]	+[b]	++++[b,c]
Spleen	Slightly enlarged (♀)[c]	Slightly enlarged (♀)[a]	n.d.	Slightly enlarged (♀)[a]	Splenomegaly[a,b,c]
Spt-GC formation	n.d.	Normal (♀ ♂)[a]	Augmented + (♀)[b]	Augmented ++ (♀)[a,b]	Augmented +++ (♀)[a,b]
% GC B cells of CD19+ splenic B cells	n.d.	No increase (♀)[a]	Increase +[b]	Increase ++ (♀)[a]	Increase +++ (♀)[a]
Absolute numbers of splenic GC B cells	n.d.	No increase (♀)[a]	n.d.	Increase + (♀)[a]	Increase ++ (♀)[a]
Increased Mortality	−[c]	−[a]	+ 5%[d]	−[a,b]	Varies from 0%[a] (and 22%[c]) to 60%[d]

[a] Kanari et al. (98).
[b] Soni et al. (163).
[c] Boross et al. (109).
[d] Li et al. (110).
n.d., not determined.

of antibody-induced nephrotoxic nephritis (NTN) that will be discussed later (89).

The production of autoantibodies by C57BL/6 mice in the absence of FcγRIIb suggests that FcγRIIb deficiency, besides modifying autoimmunity caused by other autoimmune susceptibility loci (e.g., $Slamf_{129}$, Yaa), as discussed earlier, can result in loss of tolerance in the GC. However, it is tempting to speculate that the low titers of autoantibodies, that develop with low penetrance in $Fc\gamma RIIb$ KO mice on a pure C57BL/6 background, reflect the natural occurring autoreactive B cells in the GC of a WT C57BL/6 mouse, as described earlier, that are prevented to enter the AFC pathway in the presence of FcγRIIb (178). There are indications that C57BL/6 mice are more autoimmune prone than BALB/c mice. For example, B cell receptor editing as a mechanism to maintain B cell tolerance is less effective in these mice compared to BALB/c mice (178).

The $^{NY}Fc\gamma RIIb_{B6}^{-/-}$ mouse seems to exhibit a stronger disease phenotype than the $^{Le}Fc\gamma RIIb_{B6}^{-/-}$ mouse (**Table 2**). There are several explanations for this discrepancy:

a. The strains are generated with different ES cell lines. There might be relevant genomic differences between the C57BL/6 derived ES cell lines used. This question can be answered by sequencing the $Fc\gamma RIIb$ flanking genomic regions in both mouse strains.

b. The mice have been backcrossed several generations into different C57BL/6 mouse strains. There are substantial genetic variations between the different C57BL/6 strains used in different laboratories (184).

c. Environmental factors (immune status, microbiome) play a role. The incidence of lethal disease in $Fc\gamma RIIb_{129}^{-/-}$ mice varies between different laboratories from 0% to more than 60% (98, 109, 112, 173).

d. Differences in the methods used to measure ANA. In the $^{Le}Fc\gamma RIIb_{B6}^{-/-}$ mouse ANA have been measured only by ELISA of total IgG (109), whereas in the $^{NY}Fc\gamma RIIb_{B6}^{-/-}$ mouse IgG2a and IgG2b have been measured combined with Hep-2 cell staining (163). However, a significant increase in total IgG anti-nuclear Abs compared to C57BL/6 has also been reported with the $^{NY}Fc\gamma RIIb_{B6}^{-/-}$ mouse (110).

TABLE 3 | Characteristics of GC B and T cells in $^{NY}Fc\gamma RIIb_{B6}^{-/-}$, C57BL/6 Slamf$_{129}$ congenic, and the original $Fc\gamma RIIb_{129}^{-/-}$ mice compared with WT C57BL/6 control mice.

Phenotype / Mouse strain	$Fc\gamma RIIb_{129}^{-/-}$	C57BL/6 Slamf$_{129}$ congenic	$^{NY}Fc\gamma RIIb_{B6}^{-/-}$
Increase in frequency of B220$^+$PNA^{hi} CD95^{hi} Spt-GC B cells	+ + + +	+ +	+
Increase in Splenic GC size	+ + +	+ +	+
Increase in frequency of CD4$^+$CXCR5^{hi}PD-1^{hi} GC T$_{FH}$ cells	+ + +	+	−
Increase in frequency of CD4$^+$CXCR5^{int}PD-1^{int} T$_{FH}$ cells	+ + +	+	−
Increase in CD4$^+$GL7$^+$ GC T$_{FH}$ cells	+ +	+	−
IL-21 expression in GC T$_{FH}$ cells	+ + + +	+ +	−
PD-1 expression in GC T$_{FH}$ cells	+ + + +	+ +	+ +
ICOS expression in GC T$_{FH}$ cells	+ +	−	−
Increase in frequency of GC B cells upon antigenic stimulation	n.d.	+	−
Increase in frequency of GC T$_{FH}$ cells upon antigenic stimulation	n.d.	+	−
MHC class II upregulation on GC B cells upon antigenic stimulation	n.d.	+	−
Decrease of caspase activity in DAPI^{neg}B220$^+$Fas^{hi}PNA^{hi} GC B cells	+ +	+/−	+/−

n.d., not determined (163).

The Individual Contribution of FcγRIIb Deficiency and Slamf$_{129}$ to the Phenotype of the FcγRIIb KO Mouse on Mixed 129/C57BL/6 Background

Independently, in two different laboratories congenic C57BL6 Slamf$_{129}$ mice have been generated. One was generated by intensive backcrossing of the original $Fc\gamma RIIb_{129}^{-/-}$ mouse (161) into C57BL/6 background and selection for offspring in which the Slamf locus and the FcγRIIb KO allele had been segregated (98) resulting in two congenic strains called here as C57BL/6 Slamf$_{129}$ congenic and C57BL/6 $Fc\gamma RIIb_{129}^{-/-}$ Slamf$_{B6}$ congenic, respectively. The other C57BL6 Slamf$_{129}$ congenic mice were generated by a marker-assisted speed congenic approach (163) (**Figure 1**).

The development of autoimmunity was compared between C57BL/6 $Fc\gamma RIIb_{129}^{-/-}$ Slamf$_{B6}$ congenic, C57BL/6 Slamf$_{129}$ congenic and the original $Fc\gamma RIIb_{129}^{-/-}$ mice (98) or between C57BL/6 Slamf$_{129}$ congenic, $^{NY}Fc\gamma RIIb_{B6}^{-/-}$ and the original $Fc\gamma RIIb_{129}^{-/-}$ mice (163). Both C57BL/6 $Fc\gamma RIIb_{129}^{-/-}$ Slamf$_{B6}$ congenic and C57BL/6 Slamf$_{129}$ congenic mice developed very mild disease symptoms whereas the original $Fc\gamma RIIb_{129}^{-/-}$ mice developed severe disease compared to WT C57BL/6 mice. Importantly, the phenotype of the C57BL/6 $Fc\gamma RIIb_{129}^{-/-}$ Slamf$_{B6}$ congenic mouse strain confirmed mainly the phenotype of the $^{Le}Fc\gamma RIIb_{B6}^{-/-}$ mouse [(98); **Table 2**] showing very low ANA titers and little kidney pathology compared to $Fc\gamma RIIb_{129}^{-/-}$ mice.

The development of Spt-GC B cell and T$_{FH}$ responses in C57BL/6 Slamf$_{129}$ congenic, $^{NY}Fc\gamma RIIb_{B6}^{-/-}$ and $Fc\gamma RIIb_{129}^{-/-}$ mice were carefully compared [(163); **Table 3**]. C57Bl/6 Slamf$_{129}$ congenic mice had significantly more GC B cells and T$_{FH}$ and GC T$_{FH}$ cells 12 days after immunization with OVA compared to WT C57BL/6 mice. B cells and DCs from Slamf$_{129}$ congenic mice exhibited stronger antigen presentation in in vitro assays compared to B cells and DCs from WT C57BL/6 mice. By

using a variety of in vivo and in vitro assays with naïve B cells it was found that B cell-intrinsic deficiency of FcγRIIb and expression of Slamf$_{129}$ has no effect on proliferation but promotes differentiation of naïve B cells into GC B cells as indicated by increased expression of Aicda and GL-7. The percentage of apoptotic GC B cells was significantly lower in $Fc\gamma RIIb_{129}^{-/-}$ mice compared to WT C57BL/6 mice whereas in C57BL/6 Slamf$_{129}$ congenic and $^{NY}Fc\gamma RIIb_{B6}^{-/-}$ mice this decrease was not significant. This suggests that FcγRIIb deficiency and Slamf$_{129}$ act synergistically to increase the survival of GC B cells in $Fc\gamma RIIb_{129}^{-/-}$ mice. Naïve and activated B cells from $^{NY}Fc\gamma RIIb_{B6}^{-/-}$ and to a lower extent from C57BL/6 Slamf$_{129}$ congenic mice showed an enhanced metabolic capacity compared to B cells from C57BL/6 mice. This enhancement was stronger in $Fc\gamma RIIb_{129}^{-/-}$ mice.

Taken together these observations suggest that Slamf$_{129}$ plays a predominant, and FcγRIIb deficiency a modest role in modulating the Spt-GC B cell and T$_{FH}$ responses. Some of their functions are synergistic others mutually exclusive. GC T$_{FH}$ cell responses are mainly affected by Slamf$_{129}$ [(163); **Table 3**]. By using the experimental model of the V$_H$ chain knockin strain HKIR mentioned earlier (179) it was demonstrated that B cell-specific expression of Slamf$_{129}$ is necessary for the autoreactive B cells to expand in the GC confirming previous observations in C57BL/6 Sle1 congenic mice (129).

The increased Spt-GC responses in $^{NY}Fc\gamma RIIb_{B6}^{-/-}$ and C57BL/6 Slamf$_{129}$ congenic mice were associated with the production of autoantibodies. However, the titers were much lower than in $Fc\gamma RIIb_{129}^{-/-}$ mice which had also the strongest increase in Spt-GC responses. C57BL/6 Slamf$_{129}$ congenic mice developed higher ANA titers than $^{NY}Fc\gamma RIIb_{B6}^{-/-}$ mice, staining both cytoplasm and nucleus of Hep-2 cells, whereas sera from $^{NY}Fc\gamma RIIb_{B6}^{-/-}$ mice show only cytoplasmic staining patterns (163) confirming previous results with the C57BL/6 $Fc\gamma RIIb_{129}^{-/-}$ Slamf$_{B6}$ congenic mouse strain (98). IgG2b and IgG2c ANA were significantly increased in C57BL/6 $Slamf_{129}$ congenic mice whereas only IgG2c ANA were significantly increased in $^{NY}Fc\gamma RIIb_{B6}^{-/-}$ mice. With an autoantigen array, it was shown that $Fc\gamma RIIb_{129}^{-/-}$ mice develop high titers of IgG antibodies against a large variety of autoantigens. Several of these antibodies were also present in the serum of $^{NY}Fc\gamma RIIb_{B6}^{-/-}$ mice but their titers were much lower than in $Fc\gamma RIIb_{129}^{-/-}$ mice (163). Unfortunately, sera from C57BL/6 $Slamf_{129}$ congenic mice were not tested in the autoantigen array.

Kidney pathology was absent (98) or very mild, with higher complement deposition than $^{NY}Fc\gamma RIIb_{B6}^{-/-}$ mice (163), in C57BL/6 $Slamf_{129}$ congenic mice, mild in $^{NY}Fc\gamma RIIb_{B6}^{-/-}$ or C57BL/6 $Fc\gamma RIIb_{129}^{-/-}$ $Slamf_{B6}$ congenic mice with higher IgG deposition than in C57BL/6 $Slamf_{129}$ congenic mice, and severe, with highest C3 and IgG deposition compared to the other genotypes, in $Fc\gamma RIIb_{129}^{-/-}$ mice (98, 163). In conclusion, the deficiency of FcγRIIb together with the presence of $Slamf_{129}$ results in a phenotype of the $Fc\gamma RIIb_{129}^{-/-}$ mouse with increased Spt-GC B cell responses characterized by an increase of the following parameters: metabolic activity in B cells, differentiation of B cells into a GC B cell phenotype and GC B cell survival. This is associated with loss of immune tolerance resulting in ANA production and the development of severe lupus-like disease (163). However, the underlying cellular and molecular mechanisms of these associations are not well-understood and the subject of speculation and debate with respect to the role of FcγRIIb in GC (185). This can be illustrated with the surprising observation in the $Fc\gamma RIIb_{NZB}$ KI mouse model mentioned earlier, in which FcγRIIb failed to be upregulated on activated and GC B cells resulting in enhanced early GC responses (11). Upon immunization, these KI mice showed an early and sustained increased affinity maturation of Ag-specific GC B cells. Previous models suggest that low expression of FcγRIIb reduces the BCR activation threshold resulting in less affinity maturation. However, an alternative explanation might be that low FcγRIIb expression increases the survival of bystander Ag non-specific GC B cells and, as a consequence, increases competition for T_{FH} help between Ag-specific and non-antigen specific B cells, resulting in increased affinity maturation (11).

Cell-Type-Specific *FcγRIIb* KO Mouse Models

To determine on what B cell subset(s) and on what myeloid cells FcγRIIb might be involved in a checkpoint for immune tolerance, cell-type-specific $Fc\gamma RIIb^{-/-}$ mice were generated, independently, in two different laboratories. Both the $^{Le}Fc\gamma RIIb_{B6}^{-/-}$ and $^{NY}Fc\gamma RIIb_{B6}^{-/-}$ mouse models, on a pure C57BL/6 background, were originally generated as floxed $Fc\gamma RIIb$ mice ($Fc\gamma RIIb_{B6}^{fl/fl}$) and subsequently crossed with a Cre deleter transgenic mouse to generate the germline $Fc\gamma RIIb_{B6}^{-/-}$ mice discussed earlier. In addition, the $Fc\gamma RIIb_{B6}^{fl/fl}$ mice were also crossed with a variety of cell type-specific Cre transgenic mice (**Table 4**) to generate cell-type-specific $Fc\gamma RIIb_{B6}^{-/-}$ strains that were analyzed in the following

models of diseases for which germline $Fc\gamma RIIb$ KOs are highly susceptible: (a) the induced autoimmune diseases CIA, both on permissive (immunization with chicken collagen type II) and non-permissive (immunization with bovine collagen type II) background and (b) anti-glomerular basement membrane antibody (anti-GBM) disease, (c) the spontaneous autoimmune disease lupus-like disease and (d) the non-autoimmune disease antibody-induced NTN.

Deletion of $Fc\gamma RIIb$ in all B cells of the $^{Le}Fc\gamma RIIb_{B6}^{fl/fl}$ mouse by *CD19Cre* did not increase the susceptibility of this mouse for any of the mentioned disease models. Moreover, deletion of $Fc\gamma RIIb$ on a subset of monocytes (*LysMCre*) had no effect on susceptibility for anti-GBM disease. Therefore, it was concluded that FcγRIIb deficiency on B cells or a subset of myeloid cells alone is not sufficient to increase susceptibility to anti-GBM (186). Only pan-myeloid deletion (*cEBPαCre*) of FcγRIIb increased the susceptibility of $^{Le}Fc\gamma RIIb_{B6}^{fl/fl}$ mice for CIA on the permissive background (187) and for the non-autoimmune disease NTN (89). These results suggest that for the protection against induced auto-Ab driven diseases, such as CIA, the role of FcγRIIb on B cells, as a checkpoint for immune tolerance, is less important than its role on myeloid effector cells, controlling downstream antibody effector mechanisms (187). However, it cannot be excluded that in the CIA model FcγRIIb on myeloid cells also plays a role in controlling the afferent phase of the disease, as was recently shown in Yaa^+ $^{Le}Fc\gamma RIIb_{B6}^{-/-}$ mice that will be discussed later (188).

In contrast to the results with $^{Le}Fc\gamma IIb_{B6}^{fl/fl}$ mice, deletion of FcγRIIb in all B cells (*Mb1Cre*) or in GC and post GC B cells (*Cg1Cre*) in $^{NY}Fc\gamma RIIb_{B6}^{fl/fl}$ mice resulted in increased susceptibility for CIA on the non-permissive background and permissive background, respectively. Moreover, susceptibility to CIA was also increased in DC-specific *CD11cCre/*$^{NY}Fc\gamma RIIb_{B6}^{fl/fl}$ mice indicating that FcγRIIb is involved in distinct immune tolerance controlling mechanisms (110). The reason for the discrepancy between the phenotypes of the B cell- and DC-specific $^{NY}Fc\gamma RIIb_{B6}^{-/-}$ and $^{Le}Fc\gamma IIb_{B6}^{-/-}$ mice is not known but, given the weak phenotype of the germline $^{Le}Fc\gamma RIIb_{B6}^{-/-}$ mouse, most likely the phenotype of a single cell-type-specific $^{Le}Fc\gamma RIIb_{B6}^{-/-}$ mouse is too weak to be detected with a small cohort of mice. Another partial explanation might be that the B-cell-specific Cre lines used are different. In addition, GC and post GC B cell (*Cg1Cre*) specific $^{NY}Fc\gamma RIIb_{B6}^{-/-}$ mice developed spontaneously ANA, similar to ANA in germline $^{NY}Fc\gamma RIIb_{B6}^{-/-}$ mice, whereas a deficiency in other cell types has no effect. This confirms previous results with transplantation of bone marrow from $Fc\gamma RIIb_{129}^{-/-}$ mice that the role of FcγRIIb in the spontaneous development of ANA is B cell-specific (112) and suggests that FcγRIIb on GC or post GC B cells is a checkpoint for the maintenance of immune tolerance (110) (**Table 4**).

Upon immunization with the NP-CGG model antigen $^{NY}Fc\gamma RIIb_{B6}^{-/-}$ and *Mb1Cre/*$^{NY}Fc\gamma RIIb_{B6}^{fl/fl}$ mice developed similar increased primary IgG NP-specific Ab responses compared to $^{NY}Fc\gamma RIIb_{B6}^{fl/fl}$ mice and all other cell type-specific

TABLE 4 | Disease susceptibility of cell-type-specific *FcγRIIb* KO mice.

Disease \ Mouse strain	CD19Cre: All B cells[a,b,c]	LysMCre: Subset monocytes[a,d]	cEBPαCre: pan-myeloid[b,c]	CD11cCre: DCs[c,d]	Mb1Cre: All B cells[d]	Cg1Cre: GC and post GC B cells[d]
Non-permissive bCIA[c,d]	No increase	No increase $^{NY}Fc\gamma RIIb^{fl/fl}_{B6}$ [d]	n.d.	Increase $^{NY}Fc\gamma RIIb^{fl/fl}_{B6}$ [d]	Increase $^{NY}Fc\gamma RIIb^{fl/fl}_{B6}$ [d]	No increase $^{NY}Fc\gamma RIIb^{fl/fl}_{B6}$ [d]
Permissive cCIA[c,d]	No increase $^{Le}Fc\gamma RIIb^{fl/fl}_{B6}$ [c]	n.d.	Increase $^{Le}Fc\gamma RIIb^{fl/fl}_{B6}$ [c]	No increase $^{Le}Fc\gamma RIIb^{fl/fl}_{B6}$ [c]	n.d.	Increase similar to $^{NY}Fc\gamma RIIb^{-/-}_{B6}$ [d]
KRN arthritis[d]	n.d.	Increase $^{NY}Fc\gamma RIIb^{fl/fl}_{B6}$ [d]	n.d.	n.d.	n.d.	n.d.
Anti-GBM disease[a]	No increase $^{Le}Fc\gamma RIIb^{fl/fl}_{B6}$ [a]	No increase $^{Le}Fc\gamma RIIb^{fl/fl}_{B6}$ [a]	n.d.	n.d.	n.d.	n.d.
Lupus-like disease[d]	n.d.	No ANA $^{NY}Fc\gamma RIIb^{fl/fl}_{B6}$ [d]	n.d.	No ANA $^{NY}Fc\gamma RIIb^{fl/fl}_{B6}$ [d]	No ANA $^{NY}Fc\gamma RIIb^{fl/fl}_{B6}$ [d]	ANA similar to $^{NY}Fc\gamma RIIb^{-/-}_{B6}$ [d]
NTN[b]	No increase $^{Le}Fc\gamma RIIb^{fl/fl}_{B6}$ [b]	n.d.	Increase $^{Le}Fc\gamma RIIb^{fl/fl}_{B6}$ [b]	n.d.	n.d.	n.d.
Immunization[d]	n.d.	No increase in IgG response $^{NY}Fc\gamma RIIb^{fl/fl}_{B6}$ [d]	n.d.	No increase in IgG response $^{NY}Fc\gamma RIIb^{fl/fl}_{B6}$ [d]	Increased primary/secondary IgG response $^{NY}Fc\gamma RIIb^{fl/fl}_{B6}$ [d]	Increased secondary IgG response $^{NY}Fc\gamma RIIb^{fl/fl}_{B6}$ [d]

Germline FcγRIIb KO mice showed increased susceptibility to all diseases listed in the table compared with C57BL/6 mice.
[a]*Sharp et al. (186).*
[b]*Sharp et al. (89).*
[c]*Yilmaz-Elis et al. (187).*
[d]*Li et al. (110).*
n.d., not determined.

$^{NY}Fc\gamma RIIb^{-/-}_{B6}$ mice. In contrast, secondary IgG Ab responses were increased in both $Mb1Cre/^{NY}Fc\gamma RIIb^{fl/fl}_{B6}$ and $Cg1Cre/^{NY}Fc\gamma RIIb^{fl/fl}_{B6}$ mice compared with $^{NY}Fc\gamma RIIb^{fl/fl}_{B6}$ mice. This suggests that FcγRIIb is a B cell-intrinsic negative regulator of both primary and secondary IgG responses (110).

Although individually not sufficient to induce substantial autoimmunity, epistasis between the *Yaa* locus, the $^{Le}Fc\gamma RIIb^{-/-}_{B6}$ alleles and the C57BL/6 genome results in severe lupus-like disease (109) (**Figure 1**). The cell-type-specific role of FcγRIIb in this genetic disease model was studied (188). The $Yaa^+/CD19Cre/^{Le}Fc\gamma RIIb^{fl/fl}_{B6}$ mice developed milder lupus-like disease than $Yaa^+/^{Le}Fc\gamma RIIb^{-/-}_{B6}$ mice similar to the disease in $Yaa^+/C/EBP\alpha\ Cre/^{Le}Fc\gamma RIIb^{fl/fl}_{B6}$ mice whereas $Yaa^+/CD11cCre/^{Le}Fc\gamma RIIb^{fl/fl}_{B6}$ mice stayed disease free, like $Yaa^+/^{Le}Fc\gamma RIIb^{fl/fl}_{B6}$ mice. This suggests that besides on B cells FcγRIIb on myeloid cells, but surprisingly not on DCs, contributes to the protection against spontaneous loss of immune tolerance in this mouse model. This confirms the observation with CIA in mice (110), discussed earlier, that FcγRIIb can be involved in different immune tolerance controlling mechanisms.

Strikingly, in the two strains with FcγRIIb deficient myeloid cells ($Yaa^+/^{Le}Fc\gamma RIIb^{-/-}_{B6}$ and $Yaa^+/C/EBP\alpha\ Cre/^{Le}Fc\gamma RIIb^{fl/fl}_{B6}$) but not in the strain with B cell-specific FcγRIIb deficiency ($Yaa^+/CD19Cre/^{Le}Fc\gamma RIIb^{fl/fl}_{B6}$) the frequency of peripheral Ly6C$^-$, but not Ly6C$^+$ monocytes was increased. Monocytosis, an FcRγ dependent expansion of the monocyte compartment consisting mainly of Ly6C$^-$ monocytes, is associated with the development of lupus nephritis in Yaa^+ lupus-prone mice. It has been reported that Ly6C$^+$ monocytes mature in the circulation

and are the precursors for Ly6C$^-$ monocytes (189). Deficiency of FcγRIIb most likely accelerates the maturation of monocytes in $Yaa^+/^{Le}Fc\gamma RIIb^{-/-}_{B6}$ mice. Compared to Ly6C$^+$ monocytes, mature Ly6C$^-$ monocytes express significantly higher B cell-stimulating cytokines such as BSF-3, IL-10, and IL-1β, DC markers including CD11c, CD83, Adamdec1, and the anti-apoptotic factors Bcl2 and Bcl6. This makes monocytes the most promising FcγRIIb expressing candidate myeloid cells to modulate B cell tolerance (188, 190). The transcriptome of Ly6C$^-$ monocytes suggests that they are long-lived and committed to developing into DCs.

Whether this monocyte-dependent tolerance breaking mechanism is unique for $Yaa^+/Fc\gamma RIIb^{-/-}_{B6}$ mice is not known but it is striking that also in SLE patients the serum levels of anti-dsDNA Abs highly correlate with the percentage of non-classical monocytes (191). Like mouse Ly6C$^-$ monocytes, the human counterpart CD14^{low}CD16$^+$ monocytes secrete high amounts of IL-1β in a TLR7-TLR8-MyD88–dependent manner (192).

CONCLUDING REMARKS

Forward and reverse genetics have provided convincing evidence that FcγRIIb is an important autoimmune susceptibility gene, involved in the maintenance of peripheral tolerance both in human and mice. In humans, a number of GWAS studies showed an association between a SNP *(rs1050501)* in the *FCGR2B* gene, causing a missense mutation ($FCGR2B^{T232}$) resulting in impaired FCGR2B function, and susceptibility to SLE. Meta-analyses confirmed that $FCGR2B^{T232}$ homozygosity is one of the strongest associations in SLE. Association of *rs1050501* with RA has also been reported.

In mice, the situation is more diffuse. Analysis of a variety of C57BL/6 mice congenic for the NZW and NZB haplotypes of *FcγRIIb*, with decreased expression, did not reveal clear unambiguous results with respect to the contribution of these haplotypes to the autoimmune phenotypes of these mice. The mechanism by which natural FcγRIIb variants contribute to autoimmunity is not well-understood.

The first $FcγRIIb^{-/-}$ mouse, generated by gene targeting in 129 derived ES cells and backcrossed into C57BL/6 background ($FcγRIIb_{129}^{-/-}$ mice), exhibited a surprisingly strong spontaneous autoimmune phenotype suggesting that FcγRIIb deficiency initiates loss of immune tolerance. However, independent studies with $FcγRIIb_{129}^{-/-}$ autoimmune V_H chain knockin mice pointed to a central role of FcγRIIb in a late immune tolerance checkpoint, that prevents autoimmunity by suppressing the production of autoreactive IgG from B cells, that escape negative selection in the GC and enter the AFC pathway. This should mean that FcγRIIb deficiency is mainly an amplifier of autoimmunity caused by other autoimmune susceptibility loci, rather than a primary initiator of the loss of immune tolerance. That was confirmed by the observation that $FcγRIIb^{-/-}$ mice on a pure C57BL/6 background ($FcγRIIb_{B6}^{-/-}$) have a much milder autoimmune phenotype than $FcγRIIb_{129}^{-/-}$ mice but when backcrossed into a mouse strain carrying the autoimmune susceptibility *Yaa* locus succumb to lupus-like disease. The strong autoimmune phenotype of the $FcγRIIb_{129}^{-/-}$ mouse could be explained by epistatic interactions between the C57BL/6 genome, the FcγRIIb KO allele and the 129 derived sequences (*Sle16*) flanking the *FcγRIIb* KO allele, containing the autoimmunity associated $Slamf_{129}$ (haplotype 2) gene cluster.

Spt-GC B and T_{FH} cells are activated, modestly (mainly B cells) in $FcγRIIb_{B6}^{-/-}$ mice, moderately in C57BL/6 $Slamf_{129}$ congenic mice and strongly in $FcγRIIb_{129}^{-/-}$ mice compared to Spt-GC B and T_{FH} cells in WT C57BL/6 mice. This was associated with a corresponding increase in ANA production, suggesting that FcγRIIb deficiency, besides enhancing autoimmunity caused by other autoimmune susceptibility loci, might play a modest role in the induction of the loss of immune tolerance in the GC, explaining the development with low penetrance of low ANA titers in $FcγRIIb_{B6}^{-/-}$ mice. An alternative explanation is that the low ANA titers in $FcγRIIb_{B6}^{-/-}$ mice reflect the natural background of autoreactive B cells in the GC that are prevented to enter the AFC pathway in the presence of FcγRIIb. The analysis of the development of self-reactive GC B cells and plasma cells by large scale Ig cloning from single isolated B cells, as performed with $FcγRIIb_{129}^{-/-}$ mice, should be repeated in $FcγRIIb_{B6}^{-/-}$ mice, to determine how FcγRIIb deficiency influences the frequency at which autoreactive ANA-expressing B cells participate in GC reactions, and develop in plasma cells, under physiological conditions, without the confounding effect of $Slamf_{129}$ expression.

Studies with cell-type-specific FcγRIIb deficient mice revealed that besides on B cells, FcγRIIb on DCs and monocytes can also contribute to the maintenance of immune tolerance, indicating that FcγRIIb is involved in different immune tolerance maintaining mechanisms. Series of observations suggest that on B cells impaired FcγRIIb function effects not only antibody titers but also affinity maturation and memory responses of B cells and plasma cell homeostasis associated with an increase in the production of autoantibodies. However, the underlying cellular and molecular mechanisms are not well-understood. Most likely new model systems including adoptive cell transfer and tools such as cell type-specific KO mice, to study the GC reaction, are required to answer these questions.

AUTHOR CONTRIBUTIONS

All authors listed have made a substantial, direct and intellectual contribution to the work, and approved it for publication.

FUNDING

JV was supported by Japan Society for the Promotion of Science (FY2017 JSPS invitational Fellowship for Research in Japan, L17559).

REFERENCES

1. Takai T, Li M, Sylvestre D, Clynes R, Ravetch JV. FcRγ chain deletion results in pleiotrophic effector cell defects. *Cell.* (1994) 76:519–29. doi: 10.1016/0092-8674(94)90115-5
2. Nimmerjahn F, Ravetch JV. Fc-receptors as regulators of immunity. *Adv Immunol.* (2007) 96:179–204. doi: 10.1016/S0065-2776(07)96005-8
3. Getahun A, Cambier JC. Of ITIMs, ITAMs, and ITAMis: revisiting immunoglobulin Fc receptor signaling. *Immunol Rev.* (2015) 268:66–73. doi: 10.1111/imr.12336
4. Tsao BP, Cantor RM, Kalunian KC, Chen CJ, Badsha H, Singh R, et al. Evidence for linkage of a candidate chromosome 1 region to human systemic lupus erythematosus. *J Clin Invest.* (1997) 99:725–31. doi: 10.1172/JCI119217
5. Daeron M, Latour S, Malbec O, Espinosa E, Pina P, Pasmans S, et al. The same tyrosine-based inhibition motif, in the intracytoplasmic domain of Fcγ RIIB, regulates negatively BCR-, TCR-, and FcR-dependent cell activation. *Immunity.* (1995) 3:635–46. doi: 10.1016/1074-7613(95)90134-5
6. Daeron M, Jaeger S, Du Pasquier L, Vivier E. Immunoreceptor tyrosine-based inhibition motifs: a quest in the past and future. *Immunol Rev.* (2008) 224:11–43. doi: 10.1111/j.1600-065X.2008.00666.x
7. Daeron M. Fc receptor biology. *Annu Rev Immunol.* (1997) 15:203–34. doi: 10.1146/annurev.immunol.15.1.203
8. Miettinen HM, Rose JK, Mellman I. Fc receptor isoforms exhibit distinct abilities for coated pit localization as a result of cytoplasmic domain heterogeneity. *Cell.* (1989) 58:317–27. doi: 10.1016/0092-8674(89)90846-5
9. Miettinen HM, Matter K, Hunziker W, Rose JK, Mellman I. Fc receptor endocytosis is controlled by a cytoplasmic domain determinant that actively prevents coated pit localization. *J Cell Biol.* (1992) 116:875–88. doi: 10.1083/jcb.116.4.875

10. Xiang Z, Cutler AJ, Brownlie RJ, Fairfax K, Lawlor KE, Severinson E, et al. FcγRIIb controls bone marrow plasma cell persistence and apoptosis. *Nat Immunol.* (2007) 8:419–29. doi: 10.1038/ni1440

11. Espéli M, Clatworthy MR, Bökers S, Lawlor KE, Cutler AJ, Köntgen F, et al. Analysis of a wild mouse promoter variant reveals a novel role for FcγRIIb in the control of the germinal center and autoimmunity. *J Exp Med.* (2012) 209:2307–19. doi: 10.1084/jem.20121752

12. Amezcua Vesely MC, Schwartz M, Bermejo DA, Montes CL, Cautivo KM, Kalergis AM, et al. FcγRIIb and BAFF differentially regulate peritoneal B1 cell survival. *J Immunol.* (2012) 88:4792–800. doi: 10.4049/jimmunol.1102070

13. Rudge EU, Cutler AJ, Pritchard NR, Smith KG. Interleukin 4 reduces expression of inhibitory receptors on B cells and abolishes CD22 and FcγRII-mediated B cell suppression. *J Exp Med.* (2002) 195:1079–85. doi: 10.1084/jem.20011435

14. Nimmerjahn F, Ravetch JV. Fcgγ receptors as regulators of immune responses. *Nat Rev Immunol.* (2008) 8:34–47 doi: 10.1038/nri2206

15. Starbeck-Miller GR, Badovinac VP, Barber DL, Harty JT. Cutting edge: expression of FcγRIIB tempers memory CD8 T cell function *in vivo. J Immunol.* (2014) 192:35–9. doi: 10.4049/jimmunol.1302232

16. Guilliams M, Bruhns P, Saeys Y, Hammad H, Lambrecht BN. The function of Fcγ receptors in dendritic cells and macrophages. *Nat Rev Immunol.* (2014) 14:94–108. doi: 10.1038/nri3582

17. Shushakova N, Skokowa J, Schulman J, Baumann U, Zwirner J, Schmidt RE, et al. C5a anaphylatoxin is a major regulator of activating versus inhibitory FcγRs in immune complex-induced lung disease. *J Clin Invest.* (2002) 110:1823–30. doi: 10.1172/JCI200216577

18. Skokowa J, Ali SR, Felda O, Kumar V, Konrad S, Shushakova N, et al. Macrophages induce the inflammatory response in the pulmonary Arthus reaction through Gαi2 activation that controls C5aR and Fc receptor cooperation. *J Immunol.* (2005) 174:3041–50. doi: 10.4049/jimmunol.174.5.3041

19. Snapper CM, Hooley JJ, Atasoy U, Finkelman FD, Paul WE. Differential regulation of murine B cell FcγRII expression by CD4+ T helper subsets. *J Immunol.* (1989) 143:2133–41.

20. Liu Y, Gao X, Masuda E, Redecha PB, Blank MC, Pricop L. Regulated expression of FcγR in human dendritic cells controls cross-presentation of antigen-antibody complexes. *J Immunol.* (2006) 177:8440–7. doi: 10.4049/jimmunol.177.12.8440

21. Tridandapani S, Siefker K, Teillaud JL, Carter JE, Wewers MD, Anderson CL. Regulated expression and inhibitory function of FcγRIIb in human monocytic cells. *J Biol Chem.* (2002) 277:5082–9. doi: 10.1074/jbc.M110277200

22. Tridandapani S, Wardrop R, Baran CP, Wang Y, Opalek JM, Caligiuri MA, et al. TGF-β1 Suppresses Myeloid Fcγ Receptor Function by Regulating the Expression and Function of the Common γ-Subunit. *J Immunol.* (2003) 170:4572–7. doi: 10.4049/jimmunol.170.9.4572

23. Pricop L, Redecha P, Teillaud JL, Frey J, Fridman WH, Sautes-Fridman C, et al. Differential modulation of stimulatory and inhibitory Fcγ receptors on human monocytes by Th1 and Th2 cytokines. *J Immunol.* (2001) 166:531–7. doi: 10.4049/jimmunol.166.1.531

24. Tutt AL, James S, Laversin SA, Tipton TR, Ashton-Key M, French RR, et al. Development and characterization of monoclonal antibodies specific for mouse and human Fcγ receptors. *J Immunol.* (2015) 195:5503–16. doi: 10.4049/jimmunol.1402988

25. Ganesan LP, Kim J, Wu Y, Mohanty S, Phillips GS, Birmingham DJ, et al. FcγRIIb on liver sinusoidal endothelium clears small immune complexes. *J Immunol.* (2012) 189:4981–8. doi: 10.4049/jimmunol.12 02017

26. Anderson CL, Ganesan LP, Robinson JM. The biology of the classical Fcγ receptors in non-hematopoietic cells. *Immunol Rev.* (2015) 268:236–40. doi: 10.1111/imr.12335

27. Radeke HH, Janssen-Graalfs I, Sowa EN, Chouchakova N, Skokowa J, Loscher F, et al. Opposite regulation of type II and III receptors for immunoglobulin G in mouse glomerular mesangial cells and in the induction of anti-glomerular basement membrane (GBM) nephritis. *J Biol Chem.* (2002) 277:27535–44. doi: 10.1074/jbc.M200419200

28. Ono M, Bolland S, Tempst P, Ravetch JV. Role of the inositol phosphatase SHIP in negative regulation of the immune system by the receptor Fc(γ)RIIB. *Nature.* (1996) 383:263–6. doi: 10.1038/383263a0

29. Karsten CM, Pandey MK, Figge J, Kilchenstein R, Taylor PR, Rosas M, et al. Anti-inflammatory activity of IgG1 mediated by Fc galactosylation and association of FcγRIIB and dectin-1. *Nat Med.* (2012) 18:1401–6. doi: 10.1038/nm.2862

30. Phillips NE, Parker DC. Cross-linking of B lymphocyte Fcγ receptors and membrane immunoglobulin inhibits anti-immunoglobulin-induced blastogenesis. *J Immunol.* (1984) 132:627–32.

31. Phillips NE, Parker DC. Subclass specificity of Fcγ receptor-mediated inhibition of mouse B cell activation. *J Immunol.* (1985) 134:2835–8.

32. Coggeshall KM. Inhibitory signaling by B cell FcγRIIb. *Curr Opin Immunol.* (1998) 10:306–12. doi: 10.1016/S0952-7915(98)80169-6

33. Pearse RN, Kawabe T, Bolland S, Guinamard R, Kurosaki T, Ravetch JV. SHIP recruitment attenuates FcγRIIB-induced B cell apoptosis. *Immunity.* (1999) 10:753–60. doi: 10.1016/S1074-7613(00)80074-6

34. Ashman RF, Peckham D, Stunz LL. Fc receptor off-signal in the B cell involves apoptosis. *J Immunol.* (1996) 157:5–11.

35. Daeron M, Malbec O, Latour S, Arock M, Fridman WH. Regulation of high-affinity IgE receptor-mediated mast cell activation by murine low-affinity IgG receptors. *J Clin Invest.* (1995) 95:577–85. doi: 10.1172/JCI117701

36. Clynes R, Dumitru C, Ravetch JV. Uncoupling of immune complex formation and kidney damage in autoimmune glomerulonephritis. *Science.* (1998) 279:1052–4 doi: 10.1126/science.279.5353.1052

37. Steinman RM, Hawiger D, Liu K, Bonifaz L, Bonnyay D, Mahnke K, et al. Dendritic cell function *in vivo* during the steady state: a role in peripheral tolerance. *Ann N Y Acad Sci.* (2003) 987:15–25. doi: 10.1111/j.1749-6632.2003.tb06029.x

38. Steinman RM, Hawiger D, Nussenzweig MC. Tolerogenic dendritic cells. *Annu Rev Immunol.* (2003) 21:685–711. doi: 10.1146/annurev.immunol.21.120601.141040

39. Bancherau J, Steinman RM. Dendritic cells and the control of immunity. *Nature.* (1998) 392:245–52. doi: 10.1038/32588

40. Merad M, Sathe P, Helft J, Miller J, Mortha A. The dendritic cell lineage: ontogeny and function of dendritic cells and their subsets in the steady-state and the inflamed setting. *Annu Rev Immunol.* (2013) 31:563–604. doi: 10.1146/annurev-immunol-020711-074950

41. Eisenbarth SC. Dendritic cell subsets in T cell programming: location dictates function. *Nat Rev Immunol.* (2019) 19:89–103. doi: 10.1038/s41577-018-0088-1

42. Heyman B. Antibodies as natural adjuvants. *Curr Top Microbiol Immunol.* (2014) 382:201–19. doi: 10.1007/978-3-319-07911-0_9

43. Regnault A, Lankar D, Lacabanne V, Rodriguez A, Thery C, Rescigno M, et al. Fcγ receptor-mediated induction of dendritic cell maturation and major histocompatibility complex class I-restricted antigen presentation after immune complex internalization. *J Exp Med.* (1999) 189:371–80. doi: 10.1084/jem.189.2.371

44. Sedlik C, Orbach D, Veron P, Schweighoffer E, Colucci F, Gamberale R, et al. A critical role for Syk protein tyrosine kinase in Fc receptor-mediated antigen presentation and induction of dendritic cell maturation. *J Immunol.* (2003) 170:846–52. doi: 10.4049/jimmunol.170.2.846

45. Herrada AA, Contreras FJ, Tobar JA, Pacheco R, Kalergis AM. Immune complex-induced enhancement of bacterial antigen presentation requires Fcγ receptor III expression on dendritic cells. *Proc Natl Acad Sci USA.* (2007) 104:13402–7. doi: 10.1073/pnas.0700999104

46. Yada A, Ebihara S, Matsumura K, Endo S, Maeda T, Nakamura A, et al. Accelerated antigen presentation and elicitation of humoral response *in vivo* by FcγRIIB- and FcγRI/III-mediated immune complex uptake. *Cell Immunol.* (2003) 225:21–32. doi: 10.1016/j.cellimm.2003.09.008

47. Kalergis AM, Ravetch JV. Inducing tumor immunity through the selective engagement of activating Fcγ receptors on dendritic cells. *J Exp Med.* (2002) 195:1653–9. doi: 10.1084/jem.20020338

48. Tobar JA, González PA, Kalergis AM. Salmonella escape from antigen presentation can be overcome by targeting bacteria to Fcγ receptors on dendritic cells. *J Immunol.* (2004) 173:4058–65. doi: 10.4049/jimmunol.173.6.4058

49. Schuurhuis DH, van Montfoort N, Ioan-Facsinay A, Jiawan R, Camps M, Nouta J, et al. Immune complex-loaded dendritic cells are superior to soluble immune complexes as antitumor vaccine. *J Immunol.* (2006) 176:4573–80. doi: 10.4049/jimmunol.176.8.4573

50. Boross P, van Montfoort N, Stapels DA, van der Poel CE, Bertens C, Meeldijk J, et al. FcRγ-chain ITAM signaling is critically required for cross-presentation of soluble antibody-antigen complexes by dendritic cells. *J Immunol.* (2014) 193:5506–14. doi: 10.4049/jimmunol.1302012

51. Schuurhuis DH, Ioan-Facsinay A, Nagelkerken B, van Schip JJ, Sedlik C, Melief CJ, et al. Antigen-antibody immune complexes empower dendritic cells to efficiently prime specific CD8+ CTL responses *in vivo. J Immunol.* (2002) 168:2240–6. doi: 10.4049/jimmunol.168.5.2240

52. van Montfoort N, t Hoen PA, Mangsbo SM, Camps MG, Boross P, Melief CJ, et al. Fcγ receptor IIb strongly regulates Fcγ receptor-facilitated T cell activation by dendritic cells. *J Immunol.* (2012) 189:92–101. doi: 10.4049/jimmunol.1103703

53. Rafiq K, Bergtold A, Clynes R. Immune complex-mediated antigen presentation induces tumor immunity. *J Clin Invest.* (2002) 110:71–9. doi: 10.1172/JCI15640

54. Desai DD, Harbers SO, Flores M, Colonna L, Downie MP, Bergtold A, et al. Fcγ receptor IIB on dendritic cells enforces peripheral tolerance by inhibiting effector T cell responses. *J Immunol.* (2007) 178:6217–26. doi: 10.4049/jimmunol.178.10.6217

55. Fransen MF, Benonisson H, van Maren WW, Sow HS, Breukel C, Linssen MM, et al. Restricted role for FcγR in the regulation of adaptive immunity. *J Immunol.* (2018) 200:2615–26. doi: 10.4049/jimmunol.1700429

56. Ho NI, Camps MGM, de Haas EFE, Trouw LA, Verbeek JS, Ossendorp F. C1q-dependent dendritic cell cross-presentation of *in vivo*-formed antigen-antibody complexes. *J Immunol.* (2017) 198:4235–43. doi: 10.4049/jimmunol.1602169

57. den Haan JM, Bevan MJ. Constitutive versus activation-dependent cross-presentation of immune complexes by CD8(+) and CD8(-) dendritic cells *in vivo. J Exp Med.* (2002) 196:817–27. doi: 10.1084/jem.20020295

58. Dhodapkar KM, Kaufman JL, Ehlers M, Banerjee DK, Bonvini E, Koenig S, et al. Selective blockade of inhibitory Fcγ receptor enables human dendritic cell maturation with IL-12p70 production and immunity to antibody-coated tumor cells. *ProcNatlAcadSci USA.* (2005) 102:2910–5. doi: 10.1073/pnas.0500014102

59. van Montfoort N, Camps MG, Khan S, Filippov DV, Weterings JJ, Griffith JM, et al. Antigen storage compartments in mature dendritic cells facilitate prolonged cytotoxic T lymphocyte cross-priming capacity. *ProcNatlAcadSci USA.* (2009) 106:6730–5. doi: 10.1073/pnas.0900969106

60. Garcia De Vinuesa C, Gulbranson-Judge A, Khan M, O'Leary P, Cascalho M, Wabl M, et al. Dendritic cells associated with plasmablast survival. *Eur J Immunol.* (1999) 29:3712–21. doi: 10.1002/(SICI)1521-4141(199911)29:11<3712::AID-IMMU3712>3.3.CO;2-G

61. Balazs M, Martin F, Zhou T, Kearney J. Blood dendritic cells interact with splenic marginal zone B cells to initiate T-independent immune responses. *Immunity.* (2002) 17:341–52. doi: 10.1016/S1074-7613(02)00389-8

62. Bergtold A, Desai DD, Gavhane A, Clynes R. Cell surface recycling of internalized antigen permits dendritic cell priming of B cells. *Immunity.* (2005) 23:503–14. doi: 10.1016/j.immuni.2005.09.013

63. Gilliet M, Cao W, Liu YJ. Plasmacytoid dendritic cells: sensing nucleic acids in viral infection and autoimmune diseases. *Nat Rev Immunol.* (2008) 8:594–606. doi: 10.1038/nri2358

64. Reizis B. Intracellular pathogens and CD8(+) dendritic cells: dangerous liaisons. *Immunity.* (2011) 35:153–5. doi: 10.1016/j.immuni.2011.08.003

65. Goubier A, Dubois B, Gheit H, Joubert G, Villard-Truc F, Asselin-Paturel C, et al. Plasmacytoid dendritic cells mediate oral tolerance. *Immunity.* (2008) 29:464–75. doi: 10.1016/j.immuni.2008.06.017

66. Irla M, Kupfer N, Suter T, Lissilaa R, Benkhoucha M, Skupsky J, et al. MHC class II-restricted antigen presentation by plasmacytoid dendritic cells inhibits T cell-mediated autoimmunity. *J Exp Med.* (2010) 207:1891–905. doi: 10.1084/jem.20092627

67. Flores MD, Desai DD, Downie M, Liang B, Reilly MP, McKenzie SE, et al. Dominant expression of the inhibitory FcγRIIB prevents antigen presentation by murine plasmacytoid dendritic cells. *J Immunol.* (2009) 183:7129–39. doi: 10.4049/jimmunol.0901169

68. Bjorck P, Beilhack A, Herman EI, Negrin RS, Engleman EG. Plasmacytoid dendritic cells take up opsonized antigen leading to CD4+ and CD8+ T cell activation *in vivo. J Immunol.* (2008) 181:3811–7. doi: 10.4049/jimmunol.181.6.3811

69. Benitez-Ribas D, Adema GJ, Winkels G, Klasen IS, Punt CJ, Figdor CG, et al. Plasmacytoid dendritic cells of melanoma patients present exogenous proteins to CD4_ T cells after FcγRII-mediated uptake. *J Exp Med.* (2006) 203:1629–35. doi: 10.1084/jem.20052364

70. Vollmer J, Tluk S, Schmitz C, Hamm S, Jurk M, Forsbach A, et al. Immune stimulation mediated by autoantigen binding sites within small nuclear RNAs involves Toll-like receptors 7 and 8. *J Exp Med.* (2005) 202:1575–85. doi: 10.1084/jem.20051696

71. Ronnblom L, Alm GV, Eloranta ML. Type I interferon and lupus. *Curr Opin Rheumatol.* (2009) 21:471–7. doi: 10.1097/BOR.0b013e32832e089e

72. Means TK, Latz E, Hayashi F, Murali MR, Golenbock DT, Luster AD. Human lupus autoantibody-DNA complexes activate DCs through the cooperation of CD32 and TLR9. *J Clin Invest.* (2005) 115:407–17. doi: 10.1172/JCI200523025

73. Nemazee D. Mechanisms of central tolerance for B cells. *Nat Rev Immunol.* (2017) 17:281–94. doi: 10.1038/nri.2017.19

74. Cooke MP, Heath AW, Shokat KM, Zeng Y, Finkelman FD, Linsley PS, et al. Immunoglobulin signal transduction guides the specificity of B cell-T cell interactions and is blocked in tolerant self-reactive B cells. *J Exp Med.* (1994) 179:425–38. doi: 10.1084/jem.179.2.425

75. Healy JI, Dolmetsch RE, Timmerman LA, Cyster JG, Thomas ML, Crabtree GR, et al. Different nuclear signals are activated by the B cell receptor during positive versus negative signaling. *Immunity.* (1997) 6:419–28. doi: 10.1016/S1074-7613(00)80285-X

76. Goodnow CC, Crosbie J, Jorgensen H, Brink RA, Basten A. Induction of self-tolerance in mature peripheral B lymphocytes. *Nature.* (1989) 342:385–91. doi: 10.1038/342385a0

77. Brink R, Phan TG. Self-reactive B cells in the germinal center reaction. *Annu Rev Immunol.* (2018) 36:339–57. doi: 10.1146/annurev-immunol-051116-052510

78. Akkaraju S, Canaan K, Goodnow CC. (1997). Self-reactive B cells are not eliminated or inactivated by autoantigen expressed on thyroid epithelial cells. *J.Exp.Med.* 186, 2005–2012 doi: 10.1084/jem.186.12.2005

79. Aplin BD, Keech CL, de Kauwe AL, Gordon TP, Cavill D, McCluskey J. Tolerance through indifference: autoreactive B cells to the nuclear antigen La show no evidence of tolerance in a transgenic model. *J Immunol.* (2003) 171:5890–900. doi: 10.4049/jimmunol.171.11.5890

80. El Shikh ME, El Sayed RM, Sukumar S, Szakal AK, Tew JG. Activation of B cells by antigens on follicular dendritic cells. *Trends Immunol.* (2010) 31:205–11. doi: 10.1016/j.it.2010.03.002

81. Chan TD, Wood K, Hermes JR, Butt D, Jolly CJ, Basten A, et al. Elimination of germinal-center-derived self-reactive B cells is governed by the location and concentration of self-antigen. *Immunity.* (2012) 37:893–904. doi: 10.1016/j.immuni.2012.07.017

82. Krautler NJ, Suan D, Butt D, Bourne K, Hermes JR, Chan TD, et al. Differentiation of germinal center B cells into plasma cells is initiated by high-affinity antigen and completed by Tfh cells. *J Exp Med.* (2017) 214:1259–67. doi: 10.1084/jem.20161533

83. Heesters BA, van der Poel CE, Das A, Carroll MC. Antigen presentation to B cells. *Trends Immunol.* (2016) 37:844–54. doi: 10.1016/j.it.2016.10.003

84. Tew JG, Wu J, Fakher M, Szakal AK, Qin D. Follicular dendritic cells: beyond the necessity of T cell help. *Trends Immunol.* (2001) 22:361–7. doi: 10.1016/S1471-4906(01)01942-1

85. Ravetch JV, Lanier LL. Immune inhibitory receptors. *Science.* (2000) 290:84–9. doi: 10.1126/science.290.5489.84

86. RavetchJV, Bolland S. IgG Fc receptors. *Annu Rev Immunol.* (2001) 19:275–90. doi: 10.1146/annurev.immunol.19.1.275

87. Ono M, Okada H, Bolland S, Yanagi S, Kurosaki T, Ravetch JV. Deletion of SHIP or SHP-1 reveals two distinct pathways for inhibitory signaling. *Cell.* (1997) 90:293–301. doi: 10.1016/S0092-8674(00)80337-2

88. Tzeng SJ, Bolland S, Inabe K, Kurosaki T, Pierce SK. The B cell inhibitory Fc receptor triggers apoptosis by a novel c-Abl family kinase-dependent pathway. *J Biol Chem.* (2005) 280:35247–54. doi: 10.1074/jbc.M505308200

89. Sharp PE, Martin-Ramirez J, Mangsbo SM, Boross P, Pusey CD, Touw IP, et al. FcγRIIb on myeloid cells and intrinsic renal cells rather than B cells protects from nephrotoxic nephritis. *J Immunol.* (2013) 190:340–8. doi: 10.4049/jimmunol.1202250

90. Shirai T, Hirose S, Okada T, Nishimura H. Immunology and immunopathology of the autoimmune disease of NZB and related mouse strains. In: Rihova EB, Vetvicka V, editors. *Immunological Disorders in Mice.* Boca Raton, FL: CRC Press, Inc. (1991) 95–136.

91. Reininger L, Radaszkiewicz T, Kosco M, Melchers F, Rolink AG. Development of autoimmune disease in SCID mice populated with long-term "in vitro" proliferating (NZB x NZW)F1 pre-B cells. *J Exp Med.* (1992) 176:1343–53. doi: 10.1084/jem.176.5.1343

92. Reininger L, Winkler TH, Kalberer CP, Jourdan M, Melchers F, Rolink AG. Intrinsic B cell defects in NZB and NZW mice contribute to systemic lupus erythematosus in (NZB x NZW)F1 mice. *J Exp Med.* (1996) 184:853–61. doi: 10.1084/jem.184.3.853

93. Helyer BJ, Howie JB. Renal disease associated with positive lupus erythematosus tests in a cross-bred strain of mice. *Nature.* (1963) 12:197. doi: 10.1038/197197a0

94. Theofilopoulos AN, Dixon FJ. Murine models of systemic lupus erythematosus. *Adv Immunol.* (1985) 37:269–390. doi: 10.1016/S0065-2776(08)60342-9

95. Rudofsky UH, Evans BD, Balaban SL, Mottironi VD, Gabrielsen AE. Differences in expression of lupus nephritis in New Zealand mixed H-2z homozygous inbred strains of mice derived from New Zealand black and New Zealand white mice. Origins and initial characterization. *Lab Invest.* (1993) 68:419–26.

96. Morel L, Rudofsky UH, Longmate JA, Schiffenbauer J, Wakeland EK. Polygenic control of susceptibility to murine systemic lupus erythematosus. *Immunity.* (1994) 1:219–29. doi: 10.1016/1074-7613(94)90100-7

97. Morel L, Wakeland EK. Lessons from the NZM2410 model and related strains. *Int Rev Immunol.* (2000) 19:423–46. doi: 10.3109/08830180009055506

98. Kanari Y, Sugahara-Tobinai A, Takahashi H, Inui M, Nakamura A, Hirose S, et al. Dichotomy in FcγRIIB deficiency and autoimmune-prone SLAM haplotype clarifies the roles of the Fc receptor in development of autoantibodies and glomerulonephritis. *BMC Immunol.* (2014) 24:47. doi: 10.1186/s12865-014-0047-y

99. Mohan C, Alas E, Morel L, Yang P, Wakeland EK. Genetic dissection of SLE pathogenesis. Sle1 on murine chromosome 1 leads to a selective loss of tolerance to H2A/H2B/DNA subnucleosomes. *J Clin Invest.* (1998) 101:1362–72.

100. Morel L, Croker BP, Blenman KR, Mohan C, Huang G, Gilkeson G, et al. Genetic reconstitution of systemic lupus erythematosus immunopathology with polycongenic murine strains. *Proc Natl Acad Sci USA.* (2000) 97:6670–5. doi: 10.1073/pnas.97.12.6670

101. Sobel ES, Mohan C, Morel L, Schiffenbauer J, Wakeland EK. Genetic dissection of SLE pathogenesis: adoptive transfer of Sle1 mediates the loss of tolerance by bone marrow-derived B cells. *J Immunol.* (1999) 162:2415–21.

102. Sobel ES, Satoh M, Chen Y, Wakeland EK, Morel L. The major murine systemic lupus erythematosus susceptibility locus Sle1 results in abnormal functions of both B and T cells. *J Immunol.* (2002) 169:2694–700. doi: 10.4049/jimmunol.169.5.2694

103. Jiang Y, Hirose S, Abe M, Sanokawa-Akakura R, Ohtsuji M, Mi X, et al. Polymorphisms in IgG Fc receptor IIB regulatory regions associated with autoimmune susceptibility. *Immunogenetics.* (2000) 51:429–35. doi: 10.1007/s002510050641

104. Luan JJ, Monteiro RC, Sautes C, Fluteau G, Eloy L, Fridman WH, et al. Defective FcγRII gene expression in macrophages of NOD mice: genetic linkage with up-regulation of IgG1 and IgG2b in serum. *J Immunol.* (1996) 157:4707–16.

105. Pritchard NR, Cutler AJ, Uribe S, Chadban SJ, Morley BJ, Smith KG. Autoimmune-prone mice share a promoter haplotype associated with reduced expression and function of the Fc receptor FcγRII. *Curr Biol.* (2000) 10:227–30. doi: 10.1016/S0960-9822(00)00344-4

106. Rahman ZS, Manser T. Failed up-regulation of the inhibitory IgG Fc receptor Fcγ RIIB on germinal center B cells in autoimmune-prone mice is not associated with deletion polymorphisms in the promoter region of the FcγRIIB gene. *J Immunol.* (2005) 175:1440–9. doi: 10.4049/jimmunol.175.3.1440

107. Xiu Y, Nakamura K, Abe M, Li N, Wen XS, Jiang Y, et al. Transcriptional regulation of Fcgr2b gene by polymorphic promoter region and its contribution to humoral immune responses. *J Immunol.* (2002) 169:4340–6. doi: 10.4049/jimmunol.169.8.4340

108. Rahman ZS, Niu H, Perry D, Wakeland E, Manser T, Morel L. Expression of the autoimmune Fcgr2b NZW allele fails to be upregulated in germinal center B cells and is associated with increased IgG production. *Genes Immun.* (2007) 8:604–12. doi: 10.1038/sj.gene.6364423

109. Boross P, Arandhara VL, Martin-Ramirez J, Santiago-Raber ML, Carlucci F, Flierman R, et al. The inhibiting Fc receptor for IgG, FcγRIIB, is a modifier of autoimmune susceptibility. *J Immunol.* (2011) 187:1304–13. doi: 10.4049/jimmunol.1101194

110. Li F, Smith P, Ravetch JV. Inhibitory Fcγ receptor is required for the maintenance of tolerance through distinct mechanisms. *J Immunol.* (2014) 192:3021–8. doi: 10.4049/jimmunol.1302934

111. Bygrave AE, Rose KL, Cortes-Hernandez J, Warren J, Rigby RJ, Cook HT, et al. Spontaneous autoimmunity in 129 and C57BL/6 mice-implications for autoimmunity described in gene-targeted mice. *PLoS Biol.* (2004) 2:E243. doi: 10.1371/journal.pbio.0020243

112. Bolland S, Ravetch JV. Spontaneous autoimmune disease in Fc(γ)RIIB-deficient mice results from strain-specific epistasis. *Immunity.* (2000) 13:277–85. doi: 10.1016/S1074-7613(00)00027-3

113. Bolland S, Yim YS, Tus K, Wakeland EK, Ravetch JV. Genetic modifiers of systemic lupus erythematosus in FcγRIIB$^{-/-}$ mice. *J Exp Med.* (2002) 195:1167–74. doi: 10.1084/jem.20020165

114. Jorgensen TN, Alfaro J, Enriquez HL, Jiang C, Loo WM, Atencio SA, et al. Development of Murine Lupus involves the combined genetic contribution of the *SLAM* and *FcγR* intervals within the *Nba2* autoimmune susceptibility locus. *J Immunol.* (2010) 184:775–86. doi: 10.4049/jimmunol.0901322

115. Cheung Y-H, Landolt-Marticorena C, Lajoie G, Wither JE. The Lupus phenotype in B6.NZBc1 congenic mice reflects interactions between multiple susceptibility loci and a suppressor locus. *Genes Immun.* (2011) 12:251–62. doi: 10.1038/gene.2010.71

116. Morel L, Blenman KR, Croker BP, Wakeland EK. The major murine systemic lupus erythematosus susceptibility locus, Sle1, is a cluster of functionally related genes. *Proc Natl Acad Sci USA.* (2001) 98:1787–92. doi: 10.1073/pnas.98.4.1787

117. Wandstrat AE, Nguyen C, Limaye N, Chan AY, Subramanian S, Tian XH, et al. Association of extensive polymorphisms in the SLAM/CD2 gene cluster with murine lupus. *Immunity.* (2004) 21:769–80. doi: 10.1016/j.immuni.2004.10.009

118. Veillette A. Immune regulation by SLAM family receptors and SAP-related adaptors. *Nat Rev Immunol.* (2006) 6:56–66. doi: 10.1038/nri1761

119. Schwartzberg PL, Mueller KL, Qi H, Cannons JL. SLAM receptors and SAP influence lymphocyte interactions, development and function. *Nat Rev Immunol.* (2009) 9:39–46. doi: 10.1038/nri2456

120. Sintes J, Bastos R, Engel P. *SLAM Family Receptors and Autoimmunity, Autoimmune Disorders - Pathogenetic Aspects.* Mavragani C, editor. Rijeka: InTech (2011). doi: 10.5772/20641

121. Cannons JL, Yu LJ, Jankovic D, Crotty S, Horai R, Kirby M, et al. SAP regulates T cell-mediated help for humoral immunity by a mechanism distinct from cytokine regulation. *J Exp Med.* (2006) 203:1551–65. doi: 10.1084/jem.20052097

122. Crotty S, Kersh EN, Cannons J, Schwartzberg PL, Ahmed R. SAP is required for generating long-term humoral immunity. *Nature.* (2003) 421:282–7. doi: 10.1038/nature01318

123. Ma CS, Hare NJ, Nichols KE, Dupré L, Andolfi G, Roncarolo MG, et al. Impaired humoral immunity in X-linked lymphoproliferative disease associated with defective IL-10 production by CD4+ T cells. *J Clin Invest.* (2005) 115:1049–59. doi: 10.1172/JCI200523139

124. Graham DB, Bell MP, McCausland MM, Huntoon CJ, van Deursen J, Faubion WA, et al. Ly9 (CD229)-deficient mice exhibit T cell defects yet do not share several phenotypic characteristics associated with SLAM- and SAP-deficient mice. *J Immunol.* (2006) 176:291–300. doi: 10.4049/jimmunol.176.1.291

125. Romero X, Zapater N, Calvo M, Kalko SG, de la Fuente MA, Tovar V, et al. CD229 (Ly9) lymphocyte cell surface receptor interacts homophilically through its N-terminal domain and relocalizes to the immunological synapse. *J Immunol.* (2005) 174:7033–42. doi: 10.4049/jimmunol.174.11.7033

126. Cannons JL, Qi H, Lu KT, Dutta M, Gomez-Rodriguez J, Cheng J, et al. Optimal germinal center responses require a multistage T cell:B cell adhesion process involving integrins, SLAM-associated protein, and CD84. *Immunity.* (2010) 32:253–65. doi: 10.1016/j.immuni.2010.01.010

127. Qi H, Cannons JL, Klauschen F, Schwartzberg PL, Germain RN. SAP-controlled T-B cell interactions underlie germinal centre formation. *Nature.* (2008) 455:764–9. doi: 10.1038/nature07345

128. Kumar KR, Li L, Yan M, Bhaskarabhatla M, Mobley AB, Nguyen C, et al. Regulation of B cell tolerance by the lupus susceptibility gene Ly108. *Science.* (2006) 312:1665–9. doi: 10.1126/science.1125893

129. Wong EB, Soni C, Chan AY, Domeier PP, Shwetank, Abraham T, et al. B cell-intrinsic CD84 and Ly108 maintain germinal center B cell tolerance. *J Immunol.* (2015) 194:4130–43. doi: 10.4049/jimmunol.1403023

130. Morel L, Tian XH, Croker BP, Wakeland EK. Epistatic modifiers of autoimmunity in a murine model of lupus nephritis. *Immunity.* (1999) 11:131–9. doi: 10.1016/S1074-7613(00)80088-6

131. Niederer HA, Willcocks LC, Rayner TF, Yang W, Lau YL, Williams TN, et al. Copy number, linkage disequilibrium and disease association in the FCGR locus. *Hum Mol Genet.* (2010) 19:3282–94. doi: 10.1093/hmg/ddq216

132. Breunis, WB, van Mirre E, Bruin M, Geissler J, de Boer M, Peters M, et al. Copy number variation of the activating FCGR2C gene predisposes to idiopathic thrombocytopenic purpura. *Blood.* (2008). 111:1029–38. doi: 10.1182/blood-2007-03-079913

133. Willcocks LC, Lyons PA, Clatworthy MR, Robinson JI, Yang W, Newland SA, et al. Copy number of FCGR3B, which is associated with systemic lupus erythematosus, correlates with protein expression and immune complex uptake. *J Exp Med.* (2008) 205:1573–82. doi: 10.1084/jem.20072413

134. Zhou XJ, Lv JC, Bu DF, Yu L, Yang YR, Zhao J, et al. Copy number variation of FCGR3A rather than FCGR3B and FCGR2B is associated with susceptibility to anti-GBM disease. *Int Immunol.* (2010) 22:45–51. doi: 10.1093/intimm/dxp113

135. Smith KG, Clatworthy MR. FcγRIIB in autoimmunity and infection: evolutionary and therapeutic implications. *Nat Rev Immunol.* (2010) 10:328–43. doi: 10.1038/nri2762

136. Su K, Wu J, Edberg JC, Li X, Ferguson P, Cooper GS, et al. A promoter haplotype of the immunoreceptor tyrosine-based inhibitory motif-bearing FcγRIIb alters receptor expression and associates with autoimmunity. I. Regulatory FCGR2B polymorphisms and their association with systemic lupus erythematosus. *J Immunol.* (2004) 172:7186–91. doi: 10.4049/jimmunol.172.11.7186

137. Su K, Li X, Edberg JC, Wu J, Ferguson P, Kimberly RP. A promoter haplotype of the immunoreceptor tyrosine-based inhibitory motif-bearing FcγRIIb alters receptor expression and associates with autoimmunity. II. Differential binding of GATA4 and Yin-Yang transcription factors and correlated receptor expression and function. *J Immunol.* (2004) 172:7192–9. doi: 10.4049/jimmunol.172.11.7192

138. Su K, Yang H, Li X, Gibson AW, Cafardi JM, Zhou T, et al. Expression profile of FcγRIIb on leukocytes and its dysregulation in systemic lupus erythematosus. *J Immunol.* (2007) 178:3272–80. doi: 10.4049/jimmunol.178.5.3272

139. Blank MC, Stefanescu RN, Masuda E, Marti F, King PD, Redecha PB, et al. Decreased transcription of the human FCGR2B gene mediated by the−343 G/C promoter polymorphism and association with systemic lupus erythematosus. *Hum Genet.* (2005) 117:220–7. doi: 10.1007/s00439-005-1302-3

140. Kyogoku C, Dijstelbloem HM, Tsuchiya N, Hatta Y, Kato H, Yamaguchi A, et al. Fcγ receptor gene polymorphisms in Japanese patients with systemic lupus erythematosus: contribution of FCGR2B to genetic susceptibility. *Arthritis Rheum.* (2002) 46:1242–54. doi: 10.1002/art.10257

141. Kono H, Kyogoku C, Suzuki T, Tsuchiya N, Honda H, Yamamoto K, et al. FcγRIIB Ile232Thr transmembrane polymorphism associated with human systemic lupus erythematosus decreases affinity to lipid rafts and attenuates inhibitory effects on B cell receptor signaling. *Hum Mol Genet.* (2005) 14:2881–92. doi: 10.1093/hmg/ddi320

142. Floto RA, Clatworthy MR, Heilbronn KR, Rosner DR, MacAry PA, Rankin A, et al. Loss of function of a lupus-associated FcγRIIb polymorphism through exclusion from lipid rafts. *Nat Med.* (2005) 11:1056–8. doi: 10.1038/nm1288

143. Chen JY, Wang CM, Ma CC, Luo SF, Edberg JC, Kimberly RP, et al. Association of a transmembrane polymorphism of Fcγ receptor IIb (FCGR2B) with systemic lupus erythematosus in Taiwanese patients. *Arthritis Rheum.* (2006) 54:3908–17. doi: 10.1002/art.22220

144. Siriboonrit U, Tsuchiya N, Sirikong M, Kyogoku C, Bejrachandra S, Suthipinittharm P, et al. Association of Fcγ receptor IIb and IIIb polymorphisms with susceptibility to systemic lupus erythematosus in Thais. *Tissue Antigens.* (2003) 61:374–83. doi: 10.1034/j.1399-0039.2003.00047.x

145. Chu ZT, Tsuchiya N, Kyogoku C, Ohashi J, Qian YP, Xu SB, et al. Association of Fcγ receptor IIb polymorphism with susceptibility to systemic lupus erythematosus in Chinese: a common susceptibility gene in the Asian populations. *Tissue Antigens.* (2004) 63:21–7. doi: 10.1111/j.1399-0039.2004.00142.x

146. Li X, Wu J, Carter RH, Edberg JC, Su K, Cooper GS, et al. A novel polymorphism in the Fcγ receptor IIB (CD32B) transmembrane region alters receptor signaling. *Arthritis Rheum.* (2003) 48:3242–52. doi: 10.1002/art.11313

147. Willcocks LC, Carr EJ, Niederer HA, Rayner TF, Williams TN, Yang W, et al. A defunctioning polymorphism in FCGR2B is associated with protection against malaria but susceptibility to systemic lupus erythematosus. *Proc Natl Acad Sci USA.* (2010) 107:7881–5. doi: 10.1073/pnas.0915133107

148. Lee YH, Ji JD, Song GG. Fcγ receptor IIB and IIIB polymorphisms and susceptibility to systemic lupus erythematosus and lupus nephritis: a meta-analysis. *Lupus.* (2009) 18:727–34. doi: 10.1177/0961203309104020

149. Zhu XW, Wang Y, Wei YH, Zhao PP, Wang XB, Rong JJ, et al. Comprehensive Assessment of the Association between FCGRs polymorphisms and the risk of systemic lupus erythematosus: evidence from a meta-analysis. *Sci Rep.* (2016) 6:31617. doi: 10.1038/srep31617

150. Chen JY, Wang CM, Ma CC, Hsu LA, Ho HH, Wu YJ, et al. A transmembrane polymorphism in FcγRIIb (FCGR2B) is associated with the production of anti-cyclic citrullinated peptide autoantibodies in Taiwanese RA. *Genes Immun.* (2008) 9:680–8. doi: 10.1038/gene.2008.56

151. Clatworthy MR, Willcocks L, Urban B, Langhorne J, Williams TN, Peshu N, et al. Systemic lupus erythematosus-associated defects in the inhibitory receptor FcγRIIb reduce susceptibility to malaria. *ProcNatlAcadSci USA.* (2007) 104:7169–74. doi: 10.1073/pnas.0608889104

152. Morel L. Genetics of SLE: evidence from mouse models. *Nat Rev Rheumatol.* (2010) 6:348–57. doi: 10.1038/nrrheum.2010.63

153. Cunninghame Graham DS, Vyse TJ, Fortin PR, Montpetit A, Cai YC, Lim S, et al. Association of LY9 in UK and Canadian SLE families. *Genes Immun.* (2008) 9:93–102. doi: 10.1038/sj.gene.6364453

154. Suarez-Gestal M, Calaza M, Endreffy E, Pullmann R, Ordi-Ros J, Sebastiani GD, et al. Replication of recently identified systemic lupus erythematosus genetic associations: a case-control study. *Arthritis Res Ther.* (2009) 11:R69. doi: 10.1186/ar2698

155. Suzuki A, Yamada R, Kochi Y, Sawada T, Okada Y, Matsuda K, et al. Functional SNPs in CD244 increase the risk of rheumatoid arthritis in a Japanese population. *Nat Genet.* (2008) 40:1224–9. doi: 10.1038/ng.205

156. Ota Y, Kawaguchi Y, Takagi K, Tochimoto A, Kawamoto M, Katsumata Y, et al. Single nucleotide polymorphisms of CD244 gene predispose to renal and neuropsychiatric manifestations with systemic lupus erythematosus. *Mod Rheumatol.* (2010) 20:427–31. doi: 10.1007/s10165-010-0302-x

157. Harley IT, Kaufman KM, Langefeld CD, Harley JB, Kelly JA. Genetic susceptibility to SLE: new insights from fine mapping and genome-wide association studies. *Nat Rev Genet.* (2009) 10:285–90. doi: 10.1038/nrg2571

158. Theofilopoulos AN, Kono DH, Baccala R. The multiple pathways to autoimmunity. *Nat Immunol.* (2017) 18:716–24. doi: 10.1038/ni.3731

159. Wandstrat AE, Wakeland E. The genetics of complex autoimmune diseases: non-MHC susceptibility genes. *Nat Immunol.* (2001) 2:802–9. doi: 10.1038/ni0901-802

160. Mooney MA, Nigg JT, McWeeney SK, Beth Wilmot B. Functional and genomic context in pathway analysis of GWAS data. *Trends Genet.* (2014) 30:390–400. doi: 10.1016/j.tig.2014.07.004

161. Takai T, Ono M, Hikida M, Ohmori H, Ravetch JV. Augmented humoral and anaphylactic responses in Fcγ RII-deficient mice. *Nature.* (1996) 379:346–9. doi: 10.1038/379346a0

162. Nimmerjahn F, Ravetch JV. Antibody-mediated modulation of immune responses. *Immunol Rev.* (2010) 236:265–75. doi: 10.1111/j.1600-065X.2010.00910.x

163. Soni C, Domeier PP, Wong EB, Shwetank, Khan TN, Elias MJ, et al. Distinct and synergistic roles of FcγRIIB deficiency and 129 strain-derived SLAM family proteins in the development of spontaneous germinal centers and autoimmunity. *J Autoimmun.* (2015) 63:31–46. doi: 10.1016/j.jaut.2015.06.011

164. Yuasa T, Kubo S, Yoshino T, Ujike A, Matsumura K, Ono M, et al. Deletion of fcγ receptor IIB renders H-2(b) mice susceptible to collagen-induced arthritis. *J Exp Med.* (1999) 189:187–94. doi: 10.1084/jem.189.1.187

165. Nakamura A, Yuasa T, Ujike A, Ono M, Nukiwa T, Ravetch JV, et al. Fcγ receptor IIB-deficient mice develop Goodpasture's syndrome upon immunization with type IV collagen: a novel murine model for autoimmune glomerular basement membrane disease. *J Exp Med.* (2000) 191:899–906. doi: 10.1084/jem.191.5.899

166. van den Berghe T, Hulpiau P, Martens L, Vandenbroucke RE, Van Wonterghem E, Perry SW, et al. Passenger mutations confound interpretation of all genetically modified congenic mice. *Immunity.* (2015) 43:200–9. doi: 10.1016/j.immuni.2015.06.011

167. Shlomchik MJ, Marshak-Rothstein A, Wolfowicz CB, Rothstein TL, Weigert MG. The role of clonal selection and somatic mutation in autoimmunity. *Nature.* (1987) 328:805–11. doi: 10.1038/328805a0

168. Shlomchik M, Mascelli M, Shan H, Radic MZ, Pisetsky D, Marshak-Rothstein A, et al. Anti-DNA antibodies from autoimmune mice arise by clonal expansion and somatic mutation. *J Exp Med.* (1990) 171:265–92. doi: 10.1084/jem.171.1.265

169. van Es JH, Gmelig Meyling FH, van de Akker WR, Aanstoot H, Derksen RH, Logtenberg T. Somatic mutations in the variable regions of a human IgG anti-double-stranded DNA autoantibody suggest a role for antigen in the induction of systemic lupus erythematosus. *J Exp Med.* (1991) 173:461–70. doi: 10.1084/jem.173.2.461

170. Winkler TH, Fehr H, Kalden JR. Analysis of immunoglobulin variable region genes from human IgG anti-DNA hybridomas. *Eur J Immunol.* (1992) 22:1719–28. doi: 10.1002/eji.1830220709

171. Wellmann U, Letz M, Herrmann M, Angermuller S, Kalden JR, Winkler TH. The evolution of human anti-double-stranded DNA autoantibodies. *Proc Natl Acad Sci USA.* (2005) 102:9258–63. doi: 10.1073/pnas.0500132102

172. Mietzner B, Tsuiji M, Scheid J, Velinzon K, Tiller T, Abraham K, et al. Autoreactive IgG memory antibodies in patients with systemic lupus erythematosus arise from nonreactive and polyreactive precursors. *Proc Natl Acad Sci USA.* (2008) 105:9727–32. doi: 10.1073/pnas.0803644105

173. Tiller T, Kofer J, Kreschel C, Busse CE, Riebel S, Wickert S, et al. Development of self-reactive germinal center B cells and plasma cells in autoimmune FcγRIIB-deficient mice. *J Exp Med.* (2010) 207:2767–78. doi: 10.1084/jem.20100171

174. Li H, Jiang Y, Prak EL, Radic M, Weigert M. Editors and editing of anti-DNA receptors. *Immunity.* (2001) 15:947–57. doi: 10.1016/S1074-7613(01)00251-5

175. Radic MZ, Weigert M. Genetic and structural evidence for antigen selection of anti-DNA antibodies. *Annu Rev Immunol.* (1994) 12:487–520. doi: 10.1146/annurev.iy.12.040194.002415

176. Sekiguchi DR, Jainandunsing SM, Fields ML, Maldonado MA, Madaio MP, Erikson J, et al. Chronic graft-versus-host in Ig knockin transgenic mice abrogates B cell tolerance in anti-double-stranded DNA B cells. *J Immunol.* (2002) 168:4142–53. doi: 10.4049/jimmunol.168.8.4142

177. Sekiguchi DR, Eisenberg RA, Weigert M. Secondary heavy chain rearrangement: a mechanism for generating anti-double-stranded DNA B cells. *J Exp Med.* (2003) 197:27–39. doi: 10.1084/jem.20020737

178. Fukuyama H, Nimmerjahn F, Ravetch JV. The inhibitory Fcγ receptor modulates autoimmunity by limiting the accumulation of immunoglobulin G+ anti-DNA plasma cells. *Nat Immunol.* (2005) 6:99–106. doi: 10.1038/ni1151

179. Rahman ZS, Alabyev B, Manser T. FcγRIIB regulates autoreactive primary antibody-forming cell, but not germinal center B cell, activity. *J Immunol.* (2007) 178:897–907. doi: 10.4049/jimmunol.178.2.897

180. Yajima K, Nakamura A, Sugahara A, Takai T. FcγRIIB deficiency with Fas mutation is sufficient for the development of systemic autoimmune disease. *Eur J Immunol.* (2003) 33:1020–9. doi: 10.1002/eji.200323794

181. Weisenburger T, von Neubeck B, Schneider A, Ebert N, Schreyer D, Acs A, et al. Epistatic Interactions Between Mutations of Deoxyribonuclease 1-Like 3 and the Inhibitory Fc Gamma Receptor IIB Result in Very Early and Massive Autoantibodies Against Double-Stranded DNA. *Front Immunol.* (2018) 9:1551. doi: 10.3389/fimmu.2018.01551

182. McGaha TL, Sorrentino B, Ravetch JV. Restoration of tolerance in lupus by targeted inhibitory receptor expression. *Science.* (2005) 307:590–3. doi: 10.1126/science.1105160

183. Brownlie RJ, Lawlor KE, Niederer HA, Cutler AJ, Xiang Z, Clatworthy MR, et al. Distinct cell-specific control of autoimmunity and infection by FcγRIIb. *J Exp Med.* (2008) 205:883–95. doi: 10.1084/jem.20072565

184. Simon MM, Greenaway S, White JK, Fuchs H, Gailus-Durner V, Wells S, et al. A comparative phenotypic and genomic analysis of C57BL/6J and C57BL/6N mouse strains. *Genome Biol.* (2013) 4:R82 doi: 10.1186/gb-2013-14-7-r82

185. Ravetch JV, Nimmerjahn F, Carroll MC. Fc and complement receptors. In: Alt F, Honjo T, Radbruch A, Reth M editors. *Molecular Biology of B Cells.* Cambridge: Academic Press (2015). p. 171–86. doi: 10.1016/B978-0-12-397933-9.00011-4

186. Sharp PE, Martin-Ramirez J, Boross P, Mangsbo SM, Reynolds J, Moss J, et al. Increased incidence of anti-GBM disease in Fcγ receptor 2b deficient mice, but not mice with conditional deletion of Fcgr2b on either B cells or myeloid cells alone. *Mol Immunol.* (2012) 50:49–56. doi: 10.1016/j.molimm.2011.12.007

187. Yilmaz-Elis AS, Ramirez JM, Asmawidjaja P, van der Kaa J, Mus AM, Brem MD, et al. FcγRIIb on myeloid cells rather than on B cells protects from collagen-induced arthritis. *J Immunol.* (2014) 192:5540–7. doi: 10.4049/jimmunol.1303272

188. Lin Q, Ohtsuji M, Amano H, Tsurui H, Tada N, Sato R, et al. FcγRIIb on B cells and myeloid cells modulates B cell activation and autoantibody responses via different but synergistic pathways in lupus-prone Yaa mice. *J Immunol.* (2018) 201:3199–210. doi: 10.4049/jimmunol.1701487

189. Mildner A, Giladi A, David E, Lara-Astiaso D, Lorenzo-Vivas E, Paul F, et al. Genomic characterization of murine monocytes reveals C/EBPβ transcription factor dependence of Ly6C⁻ cells. *Immunity.* (2017) 46:849–62. doi: 10.1016/j.immuni.2017.04.018

190. Hirose S, Lin Q, Ohtsuji M, Nishimura H, Verbeek JS. Monocyte subsets involved in the development of systemic lupus erythematosus and rheumatoid arthritis. *Int Immunol.* (2019) 31:dxz036. doi: 10.1093/intimm/dxz036

191. Biesen R, Demir C, Barkhudarova F, Grün JR, Steinbrich-Zollner M, Backhaus M, et al. Sialic acid-binding Ig-like lectin 1 expression in inflammatory and resident monocytes is a potential biomarker for monitoring disease activity and success of therapy in systemic lupus erythematosus. *Arthritis Rheum.* (2008) 58:1136–45. doi: 10.1002/art.23404

192. Cros J, Cagnard N, Woollard K, Patey N, Zhang SY, Senechal B, et al. Human CD14dim monocytes patrol and sense nucleic acids and viruses via TLR7 and TLR8 receptors. *Immunity.* (2010) 33:375–86. doi: 10.1016/j.immuni.2010.08.012

3

FCGR3A and FCGR2A Genotypes Differentially Impact Allograft Rejection and Patients' Survival After Lung Transplant

Pascale Paul[1,2]*, Pascal Pedini[3], Luc Lyonnet[1], Julie Di Cristofaro[4], Anderson Loundou[5], Mathieu Pelardy[3], Agnes Basire[3], Françoise Dignat-George[1,2], Jacques Chiaroni[3,4], Pascal Thomas[6], Martine Reynaud-Gaubert[7] and Christophe Picard[3,4]

[1] Department of Hematology, Hopital de la Conception, INSERM CIC-1409, Assistance Publique-Hôpitaux Marseille (AP-HM), Marseille, France, [2] INSERM 1263, INRA, C2VN, Aix-Marseille Université (AMU), INSERM, Marseille, France, [3] Établissement Français du Sang PACA-Corse 13005, Marseille, France, [4] "Biologie des Groupes Sanguins", UMR 7268 ADÉS Aix-Marseille Université/EFS/CNRS, Marseille, France, [5] Département de santé Publique - EA 3279, Assistance Publique-Hôpitaux Marseille (AP-HM), Aix-Marseille Université, Marseille, France, [6] Service de Chirurgie Thoracique et Transplantation Pulmonaire, CHU Nord Assistance Publique-Hôpitaux Marseille (AP-HM), Aix-Marseille Université, Marseille, France, [7] Service de Pneumologie et Transplantation Pulmonaire, CHU Nord Assistance Publique-Hôpitaux Marseille (AP-HM) - IHU Méditerranée Infection Aix-Marseille-Université, Marseille, France

*Correspondence:
Pascale Paul
pascale.paul@univ-amu.fr

Fc gamma receptors (FcγRs) play a major role in the regulation of humoral immune responses. Single-nucleotide polymorphisms (SNPs) of *FCGR2A* and *FCGR3A* can impact the expression level, IgG affinity and function of the CD32 and CD16 FcγRs in response to their engagement by the Fc fragment of IgG. The CD16 isoform encoded by *FCGR3A* [158V/V] controls the intensity of antibody-dependent cytotoxic alloimmune responses of natural killer cells (NK) and has been identified as a susceptibility marker predisposing patients to cardiac allograft vasculopathy after heart transplant. This study aimed to investigate whether *FCGR2A* and *FCGR3A* polymorphisms can also be associated with the clinical outcome of lung transplant recipients (LTRs). The SNPs of *FCGR2A* ([131R/H], rs1801274) and *FCGR3A* ([158V/F], rs396991) were identified in 158 LTRs and 184 Controls (CTL). The corresponding distribution of genotypic and allelic combinations was analyzed for potential links with the development of circulating donor-specific anti-HLA alloantibodies (DSA) detected at months 1 and 3 after lung transplant (LTx), the occurrence of acute rejection (AR) and chronic lung allograft dysfunction (CLAD), and the overall survival of LTRs. The *FCGR3A* [158V/V] genotype was identified as an independent susceptibility factor associated with higher rates of AR during the first trimester after LTx (HR 4.8, $p < 0.0001$, 95% CI 2.37–9.61), but it could not be associated with the level of CD16- mediated NK cell activation in response to the LTR's DSA, whatever the MFI intensity and C1q binding profiles of the DSA evaluated. The *FCGR2A* [131R/R] genotype was associated with lower CLAD-free survival of LTRs, independently of the presence of DSA at 3 months (HR 1.8, $p = 0.024$, 95% CI 1.08–3.03). Our data indicate that FCGR SNPs differentially affect the clinical outcome of

LTRs and may be of use to stratify patients at higher risk of experiencing graft rejection. Furthermore, these data suggest that in the LTx setting, specific mechanisms of humoral alloreactivity, which cannot be solely explained by the complement and CD16-mediated pathogenic effects of DSA, may be involved in the development of acute and chronic lung allograft rejection.

Keywords: Fc-gamma receptors, natural killer cells, lung transplantation, chronic lung allograft dysfunction, HLA antibodies, allograft rejection

INTRODUCTION

Lung transplantationi (LTx) remains a challenging therapeutic option for patients with end-stage pulmonary disease. Significant improvement in immunosuppressive strategies has led to decreased lung allograft loss in the early post-transplant period. When compared to other solid organ transplantation settings, LTx remains associated with the lowest survival rates with a median survival of 6 years after transplant (1). Chronic lung allograft dysfunction (CLAD) is the main cause of chronic lung allograft rejection and is characterized by an irreversible loss of lung function associated with a high prevalence of complications such as bronchiolitis obliterans syndrome (BOS) and restrictive allograft syndrome (RAS) (2). Factors that relate to the HLA mismatch, to the graft procedure (ischemia, unilateral or bilateral surgery) and initial lung disease can lead to highly variable levels of recipient immune response to the lung allograft. Inflammatory biomarkers and antibodies, occurrence of acute cellular rejection (ACR), infections/colonization, auto-immunity, and air pollution have been analyzed for their potential predictive value in anticipating development of immunological responses associated with CLAD. Toll receptors, pro-inflammatory cytokines and non-classical HLA molecules, i.e., HLA-G and HLA-E polymorphisms or haplotypes, have been associated with CLAD (3–9), but the underlying mechanisms involved in this devastating outcome of LTx in a given recipient are still poorly understood. Antibody-mediated rejection (ABMR) has been associated with a higher incidence of chronic lung allograft dysfunction (CLAD) and mortality after LTx but the specific mechanisms and histological or immunological biomarkers that allow to define the clinical ABMR entity still await further comprehension (10). Detection of preexisting or development of *de novo* donor-specific human leukocyte antigen (HLA) alloantibodies (DSAs) have been extensively investigated for their potential value as biomarkers of humoral responses that may predict adverse outcome of LTx.

Various studies suggest that the pre-transplant detection of circulating DSA is not associated with an increased risk of developing CLAD or related death if prospective cross-match testing was negative (11, 12). The pretransplant detection of DSA and antibodies directed againd non-HLA antigens such as angiotensin type 1 receptor (AT1R) and endothelin type A receptor (ETAR) is reported to have a negative impact on lung transplant outcome (13).

Early detection of *de novo* DSA detected at 1 month after LTx has been significantly associated with a worse outcome (14). Multiplex solid phase single antigen bead assay (SAFB) detection of *de novo* DSAs, notably anti-HLA DQ DSA, have also been associated with acute cellular rejection (ACR) (15) CLAD (16–18). The presence of circulating DSA at the time of lung allograft biopsy has been identified as a risk factor for graft loss (19).

Although there is more and more direct and indirect evidence regarding the role of *de novo* DSA in CLAD occurrence, the mechanisms that sustain the variable toxicity of these anti-HLA antibodies to the lung allograft are still unclear. One of the well-known cytotoxic mechanisms of DSA occurs through the IgG-mediated activation of the complement cascade that results in C4d deposition within the graft. C4d staining in lung allograft biopsies is considered as a diagnosis criteria for ABMR (10, 20–28). However, although recent evidence suggests that detection of complement-binding DSA can be associated with lung allograft failure (29), the predictive value of complement-binding DSA on LTx clinical outcome remains to be firmly demonstrated.

IgG antibodies can also activate the immune system through ligation of functional Fc gamma receptors (FcγRs). Since these receptors are expressed by a variety of immune cells, including B cells, natural killer cells, platelets, dendritic cells and macrophages, FcR receptors constitute a major checkpoint that regulates the intensity of auto- and allo-immune responsiveness of the host in response to infectious and humoral threats (30, 31). As infections and the immune alloreactivity of the recipient toward the transplant remain a leading cause of graft rejection and death during the first year after LTx, there is a need for biomarkers that may improve the monitoring of early humoral responses in LTRs (32–34) and open therapeutic perspectives to dampen antibody-driven inflammation in immunized patients (35, 36).

Polymorphisms of FcγRIIA (*FCGR2A* [131R/H], rs1801274) FcγRIIIA (*FCGR3A* [158V/F], rs396991) genes, that respectively, encode for the CD32 and CD16 receptors for the Fc segment of IgG, have an impact on the level of expression and immune function of these activating FcγRs. Various reports have highlighted the clinical relevance of these SNPs in controlling the host immune response to monoclonal antibody therapy.

Abbreviations: HLA, Human Leukocyte Antigen; LTx, Lung Transplant; LTRx, Lung Transplant Recipient; Abs, Antibodies; Ag, Antigen; DSA, Donor-Specific Antibodies; BOS, Bronchiolitis Obliterans Syndrome; CLAD, Chronic Lung Allograft Dysfunction; ADCC, Antibody dependent cell cytotoxicity; CT, Computed Tomography; RAS, Restrictive Allograft Syndrome; ABMR, Antibody Mediated Rejection; ACR, Acute Cellular Rejection; SAFB, Single-Antigen Flow Beads; D, Days; M, Month; CMV, Cytomegalovirus; MFI, Mean Fluorescence Intensity; OS, Overall Survival; DFS, Disease Free Survival; CDC, Complement-Dependent Cytotoxicity; CF, Cystic Fibrosis.

The presence of a histidine (H) rather than an arginine (R) at position 131 results in higher affinity for IgG1 and IgG2. The *FCGR2A* [131H/H] genotype has been associated with higher efficacy of Rituximab-mediated B cell depletion strategies before transplant of ABO-incompatible organs. This *FCGR2A* [131H/H] SNP has also been identified as a susceptibility marker associated with the severity of community-acquired pneumonia (37).Genetic variation in the *FCGR2A* gene has also been shown to be associated with an increased prevalence of invasive pneumococcal diseases and respiratory infections after LTx (38, 39), regardless of the site of pneumococcal infection (40). Pro-inflammatory effects associated with the *FCGR2A* [131R/R] genotype have also been reported as a consequence of activating signals that result from the dynamic interactions between CD32 and its cognate C-reactive protein (CRP) and immunoglobulin ligands.

The clinical relevance of CD16 inflammatory pathways in antibody-mediated rejection of kidney and heart allografts has also been illuminated by studies that deciphered the molecular landscape of immune and endothelial cell transcripts that associate with ABMR lesions evaluated in allograft biopsies (41–43). Ligation of the Fc domain of IgG has also been identified as a mechanism that allows CD16-dependant clearance of viral pathogens by immune NK cells (44). Recent studies suggest that the Fc fragment of DSA can indeed exert its adverse cytotoxic and inflammatory effects though a complement-independent mechanism that relies on level of expression of the NK-cell surface CD16 receptor and its affinity for the Fc fragment of alloantibodies. The intensity of host antibody dependent cell cytotoxicity (ADCC) is known to be conditioned by the capacity of NK effector cells to form conjugates with antibody-coated allogeneic cells, which is in part influenced by the *FCGR3A* [158V/F] genotype (45–47). We and others have recently shown that polymorphic variation in the *FCGR3A* genes is also likely to affect the pathogenic effects of IgG alloantibodies by controlling the level of the CD16 dependent recipient's immunological cytotoxic responses to allogeneic donor cells exposed to chronic alloantibody threat (35, 48–51).

Genotypic variation in the *FCGR3A* receptor can thus impact the strength of FcR-dependent ADCC responses of NK cells and regulate their capacity to secrete inflammatory cytokines and release CD107a/Lamp1$^+$ cytotoxic granules containing perforin and granzyme (50, 52, 53). The inter-individual variability in the functional CD16 receptor-dependent engagement by the Fc fragment of alloantibodies has been shown to condition the intensity of antibody-dependent cellular cytotoxicity (ADCC) of NK cells and the response to IgG immunotherapy.

The strength of FcR-mediated ADCC can also be affected by the isotype and glycosylation status of alloantibodies. The IgG1 and IgG3 isoforms have higher affinity for the CD16 *FCGR3A* [158V/V] variant when compared to *FCGR3A* [158F/F], thereby spurring increased effector cell activity in response to these IgG subclasses. We have shown that this high-affinity homozygous *FCGR3A* [158V/V] genotype is an independent predictor of cardiac allograft vasculopathy (48) and may be a clinically relevant underlying mechanism that sustains the level of DSA-mediated allograft injury (48–50). The recent evidence that the

NK cell infiltration of the graft can predict kidney graft failure also sustains the clinical relevance of these NK cell mediated mechanisms of allograft injury (54).

Considering the central contribution of polymorphisms affecting FcγRIIA and FcγRIIIA genes and receptor function in the individual shaping of antibody-mediated inflammatory and cytotoxic alloimmune responses of the recipient, deciphering the mechanisms and FcγR susceptibility profiles that may be associated with LTx outcome is necessary to optimize risk stratification (8).

This study thus aimed to investigate whether FcγR polymorphisms may be linked to the pathogenic mechanisms of DSA toxicity and be associated with adverse clinical complications that impair patient and allograft outcome after LTx.

MATERIALS AND METHODS

Participants and Study Design

We conducted a retrospective single-center study enrolling 158 adult patients who underwent lung transplants (LTx) at the Marseille Lung Transplant Center between December 2006 and December 2013. All patients from the French cohort (COLT, *Cohort in Lung Transplantation*, l'Institut du Thorax, INSERM UMR1087/CNRS UMR 6291, CNIL 911142) were recruited in this study. All subjects gave written informed consent in accordance with the Declaration of Helsinki. A group of 184 healthy unrelated volunteer French bone marrow donors were also recruited to constitute a control cohort, allowing the analysis of the FcγR genotype. Blood donations were collected in the "Etablissement Francais du Sang," in accordance with BSL-2 practices. A medical interview was carried out prior to blood donation to exclude donors with medical contraindications. This study was carried out in accordance with the French Public Health Code (art L1221-1), approved by an institutional ethics committee and conducted in compliance with the Good Clinical Practice Guidelines declaration of Helsinki and Istanbul.

Post-transplant Clinical Management

All recipients received a similar standardized immunosuppressive regimen in accordance with our institutional protocols. Induction therapy consisted of intravenous administration (IV) of rabbit anti-thymocyte globulins (rATG, Pasteur Merieux, Lyon, France) given for the first 3 post-operative days [except when daily lymphocyte count was below 200/mm^3, and when there were cytomegalovirus (CMV) and/or EBV mismatches (i.e., seronegative recipient and seropositive donor)] and high dose methylprednisolone (6 mg/kg/d Day 1, 2 mg/kg/d Day 2 and Day 3, and 1 mg/kg/d thereafter). The standard triple maintenance immunosuppressive regimen consisted of tacrolimus (adjusted to maintain whole blood levels varying between 12 and 14 ng/ml), mycophenolate mofetil in 5 patients (adjusted to a white blood cell count above 4,000 mm^3), and steroids (prednisone) tapered to 0.25 mg/kg/d over the first 3 months and stopped around 12 months after surgery.

According to CMV recipient positive (R+) and donor positive/recipient negative (D+/R−) status, patients received CMV prophylaxis with IV ganciclovir switch to oral valganciclovir.

Postoperatively, recipients received prophylactic or preemptive anti-infection treatment (antibiotic, antiviral, and antifungal therapies) according to their preoperative and/or concomitant infectious status.

Recipients had regular visits to the transplant center for clinical radiological and functional evaluation. At our institution, surveillance transbronchial biopsies are routinely performed at the end of the first month, or earlier if clinically indicated. All transbronchial biopsies were graded for ACR (A grade) and lymphocytic bronchiolitis (B grade) (LB) by lung transplant pathologists. ACR and LB were defined, respectively, as perivascular or peribronchial mononuclear inflammation according to the International Society for Heart and Lung Transplantation (ISHLT) criteria. Histologic appraisal of ACR and LB was conducted in accordance with accepted ISHLT standards in terms of the minimum number of biopsy samples and exclusion of opportunistic infection (27, 28). Pulmonary function tests (PFTs) were routinely conducted at our center on a monthly basis for the first 12 post-operative months, at M2 intervals in the second year and at M3 intervals thereafter. The baseline FEV_1 value was calculated as the average of the 2 best FEV_1 values at least 2 measure gap. Baseline values of total lung capacity (TLC) and FEV_1/FVC were defined as the average of the 2 measurements obtained at the same time as the best 2 FEV_1 measurements. Chronic lung allograft dysfunction (CLAD) was defined according to the standardized international criteria (55). The phenotype BOS or RAS was specified according to ISHLT guidelines (56). The following histological patterns compatible with AMR were also analyzed: (i) neutrophil capillaritis and (ii) acute lung injury with or without diffuse alveolar damage and with or without organizing pneumonia.

HLA Antibody Screening and Identification Protocol

Recipient serum samples from 2006 to 2013 were collected routinely prior to transplant, at the minimum when the patient was placed on the waiting list and before the transplant procedure (D0: Day 0) and serially after LTx (at month 1 and 3). All sera samples obtained from the 158 recipients were further assessed using Luminex single-antigen flow beads (SAFB) to determine antibody specificity using Single Antigen—One Lambda reagents (LABScreen® Single Antigen class I or LABScreen® Single Antigen class II, One Lambda, Thermo Fisher Scientific, Canoga Park, California, USA) according to the recommendations of the manufacturers. The mean fluorescence intensity (MFI) used the baseline formula proposed by the Fusion™ v 3.2 software. All beads with a normalized MFI threshold >1,000 were considered positive. Since detected circulating alloantibodies were often directed against distinct HLA class I and/or class II antigens, the cumulative mean fluorescence intensity (cMFI) of DSA was calculated as the sum of the MFI for each of the individual DSAs detected. DSA were considered to be HLA

antibodies directed against donor HLA antigen. Putative HLA-Cw and -DQA1 DSA were identified in accordance with the conventional linkage disequilibrium that is reported between HLA-B and HLA-C loci and between HLA-DQB1 and HLA-DQA1 loci, as respectively, described in the French population (57) and by supplementary extensive genotyping of HLA- genes in the recipient. Putative HLA-DR51, -DR52 and -DR53 DSA were determined in accordance with the linkage disequilibrium between DRB3, DRB4, DRB5 loci and DRB1 loci of recipient. The allelic specificities of HLA-Cw, DQA and -DR51, -DR52 and -DR53 DSA were assigned accordingly.

C1q Detection
All patients with HLA antibodies were tested for the presence of C1q. The binding level was determined by the C1qScreen™ assay per manufacturer instructions (One Lambda, Thermo Fisher Scientific, Canoga Park, California, USA). Fluorescence intensity was measured using Luminex-based LABScan™ 100 flow analyzer. C1q specific antibody specificity and binding levels were analyzed and determined through the Fusion™ v 3.2 software. C1q MFI > 1,000 was considered positive.

FCGR2A and FCGR3A Genotyping
The detection of single nucleotide polymorphisms (SNPs) allowed for the genotyping of FCGR3A ([158V/F], rs396991) and FCGR2A ([131R/H], rs1801274) as described (5, 48) using the SNAPSHOT technique. Genomic DNA was extracted from a 200-μl whole blood sample using the QIAmp Blood DNA Mini kit (Qiagen, Courtaboeuf, France) according to manufacturer instructions. A previously described homemade primer extension method (58) was used to simultaneously analyze the SNPs of the FcγR genes. The forward and reverse primers sequences were, respectively: FCGR3A-F 5′ TCCTAA TAGGTTTGGCAGTG 3′ and FCGR3A-R 5′ AAATGTTCA GAGATGCTGCT 3′, FCGR2A-F 5′ CCAGGAGGGAGAAAC CATC 3′ and FCGR2A-R 5′ CTCTTCTCCCCTCCCTACAT 3′. The extension primers are, respectively: FCGR3A_176-F: 30T-CCTACTTCTGCAGGGGGCTT and FCGR2A_166F 57T-CCAAAAGCCACACTCAAAGA. Data were analyzed using GeneMapper 4.0 with specific detection parameters. Using an in-house computer program, output files (.txt) exported from GeneMapper 4.0 were automatically formatted into files readable by the "Phenotype" application of the Gene[Rate] computer tool package (http://geneva.unige.ch/generate). For each different allele obtained, PCR products were sequenced on both strands using the BigDye Terminator v1.1 Sequencing Kit (Applied Biosystems) and analyzed on an automated fluorescence-based ABI PRISM 3130 XL genetic analyzer according to manufacturer protocol. FcR polymorphisms at these 4 loci were analyzed for allele frequencies, or homozygous or heterozygous allelic combination of FcγR alleles defining the corresponding genotype.

HLA Genotyping
Recipients and deceased donors were genotyped for low resolution HLA-A, -B, -DRB1, and -DQB1 loci by LABType® SSO (One Lambda, Thermo Fisher Scientific, Canoga Park,

California, USA) according to the manufacturer's specifications and the retrieved output was analyzed for allele identification using HLA Fusion™ v 1.2.1. Software (One Lambda, Thermo Fisher Scientific, Canoga Park, California, USA).

Phenotypic Analysis of Antibody-Dependent NK Cell Activation

Evaluation of the CD16-dependent alloreactive potential of DSA was assessed using the previously described NK cell humoral activation test (NK-CHAT) (50). The level of serum-induced CD16 engagement and the degranulating potential of NK cells was assessed by flow cytometry analysis of the level of CD16 cell surface expression within the $CD3^-CD56^+$ NK cell compartment, gated within PBMC effector cells after exposure to target B cells that had been precoated in the presence of LTRs or control sera. Effector cells used in the standardized assay were prepared from a healthy donor displaying the $FCGR3A$ [158V/V] encoding the high-affinity CD16 variant. The HLA typing of the two B cell lines used as targets were A2/A2, B44/B56, Cw1/Cw5, DR1/DR4, DR53, DQ5/DQ7 and A3/A3 B7/B35, Cw4/Cw5, DR10/DR15, DR51, DQ5/DQ6. Sera were selected for the presence of DSA recognizing a limited set of HLA antigens expressed by EBV target cell lines. Briefly, 500,000 target B cells (B-EBV cell lines expressing the cognate DSA target alloantigens detected in LTR) were incubated with control (CTL) unsensitized human male AB serum (Lonza) to block FcR, then rinsed and incubated for 15 min in the presence of 50% LTR serum [or CTL serum supplemented or not with 10 γg/ml of Rituximab IgG (positive control)] and then rinsed to remove unbound antibodies. Incubation of effector PBMC and pre-coated allogeneic B-EBV cell targets (1:1 ratio) was performed for 3 h at 37°C in presence of GolgiStop (Becton Dickinson 554724) and CD107-PC5 (Becton Dickinson 555802). Cells were then washed and labeled with CD3-ECD (Beckman Coulter A07748), CD16-PE (Beckman Coulter A07766), CD56-PC7 (Beckman Coulter A21692) for 15 min at room temperature protected from light. After 1 wash step, cells were resuspended in 500 μl PBS 2% SVF. Data acquisition and analysis was performed on a Beckman Coulter Navios cytometer. The mean fluorescence intensity of CD16 and percent of NK cells expressing Lamp1/CD107a expression was analyzed within the CD3-CD56+ NK cell subset. The NK-CHAT CD16 down regulation index (CD16DRI) was evaluated as a ratio between CD16 MFI measured on NK cells incubated with target cells in presence of effector cell autologous CTL serum/CD16 MFI of NK cells incubated with target cells and recipient serum to be tested. CD16DRI = (MFI CD16 control serum)/(MFI CD16 test serum). Alternatively, when serum at time of LTx was available for the assay, the baseline CD16 expression was evaluated in reference to the DSA negative serum collected at time of LTx. Sera containing HLA-DQ7 DSA obtained from kidney transplant recipients (KTR) with antibody-mediated rejection (ABMR) at time of diagnosis, previously described to induce high levels of CD16-dependent NK cell alloreactivity, were introduced as positive controls of the experiments, indexing the CD16 down regulation induced by LTx sera.

Statistical Analyses

Variables used to perform univariate and multivariable analyses included preoperative donor variables (donor age, sex, CMV status, HLA typing), preoperative donor–recipient matching parameters (age, sex, CMV status, and HLA mismatch), operative variables such as ischemia time, type of procedure (single vs. bilateral LTx) and preoperative and post-operative recipient variables (initial lung disease, HLA typing, pre- and post-transplant immunization status, occurrence of AR BOS, RAS, CLAD, or infectious bacterial episodes occurring during the first year post-transplant), and notably during the early post-Tx period at months 1 (M1) and 3 (M3) after LTx (**Table 1**).

Continuous variables were presented as median values and 25–75 interquartile ranges or mean ± sd according to their distribution evaluated using the Agostino & Pearson omnibus normality test performed using GraphPad Prism version 5.00 for Windows (GraphPad Software, La Jolla, California, USA). Categorical variables were presented as percentages. Fisher's exact test and the chi-square test were used to compare categorical data and t-tests or Mann Whitney tests were used for the comparison of continuous variables.

The primary endpoints of this study were overall survival (OS) and disease/CLAD-free survival (DFS). OS was defined as the interval between the date of transplant and the last follow-up visit or death. DFS was defined as the time interval from transplant to the first event: either the graft failure or diagnosis of acute rejection or CLAD in living recipients, or the death of the patient. The Kaplan-Meier method was used to estimate overall survival and rejection-free survival. The log-rank test was used to assess the univariate effects on OS and DFS. For all analyses, a 2-sided $p < 0.05$ was considered statistically significant. Variables with a $p < 0.2$ were also considered to construct multivariate regression models. Multivariate analyses were performed using Fine and Gray's proportional hazards regression model. All analyses were performed using IBM SPSS 15.0 software (SPSS Inc., Chicago, IL) and the cmprsk package (developed by Gray, June 2001) on R2.3.0 software (http://www.R-project.org).

RESULTS

Characteristics of the LTR Cohort

The demographic characteristics and clinical features of the 158 adult LTRs (median age: 42 years, 75 females and 83 males) are summarized in **Table 1**. Patients received a first LTx for cystic fibrosis (37%), emphysema (29%), pulmonary fibrosis (22%), or another diagnosis (12%). The median follow-up time was 38 months after LTx. Median survival time of the 94 patients who were alive at time of follow-up was 4.2 years. Sixty-four patients (40.5%) died during the study follow-up (median time before death 12.6 months, 25–75 interquartile range: 1.8–35.5 years) and 5 patients experienced CLAD-associated graft failure with indication of a second lung transplant or death. Among deceased patients, 32 patients died during the first year post-LTx, among which 12 patients died during the first month post-LTx and 9 between the first and third months post-LTx. Acute rejection diagnosis was confirmed in the lung transplant biopsy of 53 patients (36%), the first rejection episode occurring before the

TABLE 1 | Demographic and Clinical characteristics of LTRs.

Recipient, n	158
Recipient age at LTx (years), median(25–75)	42 (30–54)
Recipient Age ≥ 50, n (%)	54 (34)
Donor Age, median (25–75)	43 (29–54)
Male Gender, n (%)	83 (53)
Native Lung Disease	
Cystic Fibrosis, n (%)	59 (37)
Fibrosis, n (%)	35 (22)
Emphysema, n (%)	46 (29)
Other, n (%)	18 (12)
Transplantation type	
Bilateral LTx, n (%)	118 (74)
Single LTx, n (%)	36 (24)
Other, n (%)	4 (2)
CMV Risk	
CMV R- (%)	50
CMV Mismatch D+R- (%)	21
Immunization Status	
HLA Mismatch, median (25–75)	7 (6–7)
DSA M1, n	49
MFI DSAM1, median (25–75)	13,000 (5,500–18,750)
DSA M3, n	27
MFI DSA M3, median (25–75)	7,100 (3,500–13,500)
M1 DSA persisting at M3, n	21
C1q DSAM1, n	20
C1q DSAM3, n	7
Bacterial Infections	
M1, n	20
M3, n	11
First year, n	35
Transplant Outcome	
Time follow up post-LTx (months), median (25–75)	38.5 (23–62)
Rejection events	
Biopsy proven Acute rejection Day 0-M3, n (%)	41 (28)
Biopsy proven Acute rejection first year, n (%)	53 (35)
Time before Acute Rejection event (Days), median (25–75)	42 (22–179)
CLAD, n	40 (25)
Time before CLAD (months), median (25–75)	22 (13–32)
BOS, n (%)	35 (22)
RAS, n (%)	5 (3)
Allograft and Patients' Survival	
CLAD- or Graft failure-free Survival, n (%)	71 (45)
Death, n (%)	64 (40)
Time before Death (months), median (25–75)	13 (1.8–35)
Death or Graft failure with 2nd LTx, n (%)	68 (43)

Data are presented as a number and %, or median (25–75 Interquartile ranges). BOS, Bronchiolitis obliterans syndrome; RAS, restrictive allograft syndrome; CLAD, chronic lung allograft dysfunction; M1 and M3, month 1 and 3 post-LTx.

third month in 41 LTRs (occurring before the fourth month in 24 LTRs and during the third month and the twelfth month post-LTx in 11 LTRs). The occurrence of acute rejection could be associated with the presence of DSA in 49% of these patients ($n = 20$). During the study period, 40 LTRs (25%) developed CLAD, of which 35 (87%) had BOS and 5 (12%) had RAS. Seventeen of the patients with a CLAD diagnosis did not survive and 5 were considered for a second transplant procedure. CLAD-free survival of the graft was observed in 71 patients (45%) with a median disease-free survival time of 4.2 years (25–75 percentile: 3.1–5.8).

Distribution of *FCGR3A* and *FCGR2A* Polymorphisms

Genotyping of the *FCGR2A* and *FCGR3A* polymorphisms was performed in 158 LTRs and analyzed in reference to a control cohort of 184 healthy donors (CTLs) (**Figure 1**). The *FCGR2A*-H allele was detected in 75.3% of LTRs and 83.1% of CTLs ($p = 0.0734$) while the -R allele was detected in 67.7% of LTRs and in 76% of CTLs ($p = 0.0851$). Although the distribution of *FCGR2A* [131R/R] and *FCGR2A* [131H/H] was not significantly altered in LTRs, the frequency of *FCGR2A* [131H/R] was found to be significantly lower in LTRs analyzed in reference to CTLs (chi-square $p = 0.0028$). The distribution of *FCGR3A* alleles did not significantly differ between patients and controls; presence of the -F allele was detected in 81% of LTRs and in 83.7% of CTLs while the -V allele distribution was in 64.6% of LTRs and in 68.5% in CTLs. The genotype frequencies of the various genotype combinations resulting from analysis of these SNPs in the LTR and CTL cohorts are illustrated in **Figure 1**. The frequency of the *FCGR3A* [158F/F] genotype was positively correlated with the *FCGR2A* [131R/R] genotype in CTLs and in LTRs ($p = 0.008$ and $p < 0.0001$, respectively). Presence of the *FCGR2A* [131R/R] was thus significantly associated with lower rates of patients with the *FCGR3A* [158V/V] good responder genotypes in LTRs ($p = 0.038$), but this inverse correlation did not reach significance in the control cohort (**Table 2**). Analysis of the groups stratified according for FCGR SNPs did not reveal any significant difference regarding the age of the LTR and type of underlying initial lung disease. The *FCGR2A* [131H/R] SNP with was found to be associated with recipient gender ($p = 0.029$). The *FCGR2A* [131H/H] genotype was observed to be significantly more common in women LTRs (32 out of 51, $p = 0.008$).

DSA Immunization During the First 3 Months Following Lung Transplant Is Associated With FCGR Polymorphism

During the first 3 months post-transplant, 55 patients developed *de novo* circulating DSA. During the first month post-LTx (M1), DSA developed in 49 LTRs (12 HLA class I, 20 HLA class II, and 17 HLA class I and II). The median MFI of DSA detected at M1 was 7,000 for HLA Class I DSA and 12,100 for HLA Class II DSA and 12 patients (8%) exhibited high cMFI values of DSA (over the 18,750 threshold corresponding to the 75 percentile value observed for MFI analyzed at M1) (**Table 1**). Circulating DSA could be detected in 27 LTRs analyzed at month 3 (M3) post-LTx (11 HLA class I, 13 HLA class II and 3 HLA class I and II) (**Figure 2**). The development of *de novo* DSA was observed at M3 in 6 LTRs with no detectable DSA at M1 (4 HLA class I, 1

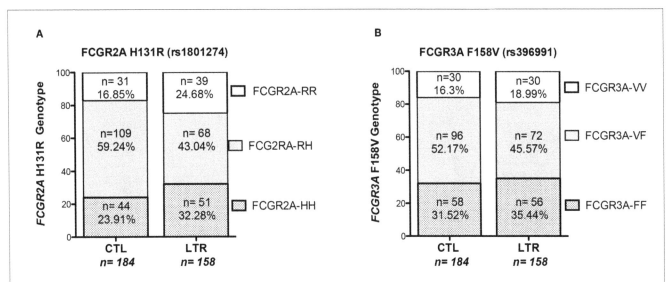

FIGURE 1 | Distribution of *FCGR3A* and *FCGR2A* genotypes in LTRs and CTLs. The proportion of the *FCGR2A* (left Panel, **A**) and *FCGR3A* (right panel, **B**) genotypes resulting from the SNP allelic combination were analyzed in a cohort of 158 LTRs and 184 CTLs recruited in southern France.

TABLE 2 | Association between the *FCGR2A* [131R/R] and FCGR3A [158V/F] genotypes observed in LTRs and CTLs.

		FCGR2A genotype LTR			
		HH $n = 51$	HR $n = 68$	RR $n = 39$	p-value FCGR2A-RR vs. FCGR3A
FCGR3A genotype	FF, $n = 56$	8	24	24	$p < 0.001$
	VF, $n = 72$	30	30	12	$p = 0.032$
	VV, $n = 30$	13	14	3	$p = 0.038$

		FCGR2A genotype CTL			
		HH $n = 44$	HR $n = 109$	RR $n = 31$	p-value FCGR2A-RR vs. FCGR3A
FCGR3A genotype	FF, $n = 58$	8	34	16	$P = 0.008$
	VF, $n = 96$	24	59	13	$p = 0.211$
	VV, $n = 30$	12	16	2	$p = 0.103$

HLA class II and 1 HLA Class I and Class II). The median MFI values of DSA detected at M1 and at M3 were, respectively, 13,000 and 7,100 (**Table 1**, **Figure 2**). DSA detected at M1 persisted at M3 in 21 LTRs (44% of DSA-positive MTR at M1) and 4 of these M3 DSA were also detectable 1 year post-transplant. HLA-DQ DSA were the only HLA class II persisting at M3. The median cMFI level of DSA detected at M1 and persisting at M3 (14,600, 25–75 percentile, 7,000–23,250) could not be linked to their persistence at M3 and did not significantly differ from the cMFI of DSA observed at M1 but undetectable at M3 (median MFI: 12,200, 25–75 percentile 4,000–16,000). Circulating DSA directed against DQ specificities were detected in 33 LTRs at M1 (median DQ-DSA MFI: 12,000 25–75 percentile 7,600–14,500) and in 14 LTRs at M3 (median 12,000, 5,000–15,850, 11 HLA-DQ DSA detected at M1 persist at M3 while 3 of the 14 HLA-DQ DSA detected at M3 were *de novo* DSA). C1q Binding DSA at

M1 were detected in 20 LTRs (2 HLA class I, 15 HLA class II, and 3 HLA class I and II) with a median cMFI of C1q-binding DSA detected at M1 of 23,000 (25–75 percentile 6,300–30,000). Seven of the 27 DSA detected at M3 were found to bind C1q (1 HLA class I, 5 class II HLA DSA and 1 HLA class I and class II), with a median cMFI of 17,150 (25–75 percentile 7,000–31,000). All C1q binding DSA detected at M3 were also detected at M1.

The *FCGR2A* [131R/R] genotype was also to found to correlate with the detection of circulating DSA at M3 ($p = 0.011$) and notably to the development of *de novo* DSA between the first and second months post-transplant (4 out of the 6 *de novo* DSA detected at M3 were genotyped as *FCGR2A* [131R/R], $p = 0.017$). *FCGR3A* [158V/V] tends to be inversely associated with the persistence of DSA at M3 ($p = 0.07$, **Table 3**), as only 1 out of the 21 patients with persistent DSA at M3 was genotyped as *FCGR3A*

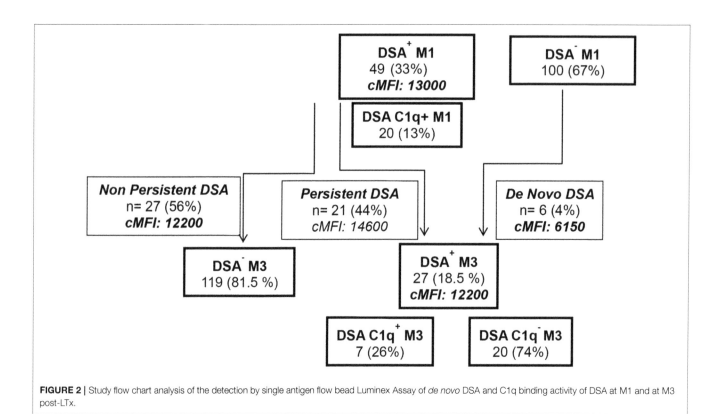

FIGURE 2 | Study flow chart analysis of the detection by single antigen flow bead Luminex Assay of *de novo* DSA and C1q binding activity of DSA at M1 and at M3 post-LTx.

TABLE 3 | Patients immunization characteristics according to the *FCGR2A* and *FCGR3A* genotypes.

	FCGR2A			FCGR3A		
	HH/RH	**RR**	*p*-value	**FF/VF**	**VV**	*p*-value
n = 158	119	39		128	30	
DSA M1, *n* = 49	33	16	0.161[t]	40	9	0.926, ns
Median MFI DSA M1	13,000	13,500	0.639, ns	12,500	13,800	0.477, ns
C1q DSA M1, *n* = 24	18	6	0.919, ns	19	5	0.869, ns
DSA M3, *n* = 27	15	12	0.011	26	1	0.024
DQ DSA M3, *n* = 14	7	7	0.022	13	1	0.225, ns
M1 DSA persisting at M3, *n* = 21	13	8	0.146[t]	20	1	0.07[t]
Median MFI DSA M3	6,300	9,500	0.494, ns	7,500	4,500	NA
C1q DSA M3, *n* = 7	5	2	0.840, ns	7	0	0.187[t]

Continuous variables are expressed as median (25–75 percentile ranges). p-values of the statistical tests comparing groups (Chi-2 or non-parametric Mann-Whitney test) were considered as significant when p-values were <0.05, tendency ([t]) when p > 0.05 and <0.2 and non-significant (ns) when p > 0.2 or NA when non-applicable. M1 and M3, month 1 and 3 post-LTx.

[158V/V]. The *FCGR3A*-F allele was significantly associated with the detection of circulating DSA at M3 (26 out of 27 LTRs with detectable circulating DSA at M3 were positive for the *FCGR3A*-F allele, *p* = 0.024) (**Table 3**).

FcGR3A and *FcGR2A* Polymorphisms Are Differentially Associated With Acute and Chronic Lung Allograft Rejection

The *FCGR3A* [158V/V] was also identified as a susceptibility genotype associated with a higher risk of acute rejection (log rank test for equality of survivor functions *p* = 0.0009,

Figure 3A). Multivariate Cox regression analysis also revealed that the susceptibility conferred by the *FCGR3A* [158V/V] genotype (OR 4.8, *p* < 0.0001, 95% CI 2.375–9.607) was independent from the development of DSA at M3 and their C1q binding activity. *FCGR2A* [131R/H] was not observed to affect the rate of acute rejection. The *FCGR2A* [131R/R] genotype was instead associated with the detection of DSA occurring in the absence of acute rejection (*p* = 0.029).

The DSA immunization status of the patient evaluated during the first year post- LTx could not be associated with CLAD. Although the number of observations was small, 4 of the 5 LTRs

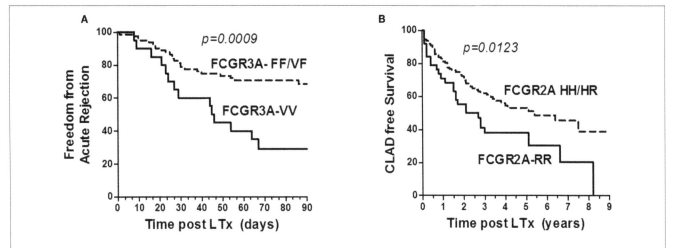

FIGURE 3 | Analysis of the influence of Fc-gamma Receptor polymorphisms on Rejection Free survival. **(A)** Impact of *FCGR3A* genotype on freedom from acute lung rejection. Kaplan–Meir Survival analysis links the *FCGR3A* [158V/V] (solid line, $n = 20$) to lower acute-rejection-free survival after 3 months post-LTx in LTRs, when compared with the *FCGR3A* [158V/F] and *FCGR3A* [158F/F] group (dashed line, $n = 81$). LTRs with the *FCGR3A* [158V/V] show an increased rate of acute rejection events occurring during the first 3 months post-LTx. **(B)** Impact of *FCGR2A* genotype on CLAD free survival. Kaplan–Meir Survival analysis links the *FCGR2A* [131R/R] (solid line, $n = 39$) to a lower CLAD-free survival rate in LTRs over time or study follow-up (years, x axis), when compared with the *FCGR2A* [131H/H] and *FCGR2A* [131R/H] group (dashed line, $n = 119$).

who developed RAS-associated CLAD were homozygous for the *FCGR3A*–FF allele ($p = 0.034$). While the *FCGR3A* [158V/F] could not be significantly associated with the risk of CLAD, *FCGR2A* [131R/R] was identified as a susceptibility marker associated with lower CLAD-free survival of LTRs ($n = 87$, logrank test for equality of survivor functions $p = 0.0123$, **Figure 3B**). Multivariate Cox regression models adjusting co-variables identified using univariate analysis further identified *FCGR2A* [131R/R] as an independent susceptibility marker associated with CLAD (OR 2.2; $p = 0.022$, 95CI 1.126–4.435) (**Table 4**). Multivariate Cox analysis further showed that the *FCGR2A* [131R/R] genotype is significantly associated with the enhanced risk of developing a composite LTx adverse outcomes (CLAD, graft failure or death), independently of other factors such as detection of DSA at M3 or native emphysema lung disease (**Table 4**).

LTx DSAs Have No Major Impact on CD16-Dependent NK Cell Cytotoxic Activation

Considering our previous finding that identifies the potential value of *FCGR3A* [158V/F] in predicting cardiac allograft vasculopathy (48), we further investigated whether the presence of association of acute rejection events with high affinity *FCGR3A* [158V/V] genotype could be associated with the DSA-mediated pathogenic effects that promote acute rejection mechanisms of lung allograft. Using the NK-cellular humoral activation test (NK-CHAT), previously designed to index the level of DSA-mediated engagement of CD16 and unravel potential ADCC-driven pathogenic effects of circulating DSA (41), we therefore aimed to investigate whether circulating DSA detected at M1 or M3 in LTRs have the potential to stimulate NK cell alloreactivity. Evaluation of the DSA-induced down regulation

of NK cell CD16 expression (CD16 Down Regulation Index or CD16DRI) was performed in a standardized NK-CHAT assay analyzing alloreactivity of NK cells toward serum-coated CD20+ B lymphocytes expressing the cognate HLA target alloantigen, using 23 serum samples obtained from 20 distinct LTRs (**Table 5**). Thirteen sera were collected at M1 and ten at M3. Four sera had detectable DSA that persisted at M3. Seven DSA at M1 and Four DSA at M3 were C1q positive.

Surprisingly, the CD16DRI values induced by the DSA+ LTx sera were very low when compared to those obtained in response to Rituximab. These CD16 DRI values could not be associated with the intensity of DSA MFI and C1q binding activity of DSA. Furthermore, the CD16DRI of LTRs (LTR 17, 18, and 20) with HLA DQ7 DSA were lower than those obtained of ABMR kidney transplant recipients (KTR) with HLA DQ7 DSA and with similar MFI (**Figure 4**).

In contrast to the results previously observed in the kidney and heart transplant setting, the association of the *FCGR3A* [158V/V] genotype with acute rejection appears to be independent of the presence of circulating DSA and the DSA MFI levels. In contrast to the KTR serum, NK-CHAT evaluation of the serum of immunized LTRs did not reveal significant alloreactive DSA toxicity and did not allow for determination of their pathogenic potential in eliciting CD16 and NK-cell cytotoxic activation.

FCGR2A Polymorphism Impacts Patients and Allograft Survival

Occurrence of acute and chronic events or infectious episodes was not shown to have a major impact on overall survival in the analyzed cohort.

Early development of DSA that persist at M3 ($n = 21$) were associated with lower graft or patient survival rates ($p = 0.002$) and were associated with the presence of the low-affinity F allelic

TABLE 4 | Univariate analysis and multivariate Cox regression analysis of risk factors associated with acute or chronic rejection events.

Risk covariables	Univariate analysis p-value	Hazard ratio	Std. Err.	z	P > z	(95% Conf.interval)		
Acute Rejection in the first 3 months post-LTx, n= 41								
FCGR3A [158 V/V]	0.003	4.8	1.70	4.39	**<0.0001**	**2.375**	–	**9.607**
Native Lung Disease Emphysema	0.037	0.4	0.18	−2.05	**0.040**	**0.173**	–	**0.961**
M3 C1q Binding DSA	0.009	4.4	2.87	2.28	**0.023**	**1.231**	–	**15.789**
Single lung Tx	0.091	2.6	0.96	2.56	**0.010**	**1.251**	–	**5.352**
FCGR3A [158 V/F]	0.003	4.4	1.54	4.29	**<0.0001**	**2.247**	–	**8.761**
Native Lung Disease Emphysema	0.037	0.4	0.17	−2.17	**0.03**	**0.161**	–	**0.909**
M3 DSA+	Ns (p = 0.251)	3.1	1.27	2.82	**0.005**	**1.417**	–	**6.917**
Single lung Tx	0.091	2.9	1.12	2.89	**0.004**	**1.419**	–	**6.243**
CLAD, n= 40								
FCGR2A [131R/R]	0.185	2.23	0.781	2.3	**0.022**	**1.126**	–	**4.435**
Native Lung Disease Emphysema	0.177	2.65	0.900	2.86	**0.004**	**1.360**	–	**5.157**
Recipient Gender: Female	0.142	1.62	0.531	1.47	0.141	0.852	–	3.080
Acute Rejection 1st Year	0.050	1.93	0.621	2.03	**0.042**	**1.024**	–	**3.625**
Composite adverse outcome: CLAD, graft loss or death n = 87								
FCGR2A [131R/R]	0.185[t]	1.8	0.475	2.3	**0.024**	**1.080**	–	**3.028**
Native Lung Disease Emphysema	0.177	2.1	0.514	2.95	**0.003**	**1.279**	–	**3.439**
M3 DSA	0.075	1.9	0.557	2.44	**0.015**	**1.145**	–	**3.080**

Covariables (risk covariables) used to explain the Lung transplant outcome primary variable (Acute Rejection, CLAD or adverse composite outcome that includes CLAD or Graft loss or death) are listed on the left column. The bold text refers to covariables that retained independent significant p-values in multivariate cox regression models.

variant of CD16. Persistence of DSA at M3 was thus lower in FCGR3A [158V/V] LTRs ($p = 0.029$). Other parameters such as high MFI DSA detected at M1 (>18,750 MFI, 75 percentile value of DSA MFI at M1 post-LTx, $p = 0.109$) or FCRGR2A [131R/R] ($p = 0.052$) tended to be associated with the risk of death. While the FCGR3A genotype could not be associated to overall survival, the FCRGR2A [131R/R] genotype was identified as a risk factor associated with the composite adverse outcome combining graft failure or patient death ($n = 68$, log rank test for equality of survivor functions $p = 0.0417$, **Figure 5**). Multivariate analysis of variables associated with death from all causes after LTx ($n = 64$, 40.5% of the LTR cohort) retained initial diseases other than cystic fibrosis ($p = 0.048$) DSA with MFI values > to the 75 percentile 18,750 MFI value for DSA detected at M1 as significant risk factors (**Table 6**). The FCRGR2A [131R/R] genotype was shown to be an independent factor associated with lower overall survival of LTRs using multivariate logistic Cox regression models (HR: 1.8, $p = 0.047$ 95% CI: 1.008–3.121, **Table 6**).

DISCUSSION

FcγR constitute a major marker of immune activation in response to infections, antibodies and CRP inflammatory ligands. Recent studies suggest that the engagement of FcR by the Fc fragment of alloantibodies can influence the cytotoxic activation level of NK cells toward the heart or kidney allograft. This study aimed to investigate whether the combined evaluation of FCGR3A [158F/V] and FCGR2A [131H/R] SNPs and biomarkers that index the level of CD16-dependent ADCC of NK cells might

also be relevant to stratify patients at higher risk of lung allograft failure.

Our results show evidence that the FCGR3A [158V/V] genotype can be identified as a genetic marker that predisposes LTRs to acute rejection, independently of their DSA immunization status. Fifteen out of thirty patients with the FCGR3A [158V/V] genotype indeed developed acute rejection during the first trimester. Since this profile has been associated with higher NK cell responsiveness, we further investigated how it may relate to the NK cell mediated cytotoxic effects of DSA toward the lung allograft. Various studies have shown that the detection of circulating DSA with an ability to ligate the C1q component and activate the complement cascade can be associated with a greater risk of acute rejection and allograft loss after heart or kidney transplant. These complement-dependent mechanisms of DSA-mediated cytotoxic effects have also been recently documented in the lung transplant setting (19, 20). As previously reported (29), all C1q DSA detected at M3 were directed toward donor HLA-DQ alloantigens and C1q positive were shown to be significantly associated with acute rejection in the study cohort. A limitation of our study is the lack of elements allowing the distinction of cellular acute rejection (ACR) from ABMR. Endothelial deposition of C4d and microvascular inflammation were shown to be reliable markers of ABMR in renal and cardiac allografts, but the clinical relevance of C4d staining within lung allograft biopsies still remains controversial for lungs. These diagnostic criteria for ABMR were not always available on a routine basis at the time of evaluation until the Banff nomenclature released more accurate histologic features that characterize lung allograft grafts biopsies of DSA-positive LTRs.

TABLE 5 | NK-CHAT: Evaluation of DSA reactivity toward B cell targets expressed in sera collected from LTR and KTR, used as positive controls for NK-CHAT.

LTR	Serum Time post-LTx	DSA HLA class I/II	MFI DSA	MFI C1q DSA	Serum induced CD107 up regulation (CD107URI)	Serum induced CD16 down regulation index (CD16DRI)	CLAD	AR	Death
LTR 1	M1	Class I	A3:8,500 B7:8,500	A3:14,000 B7: > 15,000	1	1	na	1	1
LTR 2	M1	Class I	A2:7,000 B44:3,000	A2: 3,000 B44: 10,000	1	1	1	1	0
LTR 3	M1	Class I	A2: 3,200	Negative	1	1	1	1	0
LTR 4	M1	Class I	A3: 2,300	Negative	1	1	0	0	0
LTR 5	M3	Class I	B7: 3,000	Negative	1.6	1	0	1	0
LTR 6	M1	Class I and II	A2: 3,500 DQ7: 13,000	DQ7: 10,000	0.4	1	0	0	0
	M3	Class II	DQ7: 9,000	Negative	0.5	1	0	0	0
LTR 7	M1	Class II	DQ2:10,000 DR53:3,000	Negative	3.3	1.2	na	0	1
LTR 8	M1	Class II	DQ5: 9,500	Negative	1.6	1	1	1	1
LTR 9	M1	Class II	DQ6: 10,000	Negative	1.4	1.2	0	0	0
LTR 10	M1	Class II	DQ7 > 15,000	DQ7 > 15,000	0.9	1.3	0	0	0
LTR 11	M1	Class II	DQ7:11,000 DQ9:4,000	DQ7:11,500 DQ9:11,500	0.9	1	1	0	1
LTR 12	M1	Class II	DQ7: 13,000	Negative	1.4	1.1	0	0	0
LTR 13	M3	Class II	DQ5: 14,000	DQ5: 9,000	0.9	1.4	0	0	0
LTR 14	M3	Class II	DQ5: 13,000	Negative	<1	<1	na	0	**1**
LTR 15	M3	Class II	DQ5 4,500	Negative	<1	<1	0	0	0
LTR 16	M3	Class II	DR53: 3,000	Negative	1	1	0	0	0
LTR 17	M3		DQ7: 13,400	DQ7 11,000	1	1			
LTR 18	M3	Class II	DQ7: 16,000	DQ7, 14,000	3	2.1	na	0	1
LTR 19	M1	Class II	DQ5:7,500 DQ6:6,000	DQ5: 7,000 DQ6: 6,500	1.2	<1	0	1	0
	M3	Class II	DQ5: 3,500	Negative	<1	<1			
LTR 20	M1	Class II	DQ7: 9,000	DQ7: 6,000	1.5	1.9	0	0	0
	M3	Class II	DQ7: 12,500	DQ7: 9,000	1.4	1.9			
KTR 1 ABMR	At time of ABMR	Class II	DQ7: 9,000	nt	6.5	29	na	na	na
KTR 2 ABMR	diagnoss	Class II	DQ7: 13,000	nt	7	42	na	na	na

AR, acute rejection; na, not applicable; nt, non-tested.

However, the association between the *FCGR3A* [158V/V] genotype and presence of circulating DSA at M1 or at M3 did not appear to confer a higher risk of acute rejection, whatever their MFI and their C1q binding activity status, thus suggesting that the graft damage associated with the *FCGR3A* [158V/V] genotype is independent from DSA immunization status. This finding was unexpected, as we have previously shown that the intensity of antibody-dependent CD16 activation of NK cells, indexed by the non-invasive NK-CHAT, is significantly enhanced in recipients that bear the *FCGR3A* [158V/V] genotype and constitute a relevant cytotoxic mechanism sustaining toxic effects of DSA and allograft vasculopathy (48, 50). In contrast, NK-CHAT evaluation of DSA from LTRs actually shows evidence that the engagement of CD16 by LTx DSA is low when analyzed in reference to anti-HLA class II DSA that are found in the serum of kidney transplant recipients at time of ABMR diagnosis and that exhibit comparable HLA-DQ7 specificities and MFI values.

This low potential of LTx DSA to induce CD16-mediated NK cell activation appears to be independent of their C1q binding activity and could not be associated with adverse outcome of LTx in the present study. As CD16 exhibits higher affinity for IgG1 and IgG3 alloantibodies, this failure of DSA to engage CD16 mediated cytotoxic functions may be due to the IgG2 and/or IgG4 isotypes of DSA, which have been shown to exhibit lower affinity for CD16. This finding may also indicate that the glycosylation pattern of IgG1 DSA interferes with the FcγRs-mediated recognition of the Fc fragment of IgG by immune cells or complement factors. These hypotheses are supported by the observation that only 30% of circulating DSA detected at M1 and at M3 were found to bind C1q in this study cohort and by previous findings that report high IgG4 levels in patients with cystic fibrosis lung disease (59). These data suggest that, in contrast to previous findings, the *FCGR3A* [158V/V] susceptibility genotype does not appear as a major mechanism of

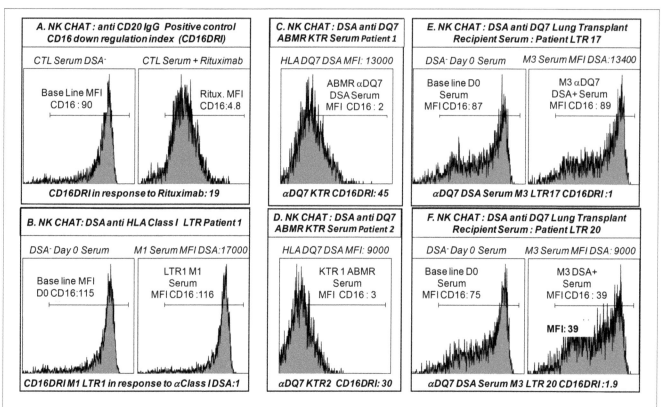

FIGURE 4 | Representative illustration of the NK-Cellular Humoral test (NK-CHAT) used to evaluate serum- and DSA- induced NK cell activation toward B cell lines expressing cognate HLA class I or HLA-DQ7 donor-specific allo-antigens. **(A)** PBMC effectors obtained from *FCGR3A* [158 V/V] CTL were exposed to B-EBV cell lines previously coated with DSA-negative serum. This allowed for evaluation of the baseline expression level of CD16 expression (CD16MFI) within the CD3-CD56+CD16+ NK cell compartment when PBMC were exposed to B cell targets. As a positive control indexing the level of IgG-induced CD16 down regulation (CD16DRI), the same B-EBV cell lines were coated in the presence of 10γ/ml Rituximab (anti CD20 IgG) prior to exposure to the effector PBMC. This allowed for calculation of the CD16 down regulation index (CD16DRI: baseline CD16MFI NK cells exposed to B cells coated with CTL DSA-negative serum/CD16 MFI of NK cells exposed to the same B targets pre-coated in presence of Rituximab). In this context, CD16DRI in response to Rituximab = 19, i.e., 90/4.8. **(B)** The CD16 DRI of NK cells was evaluated in response to the serum collected at M1 in one LTR (LTR 1, **Table 5**) with detectable levels of DSA recognizing the HLA-A3 and -B7 expressed on the B cell targets. Non-immunized serum (DSA-negative) collected from LTR 1 at time of LTx (D0) was used as the reference baseline CD16 MFI value to calculate the CD16DRI. Despite a cumulative MFI of DSA >17,000, DSA detected at M1 in LTR1 failed to induce CD16-dependent NK cell alloreactivity (CD16DRI = 1). **(C)** The CD16 DRI of NK cells was evaluated in response to the serum collected at time of ABMR diagnosis in one kidney transplant recipients (KTR 1, **Table 5**) with detectable levels of DSA recognizing the HLA-DQ7 (MFI: 13,000) expressed on the B cell targets. The CD16DRI of KTR1 (CD16DRI: 45) was greater than that observed in response to the Rituximab (CD16DRI:19, **A**). **(D)** The CD16 DRI of NK cells was evaluated in response to the serum collected at time of ABMR diagnosis in a second KTR (KTR 2, **Table 5**) with detectable levels of DSA recognizing the HLA-DQ7 (MFI: 9,000) expressed on the B cell targets. The CD16DRI of KTR1 (CD16DRI: 30) was greater than that observed in response to the Rituximab (CD16DRI:19, **A**). **(E)** The CD16 DRI of NK cells was evaluated in response to the serum collected at M3 (time of acute rejection) in a second LTR (LTR 17, **Table 5**) with detectable levels of DSA recognizing the HLA- DQ7 (MFI: 13,400) expressed on the B cell targets. Non-immunized serum (DSA-negative) collected from LTR 17 at D0 was used as the reference baseline CD16 MFI value to calculate the CD16DRI (CD16DRI = 1). The MFI DSA of LTR 17 (MFI: 13,400) was similar to the MFI DSA of ABMR KTR 1 serum as illustrated in **(C)**. **(F)** The CD16 DRI of NK cells was evaluated in response to the serum collected at M3 (time of acute rejection) in a third LTR (LTR 20, **Table 5**) with detectable levels of DSA recognizing the HLA- DQ7 (MFI DSA: 9,000) expressed on the B cell targets. The DSA-negative serum of LTR 20 collected at D0 was used as a baseline CD16 MFI value to calculate the CD16DRI (CD16DRI = 1.9). The MFI DSA of LTR 20 (MFI: 9,000) was similar to the MFI DSA of ABMR KTR 2 serum evaluated in **(D)**.

DSA-mediated lung allograft injury. CD16-dependent activation of NK cells in *FCGR3A* [158V/V] individuals that develop acute rejection may nevertheless be mediated by allo- or auto-antibodies that target non-HLA antigens and may not be revealed in the standardized NK-CHAT assay revealing CD16 cellular activation toward B lymphocyte cell targets. Several reports have indeed described ABMR lesions of the graft that occur in the absence of detectable levels of circulating DSA in the serum of kidney or heart transplant recipients. Antibodies directed against endothelial antigens or stress-induced antigens, such as

vimentin, collagen V, Kα1 tubulin, AT1R, and MICA have also been reported in transplant recipients but the role of these non-HLA antibodies in the destruction and accelerated dysfunction of lung allograft remains poorly addressed (60). These reports have nevertheless raised interest in chronic injury resulting from humoral responses targeting non-HLA antigens, as these may be underestimated by the standard monitoring of patients' immunization status which is mainly restricted to the detection of anti-HLA alloantibodies (52). While the rate of acute rejection during the first year was previously identified as a risk factor

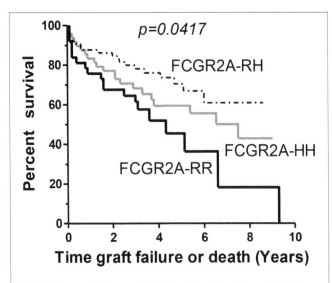

FIGURE 5 | Kaplan-Meir survival analysis of lung allograft survival stratified according to *FCGR2A* [131R/H] genotypes. The *FCGR2A* [131R/R] homozygous genotype (solid black line, *n* = 39) is associated with lower survival rates in LTRs when compared to *FCGR2A* [131H/R] (gray line, *n* = 68) or the *FCGR2A* [131H/H] (dashed line, *n* = 51).

for CLAD occurrence, occurrence of acute rejection in the first trimester could not be associated with an enhanced risk of developing chronic rejection nor with patient or graft survival in the present cohort. The F allelic variant of CD16 with low affinity for the Fc fragment of IgG was associated with the early development during the first month post-LTx of DSA that persist at M3. Persistence of DSA at M3 was thus less frequent in *FCGR3A* [158V/V] LTRs and was shown to be associated with lower survival times in LTR.

Our observations also identify a link between the presence of circulating DSA at M3 and the *FCGR2A* [131R/R] genotype, thus suggesting that FCGR2 polymorphisms may actually be associated with the persistence of harmful DSA at M3 rather than in the development of anti-HLA antibodies *per se*. The *FCGR2A* [131R/R] genotype was reported to be associated with shorter allograft survival in immunized kidney transplant recipients (KTR) (61, 62). We find that, independently of the risk associated with the *FCGR2A* [131R/R] genotype, detection and persistence of DSA at M3 constitute independent predictors of the adverse clinical composite outcome comprising CLAD or the patient's death. The persistence of DSA has been reported as a risk factor linked to BOS and to LTR death (16). A recent report showed that a majority of patients who were positive for *de novo* DSA during the first year after LTx developed BOS and were at higher risk of graft failure or death (63). In line with these reports, our study suggests that, independently of the presence of the susceptible *FCGR2A* [131R/R] genotype, the presence at M1 of DSA with high affinity for donor antigens (MFI DSA M1 > 18,750) can be identified as a risk factor associated with lower survival of LTRs.

The role of the complement-dependent pathogenicity of DSA is less well-documented in the lung transplant setting (19, 20). In a murine model of BOS, complement activation by antibodies to

HLA class I was not required for the development of obliterative airway disease (OAD) that is similar to BOS in human LTx. Interestingly, in this study, at 90 days after LTx, only one out of 5 BOS patients had C1q DSA detected by SAFB whereas 3 out of 11 stable patients had C1q DSA. However, in our study, C1q DSA detected at M1 and M3 were mostly directed against HLA class II antigenic targets (90%) and do not appear as major contributors associated with the development of CLAD.

Although this is a limitation of the study, we cannot exclude the idea that auto-antibodies that target non-HLA antigens which were associated with the development of DSA, such as autoantibodies against K-α1 tubulin (K-α1T) and collagen V (ColV) (64), can participate in the chronic FcR-dependent reaction of recipient cells toward the lung allograft. This is supported by studies that report that development of col (V)-specific TH-17 cells may contribute to the pathogenesis of BOS (25, 59). Indeed, our standardized NK-CHAT evaluation of the DSA induced NK-cell activation was conducted toward B cell lines that express cognate HLA alloantigens. As B cells may not be relevant to evaluate the deleterious impact of non-HLA alloantibodies toward the lung allograft, this is a limit that prompts further studies that uses serum-coated lung epithelial or endothelial cells targets to evaluate NK cell ADCC.

FCGR2A [131R/H] is considered to be a heritable risk factor for a variety of infectious and inflammatory autoimmune diseases, including systemic lupus erythematosus, rheumatoid arthritis, malaria, multiple sclerosis, and anti-neutrophil cytoplasmic auto-antibody positive systemic vasculitis (65). The CD32 membrane receptor is expressed by a variety of immune cells that orchestrate the humoral immune response to pathogens, including B-lymphocytes, natural killer cells, macrophages, mast cells, and neutrophils. Its capacity to recognize IgGs bound to pathogens or infected cells has a protective effect against infections. While the *FCGR2A* allelic isoforms exhibit similar affinity for IgG1, the *FCGR2A* [131H/H] is the only FcγR variant that recognizes IgG2 subclasses, thus suggesting that the capacity to sense IgG2 antibodies may lead to impairment of pathogen surveillance in patients that lack the H allele. This SNP has been shown to play a role in the susceptibility to bacterial infections as *FCGR2A* [131H/H] individuals have greater potential to mediate IgG2-dependent bacterial phagocytosis than patients genotyped as *FCGR2A* [131R/R]. A distinct SNP (rs12746613) within the *FCGR2A* gene was previously associated with a higher risk of respiratory infections and mortality after LTx, but this variant was not associated with the risk of developing CLAD (34). Unlike other studies, our analysis of the present LTR cohort did not reveal any significant association between *FCGR2A* [131R/H] and occurrence of respiratory infections or the number of infection-related deaths. This discrepancy may relate to preventive and curative treatment of bacterial infections that differ between the transplantation centers. It may also reflect a complex interaction of these FCGR genotypes that encourages the overall survival of LTR for patients that have better capacities to thwart infections and overcome early acute rejection events. The observed finding of a inverse link between the *FCGR2A* [131R/R] susceptibility genotype and presence of the FCGR3A-V allele encoding the

TABLE 6 | Univariate analysis and multivariate Cox regression analysis of variables associated with graft loss and patient death post-LTx.

Covariables	Univariate analysis p-value	Hazard ratio	Std. Err.	z	P>z	(95% Conf.interval)		
Death, All causes, n = 64								
FCGR2A [131R/R]	0.114	**1.8**	0.511	1.99	0.047	1.008	–	3.121
Native Lung Disease: Cystic Fibrosis	**0.048**	**0.5**	0.53	−2.25	0.024	0.278	–	0.915
MFI DSA M1 > 18,750 (75 percentile)	0.109	**2.7**	1.123	2.36	0.018	1.184	–	6.093
Graft loss or LTR death, n = 68								
FCGR2A [131R/R]	**0.052**	**1.85**	0.552	1.99	0.047	1.008	–	3.392
MFI DSA M1 > 18,750 (75 percentile)	0.166	**2.8**	1.259	2.29	0.022	1.159	–	6.759
RAS	**0.009**	**2.8**	1.385	2.08	0.037	1.062	–	7.384
Native Lung Disease: Cystic Fibrosis	**0.034**	0.53	0.181	−1.86	0.063	0.272	–	1.034
DSA at M1 persisting at M3	0.153	1.37	0.550	0.78	0.436	0.622	–	3.009
Bilateral Lung Transplant	0.161	0.92	0.319	−0.24	0.814	0.467	–	1.818

Covariables (risk covariables) used to explain the Lung transplant outcome primary variable (Death all cause or Graft loss/death) are listed on the left column. The bold text refers to covariables that retained independent significant p-values in multivariate cox regression models.

CD16 receptor variant with higher affinity for the IgG Fc fragment in LTRs, may in part explain a lack of association of the FcCR3A-VV genotype with DSA- mediated chronic lung allograft dysfunction. In this study, the presence of the FCGR2A [131H/H] was observed to be strongly associated with the presence of the "high IgG1 responder" FCGR3A [158V/V] genotype, and such linkage disequilibrium may in part explain how this intricate distribution of susceptible and protective FCR SNPs may participate in the complex tuning of the host immune response to early infectious and humoral challenges and may be associated with enhanced survival and lower rates of CLAD in patients who have the protective FCGR2A [131H/R or H/H] genotype, notably in female LTRs.

In addition to this protective role against pathogens, the SNP dependent affinity of CD32 for the Fc fragment of IgG and/or CRP ligands was also identified as promoting inflammation. CD32-dependent triggering of immune cells is in part conditioned by the polymorphism and the expression profile of this functional receptor at the surface of immune cells. As is expressed by most leukocytes/macrophages that infiltrate the lung graft, FCGR2A [131R/H] could also influence the acquisition of an inflammatory-activated profile that favors tissue recruitment of activated lymphocytes to the lung (66). Interestingly, the FCGR2A [131R/R] susceptible genotype identified in this study has been associated with higher CRP binding avidity for the CD32 receptor expressed at the surface of monocytes and neutrophils.

Considering the growing evidence of the key role of CRP as an inflammatory mediator involved in the development of atherosclerosis and endothelial dysfunction, it is expected that CRP may be more powerful in triggering the pro-inflammatory function of CD32-expressing cell subsets such as platelets, endothelial cells, monocytes, and leukocytes in FCGR2A [131R/R] LTRs.

In conclusion, these data highlight that FCGR2A and FCGR3A polymorphisms constitute predisposing factors that

are associated with the outcome of lung allografts. This study suggests that the combined assessment of the FCGR genotype and CRP or IgG ligands is thus an intriguing prospect to further decipher the complex mechanisms that shape the alloimmune and inflammatory responses in response to infectious and humoral threats. As shown in other organ transplant settings, our study indicates FCGR genotyping may favor early stratification of patients at risk and may create new perspectives to adapt personalized preventive and therapeutic approaches to prevent adverse outcomes of lung transplants.

ETHICS STATEMENT

All patients from the French cohort (COLT, Cohort in Lung Transplantation, l'Institut du Thorax, INSERM UMR1087/CNRS UMR 6291, CNIL 911142) were recruited in this study and gave their written informed consent to participate to the study in accordance with the Declaration of Helsinki. A group of 184 healthy unrelated of volunteer French bone marrow donors were also recruited to constitute a control cohort allowing analysis of FcγR genotype. Blood donations were collected in the Etablissement Francais du Sang, in accordance with BSL-2 practices. A medical interview was carried out prior to blood donation to exclude donors with medical contraindications. This study was carried out in accordance with the French Public Health Code (art L1221-1), approved by institutional ethics committee and conducted in compliance with the Good Clinical Practice Guidelines, declaration of Helsinki and Istanbul.

AUTHOR CONTRIBUTIONS

CP and PPa designed and coordinated the study, analyzed the data, and wrote the paper. PPe, LL, and JD performed experiments. AL contributed to the methodological and statistical analysis. MP, AB, FD-G, and JC contributed to the research design. PT and MR-G contributed to the collection of patient material and to the clinical aspects of the study.

FUNDING

This work was supported in part by Vaincre la mucoviscidose through TP1008 funding and the *Gregory Lemarchal* association.

REFERENCES

1. Chambers DC, Yusen RD, Cherikh WS, Goldfarb SB, Kucheryavaya AY, Khusch K, et al. The registry of the international society for heart and lung transplantation: thirty-fourth adult lung and heart-lung transplantation report-2017; focus theme: allograft ischemic time. *J Heart Lung Transplant.* (2017) 36:1047–59. doi: 10.1016/j.healun.2017.07.016
2. Thabut G, Mal H. Outcomes after lung transplantation. *J Thorac Dis.* (2017) 9:2684–91. doi: 10.21037/jtd.2017.07.85
3. Brugiere O, Thabut G, Krawice-Radanne I, Rizzo R, Dauriat G, Danel C, et al. Role of HLA-G as a predictive marker of low risk of chronic rejection in lung transplant recipients: a clinical prospective study. *Am J Transplant.* (2015) 15:461–71. doi: 10.1111/ajt.12977
4. Verleden SE, Vos R, Vanaudenaerde BM, Verleden GM. Chronic lung allograft dysfunction phenotypes and treatment. *J Thorac Dis.* (2017) 9:2650–9. doi: 10.21037/jtd.2017.07.81
5. Di Cristofaro J, Pelardy M, Loundou A, Basire A, Gomez C, Chiaroni J, et al. HLA-E()01:03 allele in lung transplant recipients correlates with higher chronic lung allograft dysfunction occurrence. *J Immunol Res.* (2016) 2016:1910852. doi: 10.1155/2016/1910852
6. Di Cristofaro J, Reynaud-Gaubert M, Carlini F, Roubertoux P, Loundou A, Basire A, et al. HLA-G*01:04 approximately UTR3 recipient correlates with lower survival and higher frequency of chronic rejection after lung transplantation. *Am J Transplant.* (2015) 15:2413–20. doi: 10.1111/ajt.13305
7. Gregson AL. Infectious triggers of chronic lung allograft dysfunction. *Curr Infect Dis Rep.* (2016) 18:21. doi: 10.1007/s11908-016-0529-6
8. Ruttens D, Vandermeulen E, Verleden SE, Bellon H, Vos R, Van Raemdonck DE, et al. Role of genetics in lung transplant complications. *Ann Med.* (2015) 47:106–15. doi: 10.3109/07853890.2015.1004359
9. Agbor-Enoh S, Jackson AM, Tunc I, Berry GJ, Cochrane A, Grimm D, et al. Late manifestation of alloantibody-associated injury and clinical pulmonary antibody-mediated rejection: evidence from cell-free DNA analysis. *J Heart Lung Transplant.* (2018) 37:925–32. doi: 10.1016/j.healun.2018.01.1305
10. Levine DJ, Glanville AR, Aboyoun C, Belperio J, Benden C, Berry GJ, et al. Antibody-mediated rejection of the lung: a consensus report of the International Society for Heart and Lung Transplantation. *J Heart Lung Transplant.* (2016) 35:397–406. doi: 10.1016/j.healun.2016.01.1223
11. Chin N, Paraskeva M, Paul E, Cantwell L, Levvey B, Williams T, et al. Comparative analysis of how immune sensitization is defined prior to lung transplantation. *Hum Immunol.* (2015) 76:711–6. doi: 10.1016/j.humimm.2015.09.025
12. Zazueta OE, Preston SE, Moniodis A, Fried S, Kim M, Townsend K, et al. The presence of pretransplant HLA antibodies does not impact the development of chronic lung allograft dysfunction or CLAD-related death. *Transplantation.* (2017) 101:2207–12. doi: 10.1097/TP.0000000000001494
13. Reinsmoen NL, Mirocha J, Ensor CR, Marrari M, Chaux G, Levine DJ, et al. A 3-center study reveals new insights into the impact of non-HLA antibodies on lung transplantation outcome. *Transplantation.* (2017) 101:1215–21. doi: 10.1097/TP.0000000000001389
14. Le Pavec J, Suberbielle C, Lamrani L, Feuillet S, Savale L, Dorfmuller P, et al. *De-novo* donor-specific anti-HLA antibodies 30 days after lung transplantation are associated with a worse outcome. *J Heart Lung Transplant.* (2016) 35:1067–77. doi: 10.1016/j.healun.2016.05.020
15. Lobo LJ, Aris RM, Schmitz J, Neuringer IP. Donor-specific antibodies are associated with antibody-mediated rejection, acute cellular rejection, bronchiolitis obliterans syndrome, and cystic fibrosis after lung transplantation. *J Heart Lung Transplant.* (2013) 32:70–7. doi: 10.1016/j.healun.2012.10.007
16. Roux A, Bendib Le Lan I, Holifanjaniaina S, Thomas KA, Picard C, Grenet D., et al. Characteristics of donor-specific antibodies associated with antibody-mediated rejection in lung transplantation. *Front Med.* (2017) 4:155. doi: 10.3389/fmed.2017.00155
17. Verleden SE, Vanaudenaerde BM, Emonds MP, Van Raemdonck DE, Neyrinck AP, Verleden GM, et al. Donor-specific and -nonspecific HLA antibodies and outcome post lung transplantation. *Eur Respir J.* (2017) 50:1701248. doi: 10.1183/13993003.01248-2017
18. Tikkanen JM, Singer LG, Kim SJ, Li Y, Binnie M, Chaparro C, et al. *De novo* DQ donor-specific antibodies are associated with chronic lung allograft dysfunction after lung transplantation. *Am J Respir Crit Care Med.* (2016) 194:596–606. doi: 10.1164/rccm.201509-1857OC
19. Visentin J, Chartier A, Massara L, Linares G, Guidicelli G, Blanchard E, et al. Lung intragraft donor-specific antibodies as a risk factor for graft loss. *J Heart Lung Transplant.* (2016) 35:1418–26. doi: 10.1016/j.healun.2016.06.010
20. Vandermeulen E, Lammertyn E, Verleden SE, Ruttens D, Bellon H, Ricciardi M, et al. Immunological diversity in phenotypes of chronic lung allograft dysfunction: a comprehensive immunohistochemical analysis. *Transpl Int.* (2017) 30:134–43. doi: 10.1111/tri.12882
21. Kulkarni HS, Bemiss BC, Hachem RR. Antibody-mediated rejection in lung transplantation. *Curr Transplant Rep.* (2015) 2:316–23. doi: 10.1007/s40472-015-0074-5
22. Roden AC, Maleszewski JJ, Yi ES, Jenkins SM, Gandhi MJ, Scott JP, et al. Reproducibility of Complement 4d deposition by immunofluorescence and immunohistochemistry in lung allograft biopsies. *J Heart Lung Transplant.* (2014) 33:1223–32. doi: 10.1016/j.healun.2014.06.006
23. Hachem RR, Kamoun M, Budev MM, Askar M, Ahya VN, Lee JC, et al. Human leukocyte antigens antibodies after lung transplantation: primary results of the HALT study. *Am J Transplant.* (2018) 18:2285–94. doi: 10.1111/ajt.14893
24. Kozlowski T, Weimer ET, Andreoni K, Schmitz J. C1q test for identification of sensitized liver recipients at risk of early acute antibody-mediated rejection. *Ann Transplant.* (2017) 22:518–23. doi: 10.12659/AOT.904867
25. Kauke T, Oberhauser C, Lin V, Coenen M, Fischereder M, Dick A, et al. *De novo* donor-specific anti-HLA antibodies after kidney transplantation are associated with impaired graft outcome independently of their C1q-binding ability. *Transpl Int.* (2017) 30:360–70. doi: 10.1111/tri.12887
26. Wallace WD, Li N, Andersen CB, Arrossi AV, Askar M, Berry GJ, et al. Banff study of pathologic changes in lung allograft biopsy specimens with donor-specific antibodies. *J Heart Lung Transplant.* (2016) 35:40–8. doi: 10.1016/j.healun.2015.08.021
27. Berry GJ, Burke MM, Andersen C, Bruneval P, Fedrigo M, Fishbein MC, et al. The 2013 International Society for Heart and Lung Transplantation Working Formulation for the standardization of nomenclature in the pathologic diagnosis of antibody-mediated rejection in heart transplantation. *J Heart Lung Transplant.* (2013) 32:1147–62. doi: 10.1016/j.healun.2013.08.011
28. Stewart S, Fishbein MC, Snell GI, Berry GJ, Boehler A, Burke MM, et al. Revision of the 1996 working formulation for the standardization of nomenclature in the diagnosis of lung rejection. *J Heart Lung Transplant.* (2007) 26:1229–42. doi: 10.1016/j.healun.2007.10.017
29. Brugiere O, Roux A, Le Pavec J, Sroussi D, Parquin F, Pradere P, et al. Role of C1q-binding anti-HLA antibodies as a predictor of lung allograft outcome. *Eur Respir J.* (2018) 52:1701898. doi: 10.1183/13993003.01898-2017
30. Das LK, Ide K, Tanaka A, Morimoto H, Shimizu S, Tanimine N, et al. Fc-gamma receptor 3A polymorphism predicts the incidence of urinary tract infection in kidney-transplant recipients. *Hum Immunol.* (2017) 78:357–62. doi: 10.1016/j.humimm.2017.03.006
31. Shimizu S, Tanaka Y, Tazawa H, Verma S, Onoe T, Ishiyama K, et al. Fc-gamma receptor polymorphisms predispose patients to infectious complications after liver transplantation. *Am J Transplant.* (2016) 16:625–33. doi: 10.1111/ajt.13492

32. Alsaeed M, Husain S. Infections in heart and lung transplant recipients. *Crit Care Clin.* (2019) 35:75–93. doi: 10.1016/j.ccc.2018.08.010

33. Nosotti M, Tarsia P, Morlacchi LC. Infections after lung transplantation. *J Thorac Dis.* (2018) 10:3849–68. doi: 10.21037/jtd.2018.05.204

34. Sarmiento E, Cifrian J, Calahorra L, Bravo C, Lopez S, Laporta R, et al. Monitoring of early humoral immunity to identify lung recipients at risk for development of serious infections: a multicenter prospective study. *J Heart Lung Transplant.* (2018) 37:1001–12. doi: 10.1016/j.healun.2018.04.001

35. Castro-Dopico T, Clatworthy MR. Fcgamma receptors in solid organ transplantation. *Curr Transplant Rep.* (2016) 3:284–93. doi: 10.1007/s40472-016-0116-7

36. Ivan E, Colovai AI. Human Fc receptors: critical targets in the treatment of autoimmune diseases and transplant rejections. *Hum Immunol.* (2006) 67:479–91. doi: 10.1016/j.humimm.2005.12.001

37. Meletiadis J, Walsh TJ, Choi EH, Pappas PG, Ennis D, Douglas J, et al. Study of common functional genetic polymorphisms of FCGR2A, 3A and 3B genes and the risk for cryptococcosis in HIV-uninfected patients. *Med Mycol.* (2007) 45:513–8. doi: 10.1080/13693780701390140

38. Ruttens D, Verleden SE, Goeminne PC, Vandermeulen E, Wauters E, Cox B, et al. Genetic variation in immunoglobulin G receptor affects survival after lung transplantation. *Am J Transplant.* (2014) 14:1672–7. doi: 10.1111/ajt.12745

39. De Rose V, Arduino C, Cappello N, Piana R, Salmin P, Bardessono M, et al. Fcgamma receptor IIA genotype and susceptibility to *P. aeruginosa* infection in patients with cystic fibrosis. *Eur J Hum Genet.* (2005) 13:96–101. doi: 10.1038/sj.ejhg.5201285

40. Bougle A, Max A, Mongardon N, Grimaldi D, Pene F, Rousseau C, et al. Protective effects of FCGR2A polymorphism in invasive pneumococcal diseases. *Chest.* (2012) 142:1474–81. doi: 10.1378/chest.11-2516

41. Halloran PF, Venner JM, Madill-Thomsen KS, Einecke G, Parkes MD, Hidalgo LG, et al. Review: the transcripts associated with organ allograft rejection. *Am J Transplant.* (2018) 18:785–95. doi: 10.1111/ajt.14600

42. Loupy AJ, Duong Van Huyen P, Hidalgo L, Reeve J, Racape M, Aubert O, et al. Gene expression profiling for the identification and classification of antibody-mediated heart rejection. *Circulation.* (2017) 135:917–35. doi: 10.1161/CIRCULATIONAHA.116.022907

43. Roux A, Levine DJ, Zeevi A, Hachem R, Halloran K, Halloran PF, et al. Banff lung report: current knowledge and future research perspectives for diagnosis and treatment of pulmonary antibody-mediated rejection (AMR). *Am J Transplant.* (2018) 19:21–31. doi: 10.1111/ajt.14990

44. Dai HS, Griffin N, Bolyard C, Mao HC, Zhang J, Cripe TP, et al. The Fc domain of immunoglobulin is sufficient to bridge NK cells with virally infected cells. *Immunity.* (2017) 47, 159–170.e10. doi: 10.1016/j.immuni.2017.06.019

45. Hatjiharissi E, Xu L, Santos DD, Hunter ZR, Ciccarelli BT, Verselis S, et al. Increased natural killer cell expression of CD16, augmented binding and ADCC activity to rituximab among individuals expressing the Fc{gamma}RIIIa-158 V/V and V/F polymorphism. *Blood.* (2007) 110:2561–4. doi: 10.1182/blood-2007-01-070656

46. Hussain K, Hargreaves CE, Rowley TF, Sopp JM, Latham KV, Bhatta P, et al. Impact of human FcgammaR gene polymorphisms on IgG-triggered cytokine release: Critical importance of cell assay. *Format Front Immunol.* (2019) 10:390. doi: 10.3389/fimmu.2019.00390

47. Perez-Romero CA, Sanchez IP, Naranjo-Piedrahita L, Orrego-Arango JC, Muskus-Lopez CE, Rojas-Montoya W, et al. Frequency analysis of the g.7081T>G/A and g.10872T>G polymorphisms in the FCGR3A gene (CD16A) using nested PCR and their functional specific effects. *Genes Immun.* (2019) 20:39–45. doi: 10.1038/s41435-017-0001-0

48. Paul P, Picard C, Sampol E, Lyonnet L, Di Cristofaro J, Paul-Delvaux L, et al. Genetic and functional profiling of CD16-dependent natural killer activation identifies patients at higher risk of cardiac allograft vasculopathy. *Circulation.* (2018) 137:1049–59. doi: 10.1161/CIRCULATIONAHA.117.030435

49. Arnold ML, Kainz A, Hidalgo LG, Eskandary F, Kozakowski N, Wahrmann M, et al. Functional Fc gamma receptor gene polymorphisms and donor-specific antibody-triggered microcirculation inflammation. *Am J Transplant.* (2018) 18:2261–73. doi: 10.1111/ajt.14710

50. Legris T, Picard C, Todorova D, Lyonnet L, Laporte C, Dumoulin C, et al. Antibody-dependent NK cell activation is associated with late kidney allograft dysfunction and the complement-independent alloreactive potential of donor-specific antibodies. *Front Immunol.* (2016) 7:288. doi: 10.3389/fimmu.2016.00288

51. Sablik KA, Litjens NHR, Klepper M, Betjes MGH. Increased CD16 expression on NK cells is indicative of antibody-dependent cell-mediated cytotoxicity in chronic-active antibody-mediated rejection. *Transpl Immunol.* (2019) 54:52–8. doi: 10.1016/j.trim.2019.02.005

52. Delville M, Charreau B, Rabant M, Legendre C, Anglicheau D. Pathogenesis of non-HLA antibodies in solid organ transplantation: where do we stand? *Hum Immunol.* (2016) 77:1055–62. doi: 10.1016/j.humimm.2016.05.021

53. Venner JM, Hidalgo LG, Famulski KS, Chang J, Halloran PF. The molecular landscape of antibody-mediated kidney transplant rejection: evidence for NK involvement through CD16a Fc receptors. *Am J Transplant.* (2015) 15:1336–48. doi: 10.1111/ajt.13115

54. Yazdani S, Callemeyn J, Gazut S, Lerut E, de Loor H, Wevers M, et al. Natural killer cell infiltration is discriminative for antibody-mediated rejection and predicts outcome after kidney transplantation. *Kidney Int.* (2018) 95:188–98. doi: 10.1016/j.kint.2018.08.027

55. Verleden GM, Raghu G, Meyer KC, Glanville AR, Corris P. A new classification system for chronic lung allograft dysfunction. *J Heart Lung Transplant.* (2014) 33:127–33. doi: 10.1016/j.healun.2013.10.022

56. Kapila A, Baz MA, Valentine VG, Bhorade SM. Reliability of diagnostic criteria for bronchiolitis obliterans syndrome after lung transplantation: a survey. *J Heart Lung Transplant.* (2015) 34:65–74. doi: 10.1016/j.healun.2014.09.029

57. Pedron BV, Guerin-El Khourouj V, Dalle JH, Ouachee-Chardin M, Yakouben K, Corroyez F, et al. Contribution of HLA-A/B/C/DRB1/DQB1 common haplotypes to donor search outcome in unrelated hematopoietic stem cell transplantation. *Biol Blood Marrow Transplant.* (2011) 17:1612–8. doi: 10.1016/j.bbmt.2011.03.009

58. Di Cristofaro J, Buhler S, Frassati C, Basire A, Galicher V, Baier C, et al. Linkage disequilibrium between HLA-G*0104 and HLA-E*0103 alleles in Tswa Pygmies. *Tissue Antigens.* (2011) 77:193–200. doi: 10.1111/j.1399-0039.2010.01599.x

59. Clerc A, Reynaud Q, Durupt S, Chapuis-Cellier C, Nove-Josserand R, Durieu I, et al. Elevated IgG4 serum levels in patients with cystic fibrosis. *PLoS ONE.* (2017) 12:e0181888. doi: 10.1371/journal.pone.0181888

60. Yousem SA, Zeevi A. The histopathology of lung allograft dysfunction associated with the development of donor-specific HLA antibodies. *Am J Surg Pathol.* (2012) 36:987–92. doi: 10.1097/PAS.0b013e31825197ae

61. Yuan FF, Watson N, Sullivan JS, Biffin S, Moses J, Geczy AF, et al. Association of Fc gamma receptor IIA polymorphisms with acute renal-allograft rejection. *Transplantation.* (2004) 78:766–9. doi: 10.1097/01.TP.0000132560.77496.CB

62. Arnold ML, Fuernrohr BG, Weiss KM, Harre U, Wiesener MS, Spriewald BM. Association of a coding polymorphism in Fc gamma receptor 2A and graft survival in re-transplant candidates. *Hum Immunol.* (2015) 76:759–64. doi: 10.1016/j.humimm.2015.09.034

63. Kauke T, Kneidinger N, Martin B, Dick A, Schneider C, Schramm R, et al. Bronchiolitis obliterans syndrome due to donor-specific HLA-antibodies. *Tissue Antigens.* (2015) 86:178–85. doi: 10.1111/tan.12626

64. Saini D, Weber J, Ramachandran S, Phelan D, Tiriveedhi V, Liu M, et al. Alloimmunity-induced autoimmunity as a potential mechanism in the pathogenesis of chronic rejection of human lung allografts. *J Heart Lung Transplant.* (2011) 30:624–31. doi: 10.1016/j.healun.2011.01.708

65. Zhang C, Wang W, Zhang H, Wei L, Guo S. Association of FCGR2A rs1801274 polymorphism with susceptibility to autoimmune diseases: a meta-analysis. *Oncotarget.* (2016) 7:39436–43. doi: 10.18632/oncotarget.9831

66. Fildes JE, Yonan N, Tunstall K, Walker AH, Griffiths-Davies L, Bishop P, et al. Natural killer cells in peripheral blood and lung tissue are associated with chronic rejection after lung transplantation. *J Heart Lung Transplant.* (2008) 27:203–7. doi: 10.1016/j.healun.2007.11.571

4

Understanding Fc Receptor Involvement in Inflammatory Diseases: From Mechanisms to New Therapeutic Tools

Sanae Ben Mkaddem [1,2,3,4], *Marc Benhamou* [1,2,3,4] *and Renato C. Monteiro* [1,2,3,4,5*]

[1] INSERM U1149, Centre de Recherche sur l'Inflammation, Paris, France, [2] CNRS ERL8252, Paris, France, [3] Faculté de Médecine, Université Paris Diderot, Sorbonne Paris Cité, Site Xavier Bichat, Paris, France, [4] Inflamex Laboratory of Excellence, Paris, France, [5] Service d'Immunologie, DHU Fire, Hôpital Bichat-Claude Bernard, Assistance Publique de Paris, Paris, France

Correspondence:
Renato C. Monteiro
renato.monteiro@inserm.fr

Fc receptors (FcRs) belong to the ITAM-associated receptor family. FcRs control the humoral and innate immunity which are essential for appropriate responses to infections and prevention of chronic inflammation or auto-immune diseases. Following their crosslinking by immune complexes, FcRs play various roles such as modulation of the immune response by released cytokines or of phagocytosis. Here, we review FcR involvement in pathologies leading notably to altered intracellular signaling with functionally relevant consequences to the host, and targeting of Fc receptors as therapeutic approaches. Special emphasis will be given to some FcRs, such as the FcαRI, the FcγRIIA and the FcγRIIIA, which behave like the ancient god Janus depending on the ITAM motif to inhibit or activate immune responses depending on their targeting by monomeric/dimeric immunoglobulins or by immune complexes. This ITAM duality has been recently defined as inhibitory or activating ITAM (ITAMi or ITAMa) which are controlled by Src family kinases. Involvement of various ITAM-bearing FcRs observed during infectious or autoimmune diseases is associated with allelic variants, changes in ligand binding ability responsible for host defense perturbation. During auto-immune diseases such as rheumatoid arthritis, lupus or immune thrombocytopenia, the autoantibodies and immune complexes lead to inflammation through FcR aggregation. We will discuss the role of FcRs in autoimmune diseases, and focus on novel approaches to target FcRs for resolution of antibody-mediated autoimmunity. We will finally also discuss the down-regulation of FcR functionality as a therapeutic approach for autoimmune diseases.

Keywords: immunoglobilins, Fc receptor, antibody treatment, signaling/signaling pathways, inflammatory diseases

FC RECEPTOR MODES OF ACTION

Immunoglobulin Fc receptors (FcRs) are membrane molecules expressed by several hematopoietic cells that recognize the Fc region of several immunoglobulin (Ig) classes and subclasses. We distinguish FcR for IgG (FcγRI/CD64, FcγRII/CD32, and FcγRIII/CD16), IgE (FcεRI), IgA (FcαRI/CD89), IgM (FcμR), and IgA/IgM (Fcα/μR). Several other receptors expressed on different cell types also bind Ig molecules: neonatal FcR for IgG (FcRn) on intestinal epithelium, placenta, and endothelium, low affinity FcεR (FcεRII/CD23) on B cells and macrophages, and polymeric Ig receptor (pIgR) on mucosal epithelium (1–3).

The function of antibodies depends on one hand on their ability to recognize antigenic epitopes and, on the other hand, on their dynamic flexibility and their capacity to interact with their cognate FcRs. Engagement of FcRs expressed by leukocytes initiates a number of pro-inflammatory, anti-inflammatory, and immune modulatory functions in the host adaptive immune responses leading to protection but sometimes also to disease.

Several FcRs require the Immunoreceptor Tyrosine-based Activation Motif (ITAM; with the sequence Yxx[L/I]x$_{(6-8)}$Yxx[L/I]) present in the cytoplasmic tail of the receptor or of associated subunits (FcRγ or FcεRIβ chain) to induce cell signaling. ITAM-mediated functions include phagocytosis, degranulation, antibody-dependent cellular cytotoxicity (ADCC), cytokine, lipid mediator and superoxide production, all of which depend on the cell type and on outside-in signals induced by the ligand. Engagement of the type I FcRs by immune complexes, induces receptor aggregation followed by activation and recruitment of Src family kinases (SFKs), such as Lyn and Fyn (4). The former induces the phosphorylation of the conserved tyrosines in the ITAM motif, followed by activation and recruitment of the tyrosine kinase Syk. This process activates various proteins involved in cell response, such as Phospholipase C gamma 1 (PLCγ), Bruton's tyrosine kinase (Btk), guanine nucleotide exchange factor Vav and phosphoinositide 3-kinase (PI3K). Hydrolysis of phosphatidylinositol 4,5-bisphosphate (PtdIns(4,5) P$_2$) by PLCγ generates inositol 1,4,5-trisphosphate (IP$_3$) and diacylglycerol (DAG) leading to calcium mobilization and protein kinase C (PKC) activation, respectively. Calcium influx and PKC activation promote cell responses such as degranulation and cytokine production. Vav plays also an important role in actin cytoskeleton remodeling to control phagocytosis and superoxide production by NADPH oxidase. PI3K catalyzes the phosphorylation of PtdIns(4,5)P$_2$ into PtdIns(3,4,5)P$_3$ in the plasma membrane. Pleckstrin homology domains contained in proteins such as PLCγ, GRB2-associated-binding protein 2 (Gab2), protein kinase B (PKB/Akt) and Btk, bind PtdIns(3,4,5)P$_3$ thus recruiting them at the inner leaflet of the plasma membrane promoting their phosphorylation and activation (**Figure 1,** left).

The activation of ITAM-bearing immune receptors can be retro-controlled by ITIM-bearing inhibitory FcRs such as the FcγRIIB. The ITIM motif is defined by a single [I/V/L/S]xYxx[L/V] sequence. However, inhibition of cell activation by this motif requires co-ligation between the inhibitory and heterologous activating receptors by immune complexes promoting the recruitment of inositol phosphatases (SHIP-1 and SHIP-2) (6) (**Figure 1,** Middle). Another inhibitory mechanism has been recently identified that involves ITAM itself. Indeed, following low avidity ligand interactions, ITAM-bearing FcRs induce a sustained inhibitory signal without co-ligation with heterologous receptors. This mechanism was involved in the maintenance of immune homeostasis (7–14). We named this ITAM-mediated inhibitory signal, ITAMi. It has been shown

that several low affinity receptors, such as FcαRI, FcγRIIA and FcγRIIIA, can function as such bi-functional receptors to induce either activating or inhibitory signals, a property that can be exploited to reduce the susceptibility to autoimmune and inflammatory diseases (11). Monovalent or divalent targeting of FcRs bearing an ITAM motif induced ITAMi signals that involved activation and recruitment of the Src homology region 2 domain-containing tyrosine phosphatase SHP-1 (**Figure 1,** Right). It has been demonstrated that other immunoreceptors such as the antigen receptors BCR and TCR can also associate with SHP-1 upon interaction with low avidity ligands (15, 16). Moreover, SHP-1 deficiency in hematopoietic cells favors development of various auto-immunes diseases. For example, the motheaten mice (mev/mev) which express approximately 20% wild type activity of SHP-1, develop severe immune dysregulation and autoantibody production (17).

During ITAMi signaling induced by FcRs, Lyn is essential for the phosphorylation (on tyrosine residue 536) and the activation of SHP-1 (4). It has been reported that Lyn is involved in positive and negative signals induced by antigen receptors (18, 19). Lyn plays an important role in the negative selection of B cells in the bone marrow, since the absence of Lyn was associated with a decreased B cell number in the periphery of mice. In the absence of Lyn, other SFKs, such as Fyn, act as positive regulators of BCR signaling, suggesting a loss of anergy. The opposite roles of Lyn and Fyn were recently demonstrated by *in vivo* approaches. Lyn deficiency aggravates auto/inflammatory diseases such as nephritis and arthritis, while the absence of Fyn protects against these diseases (4). Additionally, we showed that activation of leukocytes in lupus nephritis patients was associated with Fyn-activated signature, suggesting that the balance between Lyn and Fyn is dysregulated during diseases.

Another FcR that play an essential role in the transcytosis by epithelial cells of dimeric IgA, but also pentameric IgM (notably during IgA deficiencies), is called the polymeric immunoglobulin receptor (pIgR). The pIgR is internalized with its ligands by endocytosis and transcytosed from the basolateral membrane into apical side of the epithelial cell (20). The central role of this receptor is to generate secretory IgA (formed of IgA dimers linked to the extracellular domain of the pIgR, also known as secretory component) in exocrine secretions to establish host-microbiota symbiosis and to mediate the protection of mucosal surfaces against pathogens (20, 21). The Fcα/μR, the Fc receptor for IgA and IgM, may play a role in systemic and mucosal immunity. It has been shown that none of the B cells, T cells, monocyte/macrophages, or NK cells in human blood samples expressed this receptor irrespective of age, ethnic origin or gender. Its expression is restricted to B cells from germinal center, follicular dendritic cells and tonsillar cells. Although, the exact function of the Fcα/μR is not fully clarified, it may play an important role in antigen presentation and B cell selection in the germinal center responses (22).

FcRs are divided into type I and type II on the basis of the conformational state of the Ig Fc domain that interacts with the receptor (1, 23). Type I Fc receptors interact with "open," but not "closed" Ig Fc conformation (**Figure 2**). These receptors include

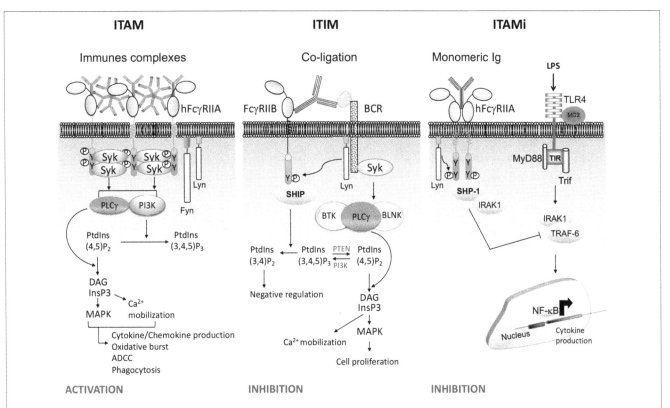

FIGURE 1 | FcR signaling (e.g., FcγRII). **(Left)**, the aggregation by an immune complex of FcR bearing ITAM motif (e.g. FcγRIIA) induces phosphorylation of the two ITAM tyrosine residues by Src kinases Lyn and Fyn responsible for recruitment and phosphorylation of Syk inducing cellular activation through PLCγ and PI3K signaling pathways. The PLCγ converts PI(4,5)P_2 into IP_3 and DAG. IP_3, a soluble inositol phosphate, leads to Ca^{2+} mobilization while DAG activate MAPK.PI3K converts PI(4,5)P_2 to PI(3,4,5)P_3 allowing recruitment of signal intermediates through their pleckstrin homology (PH) domain **(Middle)**, co-ligation between an activating heterologous receptor (e.g., the BCR) and the inhibitory FcR (i.e., FcγRIIB) induces phosphorylation of the tyrosine present within the ITIM motif by Lyn (5), leading to the phosphorylation and recruitment of phosphatases (SHIP or SHP). The phosphatases PTEN and SHIP1/2 regulate cellular levels of PI(3,4,5)P_3 by hydrolyzing it to PI(4,5)P_2 and PI(3,4)P_2, respectively. These dephosphorylations inhibit cell proliferation. **(Right)**, monovalent targeting of FcR bearing ITAM motif (e.g., FcγRIIA) induces the phosphorylation of the last tyrosine residue of the ITAM motif by Lyn responsible for transient recruitment of Syk followed by that of SHP-1 which abrogates the activation signal.

FcγRI, FcγRII, FcγRIII, FcεRI, FcαRI, FcμR, and Fcα/μR (25–29). In contrast, type II FcRs, bind preferentially Ig Fc domains in "closed" conformation. Among these are C-type lectin receptors such as FcεRII (CD23) and DC-SIGN (**Figure 3**).

For type II Fc receptors, glycosylation of the Fc domain induces a conformational change that occludes the binding site for type I Fc receptors that lies near the hinge region (open conformation) and reveals a binding site at the CH2-CH3 domain interface (closed conformation). These receptors bind antibodies in a two receptors-to-one antibody stoichiometry that may influence signal initiation (1). DC-SIGN and SIGN-R1, for example, bind secretory IgA and play an intriguing role in dendritic cells inducing IL10 and Treg-mediated tolerance (30). Signaling through these receptors, however, is not yet documented as compared to type I FcRs, with the exception of CD23. Crosslinking of CD23 on B cells activates cAMP (31) and intracellular calcium flux (32) which is associated with the activation of the SFK Fyn and of the PI3K pathway (33). These findings are in agreement with our recent data on type I FcRs (4), and indicates that Fyn also plays an activating role in B cells through type II Fc receptors.

FC RECEPTORS AND DISEASES

Gene Alleles

Several single-nucleotide polymorphisms (SNPs) have been reported in the genes encoding activating FcγRs (FcγRIIA, FcγRIIIA, and FcγRIIIB). In the gene encoding the inhibitory FcγRIIB, a SNP has been described which is associated with autoimmune diseases such as SLE and rheumatoid arthritis (RA) (34, 35). In addition to SNPs, copy-number variations (CNVs) of FcγR genes are associated with susceptibility to autoimmune disorders (34–40). Most polymorphisms concern the extracellular domains which bind to IgG, affecting the affinity between these receptors and IgG subclasses. However, no polymorphism and CNV have been clearly identified for FcγRI.

The most studied polymorphism is the one in the second Ig-like extracellular domain of the FcγRIIA that results in a point mutation of amino acid at position 131, coding for either arginine (R131) or histidine (H131). FcγRIIA-R131 binds less efficiently IgG2 than FcγRIIA-H131 (34). This *Fcgr2a* polymorphism has been described as a heritable risk factor for autoimmune and infectious diseases (41, 42). Moreover, genome-wide

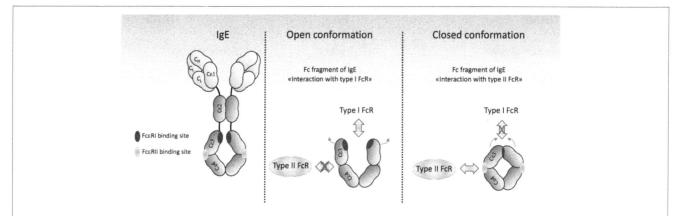

FIGURE 2 | Organization and conformational rearrangements of the IgE Fc. **(left)**, IgE and the binding sites to FcεRI (green) and to CD23 (pink) [adapted from Pennington et al. (24)] **(Middle** and **Right)**. Representation of the open and closed conformations, respectively, of the IgE Fc Cε3–4 domains, and the mutual allosteric inhibition by FcεRIα (green) and CD23 (pink).

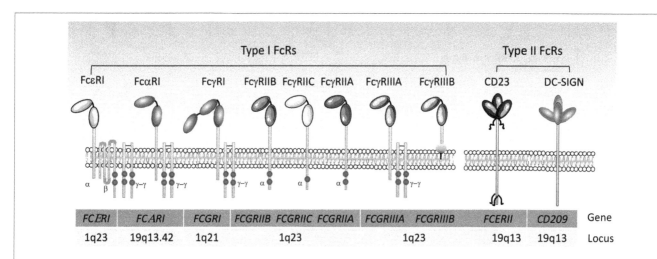

FIGURE 3 | Human type I and II Fc receptors. Schematic representation of human Fc receptors at the cell membrane and their association or not with the FcRγ-chain dimer and the FcεRIβ chain, red circles represent the tyrosine residues. The FcγRIIIB is anchored into the outer leaflet of the plasma membrane by a phosphatidylinositol-glycan (green circle).

association studies (GWAS) revealed that FcγRIIA-H131 variant is associated with higher susceptibilities to develop Kawasaki disease and ulcerative colitis (43, 44). This variant is also associated with Guillain–Barré syndrome (45), supporting that immune complexes that include IgG2 auto-antibodies are involved in inflammatory responses. In contrast, the genotype homozygous for the FcγRIIA-R131 variant-encoding gene is associated with SLE, immune thrombocytopenic purpura (ITP) and IgA nephropathy (IgAN), revealing a complex and contrasted picture for the role of IgG2-containing immune complexes in autoimmune diseases (46–48). Regarding infectious diseases, neutrophils homozygous for the gene encoding the H131 variant show a higher capacity for IgG2-mediated phagocytosis than those homozygous for the gene encoding the R131 variant (41). In agreement, patients with the R encoding allele were found to have more severe cases of Severe Acute Respiratory Syndrome infection and were more susceptible to

encapsulated microorganism infection, which was attributed to poor IgG2 binding to the R131 variant of FcγRIIA (41, 42). As mice do not express FcγRIIA homologs, transgenic mice expressing the *Fcgr2a* human gene encoding the R131 variant develop spontaneously autoimmune diseases such as pneumonitis, glomerulonephritis and RA (49, 50). Moreover, the fact that FcγRIIA-R131 expressed on the FcRγ-/- background in mice similarly develop thrombocytopenia (51) and arthritis (11, 52) indicates that pro-autoimmune signals through FcγRIIA-R131 ITAM were sufficient to induce diseases. Biochemical analyses showed that two tyrosines of FcγRIIA ITAM motif were needed to induce inflammatory signals (53). Taken together, these animal models underline the critical involvement of *Fcgr2a* polymorphism in a number of diseases.

A polymorphism has been found in the inhibitory FcγRIIB-encoding gene that leads to a single I-to-T amino acid substitution in the transmembrane domain (residue 232)

(43, 54). Human monocytes expressing the FcγRIIB-T232 failed to inhibit heterologous receptors-mediated cell activation (55). The FcγRIIB-T232 polymorphism is associated with susceptibility to develop auto-immune diseases such as SLE (42, 54, 56). However, there are some discordances concerning the SNPs in the promoter region of *Fcgr2b*, such as −386G and −120T (haplotype 2B.2), and −386C and −120A (haplotype 2B.4) variants. It has been shown that the 2B.4 SNP promoter haplotype upregulates the expression of FcγRIIB on neutrophils and monocytes that negatively correlates with lupus nephritis (46). This is in agreement with previous reports in mouse SLE-like models and suggests that FcγRIIB expression is protective in SLE (57). However, in striking contrast and in an apparent paradox, the same 2B.4 promoter haplotype was found by the same authors to correlate with SLE (46). This positive (SLE) vs. negative (lupus nephritis) paradoxical association of the 2B.4 promoter haplotype suggests multifaceted impacts of FcγRIIB in SLE that may depend on the affected cell types (e.g., monocytes vs. neutrophils). Alternatively, particular cell types expressing FcγRIIB could have aggravating or protective actions in SLE depending on which affected tissue these cells are recruited to, or on how these cells impact the systemic vs. local aspect of the disease. Thus, further investigation is necessary to elucidate the association of the promoter haplotype in disease development.

The *Fcgr3a* polymorphism is characterized by a point mutation in the codon for residue 158, encoding valine (V158) or phenylalanine (F158) in the Ig-like domain near the membrane (34–36). The FcγRIIIA-V158 variant has a higher affinity for all human IgGs than the FcγRIIIA-F158 variant (40). The FcγRIIIA-F158 is associated with susceptibility to SLE, Crohn's disease and Behçet's disease (35, 36). Although studies have also explored the association between RA and the V or F 158 variant, their results have been contradictory and this question remains unsettled (58, 59).

Several *Fcar1* polymorphisms have been found, including two in the functional promoter region of the FcαRI encoding gene (−114T/C and +56T/C relative to the major transcription start site) (60). The incidence of the −114C/C polymorphism in patients with IgAN was significantly increased compared with other chronic kidney diseases (CKD) and healthy donors (HD) (15.6 vs. 4.0% in other CKD and vs. 2.4% in HD). This *Fcar1* polymorphism in the promoter region appears to be associated with susceptibility to IgAN, suggesting the importance of FcαRI expression in this disease. A third *Fcar1* polymorphism has been described in the coding region for FcαRI, which changes codon 248 from AGC to GGC leading to G248 instead of S248 in the cytoplasmic domain of the receptor (61). Interestingly, these two different alleles demonstrate significantly different FcαRI-mediated intracellular activating signaling. The proinflammatory FcαRI-G248 variant has been associated with SLE in two ethnic groups (61). However, this *Fcar1* polymorphism was not associated with other auto-immune diseases such as systemic sclerosis, RA or IgAN (62, 63). A fourth *Fcar1* polymorphism (A/G at nt 324) was also associated with aggressive periodontitis (64). Patients displaying the nt 324 A/A allele presented polymorphonuclear neutrophil dysfunctions with a decreased phagocytosis of periodontopathic

bacteria (Porphyromonas gingivalis) as compared to patients expressing the nt 324 G/G (64).

Regarding the pIgR, it has been reported as a susceptibility gene for nasopharyngeal cancer (NPC) associated with Epstein-Barr virus (EBV) (65). This lead to a hypothesis that pIgR could be the nasopharyngeal epithelial receptor for EBV via IgA-EBV complex. Transcytosis failure due to missense C → T mutation on the *PIGR*1739 nucleotide (resulting in an A-to-V mutation near the endoproteolytic cleavage site of pIgR) could decrease the ability of pIgR to release IgA-EBV complexes, thus increasing susceptibility to develop NPC (65).

The high-affinity FcεRI is expressed by mast cells and basophils and plays an important role in allergic diseases. Several studies have identified two FcεRI polymorphisms associated with allergies. The −66T > C and/or the −315C > T are associated with atopic dermatitis, chronic urticaria, asthma, and high serum IgE levels (66–69). These polymorphisms were also associated with allergic inflammatory diseases such as atopy and nasal allergy (70, 71).

Table 1 summarizes most of described FcR alleles and their expression and functions in physiology and pathology (42–44, 46, 48, 60, 65, 66, 69, 72–83).

Alterations in FcR Expression

Several studies highlighted altered expression, structure and function of FcγRs in patients. Whereas, CD4$^+$ T cells from healthy donors fail to express significant levels of FcγR, FcγRIIA is expressed in a subpopulation of CD4$^+$ T cells in blood samples from HIV-1-positive patients and is highly enriched in inducible replication-competent proviruses suggestive of an FcγRIIA$^+$ HIV reservoir (84). Yet, in other studies, FcγRIIA expression did not selectively enrich for HIV- or SIV-infected CD4$^+$ T cells in peripheral blood or lymphoid tissue since resting FcγRIIA$^+$ CD4$^+$ T cells have <3% of the total HIV DNA amongst CD4$^+$ T cells (85, 86). Taken together, whereas FcγRIIA expression in CD4$^+$ T cells becomes a marker for HIV infection, the involvement of FcγRIIA$^+$ CD4$^+$ T cells in AIDS remains to be elucidated.

The inhibitory FcγRIIB, in contrast, is down-regulated in autoimmune diseases notably on both memory and plasma B lymphocytes of active SLE patients compared to those from healthy individuals (87). However, this down-regulation was not seen on myeloid-lineage cells. This was also observed in Hashimoto's thyroiditis (88).

High level of FcγRIIIA expression on monocytes together with that of CD14 is associated with proinflammatory cytokine profiles and higher potency in antigen presentation allowing to define monocyte subsets with distinct phenotypes and functions (89).

For FcαRI, its expression is dysregulated in patients with AIDS, ankylosing spondylitis, alcoholic liver cirrhosis, Henoch-Schonlein purpura (HSP) and IgAN (90–93). Some of these studies have shown biochemical abnormalities revealing FcαRI altered protein mobility in SDS-PAGE suggesting altered glycosylation of this receptor (90). Interestingly, mutational studies of FcαRI indicate that the N58 residue of the receptor controls IgA-binding enhancement (94). In parallel,

TABLE 1 | Human FcRs: their expression, function and allotypes.

Name	Subclass binding	Expression	Functions	Alleles	Link to diseases
FcγRI (CD64)	IgG 1/3/4	Monocytes/Macrophages Neutrophils/DCs/Mast cells	Activation	–	–
FcγRIIA (CD32a)	H_{131}:IgG 1/2/3/4 R_{131}:IgG I/(2) /3/4	Monocytes/Macrophages Neutrophils/DCs/Basophils/Mast eells/Eosinophils	Activation/inhibition	H131/R131	Kawasaki diseases (43), Ulcerative colitis (44). Childhood-onset ITP (71)/Lupus (46), IgAN (48), arthritis
FcγRIIB (CD32b)	IgG I/(2)/3/4	B cells/DCs/Mast cells/Basophils	Inhibition	Promoter−3S6C or −120/T232	Lupus (46)/lupus (42), Atopy (72)
FcγRIIC (CD32c)	IgG 1/(2)/3/4	NK cells/ Monocytes/Macrophages /Neutrophils	Activation	Q13/stopl3	Kawasaki disease (73)
FcγRIIIA (CD16)	V_{158}: IgG I(2)/3/4 F_{I58}: IgG I/(2)/3/4	NK cells/ Monocytes/Macrophages	Activation/Inhibition	V15S/F158	IgAN (48), arthritis seventy (74), childhood chronic ITP (75)/Lupus (76), arthritis (58), Crohn's disease (77)
FcγRIIIB (CD16b)	IgG 1/3/4?	Neutrophils/ Eosinophils/ Basophils	Activation		Wegener's granulomatosis (78)
FcαRI (CD89)	IgAl, IgA2, CRP	Monocytes/Macrophages Neutrophils/DCs/Kupffer cells (79)	Activation/Inhibition	114T/C	IgA nephropathy (60), AIDS, ankylosing spondylitis, alcoholic liver cirrhosis, Henoth-Schonlem purpura (HSP) (26)
FcμR	IgM	B and T lymphocytes	Inhibition/?		Chronic Lymphocytic Leukemia (CLL) (80, 81)
Fcα/μR	IgM and IgA	Germinal center B cell, Follicular dendritic cells	?		
FcεRI	IgE	Mast cells/Basophils	Activation	66T/31SC	Atopic dermatitis.ɪ asthma and chronic urticaria (66–71)
FcεRII (CD23)	IgE	B cells and macrophages	Activation	–	AIDS and B-CLL (82)
FcRn	IgG 1/2/3/4	Monocytes/Macrophages Neutrophils/DCs/endothelium/ Syncytiotrophoblasts	Recycling Transport uptake	VNTR1–5	
PlgR	plgA	Mucosal epithelium	Transcytosis	1739C to T	Nasopharyngeal cancer and infection (65)

From left to right columns: names, function, alleles that include amino acid variations in immunoglobulin domains and the transmembrane domain, cellular expression of FcRs, and diseases linked to alleles and CNVs (reference numbers are shown), and binding abilities of IgG subclasses to each FcR allele. IgAN, IgA nephropathy; CLL, chronic lymphocytic Leukemia; FcRn, neonatal Fc receptor; AIDS, acquired immune deficiency syndrome; PlgR, Polymeric immunoglobulin receptor; DCs, dendritic cells.

abnormally glycosylated IgA1 molecules (hypogalactosylation and hyposialylation on the hinge region) observed in patients with IgAN and HSP is associated with the shedding of a soluble form of FcαRI (sFcαRI), which participates in the formation of circulating IgA1 complexes (95). These IgA1-sFcαRI complexes were decreased in serum of IgAN patients with severe and progressive disease as compared to non-progressive IgAN patients (96) suggesting a kidney deposition, and hence a possible nephrotoxic action, of such complexes which is further supported by studies in IgAN patients with recurrence of the disease after kidney transplantation (97). In this study, IgA-sFcαRI complexes were decreased in the serum of patients with recurrent IgAN and sFcαRI was detected in the kidney mesangium only in patients with the recurrent disease. Direct evidence for a nephrotoxic role of IgA1-sFcαRI complexes were obtained in humanized animal models. These experimental studies were based on the fact that mouse do not have homologs of IgA1 and FcαRI. Humanized mice expressing human IgA1 and human FcαRI spontaneously develop mesangial deposits of IgA1-sFcαRI complexes (98). In the glomeruli, these complexes are captured by the transferrin receptor 1 (TfR1), which is upregulated on mesangial cells,

through interaction with polymeric (p) IgA1 and FcαRI (98, 99). Although the mechanism of TfR1 upregulation remains poorly understood, the crosslinking enzyme transglutaminase 2 has been found to be overexpressed and associated with the receptor controlling mesangial IgA1 complex deposition and renal injury (98). Polymeric IgA1 induce TfR1 expression *in vitro* on mesangial cells. Polymeric IgA1-TfR1 interaction triggers activating signals through mTOR, PI3K and ERK pathways, and phosphorylated ERK is associated with disease progression (100). Interestingly enough, in physiology TfR1-IgA1 interaction plays a role in erythropoiesis (101). Progression of IgAN to end-stage renal disease may also involve FcαRI activation on tissue macrophages surrounding hypogalactosylated IgA1-mediated mesangial lesions. Indeed, FcαRI$_{R209L}$Tg mice, with an R-to-L substitution at position 209 in the transmembrane region of FcαRI, did not develop macrophage infiltration and proteinuria (102). This mutant receptor cannot associate with the ITAM-bearing FcRγ signaling subunit (103). In agreement, only macrophages expressing wild-type FcαRI, but not those expressing FcαRI$_{R209L}$, were able to migrate to the kidney after adoptive transfer demonstrating that their chemotaxis depends on the FcRγ subunit. Of note, FcαRI can be found associated and non-associated with FcRγ on the same cells (95). Since mouse IgA and human FcαRI interaction may be sufficient to induce receptor shedding leading to IgA deposits in the kidney, we hypothesized that both receptor types could cooperate to induce disease, the FcRγ-less FcαRI allowing IgA deposits and the FcRγ-associated FcαRI promoting inflammatory cell infiltration and disease progression (102).

For FcμR (IgM receptor), deficiency in the receptor in mice revealed that this receptor plays a crucial role in B cell responses (27, 104). Mice deficient for *Fcmr* are characterized by the increase in pre-immune serum IgM, dysregulation of humoral immune responses, disturbances in B cell subpopulations, B cell proliferation alteration after BCR ligation, and autoantibody production (104, 105). Accordingly, in chronic lymphocytic leukemia (CLL), the membrane expression and the soluble form of FcμR in serum were increased. The potential mechanism proposed for the up-regulation of FcμR is that the antigen-independent self-ligation of BCR on CLL cells induces activation of Syk thus increasing the cell surface expression of FcμR. Furthermore, the IgM antibodies produced by CLL cells that had differentiated into plasma cells, recognized soluble or lymphocyte membrane self-antigens. IgM/self-antigen immune complexes would then crosslink FcμR and BCR favoring cell survival. An alternative splice variant of the soluble FcμR is increased in CLL patients, but its biological function is unclear (105, 106).

For type II FcRs, an increased expression of FcεRII on monocytes in AIDS patients has been associated with the aberrant activated phenotype of these cells during the immunopathogenesis of AIDS. Interestingly, despite the known ability of IL-10 to downregulate monocyte FcεRII expression, in AIDS the IL-10-enriched environment is not associated with the suppression of FcεRII expression on monocytes (82) indicative of an impairment of this negative regulation in patients. In B-CLL also, patients strongly express FcεRII, which is associated with B cell activation and proliferation. Moreover, altered phosphorylation of FcεRII intracellular tail were reported in B-CLL B lymphocytes (107) further supporting an active role of FcεRII in this disease.

TARGETING OF FC RECEPTORS AS THERAPEUTIC APPROACHES

Blocking/neutralizing Activating Receptor Antibodies

Both murine models and studies in patients suggest a major role of the activating FcRs in initiating and propelling immune complex-mediated inflammatory reactions. For example, human FcγRIIA transgenic mice are hypersensitive to pathogenic antibodies and develop destructive arthritic syndromes. *Ex vivo* experimentation with circulating monocytes from RA patients suggest that FcγRIIA is responsible for the production of reactive oxygen species (11, 108). Anti-receptor monoclonal antibodies, intact antibodies and antibody fragments as well as a variety of small molecules have been designed to interact with the Ig-binding domains in activating FcRs. Some of these approaches have shown encouraging results when tested *in*

vitro or *in vivo* for blocking immune complex-mediated cell effects and inflammation. Recently, we have demonstrated that divalent targeting of FcγRIIA by anti-hFcγRII F(ab)'2 fragments ameliorates RA-associated inflammation. This therapeutic effect was mediated by the induction of inhibitory ITAM (ITAMi) signaling through the activation of SHP-1. Moreover, treatment of inflammatory synovial cells from RA patients by F(ab')2 fragment of hFcγRIIA-specific antibody inhibited production of reactive oxygen species associated with the induction of FcγRIIA-mediated ITAMi signaling. These data suggest that targeting of hFcγRIIA by specific antibody such as clone IV.3 mAb could ameliorate RA-associated inflammation (11). Anti-FcαRI Fab and F(ab)'2 fragments also have demonstrated efficiency on RA (109). Interestingly, in autoimmune blistering skin diseases that involve interaction between IgA autoantibodies and the neutrophil FcαRI, targeting FcαRI by blocking peptides or antibodies prevents neutrophil migration and tissue damage *ex-vivo* (110, 111).

In allergy, treatment by anti-IgE antibodies has been considered a therapeutic option for a long time. The recombinant anti-IgE humanized monoclonal antibody-E25, named "omalizumab," is now used in several clinical trials and shows efficacy against IgE-mediated allergic reactions (112, 113) through inhibition of IgE binding to FcεRI on the surface of mast cells and basophils (113).

The above-described upregulation of FcμR expression in CLL cells is of significant clinical interest. It can be easily evaluated by flow cytometry on cells and, additionally, the levels of soluble FcμR may correlate with disease progression. Thus, it may be used as a new biomarker for CLL (106). FcμR is a good target also because it is involved in the pathogenesis of CLL and in the progression of the disease through support of leukemic cell survival (80). Hence, disrupting CLL survival signals might be achieved through FcμR therapeutic targeting. However, a large cohort of CLL patients will be required to validate these two applications (106).

IVIG

Intravenous immunoglobulins (IVIG) are harvested from the pooled plasma of 3,000 to 100,000 healthy donors. They consist of over 95% IgGs with a subclass distribution corresponding to that found in normal human serum (114). IVIG is used in treatment of several immunodeficiency diseases including idiopathic thrombocytopenic purpura (ITP), Kawasaki disease, and neurologic diseases such as Guillain–Barre syndrome, chronic inflammatory demyelinating polyneuropathy, myasthenia gravis, sclerosis, and autoimmune encephalitis (115). In ITP patients, administration of IVIG can efficiently attenuate platelet clearance from the circulation. The first proposed mechanism was the competitive blockage of the activating FcγRs on myeloid cells by IVIG, which in turn decreases autoantibody-mediated platelet phagocytosis and ADCC against platelets (116). Furthermore, in pediatric ITP patients, intravenous administration of the Fcγ fragments prepared from IVIG resulted in a rapid recovery in platelet counts (117) further indicating the role of FcγRs in IVIG action. Another IVIG anti-inflammatory mechanism involves saturation of FcRn, the IgG recycling receptor (118). FcRn plays an important role in the maintenance of IgG half-life. Therefore, inhibition of autoantibody activity can be induced by the alteration of their interaction with FcRn, impairing their half-life and accelerating their clearing from the circulation. IVIG by competing with autoantibodies for FcRn binding could therefore facilitate their clearing.

A role for the inhibitory FcγRIIB has been proposed to be exclusive in IVIG action to explain their Fc dependent effect (118). This statement was based notably on studies showing a decreased anti-inflammatory effect of IVIG in FcγRIIB-deficient animals. In other studies, a role for FcγRIII in IVIG-mediated inhibition has been reported (119) although the mechanism of action was not clearly established. Recently, we reported that IVIG can control inflammatory responses by ITAMi signaling through FcγRIIA and FcγRIII (10, 11). These data are based on the *in vitro* targeting of FcγRIIA and FcγRIII by IVIG at the physiological concentration of IgG showing an inhibitory effect on endocytosis. This was confirmed by targeting FcγRIIA or FcγRIII with F(ab′)2 fragments of specific antibodies. These results were further supported *in vivo* in mice by targeting these receptors with IVIG or with specific antibodies and this inhibitory effect was abolished in receptor-deficient mice (10, 11). Therefore, IVIG could use a combination of non-exclusive mechanisms to promote protection against auto-immune diseases. Although IVIG is well tolerated, some patients develop immediate or delayed adverse effects depending on the time occurrence. The Flu-like symptoms such as fever, fatigue and nausea are the most frequent adverse effects. For the delayed adverse effects, the most frequent are thrombotic events, neurological disorders and renal failure. These delayed adverse effects are rare but dangerous (120). The majority of adverse effects are associated with high doses of immunoglobulins; thus, determining individual dosages to guarantee the efficacy of therapy and minimize adverse effects is an urgent goal.

Treatment with highly purified serum monomeric IgA (mIgA) decreases cell activation through FcαRI-FcRγ-mediated ITAMi signaling (109). Human mIgA or anti-FcαRI Fab fragments were used to prevent or treat collagen antibody-induced arthritis in FcαRI-transgenic mice. mIgA treatment decreased significantly leukocyte infiltration to the inflamed joints of mice, which was associated with SHP-1 phosphorylation at Y536 residue in joint tissue cells. Moreover, mIgA reversed the activating ITAM to ITAMi signature and the state of inflammation in the synovial fluid isolated from RA patients (109). Of note, protection was also achieved with human serum IgA (4). These findings open new avenues to develop the concept of IVIgA as a new treatment option for inflammatory and auto-immune diseases.

Engagement of the Inhibitory FcγRIIB (Agonist)

The only FcR containing an inhibitory ITIM motif, FcγRIIB, serves as a critical negative regulator in immune complex driven reactions. In mice lacking FcγRIIB auto-immune symptoms are exacerbated, and a partial restoration of FcγRIIB expression in B cells rescued mice from developing an SLE-like phenotype (57, 121). Several FcγRIIB specific mAbs have now been developed (122, 123), one of which, mAb2B6, has been chimerized and humanized to direct myeloid-cytotoxicity against B cells (123).

These antibodies have the potential to serve as novel immune suppressors in auto-immunity either by blocking B cell activation or by targeting their destruction. In addition, they may have an advantage over CD20 antibodies for their ability to target plasma cells (124).

Targeting FcRn

Blocking FcRn-IgG interaction to decrease circulating IgG levels is one strategy to treat auto-immune disease (118). In the absence of interaction with FcRn, IgG would be degraded in lysosomes more quickly instead of being recycled back into circulation. One straightforward method would be to use recombinant soluble human FcRn to compete with membrane FcRn for IgG. Another approach to block IgG-FcRn binding would be through engineered "bait" IgG which occupy FcRn thus preventing binding of endogenous IgG. Such "bait" antibodies have been generated with a much higher affinity for FcRn at both acidic and neutral pH, thereby providing effective occupancy of FcRn, competing with, and resulting in, degradation of endogenous IgG. These antibodies are also called "Abdegs": antibodies that enhance IgG degradation (125).

An FcRn-specific blocking mAb would also provide interference with FcRn-IgG interaction. One such mAb, 1G3, was examined in rat passive and active models of myasthenia gravis, a prototypical antibody-mediated auto-immune disease (126). Treatment by 1G3 mAb resulted in amelioration of disease symptoms in a dose-dependent manner together with greatly reduced levels of pathogenic antibody in the serum.

Other Future Strategies to Target FcR-Effectors to Treat Auto-Immune/Inflammatory Diseases

Targeting of FcRs by monomeric immunoglobulins or by F(ab′)2 fragments of specific antibodies, induces ITAMi signaling which involved the recruitment of Lyn, but not Fyn. The Src kinase Lyn, leads to partial phosphorylation of the ITAM motif on tyrosine residues (11), and to the conformational change of SHP-1 that allows its recruitment through its SH2 domains to ITAM phosphotyrosine residues (127). This recruitment induces a Lyn-dependent phosphorylation of SHP-1 on Y536 and to SHP-1 phosphatase activity that inhibits the recruitment of various proteins induced by heterologous receptors (52). In contrast, multivalent crosslinking of immunoreceptors by immune complexes induces the recruitment of both Src kinases Lyn and Fyn to the receptor leading to full phosphorylation of the tyrosine residues present in the ITAM motif. This leads to the activation and the recruitment of the kinase Syk. In parallel, Fyn initiates a signaling pathway involving a PI3K-PKCα axis leading the inactivation of SHP-1 through the phosphorylation of its S591 residue barring its recruitment to the plasma membrane (128). Since S591 phosphorylation on SHP-1 keeps the phosphatase in a closed conformation (127), our recent study showed that the phosphorylation of SHP-1 on S591 residue by Fyn axis renders the Y536 residue inaccessible to Lyn. In agreement, the absence of Fyn favors the phosphorylation of SHP-1 on Y536 by Lyn, despite the crosslinking of FcγRIIA (4). These results suggest that the selective absence or inhibition of Fyn may abolish inflammation during auto-immune and proinflammatory diseases. Taken together, inhibition of Fyn or of the molecules which are upstream or downstream this SFK reverses inflammation during auto-immune and inflammatory diseases and thus, could be a new therapeutic strategy to decrease the activating ITAM signaling in these diseases. Along these lines, inhibition of PI3K (a major player of the Fyn-PI3K-PKCα axis (4)) prevents RA and lupus nephritis progression in mouse models (129). However, it should be mentioned that since Fyn is essential for activating ITAM signals (i.e., phagocytosis), the inhibition of this SFK may favor infections. Moreover, Fyn plays also other roles independently of FcRs. It has been shown that the absence of Fyn impaired multipolar-bipolar transition of newly generated neurons and neurite formation during the early phase of migration. Additionally, inhibition of Fyn decreased the branching number of the migrating cortical neurons (130). Another important hurdle is that Lyn and Fyn present a high homology and there are currently no selective inhibitory drugs. Therefore, Fyn does not appear as the best target to treat auto-immune and pro-inflammatory diseases. Identification of new targets which are downstream of Fyn and which are expressed specifically by immune cells involved in auto-immune diseases will permit development of new therapeutic strategies for auto-immune diseases that involve FcR.

CONCLUSION

Fc receptors may be responsible for diseases when dysregulated in spite of their physiologic protective function. Unraveling all aspects (expression, function, regulation) of FcR biology should help to define approaches to correct the first and to wield the second to restore homeostasis thus representing new hopes for innovative anti-inflammatory strategies. Progress in these two aspects is currently well underway, already proposing new potent therapeutic tools. The future in this field is a promise of scientific excitement.

AUTHOR CONTRIBUTIONS

SB and RM wrote this review. MB has critically read the manuscript.

FUNDING

This work was funded by Inserm, by the Agence Nationale de la Recherche (ANR grants JC -17-CE17-0002-01, ANR PRC - 18-CE14-0002-01), and also by LabEx Inflamex (ANR-11-IDEX-0005-02). RM was supported by ≪ Equipe ≫ program of the Fondation pour la recherche médicale (FRM).

REFERENCES

1. Pincetic A, Bournazos S, DiLillo DJ, Maamary J, Wang TT, Dahan R, et al. Type I and type II Fc receptors regulate innate and adaptive immunity. *Nat Immunol.* (2014) 15:707–16. doi: 10.1038/ni.2939

2. Bruhns P, Jonsson F. Mouse and human FcR effector functions. *Immunol Rev.* (2015) 268:25–51. doi: 10.1111/imr.12350

3. Kubagawa H, Kubagawa Y, Jones D, Nasti TH, Walter MR, Honjo K. The old but new IgM Fc receptor (FcmuR). *Curr Top Microbiol Immunol.* (2014) 382:3–28. doi: 10.1007/978-3-319-07911-0_1

4. Mkaddem SB, Murua A, Flament H, Titeca-Beauport D, Bounaix C, Danelli L, et al. Lyn and Fyn function as molecular switches that control immunoreceptors to direct homeostasis or inflammation. *Nat Commun.* (2017) 8:246. doi: 10.1038/s41467-017-00294-0

5. Malbec O, Fong DC, Turner M, Tybulewicz VL, Cambier JC, Fridman WH, et al. Fc epsilon receptor I-associated lyn-dependent phosphorylation of Fc gamma receptor IIB during negative regulation of mast cell activation. *J Immunol.* (1998) 160:1647–58.

6. Bolland S, Ravetch JV. Inhibitory pathways triggered by ITIM-containing receptors. *Adv Immunol.* (1999) 72:149–77. doi: 10.1016/S0065-2776(08)60019-X

7. Pasquier B, Launay P, Kanamaru Y, Moura IC, Pfirsch S, Ruffie C, et al. Identification of FcalphaRI as an inhibitory receptor that controls inflammation: dual role of FcRgamma ITAM. *Immunity.* (2005) 22:31–42. doi: 10.1016/j.immuni.2004.11.017

8. Pinheiro da Silva F, Aloulou M, Skurnik D, Benhamou M, Andremont A, Velasco IT, et al. CD16 promotes *Escherichia coli* sepsis through an FcR gamma inhibitory pathway that prevents phagocytosis and facilitates inflammation. *Nat Med.* (2007) 13:1368–74. doi: 10.1038/nm1665

9. Kanamaru Y, Pfirsch S, Aloulou M, Vrtovsnik F, Essig M, Loirat C, et al. Inhibitory ITAM signaling by Fc alpha RI-FcR gamma chain controls multiple activating responses and prevents renal inflammation. *J Immunol.* (2008) 180:2669–78. doi: 10.4049/jimmunol.180.4.2669

10. Aloulou M, Ben Mkaddem S, Biarnes-Pelicot M, Boussetta T, Souchet H, Rossato E, et al. IgG1 and IVIg induce inhibitory ITAM signaling through FcgammaRIII controlling inflammatory responses. *Blood.* (2012) 119:3084–96. doi: 10.1182/blood-2011-08-376046

11. Ben Mkaddem S, Hayem G, Jonsson F, Rossato E, Boedec E, Boussetta T, et al. Shifting FcgammaRIIA-ITAM from activation to inhibitory configuration ameliorates arthritis. *J Clin Invest.* (2014) 124:3945–59. doi: 10.1172/JCI74572

12. Iborra S, Martinez-Lopez M, Cueto FJ, Conde-Garrosa R, Del Fresno C, Izquierdo HM, et al. Leishmania uses mincle to target an inhibitory ITAM signaling pathway in dendritic cells that dampens adaptive immunity to infection. *Immunity.* (2016) 45:788–801. doi: 10.1016/j.immuni.2016.09.012

13. Getahun A, Cambier JC. Of ITIMs, ITAMs, and ITAMis: revisiting immunoglobulin Fc receptor signaling. *Immunol Rev.* (2015) 268:66–73. doi: 10.1111/imr.12336

14. Blank U, Launay P, Benhamou M, Monteiro RC. Inhibitory ITAMs as novel regulators of immunity. *Immunol Rev.* (2009) 232:59–71. doi: 10.1111/j.1600-065X.2009.00832.x

15. Stefanova I, Hemmer B, Vergelli M, Martin R, Biddison WE, Germain RN. TCR ligand discrimination is enforced by competing ERK positive and SHP-1 negative feedback pathways. *Nat Immunol.* (2003) 4:248–54. doi: 10.1038/ni895

16. Getahun A, Beavers NA, Larson SR, Shlomchik MJ, Cambier JC. Continuous inhibitory signaling by both SHP-1 and SHIP-1 pathways is required to maintain unresponsiveness of anergic B cells. *J Exp Med.* (2016) 213:751–69. doi: 10.1084/jem.20150537

17. Abram CL, Roberge GL, Pao LI, Neel BG, Lowell CA. Distinct roles for neutrophils and dendritic cells in inflammation and autoimmunity in motheaten mice. *Immunity.* (2013) 38:489–501. doi: 10.1016/j.immuni.2013.02.018

18. Chan VW, Lowell CA, DeFranco AL. Defective negative regulation of antigen receptor signaling in Lyn-deficient B lymphocytes. *Curr Biol.* (1998) 8:545–53. doi: 10.1016/S0960-9822(98)70223-4

19. Lowell CA. Src-family kinases: rheostats of immune cell signaling. *Mol Immunol.* (2004) 41:631–43. doi: 10.1016/j.molimm.2004.04.010

20. Apodaca G, Bomsel M, Arden J, Breitfeld PP, Tang K, Mostov KE. The polymeric immunoglobulin receptor. a model protein to study transcytosis. *J Clin Invest.* (1991) 87:1877–82. doi: 10.1172/JCI115211

21. Donaldson GP, Ladinsky MS, Yu KB, Sanders JG, Yoo BB, Chou WC, et al. Gut microbiota utilize immunoglobulin A for mucosal colonization. *Science.* (2018) 360:795–800. doi: 10.1126/science.aaq0926

22. Kikuno K, Kang DW, Tahara K, Torii I, Kubagawa HM, Ho KJ, et al. Unusual biochemical features and follicular dendritic cell expression of human Fcalpha/mu receptor. *Eur J Immunol.* (2007) 37:3540–50. doi: 10.1002/eji.200737655

23. Ahmed AA, Giddens J, Pincetic A, Lomino JV, Ravetch JV, Wang LX, et al. Structural characterization of anti-inflammatory immunoglobulin G Fc proteins. *J Mol Biol.* (2014) 426:3166–3179. doi: 10.1016/j.jmb.2014.07.006

24. Pennington LF, Tarchevskaya S, Brigger D, Sathiyamoorthy K, Graham MT, Nadeau KC, et al. Structural basis of omalizumab therapy and omalizumab-mediated IgE exchange. *Nat Commun.* (2016) 7:11610. doi: 10.1038/ncomms11610

25. Hogarth PM. Fc receptors are major mediators of antibody based inflammation in autoimmunity. *Curr Opin Immunol.* (2002) 14:798–802. doi: 10.1016/S0952-7915(02)00409-0

26. Monteiro RC, Van De Winkel JG. IgA Fc receptors. *Annu Rev Immunol.* (2003) 21:177–204. doi: 10.1146/annurev.immunol.21.120601.141011

27. Kubagawa H, Oka S, Kubagawa Y, Torii I, Takayama E, Kang DW, et al. Identity of the elusive IgM Fc receptor (FcmuR) in humans. *J Exp Med.* (2009) 206:2779–93. doi: 10.1084/jem.20091107

28. Shibuya A, Sakamoto N, Shimizu Y, Shibuya K, Osawa M, Hiroyama T, et al. Fc alpha/mu receptor mediates endocytosis of IgM-coated microbes. *Nat Immunol.* (2000) 1:441–6. doi: 10.1038/80886

29. Daeron M. Fc receptors as adaptive immunoreceptors. *Curr Top Microbiol Immunol.* (2014) 382:131–64. doi: 10.1007/978-3-319-07911-0_7

30. Diana J, Moura IC, Vaugier C, Gestin A, Tissandie E, Beaudoin L, et al. Secretory IgA induces tolerogenic dendritic cells through SIGNR1 dampening autoimmunity in mice. *J Immunol.* (2013) 191:2335–43. doi: 10.4049/jimmunol.1300864

31. Paul-Eugene N, Kolb JP, Abadie A, Gordon J, Delespesse G, Sarfati M, et al. Ligation of CD23 triggers cAMP generation and release of inflammatory mediators in human monocytes. *J Immunol.* (1992) 149:3066–71.

32. Kolb JP, Abadie A, Paul-Eugene N, Capron M, Sarfati M, Dugas B, et al. Ligation of CD23 triggers cyclic AMP generation in human B lymphocytes. *J Immunol.* (1993) 150:4798–809.

33. Chan MA, Gigliotti NM, Matangkasombut P, Gauld SB, Cambier JC, Rosenwasser LJ. CD23-mediated cell signaling in human B cells differs from signaling in cells of the monocytic lineage. *Clin Immunol.* (2010) 137:330–6. doi: 10.1016/j.clim.2010.08.005

34. Hargreaves CE, Rose-Zerilli MJ, Machado LR, Iriyama C, Hollox EJ, Cragg MS, et al. Fcgamma receptors: genetic variation, function, and disease. *Immunol Rev.* (2015) 268:6–24. doi: 10.1111/imr.12341

35. Gillis C, Gouel-Cheron A, Jonsson F, Bruhns P. Contribution of human fcgammars to disease with evidence from human polymorphisms and transgenic animal studies. *Front Immunol.* (2014) 5:254. doi: 10.3389/fimmu.2014.00254

36. Li X, Gibson AW, Kimberly RP. Human FcR polymorphism and disease. *Curr Top Microbiol Immunol.* (2014) 382:275–302 doi: 10.1007/978-3-319-07911-0_13

37. Zhou XJ, Lv JC, Bu DF, Yu L, Yang YR, Zhao J, et al. Copy number variation of FCGR3A rather than FCGR3B and FCGR2B is associated with susceptibility to anti-GBM disease. *Int Immunol.* (2010) 22:45–51. doi: 10.1093/intimm/dxp113

38. Fanciulli M, Norsworthy PJ, Petretto E, Dong R, Harper L, Kamesh L, et al. FCGR3B copy number variation is associated with susceptibility to systemic, but not organ-specific, autoimmunity. *Nat Genet.* (2007) 39:721–3. doi: 10.1038/ng2046

39. Takai T. Roles of Fc receptors in autoimmunity. *Nat Rev Immunol.* (2002) 2:580–92. doi: 10.1038/nri856

40. Bruhns P, Iannascoli B, England P, Mancardi DA, Fernandez N, Jorieux S, et al. Specificity and affinity of human Fcgamma receptors and their polymorphic variants for human IgG subclasses. *Blood.* (2009) 113:3716–25. doi: 10.1182/blood-2008-09-179754

41. Sanders LA, Feldman RG, Voorhorst-Ogink MM, de Haas M, Rijkers GT, Capel PJ, et al. Human immunoglobulin G (IgG) Fc receptor IIA (CD32) polymorphism and IgG2-mediated bacterial phagocytosis by neutrophils. *Infect Immun.* (1995) 63:73–81.

42. Kyogoku C, Dijstelbloem HM, Tsuchiya N, Hatta Y, Kato H, Yamaguchi A, et al. Fcgamma receptor gene polymorphisms in Japanese patients with systemic lupus erythematosus: contribution of FCGR2B to genetic susceptibility. *Arthritis Rheum.* (2002) 46:1242–54. doi: 10.1002/art.10257

43. Onouchi Y, Ozaki K, Burns JC, Shimizu C, Terai M, Hamada H, et al. Japan kawasaki disease genome U. S. K. Consortium DG. A genome-wide association study identifies three new risk loci for Kawasaki disease. *Nat Genet.* (2012) 44:517–21. doi: 10.1038/ng.2220

44. Asano K, Matsushita T, Umeno J, Hosono N, Takahashi A, Kawaguchi T, et al. A genome-wide association study identifies three new susceptibility loci for ulcerative colitis in the Japanese population. *Nat Genet.* (2009) 41:1325–9. doi: 10.1038/ng.482

45. van der Pol WL, van den Berg LH, Scheepers RH, van der Bom JG, van Doorn PA, van Koningsveld R, et al. IgG receptor IIa alleles determine susceptibility and severity of Guillain-Barre syndrome. *Neurology.* (2000) 54:1661–5. doi: 10.1212/WNL.54.8.1661

46. Tsang ASMW, Nagelkerke SQ, Bultink IE, Geissler J, Tanck MW, Tacke CE, et al. Fc-gamma receptor polymorphisms differentially influence susceptibility to systemic lupus erythematosus and lupus nephritis. *Rheumatology (Oxford).* (2016) 55:939–48. doi: 10.1093/rheumatology/kev433

47. Qiao J, Al-Tamimi M, Baker RI, Andrews RK, Gardiner EE. The platelet Fc receptor, FcgammaRIIa. *Immunol Rev.* (2015) 268:241–52. doi: 10.1111/imr.12370

48. Tanaka Y, Suzuki Y, Tsuge T, Kanamaru Y, Horikoshi S, Monteiro RC, et al. FcgammaRIIa-131R allele and FcgammaRIIIa-176V/V genotype are risk factors for progression of IgA nephropathy. *Nephrol Dial Transplant.* (2005) 20:2439–45. doi: 10.1093/ndt/gfi043

49. McKenzie SE, Taylor SM, Malladi P, Yuhan H, Cassel DL, Chien P, et al. The role of the human Fc receptor Fc gamma RIIA in the immune clearance of platelets: a transgenic mouse model. *J Immunol.* (1999) 162:4311–8.

50. Tan Sardjono C, Mottram PL, van de Velde NC, Powell MS, Power D, Slocombe RF, et al. Development of spontaneous multisystem autoimmune disease and hypersensitivity to antibody-induced inflammation in Fcgamma receptor IIa-transgenic mice. *Arthritis Rheum.* (2005) 52:3220–9. doi: 10.1002/art.21344

51. Reilly AF, Norris CF, Surrey S, Bruchak FJ, Rappaport EF, Schwartz E, et al. Genetic diversity in human Fc receptor II for immunoglobulin G: Fc gamma receptor IIA ligand-binding polymorphism. *Clin Diagn Lab Immunol.* (1994) 1:640–4.

52. Pfirsch-Maisonnas S, Aloulou M, Xu T, Claver J, Kanamaru Y, Tiwari M, et al. Inhibitory ITAM signaling traps activating receptors with the phosphatase SHP-1 to form polarized "inhibisome" clusters. *Sci Signal.* (2011) 4:ra24. doi: 10.1126/scisignal.2001309

53. Pietersz GA, Mottram PL, van de Velde NC, Sardjono CT, Esparon S, Ramsland PA, et al. Inhibition of destructive autoimmune arthritis in FcgammaRIIa transgenic mice by small chemical entities. *Immunol Cell Biol.* (2009) 87:3–12. doi: 10.1038/icb.2008.82

54. White AL, Beers SA, Cragg MS. FcgammaRIIB as a key determinant of agonistic antibody efficacy. *Curr Top Microbiol Immunol.* (2014) 382:355–72. doi: 10.1007/978-3-319-07911-0_16

55. Floto RA, Clatworthy MR, Heilbronn KR, Rosner DR, MacAry PA, Rankin A, et al. Loss of function of a lupus-associated FcgammaRIIb polymorphism through exclusion from lipid rafts. *Nat Med.* (2005) 11:1056–8. doi: 10.1038/nm1288

56. Espeli M, Smith KG, Clatworthy MR. FcgammaRIIB and autoimmunity. *Immunol Rev.* (2016) 269:194–211. doi: 10.1111/imr.12368

57. McGaha TL, Sorrentino B, Ravetch JV. Restoration of tolerance in lupus by targeted inhibitory receptor expression. *Science.* (2005) 307:590–3. doi: 10.1126/science.1105160

58. Morgan AW, Griffiths B, Ponchel F, Montague BM, Ali M, Gardner PP, et al. Fcgamma receptor type IIIA is associated with rheumatoid arthritis in two distinct ethnic groups. *Arthritis Rheum.* (2000) 43:2328–34. doi: 10.1002/1529-0131(200010)43:10<2328::AID-ANR21>3.0.CO;2-Z

59. Nieto A, Pascual M, Caliz R, Mataran L, Martin J. Association of Fcgamma receptor IIIA polymorphism with rheumatoid arthritis: comment on the article by Morgan et al. *Arthritis Rheum.* (2002) 46:556–9. doi: 10.1002/art.10122

60. Tsuge T, Shimokawa T, Horikoshi S, Tomino Y, Ra C. Polymorphism in promoter region of Fcalpha receptor gene in patients with IgA nephropathy. *Hum Genet.* (2001) 108:128–33. doi: 10.1007/s004390100458

61. Wu J, Ji C, Xie F, Langefeld CD, Qian K, Gibson AW, et al. FcalphaRI (CD89) alleles determine the proinflammatory potential of serum IgA. *J Immunol.* (2007) 178:3973–82. doi: 10.4049/jimmunol.178.6.3973

62. Broen JC, Coenen MJ, Rueda B, Witte T, Padyukov L, Klareskog L, et al. The functional polymorphism 844 A>G in FcalphaRI (CD89) does not contribute to systemic sclerosis or rheumatoid arthritis susceptibility. *J Rheumatol*. (2011) 38:446–9. doi: 10.3899/jrheum.100427

63. Maillard N, Thibaudin L, Abadja F, Masson I, Garraud O, Berthoux F, et al. Single nucleotidic polymorphism 844 A->G of FCAR is not associated with IgA nephropathy in Caucasians. *Nephrol Dial Transplant*. (2012) 27:656–60. doi: 10.1093/ndt/gfr246

64. Kaneko S, Kobayashi T, Yamamoto K, Jansen MD, van de Winkel JG, Yoshie H. A novel polymorphism of FcalphaRI (CD89) associated with aggressive periodontitis. *Tissue Antigens*. (2004) 63:572–7. doi: 10.1111/j.0001-2815.2004.0228.x

65. Hirunsatit R, Kongruttanachok N, Shotelersuk K, Supiyaphun P, Voravud N, Sakuntabhai A, et al. Polymeric immunoglobulin receptor polymorphisms and risk of nasopharyngeal cancer. *BMC Genet*. (2003) 4:3. doi: 10.1186/1471-2156-4-3

66. Hasegawa M, Nishiyama C, Nishiyama M, Akizawa Y, Mitsuishi K, Ito T, et al. A novel−66T/C polymorphism in Fc epsilon RI alpha-chain promoter affecting the transcription activity: possible relationship to allergic diseases. *J Immunol*. (2003) 171:1927–33. doi: 10.4049/jimmunol.171.4.1927

67. Potaczek DP, Sanak M, Mastalerz L, Setkowicz M, Kaczor M, Nizankowska E, et al. The alpha-chain of high-affinity receptor for IgE (FcepsilonRIalpha) gene polymorphisms and serum IgE levels. *Allergy*. (2006) 61:1230–3. doi: 10.1111/j.1398-9995.2006.01195.x

68. Kim SH, Ye YM, Lee SK, Park HS. Genetic mechanism of aspirin-induced urticaria/angioedema. *Curr Opin Allergy Clin Immunol*. (2006) 6:266–70. doi: 10.1097/01.all.0000235899.57182.d4

69. Zhou J, Zhou Y, Lin LH, Wang J, Peng X, Li J, et al. Association of polymorphisms in the promoter region of FCER1A gene with atopic dermatitis, chronic uticaria, asthma, and serum immunoglobulin E levels in a Han Chinese population. *Hum Immunol*. (2012) 73:301–5. doi: 10.1016/j.humimm.2011.12.001

70. Zhang X, Zhang W, Qiu D, Sandford A, Tan WC. The E237G polymorphism of the high-affinity IgE receptor beta chain and asthma. *Ann Allergy Asthma Immunol*. (2004) 93:499–503. doi: 10.1016/S1081-1206(10)61419-6

71. Yang HJ, Zheng L, Zhang XF, Yang M, Huang X. Association of the MS4A2 gene promoter C-109T or the 7th exon E237G polymorphisms with asthma risk: a meta-analysis. *Clin Biochem*. (2014) 47:605–11. doi: 10.1016/j.clinbiochem.2014.01.022

72. Wu J, Lin R, Huang J, Guan W, Oetting WS, Sriramarao P, et al. Functional Fcgamma receptor polymorphisms are associated with human allergy. *PLoS ONE*. (2014) 9:e89196. doi: 10.1371/journal.pone.0089196

73. van der Heijden J, Breunis WB, Geissler J, de Boer M, van den Berg TK, Kuijpers TW. Phenotypic variation in IgG receptors by nonclassical FCGR2C alleles. *J Immunol*. (2012) 188:1318–24. doi: 10.4049/jimmunol.1003945

74. Lee YH, Ji JD, Song GG. Associations between FCGR3A polymorphisms and susceptibility to rheumatoid arthritis: a metaanalysis. *J Rheumatol*. (2008) 35:2129–35. doi: 10.3899/jrheum.080186

75. Carcao MD, Blanchette VS, Wakefield CD, Stephens D, Ellis J, Matheson K, et al. Fcgamma receptor IIa and IIIa polymorphisms in childhood immune thrombocytopenic purpura. *Br J Haematol*. (2003) 120:135–41. doi: 10.1046/j.1365-2141.2003.04033.x

76. Koene HR, Kleijer M, Swaak AJ, Sullivan KE, Bijl M, Petri MA, et al. The Fc gammaRIIIA-158F allele is a risk factor for systemic lupus erythematosus. *Arthritis Rheum*. (1998) 41:1813–8. doi: 10.1002/1529-0131(199810)41:10<1813::AID-ART13>3.0.CO;2-6

77. Moroi R, Endo K, Kinouchi Y, Shiga H, Kakuta Y, Kuroha M, et al. FCGR3A-158 polymorphism influences the biological response to infliximab in Crohn's disease through affecting the ADCC activity. *Immunogenetics*. (2013) 65:265–71. doi: 10.1007/s00251-013-0679-8

78. Kelley JM, Monach PA, Ji C, Zhou Y, Wu J, Tanaka S, et al. IgA and IgG antineutrophil cytoplasmic antibody engagement of Fc receptor genetic variants influences granulomatosis with polyangiitis. *Proc Natl Acad Sci U.S.A.* (2011) 108:20736–41. doi: 10.1073/pnas.1109227109

79. van Egmond M, van Garderen E, van Spriel AB, Damen CA, van Amersfoort ES, van Zandbergen G, et al. FcalphaRI-positive liver Kupffer cells: reappraisal of the function of immunoglobulin A in immunity. *Nat Med*. (2000) 6:680–5. doi: 10.1038/76261

80. Pallasch CP, Schulz A, Kutsch N, Schwamb J, Hagist S, Kashkar H, et al. Overexpression of TOSO in CLL is triggered by B-cell receptor signaling and associated with progressive disease. *Blood*. (2008) 112:4213–9. doi: 10.1182/blood-2008-05-157255

81. Hitoshi Y, Lorens J, Kitada SI, Fisher J, LaBarge M, Ring HZ, et al. Toso, a cell surface, specific regulator of Fas-induced apoptosis in T cells. *Immunity*. (1998) 8:461–71. doi: 10.1016/S1074-7613(00)80551-8

82. Miller LS, Atabai K, Nowakowski M, Chan A, Bluth MH, Minkoff H, et al. Increased expression of CD23 (Fc(epsilon) receptor II) by peripheral blood monocytes of aids patients. *AIDS Res Hum Retroviruses*. (2001) 17:443–52. doi: 10.1089/088922201750102544

83. Morgan AW, Keyte VH, Babbage SJ, Robinson JI, Ponchel F, Barrett JH, et al. FcgammaRIIIA-158V and rheumatoid arthritis: a confirmation study. *Rheumatology (Oxford)*. (2003) 42:528–33. doi: 10.1093/rheumatology/keg169

84. Descours B, Petitjean G, Lopez-Zaragoza JL, Bruel T, Raffel R, Psomas C, et al. CD32a is a marker of a CD4 T-cell HIV reservoir harbouring replication-competent proviruses. *Nature*. (2017) 543:564–567. doi: 10.1038/nature21710

85. Abdel-Mohsen M, Kuri-Cervantes L, Grau-Exposito J, Spivak AM, Nell RA, Tomescu C, et al. CD32 is expressed on cells with transcriptionally active HIV but does not enrich for HIV DNA in resting T cells. *Sci Transl Med*. (2018) 10:eaar6759. doi: 10.1126/scitranslmed.aar6759.

86. Badia R, Ballana E, Castellvi M, Garcia-Vidal E, Pujantell M, Clotet B, et al. CD32 expression is associated to T-cell activation and is not a marker of the HIV-1 reservoir. *Nat Commun*. (2018) 9:2739. doi: 10.1038/s41467-018-05157-w

87. Su K, Yang H, Li X, Li X, Gibson AW, Cafardi JM, et al. Expression profile of FcgammaRIIb on leukocytes and its dysregulation in systemic lupus erythematosus. *J Immunol*. (2007) 178:3272–80. doi: 10.4049/jimmunol.178.5.3272

88. Liu Y, Gong Y, Qu C, Zhang Y, You R, Yu N, et al. CD32b expression is down-regulated on double-negative memory B cells in patients with Hashimoto's thyroiditis. *Mol Cell Endocrinol*. (2017) 440:1–7. doi: 10.1016/j.mce.2016.11.004

89. Wong KL, Yeap WH, Tai JJ, Ong SM, Dang TM, Wong SC. The three human monocyte subsets: implications for health and disease. *Immunol Res*. (2012) 53:41–57. doi: 10.1007/s12026-012-8297-3

90. Grossetete B, Launay P, Lehuen A, Jungers P, Bach JF, Monteiro RC. Down-regulation of Fc alpha receptors on blood cells of IgA nephropathy patients: evidence for a negative regulatory role of serum IgA. *Kidney Int*. (1998) 53:1321–35.

91. Grossetete B, Viard JP, Lehuen A, Bach JF, Monteiro RC. Impaired Fc alpha receptor expression is linked to increased immunoglobulin A levels and disease progression in HIV-1-infected patients. *AIDS*. (1995) 9:229–34. doi: 10.1097/00002030-199509030-00003

92. Silvain C, Patry C, Launay P, Lehuen A, Monteiro RC. Altered expression of monocyte IgA Fc receptors is associated with defective endocytosis in patients with alcoholic cirrhosis. Potential role for IFN-gamma. *J Immunol*. (1995) 155:1606–18.

93. Berthelot L, Jamin A, Viglietti D, Chemouny JM, Ayari H, Pierre M, et al. Value of biomarkers for predicting immunoglobulin A vasculitis nephritis outcome in an adult prospective cohort. *Nephrol Dial Transplant*. (2017) 33:1579–90. doi: 10.1093/ndt/gfx300

94. Xue J, Zhao Q, Zhu L, Zhang W. Deglycosylation of FcalphaR at N58 increases its binding to IgA. *Glycobiology*. (2010) 20:905–15. doi: 10.1093/glycob/cwq048

95. Monteiro RC. Recent advances in the physiopathology of IgA nephropathy. *Nephrol Ther*. (2018) 14(Suppl 1):S1–8. doi: 10.1016/j.nephro.2018.02.004

96. Vuong MT, Hahn-Zoric M, Lundberg S, Gunnarsson I, van Kooten C, Wramner L, et al. Association of soluble CD89 levels with disease progression but not susceptibility in IgA nephropathy. *Kidney Int*. (2010) 78:1281–7. doi: 10.1038/ki.2010.314

97. Berthelot L, Robert T, Vuiblet V, Tabary T, Braconnier A, Drame M, et al. Recurrent IgA nephropathy is predicted by altered glycosylated IgA, autoantibodies and soluble CD89 complexes. *Kidney Int*. (2015) 88:815–22. doi: 10.1038/ki.2015.158

98. Berthelot L, Papista C, Maciel TT, Biarnes-Pelicot M, Tissandie E, Wang PH, et al. Transglutaminase is essential for IgA nephropathy development acting through IgA receptors. *J Exp Med.* (2012) 209:793–806. doi: 10.1084/jem.20112005

99. Moura IC, Centelles MN, Arcos-Fajardo M, Malheiros DM, Collawn JF, Cooper MD, et al. Identification of the transferrin receptor as a novel immunoglobulin (Ig)A1 receptor and its enhanced expression on mesangial cells in IgA nephropathy. *J Exp Med.* (2001) 194:417–25. doi: 10.1084/jem.194.4.417

100. Tamouza H, Chemouny JM, Raskova Kafkova L, Berthelot L, Flamant M, Demion M, et al. The IgA1 immune complex-mediated activation of the MAPK/ERK kinase pathway in mesangial cells is associated with glomerular damage in IgA nephropathy. *Kidney Int.* (2012) 82:1284–96. doi: 10.1038/ki.2012.192

101. Coulon S, Dussiot M, Grapton D, Maciel TT, Wang PH, Callens C, et al. Polymeric IgA1 controls erythroblast proliferation and accelerates erythropoiesis recovery in anemia. *Nat Med.* (2011) 17:1456–65. doi: 10.1038/nm.2462

102. Kanamaru Y, Arcos-Fajardo M, Moura IC, Tsuge T, Cohen H, Essig M, et al. Fc alpha receptor I activation induces leukocyte recruitment and promotes aggravation of glomerulonephritis through the FcR gamma adaptor. *Eur J Immunol.* (2007) 37:1116–28. doi: 10.1002/eji.200636826

103. Launay P, Patry C, Lehuen A, Pasquier B, Blank U, Monteiro RC. Alternative endocytic pathway for immunoglobulin A Fc receptors (CD89) depends on the lack of FcRgamma association and protects against degradation of bound ligand. *J Biol Chem.* (1999) 274:7216–25. doi: 10.1074/jbc.274.11.7216

104. Honjo K, Kubagawa Y, Suzuki Y, Takagi M, Ohno H, Bucy RP, et al. Enhanced auto-antibody production and Mott cell formation in FcmuR-deficient autoimmune mice. *Int Immunol.* (2014) 26:659–72. doi: 10.1093/intimm/dxu070

105. Ouchida R, Mori H, Hase K, Takatsu H, Kurosaki T, Tokuhisa T, et al. Critical role of the IgM Fc receptor in IgM homeostasis, B-cell survival, and humoral immune responses. *Proc Natl Acad Sci USA.* (2012) 109:E2699–706. doi: 10.1073/pnas.1210706109

106. Li FJ, Kubagawa Y, McCollum MK, Wilson L, Motohashi T, Bertoli LF, et al. Enhanced levels of both the membrane-bound and soluble forms of IgM Fc receptor (FcmuR) in patients with chronic lymphocytic leukemia. *Blood.* (2011) 118:4902–9. doi: 10.1182/blood-2011-04-350793

107. Madarova M, Mucha R, Hresko S, Makarova Z, Gdovinova Z, Szilasiova J, et al. Identification of new phosphorylation sites of CD23 in B-cells of patients with chronic lymphocytic leukemia. *Leuk Res.* (2018) 70:25–33. doi: 10.1016/j.leukres.2018.05.002

108. Tsuboi N, Asano K, Lauterbach M, Mayadas TN. Human neutrophil Fcgamma receptors initiate and play specialized nonredundant roles in antibody-mediated inflammatory diseases. *Immunity.* (2008) 28:833–46. doi: 10.1016/j.immuni.2008.04.013

109. Rossato E, Ben Mkaddem S, Kanamaru Y, Hurtado-Nedelec M, Hayem G, Descatoire V, et al. Reversal of arthritis by human monomeric IgA through the receptor-mediated SH2 domain-containing phosphatase 1 Inhibitory pathway. *Arthritis Rheumatol.* (2015) 67:1766–77. doi: 10.1002/art.39142

110. van der Steen LP, Bakema JE, Sesarman A, Florea F, Tuk CW, Kirtschig G, et al. Blocking Fcalpha receptor I on granulocytes prevents tissue damage induced by IgA autoantibodies. *J Immunol.* (2012) 189:1594–601. doi: 10.4049/jimmunol.1101763

111. Heineke MH, van der Steen LPE, Korthouwer RM, Hage JJ, Langedijk JP M, Benschop JJ, et al. Peptide mimetics of immunoglobulin A (IgA) and FcalphaRI block IgA-induced human neutrophil activation and migration. *Eur J Immunol.* (2017) 47:1835–45. doi: 10.1002/eji.201646782

112. Jardieu PM, Fick RB, Jr. IgE inhibition as a therapy for allergic disease. *Int Arch Allergy Immunol.* (1999) 118:112–5 (1999) doi: 10.1159/000024043

113. Milgrom H, Fick RB Jr, Su JQ, Reimann JD, Bush RK, Watrous ML, et al. Treatment of allergic asthma with monoclonal anti-IgE antibody. rhuMAb-E25 Study Group. *N Engl J Med.* (1999) 341:1966–73. doi: 10.1056/NEJM199912233412603

114. Kazatchkine MD, Kaveri SV. Immunomodulation of autoimmune and inflammatory diseases with intravenous immune globulin. *N Engl J Med.* (2001) 345:747–55. doi: 10.1056/NEJMra993360

115. Pecoraro A, Crescenzi L, Granata F, Genovese A, Spadaro G. Immunoglobulin replacement therapy in primary and secondary antibody deficiency: the correct clinical approach. *Int Immunopharmacol.* (2017). 52:136–42. doi: 10.1016/j.intimp.2017.09.005

116. Jin F, Balthasar JP. Mechanisms of intravenous immunoglobulin action in immune thrombocytopenic purpura. *Hum Immunol.* (2005) 66:403–10. doi: 10.1016/j.humimm.2005.01.029

117. Debre M, Bonnet MC, Fridman WH, Carosella E, Philippe N, Reinert P, et al. Infusion of Fc gamma fragments for treatment of children with acute immune thrombocytopenic purpura. *Lancet.* (1993) 342:945–9. doi: 10.1016/0140-6736(93)92000-J

118. Nimmerjahn F, Ravetch JV. Anti-inflammatory actions of intravenous immunoglobulin. *Annu Rev Immunol.* (2008) 26:513–33. doi: 10.1146/annurev.immunol.26.021607.090232

119. Siragam V, Crow AR, Brinc D, Song S, Freedman J, Lazarus AH. Intravenous immunoglobulin ameliorates ITP via activating Fc gamma receptors on dendritic cells. *Nat Med.* (2006) 12:688–92. doi: 10.1038/nm1416

120. Epstein JS, Zoon KC. Important drug warning: immune globulin intravenous (human) (IGIV) products. *Neonatal Netw.* (2000) 19:60–2.

121. Bolland S, Ravetch JV. Spontaneous autoimmune disease in Fc(gamma)RIIB-deficient mice results from strain-specific epistasis. *Immunity.* (2000) 13:277–85. doi: 10.1016/S1074-7613(00)00027-3

122. van Mirre E, van Royen A, Hack CE. IVIg-mediated amelioration of murine ITP via FcgammaRIIb is not necessarily independent of SHIP-1 and SHP-1 activity. *Blood.* (2004) 103:1973. doi: 10.1182/blood-2003-11-3933

123. Veri MC, Gorlatov S, Li H, Burke S, Johnson S, Stavenhagen J, et al. Monoclonal antibodies capable of discriminating the human inhibitory Fcgamma-receptor IIB (CD32B) from the activating Fcgamma-receptor IIA (CD32A): biochemical, biological and functional characterization. *Immunology.* (2007) 121:392–404. doi: 10.1111/j.1365-2567.2007.02588.x

124. Xiang Z, Cutler AJ, Brownlie RJ, Fairfax K, Lawlor KE, Severinson E, et al. FcgammaRIIb controls bone marrow plasma cell persistence and apoptosis. *Nat Immunol.* (2007) 8:419–29. doi: 10.1038/ni1440

125. Vaccaro C, Zhou J, Ober RJ, Ward ES. Engineering the Fc region of immunoglobulin G to modulate *in vivo* antibody levels. *Nat Biotechnol.* (2005) 23:1283–8. doi: 10.1038/nbt1143

126. Liu L, Garcia AM, Santoro H, Zhang Y, McDonnell K, Dumont J, et al. Amelioration of experimental autoimmune myasthenia gravis in rats by neonatal FcR blockade. *J Immunol.* (2007) 178:5390–8. doi: 10.4049/jimmunol.178.8.5390

127. Zhang Z, Shen K, Lu W, Cole PA. The role of C-terminal tyrosine phosphorylation in the regulation of SHP-1 explored via expressed protein ligation. *J Biol Chem.* (2003) 278:4668–74. doi: 10.1074/jbc.M210028200

128. Jones ML, Craik JD, Gibbins JM, Poole AW. Regulation of SHP-1 tyrosine phosphatase in human platelets by serine phosphorylation at its C terminus. *J Biol Chem.* (2004) 279:40475–83. doi: 10.1074/jbc.M402970200

129. Camps M, Ruckle T, Ji H, Ardissone V, Rintelen F, Shaw J, et al. Blockade of PI3Kgamma suppresses joint inflammation and damage in mouse models of rheumatoid arthritis. *Nat Med.* (2005) 11:936–43. doi: 10.1038/nm1284

130. Huang Y, Li G, An L, Fan Y, Cheng X, Li X, et al. Fyn regulates multipolar-bipolar transition and neurite morphogenesis of migrating neurons in the developing neocortex. *Neuroscience.* (2017) 352:39–51. doi: 10.1016/j.neuroscience.2017.03.032

5

Concurrent Exposure of Neutralizing and Non-Neutralizing Epitopes on a Single HIV-1 Envelope Structure

Krishanu Ray [1,2]*, Meron Mengistu [1,3], Chiara Orlandi [1,3], Marzena Pazgier [1,2], George K. Lewis [1,4] and Anthony L. DeVico [1,3]

[1] Institute of Human Virology, University of Maryland School of Medicine, Baltimore, MD, United States, [2] Department of Biochemistry and Molecular Biology, University of Maryland School of Medicine, Baltimore, MD, United States, [3] Department of Medicine, University of Maryland School of Medicine, Baltimore, MD, United States, [4] Department of Microbiology and Immunology, University of Maryland School of Medicine, Baltimore, MD, United States

Correspondence:
Krishanu Ray
kray@som.umaryland.edu

The trimeric envelope spikes on the HIV-1 virus surface initiate infection and comprise key targets for antiviral humoral responses. Circulating virions variably present intact envelope spikes, which react with neutralizing antibodies; and altered envelope structures, which bind non-neutralizing antibodies. Once bound, either type of antibody can enable humoral effector mechanisms with the potential to control HIV-1 infection *in vivo*. However, it is not clear how the presentation of neutralizing vs. non-neutralizing epitopes defines distinct virus populations and/or envelope structures on single particles. Here we used single-virion fluorescence correlation spectroscopy (FCS), fluorescence resonance energy transfer (FRET), and two-color coincidence FCS approaches to examine whether neutralizing and non-neutralizing antibodies are presented by the same envelope structure. Given the spatial requirements for donor-acceptor energy transfer ($\leq$10 nm), FRET signals generated by paired neutralizing and non-neutralizing fluorescent Fabs should occur via proximal binding to the same target antigen. Fluorescent-labeled Fabs of the neutralizing anti-gp120 antibodies 2G12 and b12 were combined with Fabs of the non-neutralizing anti-gp41 antibody F240, previously thought to mainly bind gp41 "stumps." We find that both 2G12-F240 and/or b12-F240 Fab combinations generate FRET signals on multiple types of virions in solution. FRET efficiencies position the neutralizing and non-neutralizing epitopes between 7.1 and 7.8 nm apart; potentially fitting within the spatial dimensions of a single trimer-derived structure. Further, the frequency of FRET detection suggests that at least one of such structures occurs on the majority of particles in a virus population. Thus, there is frequent, overlapping presentation of non-neutralizing and neutralizing epitope on freely circulating HIV-1 surfaces. Such information provides a broader perspective of how anti-HIV humoral immunity interfaces with circulating virions.

Keywords: single HIV-1 virion, epitope exposure, neutralizing and non-neutralizing epitopes, two-color coincidence fluorescence correlation spectroscopy (FCS), FRET-FCS

INTRODUCTION

Intensive efforts are underway to develop preventive vaccines and therapeutic strategies based on humoral immunity against the HIV-1 envelope (Env). Such efforts logically consider directing antibody responses toward replication competent viral particles. Success in this regard demands an understanding of the epitope patterns expressed by virions and virus populations. On HIV-1 particles, the virus envelope spike is a heavily glycosylated trimer of three heterodimers containing gp120 surface subunits and gp41 transmembrane proteins. Gp120 binds the host cell receptor CD4 and a co-receptor, which triggers gp41 to mediate membrane fusion and viral entry. These antigens exhibit high variability in sequence and structure, driven by and allowing escape from immune pressure (1–13). At the same time, Env antigens can express highly conserved epitopes of various types, e.g., within glycan domains; within the CD4 or co-receptor binding sites; or on gp41. These epitopes are highly attractive targets for vaccine design as human antibodies (bNAbs) against them can be very broadly neutralizing (14–16) and provide potent sterilizing protection against SHIV challenge in macaque infection models (17–19).

The most highly conserved, functional and immutable Env epitopes are not neutralizing, often because they are structurally occluded on free trimers (20–22). Many of these epitopes are exposed as a consequence of natural virus-cell attachment mechanisms (21–23) but it is unclear how they are presented by free virions. One possibility is that non-neutralizing epitopes are expressed on "aberrant," non-functional envelope structures (24–26). Even if disconnected from productive attachment and entry processes, such structures could still mediate antiviral immunity if they appear on replication competent virions. Previous studies showed that non-neutralizing humoral responses directed against non-HIV antigens placed on functional virions mediated protection from SIV or HIV-1 infection in macaque and humanized mouse models, respectively (27–31). Thus, the presence and nature of any Env structure appearing in a virus population warrants careful evaluation in the context of antiviral immunity.

Numerous attempts have been made to characterize the prevalence of non-neutralizing vs. neutralizing epitope presentation in populations of HIV-1 virions and/or to partition HIV-1 virion populations into replication-competent vs. non-functional particles based on differential epitope presentations (9, 25, 26, 32–35). Such work has relied heavily on some manner of virion capture by anti-Env antibodies bound to a substrate. In general, findings from this approach have suggested that virus preparations can contain subpopulations of virions presenting variable mixtures of neutralizing and non-neutralizing epitopes. Subpopulations favoring non-neutralizing epitopes (presumably harboring a large amount of defective or degraded envelope) tend to be poorly- or non-infectious. Although useful, capture systems inform the nature of virions after some sort of adsorption procedure. Associated caveats include altered immunoreactivity patterns caused by the process of substrate attachment; altered virion characteristics caused by the capture manipulations. With some techniques, captured material may represent aggregates of particles as well as single virions. Moreover, capture methods cannot directly reveal whether individual virions present neutralizing and non-neutralizing epitopes on common surface structures, and/or show how frequently such scenarios occur within a virion population.

Previously we developed an analytical method based on fluorescence correlation spectroscopy (FCS) that allows the direct evaluation of mAb binding to HIV-1 virions continuously in solution (36). More recently we adapted this method to enable dual color detection of two different fluorescent-labeled mAbs bound to a single virion as well as detection of Förster resonance energy transfer (FRET) from fluorophores closely localized on single Env spikes. These tools can be used to investigate the relative presentation of neutralizing and non-neutralizing epitopes in virion populations and/or single spikes on an individual particle.

In the present study, the broadly cross-reactive, non-neutralizing F240 epitope (37) in the "Cluster I" domain of gp41 served as the focal point for our experiments. The F240 epitope is located within the immunodominant disulfide loop region of gp41 (38, 39), which is commonly immunoreactive on the surfaces of free virions (33, 34, 36, 40, 41). Although the F240 epitope is occluded on intact Env trimers, it seems to be exposed on undefined Env structures in which gp41 is oxidized (41). Passive transfer of mAb F240 exhibited a marginal degree of protective efficacy against SHIV challenge in macaques (42); a mAb against a related Cluster I epitope, 246D, mediated protection against HIV-1 infection in humanized mice (31); another related mAb, 7B2, (41) reduced the number of transmitted/founder SHIV variants in passively immunized macaques (43). Here we report that the antibodies directed against the F240 epitope and neutralizing gp120 epitopes bind concurrently to single virions via a shared Env-derived structure. Further, our data suggest that most particles in a virus population harbor such structures.

MATERIALS AND METHODS

HIV-1 Pseudovirus Production

HIV-1 BaL and HIV-1 JRFL pseudoviruses were generated by co-transfection of HEK293T cells with an Env-deficient HIV-1 backbone plasmid pNL4-3-ΔE-EGFP along with Env-expression plasmids (44, 45) pHIV-1-BaL 0.1 (obtained through the AIDS Research and Reference Reagent Program, Division of AIDS, NIAID) and pCAGGS-JRFL (kindly provided by J. Binley, Torrey Pines Institute of Molecular Studies, San Diego, CA). Transfections were accomplished using FuGENE 6 (Roche, Indianapolis, IN) transfection reagent at a 3:1 reagent-DNA ratio. To produce the infectious molecular clone of transmitted/founder (T/F) HIV-1 AD17 virus (46), HEK293T cells were transfected with the AD17 plasmid (kindly provided by B. Hahn, University of Pennsylvania) at a FuGENE-to-DNA ratio of 3:1. Virions-containing supernatant was harvested after 3 days, and concentrated about 10-fold by incubating with PEG-it™ virus precipitation solution (System Biosciences, Mountain View, CA) for 18 h at 4°C as recommended by vendor.

The antigen content of all virion preparations was quantified using p24 and gp120 antigen capture ELISAs. Infectivity was established using standardized procedures (47) and quantified as function of TCID$_{50}$ in TZM-bl cells. HIV-1 BaL and HIV-1 JRFL pseudoviruses with gp120 to p24 ratio of 1:10–1:50, and 200,000–500,000 TCID50/mL; HIV-1 AD17 T/F with gp120 to p24 ratio of 1:200, and 600,000 to 1,000,000 TCID50/mL were used for FCS measurements. The Aldrithiol-2 (AT-2) inactivated (48, 49) HIV-1 BaL virus produced in SupT1-CCR5 CL.30 cells was generously provided by Dr. Jeff Lifson (AIDS Vaccine Program/NCI, Frederick, MD). pEGFP-Vpr (cat# 11386 from Dr. Warner C. Greene) plasmid (50) obtained through the AIDS Research and Reference Reagent Program, Division of AIDS, NIAID, NIH, was used to generate fluorescent HIV-1 BaL pseudoviruses.

Antibodies

mAbs b12, 2G12, PG9, and F240 were purchased from Polymun Scientific (Vienna, Austria). mAbs 17b and N49P7 (14) were expressed from plasmid clones in HEK293T cells using an IgG1 backbone for heavy-chain variable regions and either a κ- or λ-chain expression vector for light-chain variable regions. mAbs were purified from culture supernatants by protein-A chromatography. Fabs of b12, 2G12, PG9, N49P7 or F240 were prepared from purified IgG (10 mg/ml) by proteolytic digestion with immobilized papain (Pierce, Rockford, IL) and purified using protein A (GE Healthcare, Piscataway, NJ), followed by gel filtration chromatography on a Superdex 200 16/60 column (GE Healthcare, Piscataway, NJ). All mAbs or Fabs were fluorescently labeled and purified with Alexa 488, 568, or 647 monoclonal Antibody Labeling Kit (Invitrogen, Molecular Probes, Eugene, OR). Briefly, the Alexa dye has a succinimidyl ester moiety that reacts efficiently with primary amines of antibody to form stable dye-protein conjugates. Each labeling reaction was performed with 100 μg of a mAb or Fab. The labeled antibody was separated from unreacted dye by centrifugation through a spin column at 1,100x g for 5 min. Recovered antibodies were dialyzed against phosphate buffered saline as necessary. Labeled mAbs or Fabs were quantified by a UV-vis spectrometer (Nanodrop 2000, Thermo-Scientific, Wilmington, DE). Dye to protein ratios were determined by measuring absorbance at 280 nm (protein) vs. absorbance at corresponding wavelength for Alexa 488, 568, or 647. Conjugated mAbs or Fabs used in our experiments had an optimal dye to protein ratio in the range of 1–2 dye per molecule of mAb or Fab.

Two-Color Fluorescence Correlation Spectroscopy

Fluorescence Correlation Spectroscopy (FCS) is a methodology that allows real-time detection of multiple protein-protein interactions in solution, by measuring diffusion and reaction kinetics of fluorescently-labeled biomolecules (51). Two-color FCS (52) has been used to monitor two different mAbs bound to HIV-1 virions. The binding of Alexa 488 or 647-labeled mAbs b12, 2G12, 17b, F240, and anti-RSV antibody, Synagis (negative control) to HIV-1 virions was monitored by tracking diffusion of their fluorescent label across the observation area, where unbound antibodies will diffuse much faster than those that

bound viral particles as described in Ray et al. (36). Briefly, HIV-1 BaL pseudovirions were diluted to 10 μg/mL p24 equivalent in a 100-μL reaction volume (gp120:p24 ratio of 1:50), and were first incubated with 100 μg/mL non-specific IgG1 (1.5 μL of a 7 mg/mL stock) for 90 min at 37°C to block non-specific binding. Then 1 μL of the test Alexa conjugated mAbs (2 μg/mL of each mAb) was introduced and allowed to interact with pseudovirions for 90 min at 37°C. For spectroscopic measurements, 11 μL of the reaction mixture was loaded onto an FCS slide reservoir, sealed, then placed on a time-resolved confocal microscope (ISS Q2) with a high numerical aperture (NA = 1.2) water objective (60x magnification). The excitation source was a Fianium SC-400 super-continuum laser. NKT super-select acousto-optical tunable filter (AOTF) filter was used to select the excitation wavelengths. The beam after AOTF was passed through narrow bandpass clean-up filters. The samples were excited with two coincident excitation at 470 and 635 nm, and fluorescence signals from the Alexa 488 (A488) or Alexa 647 (A647) mAbs were collected in two separate detection channels in the 500–550 nm and 650–720 nm region over 60 s in a constant detection volume (~1 fL) that is continuously replenished. ISS Vista vision software was used to generate the autocorrelation function of the fluorescent fluctuations of the Alexa labeled mAbs. The autocorrelation function of fluorescence intensities is given by the product of the mAb intensity at time t, $I(t)$ with the intensity after a delay time τ, $I(t+\tau)$, typically in the range from 10^{-2} to 10^2 ms, averaged over the 60 s of measurement.

For experiments in which only the conjugated mAbs and no virions were present, the autocorrelation function was fitted with a single species diffusion model equation. Diffusion coefficients of the fluorescent species under these conditions were routinely determined to be 60 μm^2/s. These values matched what was predicted for 150 kD IgG molecules in solution. In reactions with mAbs and virions, the autocorrelation was fit to a two-species diffusion model. In this operation, one species had the unbound mAb diffusion coefficient of 60 μm^2/s, and the second a diffusion coefficient of 6 μm^2/s, matching the predicted behavior of fluorescent mAbs bound to a 100 nm retroviral particle. The fitting equations were also used to determine the percentage of total mAb exhibiting the slower diffusion rate in reactions with virions. The mathematical derivation and application of the equations is described in (36). The cross-correlation measures (52, 53) between the two separate detection channels determined if two signal intensities were correlated; i.e., fluctuated in concert or independently. Only pairs of co-incident photon counts from two distinct channels (500–550 and 650–720 nm in the present case) will show positive correlation amplitude. Only dual-color cross-correlation data of two different antibodies in the presence of HIV-1 virion showing positive correlation amplitude were taken as evidence that two different antibodies bound to the same virion particle.

Characterization of Single Virion FCS Measures

As dual-label FRET measures cannot distinguish the number of targets based on signal intensity, they are most clearly interpreted when there are limiting amount of virions in the focal volume. This situation can be favored by appropriate dilutions of the virus stock. In theory, the amount of p24 in a virus preparation may be used for this purpose, assuming 10^4 virus particles per picogram of p24 (54, 55). To better determine how p24 measures could be used in this manner with our virus preparations, we generated HIV-1 BaL pseudoviruses using the usual methods, but also containing an eGFP.Vpr fluorescent marker. The eGFP.Vpr HIV-1 BaL stock contained $3\,\mu g/ml$ of p24, which based on 10^4 virus particles/picogram of p24 (54, 55), converts to 3×10^7 particles/μL or roughly 0.03 virus particle per femtoliter assuming that virions are evenly dispersed. Serially dilutions of virus were then analyzed by FCS (**Figure S1**), which detected the eGFP.Vpr signal and thereby quantified the number of particles in the focal volume at any one time. The number of fluorescent virions were determined by fitting the autocorrelation plot and extracting the correlation amplitude G(0) (51, 53). The number of molecules detected in the FCS focal volume is inverse of the correlation amplitude (51, 53). The diffusion coefficient of the eGFP.Vpr HIV-1 BaL pseudoviruses signals (5 $\mu m^2/s$) matched those previously determined for single pseudovirus particles (36). As shown in **Figure S1**, there was the expected linear relationship between p24 concentration and number of virions measured by FCS. Notably, the FCS analyses detected substantially more virions in the focal volume than what was predicted by p24 measures (for example, although $3\,\mu g/ml$ was predicted to translate into 1 virion/33fL; FCS indicated there was 1 virion/1.6 fL). FRET-FCS can only be performed with unlabeled virions as the signal from the eGFP fluorescent virion will interfere with the signal from fluorescent tagged mAbs or Fabs. Thus, a conversion factor was determined and used for experiments with other unlabeled viruses (see below) to normalize p24 concentrations to the probable numbers of virions ($\sim$1.5) being seen in the FCS focal volume of 1fL.

FRET-FCS Measurements

For FRET measurements, the Fabs (b12, 2G12, PG9, N49P7 or F240) were labeled with either donor (Alexa 488) or acceptor (Alexa 568) probes (Invitrogen mAb labeling kit). Dye-to-protein ratios were determined by measuring absorbance at 280 nm (protein) vs. 488 or 577 nm (dye). The dye-to-protein ratios were between 1 and 2. We specifically aimed to keep this low label of dye labeling as we are using a single molecule fluorescence method and minimally perturb the functionality of the protein. FRET measurements were performed in a confocal microscope (ISS Q2) equipped with a supercontinuum laser and AOTF in order to excite the molecules during its diffusion through the confocal volume. ISS Vistavision software was used to generate the FRET histogram and further analyses. FRET measurements were performed after forming complex with the HIV-1 BaL, HIV-1 JRFL, AT-2 inactivated HIV-1 BaL or HIV-1 AD17 T/F virions with donor-labeled Fab and acceptor labeled Fab. The number of virions at any given time was around 1.5 particle in the 1fL focal volume as described above.

Fluorescence responses from the donor and the acceptor molecules were separated by a dichroic beam splitter and detected by two avalanche photodiode detectors (APD) using the method of time-correlated single photon counting and the Time-Tagged Time-Resolved (TTTR) mode of the Becker and Hickl SPC-150

module. High quality bandpass (Chroma) filters were used for laser clean-up and recording donor and acceptor fluorescence in two separate detection channels. The collected single photon data was binned by 3.4 ms (corresponding to the diffusion time of the 100 nm diameter virion particle) in each channel (donor or acceptor), which resulted in intensity-time traces recorded for 120 s. Threshold values in each channel were used to identify the single molecule bursts from the corresponding background signal level. Fluorescence bursts were recorded simultaneously in donor and acceptor channels and FRET efficiencies were calculated using $E = I_A/(I_A + \gamma I_D)$ where I_D and I_A are the sums of donor counts and acceptor counts for each burst, taking into account the possible difference in the detection efficiency (γ) in two separate channels (56–60). The analyses revealed fractional quantity of FRET efficiency events for a specified bin and recorded time of the donor-acceptor intensity traces. For a measurement time of 120 s and sampling frequency of 300, total number of 36,000 events can be possibly obtained. It is important to note that an event is likely no more than two virions in the FCS observation volume of 1fL based on input concentration of p24 as shown in **Figure S1**. For each sample containing donor Fabs, acceptor Fabs and HIV-1 virions, fractions of FRET events relating to the total possible events for a given bin time or sampling frequency and measurement time were determined and subsequently the number of occurrences vs. FRET efficiency histogram plots were generated. The donor-to-acceptor distance (r) in terms of efficiency of energy transfer (E) and Förster Distance (R_0) is given by $r = R_0\ [1/E - 1]^{1/6}$. We have used the value of R_0 of 6.2 nm for the Alexa 488 (donor) and Alexa 568 (acceptor) pair for estimating the donor-to-acceptor distances. In addition to FRET measurements we have also performed FCS measurements to assess the *in vitro* binding of Fab fragments to HIV-1 virions. Consequently, we determined the translational diffusion coefficients of Alexa 488 or 568 labeled Fabs and the corresponding bound virion complexes from FCS measurements. The FCS measurements and analyses were performed as previously reported (21, 36, 57–60).

Assembly of Structural Models of b12 and 2G12 Bound to HIV Env

The model was assembled based on the available CryoEM structure of the virion associated HIV-1 trimer complexed with b12 Fab [PDB: 3DNL, (61)] and crystallographic structure of 2G12 Fab bound to $Man_9GlcNAc_2$ [PDB code: 6N2X, (62)]. 2G12 Fab was modeled into the b12 Fab-HIV-1 trimer by superimposition of the $Man_9GlcNAc_2$ moiety of the 2G12 Fab-$Man_9GlcNAc_2$ complex to the trimer at N-linked glycan at position 332 (62). The distances are measured from the center of each variable domain of Fab.

RESULTS

Previously we used FCS and fluorescent labeled proteins to examine the binding of individual anti-envelope mAbs or sCD4 to HIV-1 particles representing various strains with all reactants

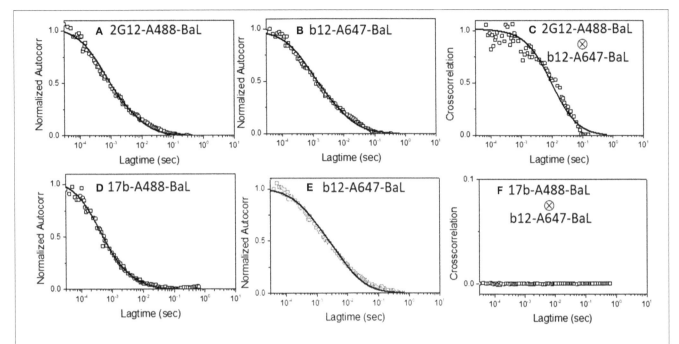

FIGURE 1 | Dual-color correlation curves of **(A–C)** 2G12-A488 and b12-A647 and **(D–F)** 17b-A488 and b12-A647 with HIV-1 BaL virions. **(A,D)** show autocorrelation plots of Alexa 488 labeled mAbs. **(B,E)** show autocorrelation plots of Alexa 647 labeled mAbs. **(C,F)** show cross-correlation curves of b12-A647 and 2G12-A488 or b12-A647 and 17b-A488 with HIV-1 BaL virions. Two color excitation wavelengths at 470 and 635 nm were used. All experiments were repeated three times with similar results.

in solution (21, 36, 41). These studies showed that the Alexa - labeled anti-gp120 bNAbs 2G12 (63) and b12 (64), and the non-neutralizing anti-gp41 mAb F240 (37, 41), bound efficiently and consistently to virions (21, 36). However, these studies did not address whether two antibodies, each of different specificity, bind to the same virion or to the same Env structure on a particle surface. We reasoned that dual color detection and FRET-FCS should afford a means to address this question.

Epitope Exposure on Single Virions by Dual Color FCS

We first applied the dual color detection method to explore the binding of two different mAbs to single HIV-1 BaL pseudovirus particles. We employed anti-envelope mAbs including b12 [a broadly neutralizing CD4 binding site antibody (64)], 2G12 [against a carbohydrate cluster on gp120 (63)], and F240 [against a cluster 1 epitope in gp41 (37, 41)] labeled with either Alexa 488 or Alexa 647. Monoclonal antibody 17b was tested as a negative control. This mAb recognizes a CD4-induced epitope on gp120 (65), binds weakly to HIV-1 BaL in the absence of sCD4, and partially competes with b12 for gp120 binding due to partial epitope overlap (20, 66). Thus, mAbs 17b and b12 are unlikely to bind the same virion except through non-specific processes. **Figure 1** shows the dual-color FCS measurements of Alexa-488 labeled 2G12 and Alexa-647 labeled b12 binding. Autocorrelation plots (**Figures 1A,B**) showed that in the reaction 42 and 45% of b12 or 2G12 mAbs, respectively, adopted the slower diffusion coefficient (6 $\mu m^2/s$) marking virion-bound mAb. Similar binding efficiencies for these mAbs were reported previously

(36). Importantly, cross-correlation analyses (51, 53) (**Figure 1C**) of signals simultaneously detected in the two channels could also be fitted to the same single diffusion coefficient 6 $\mu m^2/s$. Such findings reflect that both 2G12 and b12 being bound to the same object, having the size of a retrovirus particle. In comparison, analyses of b12-A647 and 17b-A488 mixed with HIV-1 BaL virions showed no cross-correlation in binding signals (**Figures 1D–F**). Taken together, the data obtained with mAb pairs 2G12 and b12 indicated that the dual color coincidence FCS assay system could reflect the epitope exposure patterns on virus particles in solution.

A second set of experiments examined whether a single virion binds 2G12 neutralizing mAbs along with mAb F240. In these experiments, mAb F240 was labeled with Alexa-488 and mAb 2G12 with Alexa-647, the targets were again HIV-1 BaL pseudoviruses. **Figure 2** shows the dual-color FCS measurements of Alexa-488 labeled F240 and Alexa-647 labeled 2G12 binding to HIV-1 BaL virions. Autocorrelation plots (**Figures 2A,B**) showed that in the reaction 35 and 45% of F240 or 2G12 mAbs, respectively, adopted the slower diffusion coefficient (6 $\mu m^2/s$) marking virion-bound mAb. Similar binding profiles of fluorescently labeled F240 or 2G12 to HIV-1 BaL were reported previously (36). As in the experiments pairing 2G12 with b12 (**Figure 1**), cross-correlation analyses showed simultaneous signal detection in the two channels (**Figure 2C**) fitting a single diffusion coefficient of ~6 $\mu m^2/s$, indicating that 2G12 and F240 bound to the same virion particle. To verify these results further, the binding of both 2G12 and F240 mAbs was assessed with AT-2 inactivated HIV-1 BaL virions produced and

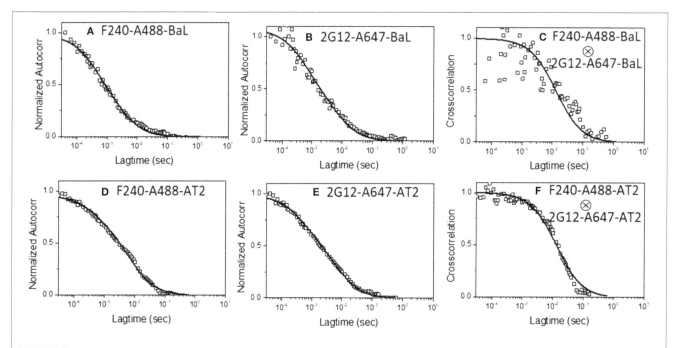

FIGURE 2 | Dual-color correlation curves of F240-A488 and 2G12-A647 with **(A–C)** HIV-1 BaL, and **(D–F)** AT-2 HIV-1 BaL virions. **(A,D)** show autocorrelation plots for F240-A488 with HIV-1 BaL and AT-2 HIV-1 BaL virions; **(B,E)** show autocorrelation plots of 2G12-A647 with HIV-1 BaL, and AT-2 HIV-1 BaL virions; **(C,F)** show cross-correlation curves of F240-A488 and 2G12-A647 with HIV-1 BaL and AT-2 HIV-1 BaL virions. The experiment was repeated three times with similar results.

purified in a different manner (41, 49). Similar auto-correlation (**Figures 2D,E**) and cross-correlation (**Figure 2F**) profiles were observed with Alexa-488 labeled F240 and Alexa-647 labeled 2G12 binding to AT-2 inactivated HIV-1 BaL virions.

Epitope Exposure on Individual Env Structures on HIV-1 Virions by FRET-FCS

Having determined that the above mAb pairs concurrently bind single virus particles, we next examined whether combinations of the above antibodies were attaching to the same Env structure on the virion. The FRET-FCS method relies on standard dipole-dipole interactions between paired donor and acceptor fluorophores, which occurs within the distance range of 2–10 nm. Thus, paired fluorescent mAbs will not create FRET signals unless they bind to tightly localized epitopes. To mitigate spatial differences caused by the probe length (i.e., whole IgG) and more precisely estimate the donor-acceptor distances, the FRET-FCS experiments employed labeled Fab fragments. The use of Fabs also enabled interpretations of FRET data vs. available structural data for Fab-Env complexes. The fluorophores pairs used in all experiments were Alexa-488 (A488 donor) and Alexa-568 (A568 acceptor). The test viruses (see below) were used at final concentrations of 10 μg/ml, which, based on relationship shown in **Figure S1**, was predicted to produce roughly 1.5 virions in the focal volume at any time.

The FRET-FCS system was first applied toward analyses of neutralizing epitopes. Reaction mixtures were constructed with fluorescent labeled 2G12 (A488 donor) and b12 (A568 acceptor) Fabs and HIV-1 BaL virions (see methods). As shown in **Figure 3**, FRET signals from the acceptor probe were indeed

detected, following a diffusion coefficient of 6 μm^2/s clearly distinguished from the ~80 μm^2/s value expected for an unbound Fab. The FRET signals fit a Gaussian profile with a mean FRET efficiency of ~25% (**Figure 3A**). These data indicated that the two Fabs occupied a highly localized space on bound virions. FRET efficiency was not biased by the donor/acceptor labeling configuration as swapping the donor-acceptor labeling between b12 Fabs and 2G12 Fabs yielded highly similar measures (**Figure 3B**). According to Forster's equation (see methods) the calculated mean FRET efficiencies were consistent with a situation where the donor and acceptor Fabs bound to virions at an average distance of 7.4 nm apart. To validate these findings, we used existing structural information (61, 67) to model (see methods) the binding of 2G12 and b12 Fabs to a single HIV-1 trimer (**Figure 4**). This exercise predicts that the Fabs would be spaced ~7.1 nm apart if bound to the same protomer and ~7.4 nm apart if each is bound to a different protomer in the same trimer. In either case, the modeling predictions closely match those calculated from the FRET efficiencies. However, it must be noted that the Alexa conjugation chemistry does not place fluorophores at single, specified positions along the length of Fabs. Thus, FRET efficiencies, and derivative donor-acceptor distances, reflect aggregate measures of spatial ranges between paratopes and fluorophores on the two Fab probes. Given that Fabs are ~3 nm long, up to 3 nm in extra distance between epitopes could be added when fluorophores are positioned at maximum distances from paratopes on each probe. However, even in this extreme situation the two epitopes can still be placed within the spatial constraints of a single trimer.

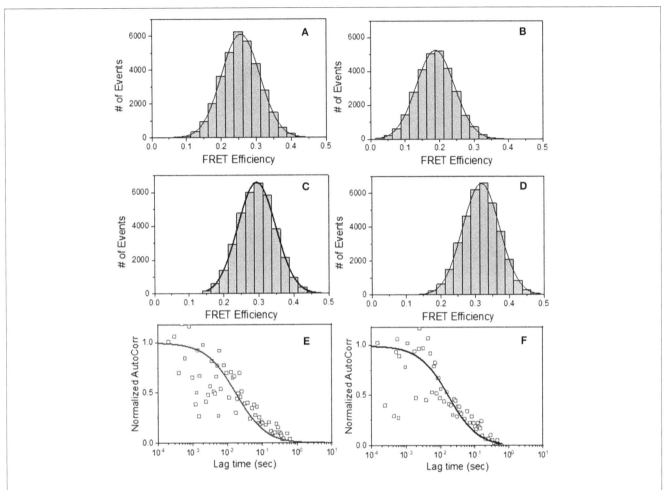

FIGURE 3 | FRET histograms of **(A)** b12 Fab-A488 and 2G12 Fab-A568 **(B)** 2G12 Fab-A488 and b12 Fab-A568, **(C)** b12 Fab-A488 and F240 Fab-A568 and **(D)** F240 Fab-A488 and b12 Fab-A568 with HIV-1 BaL virions. The solid lines in **(A–D)** are fit with a Gaussian distribution to the experimental FRET histogram data. Autocorrelation plots of the acceptor channel for **(E)** b12 Fab-A488 and 2G12 Fab-A568 and **(F)** b12 Fab-A488 and F240 Fab-A568 with HIV-1 BaL virions. The solid lines in **(E,F)** represent the fit to the experimental data. All experiments were repeated three times with similar results.

The prevalence of the above associations in the virus population was considered by comparing the events that exhibited any degree of FRET signal (**Figures 3A,B**) to the total number of events possibly observed under the reaction conditions used (see methods for calculation). These analyses indicated that in reactions with b12 Fab-A488 and 2G12 Fab-A568 or 2G12 Fab-A488 and b12 Fab-A568, donor-acceptor pairs, FRET signals covered 70–75% of the total possible observable events under the experimental system. Taken together, the data indicated that b12 and 2G12 Fabs bound to a single Env structure presented by the majority of particles observed in the FCS system.

We next applied FRET-FCS to reaction mixtures containing Fab fragments of b12 and F240 mixed with the HIV-1 BaL virions. The labeling of the two Fabs (A488 donor vs. A568 acceptor) were reciprocally interchanged to confirm that any FRET measures were not biased by the donor/acceptor labeling strategy. Moreover, FRET signals were not detected in reactions with donor (A488) and acceptor (A568) labeled Fabs in the

absence of HIV-1 virions (data not shown). This was expected, as there was no reason for the Fabs to remain in association outside of random diffusion such that a FRET signal could be generated. As shown in **Figure 3**, FRET signals were again detected when combinations of b12 Fab-A488 and F240 Fab-A568 (Panel C) or F240 Fab-A488 and b12 Fab-A568 (Panel D) were mixed with HIV-1 BaL. Single diffusion coefficients calculated for the acceptor channel were 6 $\mu m^2/s$, consistent with signals emanating from objects with the size of HIV virions (**Figures 3E,F**). As above, the number of events that exhibited any degree of FRET signal (**Figures 3C,D**) were compared to the total number of events possibly observed in the system considering the recording time and sampling frequency (see methods). The analyses showed that in reactions with b12 Fab-A488 and F240 Fab-A568 or F240 Fab-A488 and b12 Fab-A568 donor-acceptor pairs, FRET signals covered 75 and 72% of the total possible observable events in the system. Gaussian fitting to the FRET histogram data (**Figures 3C,D**) reflected FRET efficiencies of 30–35% regardless of dye pairing. This in turn

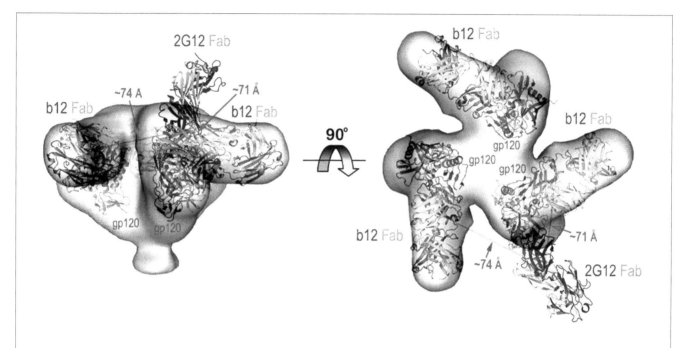

FIGURE 4 | Molecular model for b12 and 2G12 Fabs bound to the same HIV-1 trimer. The model was built using cryoEM structure of the virion associated HIV-1 trimer complexed with b12 Fab and 2G12 Fab-Man$_9$GlcNAc$_2$ complex as described in Methods. The relative distances (shown as red dotted lines) between the Fabs were measured from the centers of variable domains of each Fab. Molecular surface is displayed over the HIV-trimer and Fabs are shown in ribbon diagrams.

indicates that b12 Fab and F240 Fab bind in close proximity; ~7.1 nm apart (in the range of 6.6–8 nm) on some sort of gp120-gp41 complex.

Similar experiments were carried out with 2G12 Fab-A488 and F240 Fab-A568 pairs. **Figure 5A** shows the FRET histogram of the Fabs with HIV-1 BaL virions. Again, the histogram plot reflected 30% FRET efficiency and Fab positions ~7.1 nm apart (in the range of 6.4–8.1 nm). The FCS auto-correlation curve in the acceptor channel exhibited only a single diffusion corresponding to a HIV-1 BaL virion. To determine whether the FRET-FCS measures with HIV-1 BaL virions were generalizable, additional experiments were conducted in which the targets were either AT-2 inactivated HIV-1 BaL virus (produced in SupT1-CCR5 CL.30 cells) (41, 49) or a transmitted founder (T/F) infectious molecular clone (AD17) produced in HEK293T cells (36). As shown in **Figure 5**, both viruses exhibited FRET signals when reacted with 2G12 Fab-A488 and F240-Fab-A568 donor-acceptor pairs. The FRET pattern with the AT-2 inactivated HIV-1 BaL (**Figure 5C**), and predicted binding distance of the Fabs were comparable to what was detected with the HIV-1 BaL pseudovirus (**Figure 5A**). Between the two viruses, a slightly lower FRET efficiency was observed for HIV-1 AD17 (**Figure 5B**). One possible explanation is that HIV-1 BaL and AD17 present slightly different gp120-gp41 surface structures coincidently reactive with both Fab F240 and Fab 2G12. In any case, FRET-linked concurrent binding of the Fabs comprised 66, 58, and 58% of the total possible events in the system (see methods) for the HIV-1 BaL; HIV-1 AD17 or AT-2 inactivated HIV-1 BaL virions, respectively. These FRET-reactive fractions

of the virus population were lower than what was observed with co-localized binding of b12 and F240 Fabs (see above).

HIV-1 BaL is a "tier 1b" virus, meaning it has a relatively "open" Env structure more sensitive to neutralization by a wider variety of anti-Env mAbs. Thus, we performed additional FRET-FCS experiments with a tier-2, CCR5 tropic JRFL pseudovirus; i.e., one expressing a "closed" Env structure resistant to neutralization by most mAbs. Reactions were run with fluorescent labeled neutralizing Fabs of 2G12, b12, N49P7 [a CD4 binding site potent broadly neutralizing mAb (14)] and PG9 [a potent broadly neutralizing mAb targeted to quaternary structure in the V1-V2 loops of gp120 (68–70)] along with F240 Fab. The PG9 gp120 epitope is predicted to be at a substantial distance (~9 nm) from F240 in a single trimer, approaching the limit where FRET becomes undetectable. Nevertheless, PG9 Fab was tested as it interacts with two gp120 protomers in the trimer (68–70) and thus could inform the nature of the target antigen. Specifically, any FRET between PG9 and F240 Fab pairs could indicate the presence of two gp120s in the cognate Env structure. As shown in **Figure 6**, FRET signals were detected when combinations of 2G12 Fab-A488 and F240 Fab-A568 (Panel A); b12 Fab-A488 and F240 Fab-A568 (Panel B) were reacted with HIV-1 JRFL. The average FRET efficiencies for the 2G12-F240 and b12-F240 combinations were 25 and 20%, respectively similar to those observed with the tier-1 HIV-1 BaL virions. Accordingly, the calculated average distances for the 2G12-F240 and b12-F240 Fab pair combinations with HIV-1 BaL virion were 7.4 and 7.8 nm, respectively. FRET signals for the 2G12-F240 and b12-F240 Fab pairs with HIV-1 JRFL virions

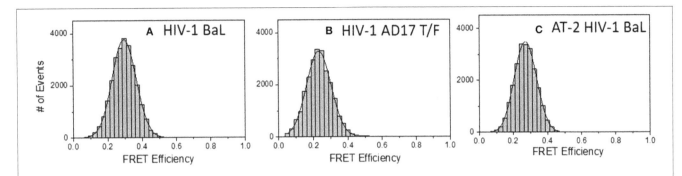

FIGURE 5 | FRET histograms of 2G12 Fab-A488 and F240 Fab-A568 reacted with different virus types: **(A)** HIV-1 BaL, **(B)** HIV-1 AD17 transmitted/founder, and **(C)** AT-2 HIV-1 BaL. The solid lines in **(A–C)** are fit with a Gaussian distribution to the experimental FRET histogram data. All measurements were repeated three times with similar results.

comprised 54 and 61% of the total possible observable events in the system.

FRET signals and efficiencies of 20% between N49P7 Fab-A488 and F240 Fab-A568 with HIV-1 JRFL virions (**Figure 6C**) reflected an average distance of 7.8 nm (in the range of 6.6–8.6 nm) between the two Fabs. This distance is similar to the average distance observed with b12-F240 Fab pairs, as expected, considering both b12 and N49P7 are CD4bs mAbs. FRET signals for the N49P7-F240 Fabs with HIV-1 JRFL virions comprised 56% of the total possible observable events in the system. The histogram for the combinations of PG9 Fab-A488 and F240 Fab-A568 mixed with HIV-1 JRFL (**Figure 6D**) reflected a FRET efficiency of about 10% for PG9-F240 pairs suggesting an average distance of 9 nm (in the range of 7.5–9.5 nm) between the two Fabs. As noted above, this result is in accordance with the available structural information of the distance between the PG9 epitope in the V1-V2 region of gp120 and F240 epitope in gp41 (41, 68–70). Notably, FRET signals from the PG9-F240 Fabs with HIV-1 JRFL virions comprised only 32% of the total possible observable events. The fit to autocorrelation plots (**Figures 6E–H**) for the acceptor channel for all the neutralizing and non-neutralizing Fab combinations showed single diffusion coefficients of 6 μm^2/s, consistent with signals emanating from objects with the size of HIV-1 virions.

DISCUSSION

Our previous FCS experiments showed that neutralizing mAbs 2G12, b12, and PG9; and the non-neutralizing anti-gp41mAb F240, bind often and efficiently to various pseudoviruses and full length infectious molecular clones produced in different ways (36). However, those analyses did not distinguish whether each mAb bound a specific subset of virions, nor did they reflect how individual virions react with multiple mAb specificities. Under the FCS conditions used here, we were able to make such determinations as each measured fluorescence event stemmed from roughly 1–2 particles in the focal volume being assayed (**Figure S1**). The diffusion coefficients of the collected signals further affirmed that they arose from objects the size of retroviral particles.

Dual color FCS established that the neutralizing mAbs 2G12 and b12 concurrently bound the majority of individual HIV-1 BaL pseudovirions in the population (**Figure 1**), and frequently enabled FRET signals (**Figure 3**) indicating occupancy of the same functional trimer, consistent with structural predictions obtained by *in silico* modeling (**Figure 4**). Observations of neutralizing antibodies bind concurrently to the same trimer are not particularly surprising from a virological standpoint; but the data as such support the utility of the approach. Moving to FRET analyses of other epitopes, a more unexpected yet consistent observation was the concurrent and highly localized binding of F240 Fab and 2G12 Fab to HIV-1 BaL and JRFL viruses; AT-2 inactivated HIV-1 BaL virions from another source; and the HIV-1 AD17 T/F molecular clone (**Figures 5, 6**). We also detected tightly localized binding of F240 Fab and N49P7 or PG9 Fab on the Tier 2 HIV-1 JRFL pseudoviruses (**Figure 6**).

The F240 epitope is occluded on intact Env trimers (41) and is often assumed to reside only on gp41 "stumps" on the virion surface (26). We cannot eliminate the possibility that some virions present such gp41 structures. Nevertheless, our data suggest the existence of another, previously unexpected type of Env structure that expresses the F240 epitope within 10 nm of a variety of broadly neutralizing sites, spaced to avoid steric competition between cognate Fabs. It seems implausible that multiple Env-derived structures (e.g., a gp41 "stump" and non-specifically adsorbed gp120 monomers of some sort) could develop a surface structure comprising the epitope positioning we measured. A more likely possibility is that the F240 and gp120 epitopes are co-located on a misfolded or partially denatured trimer segment that remains membrane-anchored, retains one or more gp120 protomers, and exposes the gp41 Cluster I domain. Detection of FRET with F240 and PG9 Fabs suggests the presence of two closely spaced gp120 protomers in the target antigen. However, FRET signals for these Fabs were detected less often (roughly 30%) among the total possible observable events, compared to the other epitope pairs. One explanation for the difference is that F240 and PG9 are co-expressed on a relatively infrequent structure, compared to a more common one expressing F240 with 2G12, b12, or N49P7. Another explanation could be

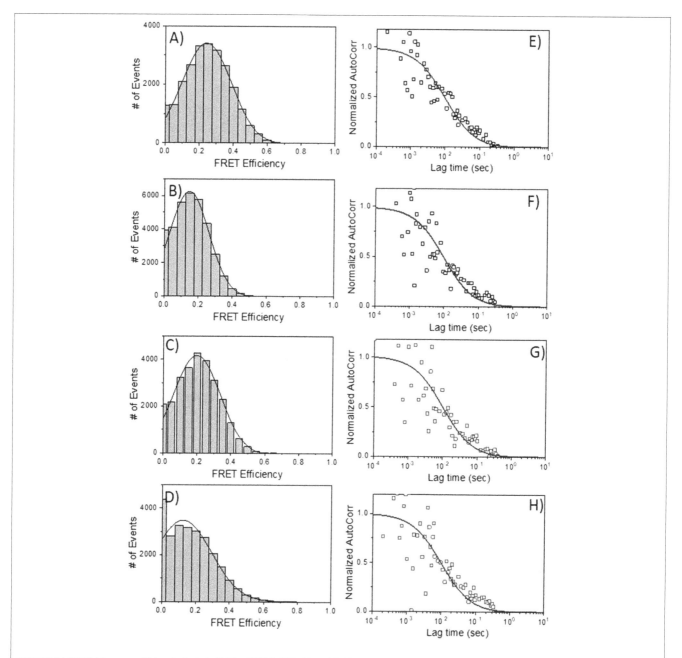

FIGURE 6 | FRET histograms of Fab pairs tested with Tier 2 HIV-1 JRFL virions. **(A)** 2G12 Fab-A488 and F240 Fab-A568; **(B)** b12 Fab-A488 and F240 Fab-A568; **(C)** N49P7 Fab-A488 and F240 Fab-A568 and **(D)** PG9 Fab-A488 and F240 Fab-A568. The solid lines in **(A–D)** are fit with a Gaussian distribution to the experimental FRET histogram data. Autocorrelation plots of the acceptor channel for **(E)** 2G12 Fab-A488 and F240 Fab-A568; **(F)** b12 Fab-A488 and F240 Fab-A568; **(G)** N49P7 Fab-A488 and F240 Fab-A568 and **(H)** PG9 Fab-A488 and F240 Fab-A568 with HIV-1 JRFL virions. The solid lines in **(E–H)** represent the fit to the experimental data. All measurements were repeated three times with similar results.

dynamic and heterogeneous positioning of PG9 Fab vs. F240 Fab, sometimes outside the FRET window, within the virion population. **Figure 7** summarizes potential scenarios for F240 and neutralizing anti-gp120 epitope presentation on virions that are consistent with the FCS data considered above. It must be noted that these sorts of Env antigens have not been apparent via virion capture approaches. One possible explanation is that the gp120-gp41 interactions in these structures are too

fragile to withstand the capture process without experiencing further degradation.

Humoral immunity includes multiple Fab- and/or Fc-driven mechanisms capable of suppressing viral infections. Thus, any conserved viral epitopes on replication-competent viruses, even if non-neutralizing, are potential points of vulnerability. Humoral responses against influenza and Ebola viruses are important cases in point, where protection from infection by

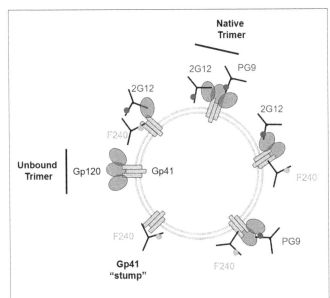

FIGURE 7 | Array of some possible structures on virion surfaces including ones that could co-express F240 and neutralizing epitopes. 2G12 and PG9 epitopes are shown as examples of the latter.

non-neutralizing antibodies has been repeatedly demonstrated (71–75). In the HIV-1 system, non-neutralizing epitopes are often considered in the context of aberrant Env structures (e.g., gp41 "stumps") on replication-defective particles while broadly neutralizing epitopes are often taken as a marker for replication-competent virions (9, 25, 26, 33, 34). However, our investigation of unadulterated, single virions in solution reveals that there is overlapping expression of both sorts of epitopes on the same virion and even on the same surface Env structures. Further, this overlap can be apparent on the majority of virions in a population. Such data point toward the potential value of developing vaccines that elicit polyclonal anti-Env responses comprising both neutralizing and non-neutralizing antibodies, which in concert may guide multiple effector mechanisms to viruses or virus infected cells.

Going a step further, our data provide a virological basis for considering whether and how certain non-neutralizing responses alone may effectively block infection, by vaccination or other preventive measure targeting gp41. In various animal models

of HIV-1 infection, antibodies to F240 and related/overlapping Cluster I epitopes on gp41 have already been linked to varying degrees of resistance (31, 42, 43, 76, 77). Our data indicate that such *in vivo* effects may involve selective activity against virions, particularly given other evidence that Cluster I epitopes are poorly expressed on infected cells (41). Vaccines that generate such responses, particularly at points of mucosal exposure, merit exploration and may now be developed using new information concerning Env structures on free virions.

AUTHOR CONTRIBUTIONS

KR designed the research, performed experiments, analyzed the data, and wrote the manuscript. MM and CO performed experiments. MP performed structural modeling. GL analyzed the data. AD designed the research, analyzed data, and wrote the manuscript.

ACKNOWLEDGMENTS

Research reported in this publication was supported by the National Institute of General Medical Sciences and National Institute of Allergy and Infectious Diseases, of the National Institutes of Health under Award Numbers (R01 GM117836 and R01 GM117836-S1 to KR) and (P01 AI120756 to AD). The content is solely the responsibility of the authors and does not necessarily represent the official views of the National Institutes of Health.

SUPPLEMENTARY MATERIAL

Figure S1 | Number of fluorescent eGFP.vpr HIV-1 BAL virions in the FCS focal volume (~1 fL) as a function of input p24 concentration. The measurements were performed in triplicates and average values are shown. Error bars indicate standard deviations.

REFERENCES

1. Kwong PD, Wyatt R, Robinson J, Sweet RW, Sodroski J, Hendrickson WA. Structure of an HIV gp120 envelope glycoprotein in complex with the CD4 receptor and a neutralizing human antibody. *Nature.* (1998) 393:648–59. doi: 10.1038/31405
2. Leonard CK, Spellman MW, Riddle L, Harris RJ, Thomas JN, Gregory TJ. Assignment of intrachain disulfide bonds and characterization of potential glycosylation sites of the type 1 recombinant human immunodeficiency virus envelope glycoprotein (gp120) expressed in Chinese hamster ovary cells. *J Biol Chem.* (1990) 265:10373–82.
3. Wei X, Decker JM, Wang S, Hui H, Kappes JC, Wu X, et al. Antibody neutralization and escape by HIV-1. *Nature.* (2003) 422:307–12. doi: 10.1038/nature01470
4. Hahn BH, Gonda MA, Shaw GM, Popovic M, Hoxie JA, Gallo RC, et al. Genomic diversity of the acquired immune deficiency syndrome virus HTLV-III: different viruses exhibit greatest divergence in their envelope genes. *Proc Natl Acad Sci USA.* (1985) 82:4813–7. doi: 10.1073/pnas.82.14.4813
5. Hartley O, Klasse PJ, Sattentau QJ, Moore JP. V3: HIV's switch-hitter. *AIDS Res Hum Retroviruses.* (2005) 21:171–89. doi: 10.1089/aid.2005.21.171
6. Saag MS, Hahn BH, Gibbons J, Li Y, Parks ES, Parks WP, et al. Extensive variation of human immunodeficiency virus type-1 *in vivo. Nature.* (1988) 334:440–4. doi: 10.1038/334440a0
7. Wyatt R, Kwong PD, Desjardins E, Sweet RW, Robinson J, Hendrickson WA, et al. The antigenic structure of the HIV gp120 envelope glycoprotein. *Nature.* (1998) 393:705–11. doi: 10.1038/31514

8. Burton DR, Stanfield RL, Wilson IA. Antibody vs. HIV in a clash of evolutionary titans. *Proc Natl Acad Sci USA.* (2005) 102:14943–8. doi: 10.1073/pnas.0505126102

9. Arakelyan A, Fitzgerald W, King DF, Rogers P, Cheeseman HM, Grivel JC, et al. Flow virometry analysis of envelope glycoprotein conformations on individual HIV virions. *Sci Rep.* (2017) 7:948. doi: 10.1038/s41598-017-00935-w

10. Fung MS, Sun CR, Gordon WL, Liou RS, Chang TW, Sun WN, et al. Identification and characterization of a neutralization site within the second variable region of human immunodeficiency virus type 1 gp120. *J Virol.* (1992) 66:848–56.

11. Putney SD, Matthews TJ, Robey WG, Lynn DL, Robert-Guroff M, Mueller WT, et al. HTLV-III/LAV-neutralizing antibodies to an E. coli-produced fragment of the virus envelope. *Science.* (1986) 234:1392–5. doi: 10.1126/science.2431482

12. Rusche JR, Javaherian K, McDanal C, Petro J, Lynn DL, Grimaila R, et al. Antibodies that inhibit fusion of human immunodeficiency virus-infected cells bind a 24-amino acid sequence of the viral envelope, gp120. *Proc Natl Acad Sci USA.* (1988) 85:3198–202. doi: 10.1073/pnas.85.9.3198

13. Sattentau QJ. Neutralization of HIV-1 by antibody. *Curr Opin Immunol.* (1996) 8:540–5. doi: 10.1016/S0952-7915(96)80044-6

14. Sajadi MM, Dashti A, Rikhtegaran Tehrani Z, Tolbert WD, Seaman MS, Ouyang X, et al. Identification of near-pan-neutralizing antibodies against HIV-1 by deconvolution of plasma humoral responses. *Cell.* (2018) 173:1783–95 e14. doi: 10.1016/j.cell.2018.03.061

15. Zhou T, Georgiev I, Wu X, Yang ZY, Dai K, Finzi A, et al. Structural basis for broad and potent neutralization of HIV-1 by antibody VRC01. *Science.* (2010) 329:811–7. doi: 10.1126/science.1192819

16. Sok D, Burton DR. Recent progress in broadly neutralizing antibodies to HIV. *Nat Immunol.* (2018) 19:1179–88. doi: 10.1038/s41590-018-0235-7

17. Moldt B, Rakasz EG, Schultz N, Chan-Hui PY, Swiderek K, Weisgrau KL, et al. Highly potent HIV-specific antibody neutralization in vitro translates into effective protection against mucosal SHIV challenge in vivo. *Proc Natl Acad Sci USA.* (2012) 109:18921–5. doi: 10.1073/pnas.1214785109

18. Pauthner MG, Nkolola JP, Havenar-Daughton C, Murrell B, Reiss SM, Bastidas R, et al. Vaccine-induced protection from homologous tier 2 SHIV challenge in nonhuman primates depends on serum-neutralizing antibody titers. *Immunity.* (2019) 50:241–52 e6. doi: 10.1016/j.immuni.2018.11.011

19. Hessell AJ, Rakasz EG, Poignard P, Hangartner L, Landucci G, Forthal DN, et al. Broadly neutralizing human anti-HIV antibody 2G12 is effective in protection against mucosal SHIV challenge even at low serum neutralizing titers. *PLoS Pathog.* (2009) 5:e1000433. doi: 10.1371/journal.ppat.1000433

20. DeVico AL. CD4-induced epitopes in the HIV envelope glycoprotein, gp120. *Curr HIV Res.* (2007) 5:561–71. doi: 10.2174/157016207782418560

21. Mengistu M, Ray K, Lewis GK, DeVico AL. Antigenic properties of the human immunodeficiency virus envelope glycoprotein gp120 on virions bound to target cells. *PLoS Pathog.* (2015) 11:e1004772. doi: 10.1371/journal.ppat.1004772

22. Guan Y, Pazgier M, Sajadi MM, Kamin-Lewis R, Al-Darmarki S, Flinko R, et al. Diverse specificity and effector function among human antibodies to HIV-1 envelope glycoprotein epitopes exposed by CD4 binding. *Proc Natl Acad Sci USA.* (2013) 110:E69–78. doi: 10.1073/pnas.1217609110

23. Mengistu M, Tang AH, Foulke JS Jr, Blanpied TA, Gonzalez MW, Spouge JL, et al. Patterns of conserved gp120 epitope presentation on attached HIV-1 virions. *Proc Natl Acad Sci USA.* (2017) 114:E9893–902. doi: 10.1073/pnas.1705074114

24. Herrera C, Spenlehauer C, Fung MS, Burton DR, Beddows S, Moore JP. Nonneutralizing antibodies to the CD4-binding site on the gp120 subunit of human immunodeficiency virus type 1 do not interfere with the activity of a neutralizing antibody against the same site. *J Virol.* (2003) 77:1084–91. doi: 10.1128/JVI.77.2.1084-1091.2003

25. Poignard P, Moulard M, Golez E, Vivona V, Franti M, Venturini S, et al. Heterogeneity of envelope molecules expressed on primary human immunodeficiency virus type 1 particles as probed by the binding of neutralizing and nonneutralizing antibodies. *J Virol.* (2003) 77:353–65. doi: 10.1128/JVI.77.1.353-365.2003

26. Moore PL, Crooks ET, Porter L, Zhu P, Cayanan CS, Grise H, et al. Nature of nonfunctional envelope proteins on the surface of human immunodeficiency virus type 1. *J Virol.* (2006) 80:2515–28. doi: 10.1128/JVI.80.5.2515-2528.2006

27. Stott EJ, Chan WL, Mills KH, Page M, Taffs F, Cranage M, et al. Preliminary report: protection of cynomolgus macaques against simian immunodeficiency virus by fixed infected-cell vaccine. *Lancet.* (1990) 336:1538–41. doi: 10.1016/0140-6736(90)93310-L

28. Mills KH, Page M, Chan WL, Kitchin P, Stott EJ, Taffs F, et al. Protection against SIV infection in macaques by immunization with inactivated virus from the BK28 molecular clone, but not with BK28-derived recombinant env and gag proteins. *J Med Primatol.* (1992) 21:50–8.

29. Stott EJ. Anti-cell antibody in macaques. *Nature.* (1991) 353:393. doi: 10.1038/353393a0

30. Page M, Quartey-Papafio R, Robinson M, Hassall M, Cranage M, Stott J, et al. Complement-mediated virus infectivity neutralisation by HLA antibodies is associated with sterilising immunity to SIV challenge in the macaque model for HIV/AIDS. *PLoS ONE.* (2014) 9:e88735. doi: 10.1371/journal.pone.0088735

31. Horwitz JA, Bar-On Y, Lu CL, Fera D, Lockhart AK, Lorenzi CC, et al. Non-neutralizing antibodies alter the course of HIV-1 infection in vivo. *Cell.* (2017) 170:637–48 e10. doi: 10.1016/j.cell.2017.06.048

32. Leaman DP, Kinkead H, Zwick MB. In-solution virus capture assay helps deconstruct heterogeneous antibody recognition of human immunodeficiency virus type 1. *J Virol.* (2010) 84:3382–95. doi: 10.1128/JVI.02363-09

33. Liu P, Williams LD, Shen X, Bonsignori M, Vandergrift NA, Overman RG, et al. Capacity for infectious HIV-1 virion capture differs by envelope antibody specificity. *J Virol.* (2014) 88:5165–70. doi: 10.1128/JVI.03765-13

34. Stieh DJ, King DF, Klein K, Aldon Y, McKay PF, Shattock RJ. Discrete partitioning of HIV-1 Env forms revealed by viral capture. *Retrovirology.* (2015) 12:81. doi: 10.1186/s12977-015-0207-z

35. Herrera C, Klasse PJ, Michael E, Kake S, Barnes K, Kibler CW, et al. The impact of envelope glycoprotein cleavage on the antigenicity, infectivity, and neutralization sensitivity of Env-pseudotyped human immunodeficiency virus type 1 particles. *Virology.* (2005) 338:154–72. doi: 10.1016/j.virol.2005.05.002

36. Ray K, Mengistu M, Yu L, Lewis GK, Lakowicz JR, DeVico AL. Antigenic properties of the HIV envelope on virions in solution. *J Virol.* (2014) 88:1795–808. doi: 10.1128/JVI.03048-13

37. Cavacini LA, Emes CL, Wisnewski AV, Power J, Lewis G, Montefiori D, et al. Functional and molecular characterization of human monoclonal antibody reactive with the immunodominant region of HIV type 1 glycoprotein 41. *AIDS Res Hum Retroviruses.* (1998) 14:1271–80. doi: 10.1089/aid.1998.14.1271

38. Xu JY, Gorny MK, Palker T, Karwowska S, Zolla-Pazner S. Epitope mapping of two immunodominant domains of gp41, the transmembrane protein of human immunodeficiency virus type 1, using ten human monoclonal antibodies. *J Virol.* (1991) 65:4832–8.

39. Tyler DS, Stanley SD, Zolla-Pazner S, Gorny MK, Shadduck PP, Langlois AJ, et al. Identification of sites within gp41 that serve as targets for antibody-dependent cellular cytotoxicity by using human monoclonal antibodies. *J Immunol.* (1990) 145:3276–82.

40. Cavacini LA, Duval M, Robinson J, Posner MR. Interactions of human antibodies, epitope exposure, antibody binding and neutralization of primary isolate HIV-1 virions. *AIDS.* (2002) 16:2409–17. doi: 10.1097/00002030-200212060-00005

41. Gohain N, Tolbert WD, Orlandi C, Richard J, Ding S, Chen X, et al. Molecular basis for epitope recognition by non-neutralizing anti-gp41 antibody F240. *Sci Rep.* (2016) 6:36685. doi: 10.1038/srep36685

42. Burton DR, Hessell AJ, Keele BF, Klasse PJ, Ketas TA, Moldt B, et al. Limited or no protection by weakly or nonneutralizing antibodies against vaginal SHIV challenge of macaques compared with a strongly neutralizing antibody. *Proc Natl Acad Sci USA.* (2011) 108:11181–6. doi: 10.1073/pnas.1103012108

43. Santra S, Tomaras GD, Warrier R, Nicely NI, Liao HX, Pollara J, et al. Human non-neutralizing HIV-1 envelope monoclonal antibodies limit the number of founder viruses during SHIV mucosal infection in rhesus macaques. *PLoS Pathog.* (2015) 11:e1005042. doi: 10.1371/journal.ppat.1005042

44. Binley JM, Cayanan CS, Wiley C, Schulke N, Olson WC, Burton DR. Redox-triggered infection by disulfide-shackled human

immunodeficiency virus type 1 pseudovirions. *J Virol*. (2003) 77:5678–84. doi: 10.1128/JVI.77.10.5678-5684.2003

45. Li Y, Svehla K, Mathy NL, Voss G, Mascola JR, Wyatt R. Characterization of antibody responses elicited by human immunodeficiency virus type 1 primary isolate trimeric and monomeric envelope glycoproteins in selected adjuvants. *J Virol*. (2006) 80:1414–26. doi: 10.1128/JVI.80.3.1414-1426.2006

46. Li H, Bar KJ, Wang S, Decker JM, Chen Y, Sun C, et al. High multiplicity infection by HIV-1 in men who have sex with men. *PLoS Pathog*. (2010) 6:e1000890. doi: 10.1371/journal.ppat.1000890

47. Li M, Salazar-Gonzalez JF, Derdeyn CA, Morris L, Williamson C, Robinson JE, et al. Genetic and neutralization properties of subtype C human immunodeficiency virus type 1 molecular env clones from acute and early heterosexually acquired infections in Southern Africa. *J Virol*. (2006) 80:11776–90. doi: 10.1128/JVI.01730-06

48. Rossio JL, Esser MT, Suryanarayana K, Schneider DK, Bess JW Jr, Vasquez GM, et al. Inactivation of human immunodeficiency virus type 1 infectivity with preservation of conformational and functional integrity of virion surface proteins. *J Virol*. (1998) 72:7992–8001.

49. Miller E, Spadaccia M, Sabado R, Chertova E, Bess J, Trubey CM, et al. Autologous aldrithiol-2-inactivated HIV-1 combined with polyinosinic-polycytidylic acid-poly-L-lysine carboxymethylcellulose as a vaccine platform for therapeutic dendritic cell immunotherapy. *Vaccine*. (2015) 33:388–95. doi: 10.1016/j.vaccine.2014.10.054

50. Schaeffer E, Geleziunas R, Greene WC. Human immunodeficiency virus type 1 Nef functions at the level of virus entry by enhancing cytoplasmic delivery of virions. *J Virol*. (2001) 75:2993–3000. doi: 10.1128/JVI.75.6.2993-3000.2001

51. Hess ST, Huang S, Heikal AA, Webb WW. Biological and chemical applications of fluorescence correlation spectroscopy: a review. *Biochemistry*. (2002) 41:697–705. doi: 10.1021/bi0118512

52. Bacia K, Kim SA, Schwille P. Fluorescence cross-correlation spectroscopy in living cells. *Nat Methods*. (2006) 3:83–9. doi: 10.1038/nmeth822

53. Schwille P, Meyer-Almes FJ, Rigler R. Dual-color fluorescence cross-correlation spectroscopy for multicomponent diffusional analysis in solution. *Biophys J*. (1997) 72:1878–86. doi: 10.1016/S0006-3495(97)78833-7

54. Summers MF, Henderson LE, Chance MR, Bess JW Jr, South TL, Blake PR, Sagi I, et al. Nucleocapsid zinc fingers detected in retroviruses: EXAFS studies of intact viruses and the solution-state structure of the nucleocapsid protein from HIV-1. *Protein Sci*. (1992) 1:563–74. doi: 10.1002/pro.5560010502

55. Tang S, Zhao J, Wang A, Viswanath R, Harma H, Little RF, et al. Characterization of immune responses to capsid protein p24 of human immunodeficiency virus type 1 and implications for detection. *Clin Vaccine Immunol*. (2010) 17:1244–51. doi: 10.1128/CVI.00066-10

56. Schuler B, Lipman EA, Eaton WA. Probing the free-energy surface for protein folding with single-molecule fluorescence spectroscopy. *Nature*. (2002) 419:743–7. doi: 10.1038/nature01060

57. Ray K, Sabanayagam CR, Lakowicz JR, Black LW. DNA crunching by a viral packaging motor: compression of a procapsid-portal stalled Y-DNA substrate. *Virology*. (2010) 398:224–32. doi: 10.1016/j.virol.2009.11.047

58. Dixit A, Ray K, Lakowicz JR, Black LW. Dynamics of the T4 bacteriophage DNA packasome motor: endonuclease VII resolvase release of arrested Y-DNA substrates. *J Biol Chem*. (2011) 286:18878–89. doi: 10.1074/jbc.M111.222828

59. Dixit AB, Ray K, Black LW. Compression of the DNA substrate by a viral packaging motor is supported by removal of intercalating dye during translocation. *Proc Natl Acad Sci USA*. (2012) 109:20419–24. doi: 10.1073/pnas.1214318109

60. Gohain N, Tolbert WD, Acharya P, Yu L, Liu T, Zhao P, et al. Cocrystal structures of antibody N60-i3 and antibody JR4 in complex with gp120 define more cluster A epitopes involved in effective antibody-dependent effector function against HIV-1. *J Virol*. (2015) 89:8840–54. doi: 10.1128/JVI.01232-15

61. Liu J, Bartesaghi A, Borgnia MJ, Sapiro G, Subramaniam S. Molecular architecture of native HIV-1 gp120 trimers. *Nature*. (2008) 455:109–13. doi: 10.1038/nature07159

62. Calarese DA, Scanlan CN, Zwick MB, Deechongkit S, Mimura Y, Kunert R, et al. Antibody domain exchange is an immunological solution to carbohydrate cluster recognition. *Science*. (2003) 300:2065–71. doi: 10.1126/science.1083182

63. Calarese DA, Lee HK, Huang CY, Best MD, Astronomo RD, Stanfield RL, et al. Dissection of the carbohydrate specificity of the broadly neutralizing anti-HIV-1 antibody 2G12. *Proc Natl Acad Sci USA*. (2005) 102:13372–7. doi: 10.1073/pnas.0505763102

64. Burton DR, Pyati J, Koduri R, Sharp SJ, Thornton GB, Parren PW, et al. Efficient neutralization of primary isolates of HIV-1 by a recombinant human monoclonal antibody. *Science*. (1994) 266:1024–7. doi: 10.1126/science.7973652

65. Sullivan N, Sun Y, Sattentau Q, Thali M, Wu D, Denisova G, et al. CD4-Induced conformational changes in the human immunodeficiency virus type 1 gp120 glycoprotein: consequences for virus entry and neutralization. *J Virol*. (1998) 72:4694–703.

66. Bublil EM, Yeger-Azuz S, Gershoni JM. Computational prediction of the cross-reactive neutralizing epitope corresponding to the [corrected] monclonal [corrected] antibody b12 specific for HIV-1 gp120. *Faseb J*. (2006) 20:1762–74. doi: 10.1096/fj.05-5509rev

67. Lee JH, Ozorowski G, Ward AB. Cryo-EM structure of a native, fully glycosylated, cleaved HIV-1 envelope trimer. *Science*. (2016) 351:1043–8. doi: 10.1126/science.aad2450

68. Walker LM, Phogat SK, Chan-Hui PY, Wagner D, Phung P, Goss JL, et al. Broad and potent neutralizing antibodies from an African donor reveal a new HIV-1 vaccine target. *Science*. (2009) 326:285–9. doi: 10.1126/science.1178746

69. McLellan JS, Pancera M, Carrico C, Gorman J, Julien JP, Khayat R, et al. Structure of HIV-1 gp120 V1/V2 domain with broadly neutralizing antibody PG9. *Nature*. (2011) 480:336–43. doi: 10.1038/nature10696

70. Wang H, Gristick HB, Scharf L, West AP, Galimidi RP, Seaman MS, et al. Asymmetric recognition of HIV-1 Envelope trimer by V1V2 loop-targeting antibodies. *Elife*. (2017) 6:27389. doi: 10.7554/eLife.27389

71. Arunkumar GA, Ioannou A, Wohlbold TJ, Meade P, Aslam S, Amanat F, et al. Broadly cross-reactive, non-neutralizing antibodies against the influenza B virus hemagglutinin demonstrate effector function dependent protection against lethal viral challenge in mice. *J Virol*. (2019) 93:e01696-18 doi: 10.1128/JVI.01696-18

72. Saphire EO, Schendel SL, Fusco ML, Gangavarapu K, Gunn BM, Wec AZ, et al. Systematic analysis of monoclonal antibodies against ebola virus GP defines features that contribute to protection. *Cell*. (2018) 174:938–52 e13. doi: 10.1016/j.cell.2018.07.033

73. Gunn BM, Yu WH, Karim MM, Brannan JM, Herbert AS, Wec AZ, et al. A role for Fc function in therapeutic monoclonal antibody-mediated protection against ebola virus. *Cell Host Microbe*. (2018) 24:221–33 e5. doi: 10.1016/j.chom.2018.07.009

74. Saphire EO, Schendel SL, Gunn BM, Milligan JC, Alter G. Antibody-mediated protection against Ebola virus. *Nat Immunol*. (2018) 19:1169–78. doi: 10.1038/s41590-018-0233-9

75. Thulin NK, Wang TT. The role of Fc gamma receptors in broad protection against influenza viruses. *Vaccines*. (2018) 6:30036. doi: 10.3390/vaccines6030036

76. Smith AJ, Wietgrefe SW, Shang L, Reilly CS, Southern PJ, Perkey KE, et al. Live simian immunodeficiency virus vaccine correlate of protection: immune complex-inhibitory Fc receptor interactions that reduce target cell availability. *J Immunol*. (2014) 193:3126–33. doi: 10.4049/jimmunol.1400822

77. Li Q, Zeng M, Duan L, Voss JE, Smith AJ, Pambuccian S, et al. Live simian immunodeficiency virus vaccine correlate of protection: local antibody production and concentration on the path of virus entry. *J Immunol*. (2014) 193:3113–25. doi: 10.4049/jimmunol.1400820

6

The Human FcγRII (CD32) Family of Leukocyte FcR in Health and Disease

Jessica C. Anania [1,2], Alicia M. Chenoweth [1,2], Bruce D. Wines [1,2,3] and P. Mark Hogarth [1,2,3]*

[1] Centre for Biomedical Research, Burnet Institute, Melbourne, VIC, Australia, [2] Department of Immunology and Pathology, Central Clinical School, Monash University, Melbourne, VIC, Australia, [3] Department of Pathology, The University of Melbourne, Melbourne, VIC, Australia

*Correspondence:
P. Mark Hogarth
mark.hogarth@burnet.edu.au

FcγRs have been the focus of extensive research due to their key role linking innate and humoral immunity and their implication in both inflammatory and infectious disease. Within the human FcγR family FcγRII (activatory FcγRIIa and FcγRIIc, and inhibitory FcγRIIb) are unique in their ability to signal independent of the common γ chain. Through improved understanding of the structure of these receptors and how this affects their function we may be able to better understand how to target FcγR specific immune activation or inhibition, which will facilitate in the development of therapeutic monoclonal antibodies in patients where FcγRII activity may be desirable for efficacy. This review is focused on roles of the human FcγRII family members and their link to immunoregulation in healthy individuals and infection, autoimmunity and cancer.

Keywords: Fc receptor, FcγR, inflammation, infection, autoimmunity, cancer, mAb therapeutics

INTRODUCTION

Fc receptors are, by definition, receptors for the Fc portion of immunoglobulins (Ig). These have been traditionally viewed primarily as cell surface receptors for Ig and whose interaction drives a surprisingly diverse range of responses mostly within the immune system or related to the physiology of antibodies in immunity.

Receptors for IgM, IgA, IgG, and IgE have been defined over the last 40 years with the majority of research focused on the receptors found on leukocytes. These receptors induce or regulate leukocyte effector functions during the course of immune responses. It is noteworthy, and also beyond the scope of this review, that a limited number and type of Fc receptors are also expressed on cells outside the immune system where they affect or participate in physiology of antibody function.

In humans, the largest grouping of Fc receptors is the "leukocyte Fc receptors" expressed primarily on effector cells. Their ectodomains bind ligand, the IgG antibody Fc region, and belong to the Ig-superfamily. They include the high affinity IgE receptor FcεRI and the distantly related IgA receptor FcαRI, but the largest group are the IgG receptors or the FcγRs which themselves comprise several groups—FcγRI, the high affinity IgG receptor, the FcγRII family (FcγRIIA, FcγRIIB, FcγRIIC), and the FcγRIII family (1, 2).

THE HUMAN FcγRII (CD32) FAMILY OF LEUKOCYTE FCR
General Comments

The human FcγRII family (also known as CD32 in the Cluster of Differentiation nomenclature) consists of a family of primarily cell membrane receptor proteins. They are encoded by the mRNA splice variants of three highly related genes—*FCGR2A*, *FCGR2B*, and *FCGR2C*, which arose by recombination of the *FCGR2A* and *FCGR2B* genes (3).

All members of the FcγRII family are integral membrane glycoproteins and contain conserved extracellular domains, exhibiting an overall 85% amino acid identity (3, 4). The high degree of amino acid and DNA identity has posed challenges in the analysis of receptor function using monoclonal antibody or nucleic acid based methods. Thus, some caution should be exercised when analyzing literature or interpreting experimental data. The encoded products of the three genes are low-affinity receptors that are defined practically as interacting poorly with monomeric IgG, i.e., micromolar affinity (5, 6), but when arrayed on the cell surface, they avidly bind multivalent complexes of IgG, e.g., immune complexes.

The FcγRIIA (also FcγRIIC) and FcγRIIB proteins have opposing cellular functions. FcγRIIA proteins are activating-type Fc receptors. In contrast, FcγRIIB is a key immune checkpoint that modulates the action of activating-type Fc receptors and the antigen receptor of B cells. When expressed, the FcγRIIC proteins retain the activating function of the cytoplasmic tail of FcγRIIA and the binding specificity of FcγRIIB ectodomains.

The focus of this review is the FcγRII family and their actions as receptors for immunoglobulins. It should be noted that FcγRIIA also acts as a receptor for pentraxins, a product of innate immunity that is important in infection and inflammation and which has been recently reviewed elsewhere (7). Since much of the biology of the Fc receptors has been determined in the mouse, it is noteworthy that the human and mouse FcR families differ significantly, with FcγRIIB being the only FcγRII forms in the mouse. Also, although the human and mouse FcγRIIB homologs are highly conserved, there are differences in their splice variants in the two species (see below). Importantly, cellular expression can also vary between humans and mice.

Human FcγRII gene polymorphism, mRNA splicing, and copy number variation (CNV) further diversifies the potential biological consequences of IgG interactions with the FcγRII receptor proteins. These properties and roles of each group of FcγRII proteins are reviewed in detail in the following sections.

PROPERTIES OF FcγRIIA

Molecular Structure

The human FcγRIIA proteins were originally defined by cross-species gene cloning (8). They are encoded by the *FCGR2A* gene (**Figure 1**) and are comprised of eight exons; two encoding the 5′ UTR, and leader sequence and the N-terminus of the mature protein; one exon for each of the two Ig-like domains of the extracellular region; one exon for the transmembrane domain; and three exons encoding the cytoplasmic tail and 3′ UTR (3). Three mRNA transcripts, two of which encode membrane proteins, arise by alternative splicing of the mRNA (**Figure 1**).

The most extensively characterized form is the canonical 40 kDa integral membrane protein, FcγRIIA1, that contains all but the first (C1*) cytoplasmic sequence (3, 4, 8–10). A second, but relatively rare, membrane form has been recently described (11, 12). FcγRIIA3 is identical in sequence to the canonical FcγRIIA1, with the notable exception of a 19-amino acid insert in its cytoplasmic tail, arising from the inclusion of the C1* exon which was believed previously to be a vestigial or cryptic exon (4).

This insertion is highly homologous (18/19-amino acids) to the insertion present in the cytoplasmic tail of inhibitory FcγRIIB1 (11–13). mRNA splicing that successfully gives rise to FcγRIIA3 is associated with an *FCGR2A*[c.7421871A>G] SNP that creates a splice acceptor site, which greatly increases the inclusion of the C1* exon (11).

An unusual mRNA has been reported that lacks the transmembrane exon resulting in a potentially secreted 32 kDa polypeptide (14). This FcγRIIA2 form is not extensively characterized and its physiology is uncertain. However, it raises the possibility that naturally occurring soluble forms may act as modulators of immune complex-induced activation and inflammation and it is noteworthy that recombinant soluble FcγRIIA inhibits immune complex-induced activation of inflammatory cells *in vitro* and *in vivo* (9).

Cellular Expression

The FcγRIIA proteins are unique to primates (15, 16). FcγRIIA1 is the most widespread and abundant of all FcγR, present on Langerhans cells, platelets and all leukocytes, with the exception of most lymphocytes (**Table 1**) (1, 16, 17). FcγRIIA3 is expressed by neutrophils and monocytes (11) and FcγRIIA2 mRNA is present in platelets, megakaryocytes, and Langerhans cells (14). The levels of FcγRIIA expression are influenced by cytokine exposure. Interferon (IFN)-γ, interleukin (IL)-3, IL-6, IFN-γ, C5a, prostaglandin-E (PGE), and dexamethasone increase expression, but IL-4, tumor necrosis factor (TNF)-α, and TNF-β reduce expression (18–21). There are also reports of FcγRII induction on CD4 and CD8 T cells upon mitogen or TCR stimulation. Both FcγRIIA and FcγRIIB are reported to be expressed on activated CD4 T cells (22, 23).

FcγRIIA Signaling ITAM Activation vs. ITAM Inhibition

Like other activating-type immunoreceptors, FcγRIIA and FcγRIIC signal via the Immunoreceptor Tyrosine-based Activation Motif (ITAM) pathway (24–26) with a major structural difference. In the case of all other activating-type immunoreceptors—which includes the antigen receptors as well as the activating type FcR, e.g., FcεRI, FcγRIIIA—the ligand binding chain and the signaling subunits are encoded in separate polypeptides e.g., FcγRIIIA and the common FcR-γ chain dimer. The assembly of a functional signaling complex requires their non-covalent association (17). However, in the case of FcγRIIA and FcγRIIC, the ITAM is present in its own IgG binding chain. Furthermore, the FcγRIIA ITAM is unusual in that it does not fit the canonical ITAM consensus sequence and includes three additional aspartic residues (**Table 2**), although how this affects FcγRII function remains unknown (13). ITAM signaling is essential for FcγRIIA-dependent phagocytosis and the induction of cytokine secretion induced by its aggregation by immune complexes. Such high stoichiometry aggregation of receptors results in receptor-associated src family kinase, particularly Fyn (27), mediated phosphorylation of the two tyrosines of the ITAM and the recruitment of Syk and the propagation of activatory signaling pathways. In human FcγRIIA transgenic mice, Fyn deficiency is protective in models of FcγR dependent nephritis

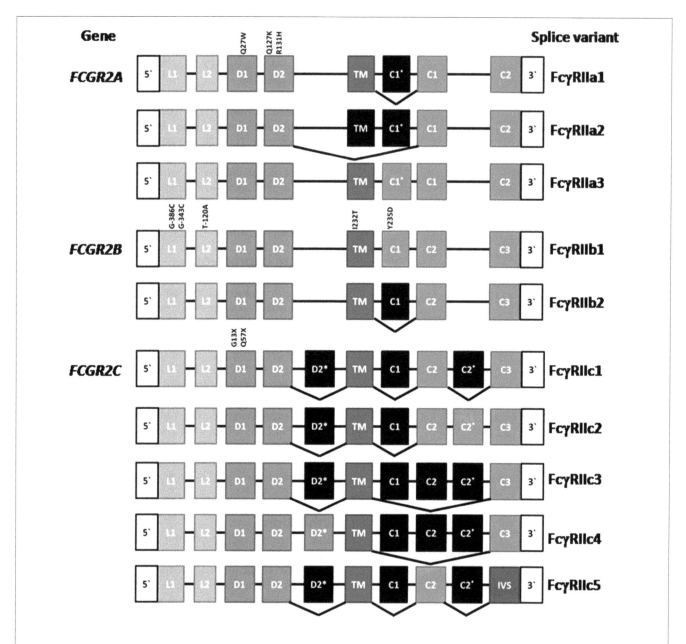

FIGURE 1 | Composition of *FCGR2A*, *FCGR2B*, and *FCGR2C* and their splice variants. Leader (L), ectodomain (D), transmembrane (TM) cytoplasmic tail (c), and intervening sequence (IVS). Expressed exons are illustrated in color, while spliced exons (selectively expressed) are represented in black. The location and position number of amino acids affected by well characterized polymorphisms are shown above the exons except for the *FCGR2B* leader exons where the nucleotide positions are given. See text for references.

and arthritis, indicating a pivotal pro-inflammatory role for Fyn kinase in ITAM signaling (27).

Since the original characterization of the activating role of ITAM pathway was described, it is now apparent that ITAMs can under certain circumstances mediate inhibitory or modulating function termed ITAMi (inhibitory ITAM) (28, 29). Under conditions of low stoichiometric interaction, the receptor-associated src family kinase Lyn phosphorylates only one of the two tyrosine residues (mono-tyrosine phosphorylation) within the ITAM, with two juxtaposed receptors presenting mono-phosphylated-ITAMs to recruit the two SH2 domains of the SH2-domain containing protein tyrosine phosphatase 1 (SHP-1). This interaction is not dissimilar to SHP1 binding via its dual SH2 domains to inhibitory immunoreceptors with dual ITIMs (30). Then Lyn phosphorylation of Tyr^{536} of SHP-1 positively regulates SHP-1 phosphatase activity resulting in the inhibition of cell activation (27). Animal studies suggest that the ITAMi effect ameliorates pathological inflammatory responses and may also be important in controlling "baseline" receptor activation. This ITAMi effect is not unique to the unusual

TABLE 1 | Leukocyte Expression of FcγRII forms.

Cell type	FcγRIIA	FcγRIIB	FcγRIIC[a]
T cells	i[b]	i[b]	?
B cells	−	+++	+
NK cells	−	−[c]	+
Macrophages	+++	++	?
Monocytes	+++	+	?
Neutrophils	+++	+	?
Eosinophils	++	•	•
Basophils	++	+++	−
Mast cells	++	−[d]	−
Platelets	++	−	−

+++ High, ++ Moderate, + Low, or − No expression. • no data.
[a]Expressed only in ~20% of humans;
[b]Expression induced in some T cell subpopulations;
[c]Expressed as a result of promoter modification related to FcγRIIC allelism.
[d]Conflicting results.

TABLE 2 | Sequence comparison of ITAMs of activating type FcγR.

Receptor ITAM	Consensus[a]
FcR-γ chain	**Y**TG**L** STRN−−−QET **Y**ET**L**
FcγRIIA and Fcγ IIC	**Y**MT**L** NPRAPTDDDKNI **Y**LT**L**

[a]Bold letters in FcRγ chain and FcγRIIA sequences indicate the critical Tyr and Leu residues of the ITAM consensus motif YxxL/I (6–12) YxxL.

FcγRIIA ITAM (29) as it has been also described for FcαRI (31, 32) and FcγRIIIA (33), both of which signal through the common FcR-γ chain dimer which contains canonical ITAMs.

Cellular Responses

FcγRIIA aggregation by IgG cross-linking initiates a variety of effector responses, depending on cellular expression which is affected by the local cytokine environment, and cross-talk between other FcR and TLR (34, 35). Internalization via both endocytosis and phagocytosis can be mediated by FcγRIIA in cell lines, i.e., ts20 (36, 37), COS-1 (38), U937 (39) as well as in primary human cells i.e., neutrophils (40, 41), monocytes (40), platelets (40, 42), and macrophages (43). FcγR phagocytosis requires ITAM activation, which also initiates the ubiquitin conjugation system. Conversely, endocytosis is dependent only on ubiquitination and clathrin, not ITAM phosphorylation (36, 37).

The internalization of antigen: antibody immune complexes by FcγR on antigen presenting cells (especially dendritic cells) is an important part of antigen presentation for the development of effective immune responses. This process also increases the efficiency of T cell activation particularly in response to low concentrations of antigen (44). The role of human FcγR in antigen presentation is well documented in *in vitro* systems and it appears that all FcγR are important at some level (45–47). However, more recent analyses have shown FcγRIIA is the major receptor in the development of so-called "vaccinal effects"

of monoclonal antibody therapy in cancer. It appears that the therapeutic antibodies targeting cancer cells can induce a long lasting protective response beyond the acute therapeutic phase of the therapy (48).

FcγRIIA1 activates neutrophils and other myeloid effector cells for direct killing of IgG-opsonized target cells including tumor cells and virus-infected cells (49). Also, FcγRIIA binding of IgG immune complexes triggers granulocytes to release inflammatory mediators such as prostaglandins, lysosomal enzymes, and reactive oxygen species, as well as cytokines including IFNγ, TNFα, IL-1, and IL-6 (50, 51). The FcγRIIA3 splice variant form is an even more potent activator of human neutrophils than FcγRIIA1, and is responsible for some severe adverse reactions to immunoglobulin replacement therapy (11). The mechanistic basis of this potency relates to its longer retention time in the cell membrane and the consequential enhanced ITAM signaling (12). Whilst this enhanced potency may present a risk factor for hypersensitivity to immunoglobulin replacement therapy, it may provide some benefit for protection against infection.

The limited number of studies of FcγRII expression of human T cells suggest FcγRII crosslinking on TCR-stimulated CD4 T cells enhances proliferation and cytokine secretion, suggesting an activating function of FcγRIIA (22, 23). The nature of FcγRIIA expression on CD4 T cells is not straightforward nor completely characterized. Purified CD4 T cells when stimulated with anti-CD3/CD28 induced surface expression of FcγRII on 10% of cells and intracellular expression in 50%. In contrast, unstimulated cells express little FcγRII (23). Imaging of FcγRII-expressing CD4 T cells sorted from unstimulated normal peripheral blood mononuclear cells, or those from HIV-1+ individuals shows cells displaying punctate FcγRIIA staining (23) or discrete patches of B cell membrane. These B cell membrane patches include FcγRIIB and CD19 markers (52), consistent with possible trogocytosis by the activated T cell from the B cell. Similarly, FcγRIIIA is also expressed on activated CD4 T cells, and this expression appears to be both intrinsic upon cell activation and acquired by trogocytosis of APC membrane (53).

FcγRIIA plays an important role in the normal physiology of platelet activation, adhesion, and aggregation following vessel injury (54). More recent studies indicate FcγRIIA associates with glycoprotein (GP) Ib-IX-V on platelets and can thereby be indirectly stimulated by von Willebrand factor (VWF) or after stimulation of G-protein-coupled receptors (GPCRs) (54). Interestingly, FcγRIIA signaling on platelets is regulated by proteolytic cleavage of the cytoplasmic tail, or "de-ITAM-ising" (55).

PROPERTIES OF FcγRIIB

Molecular Structure

Initially, FcγRIIB was discovered in the mouse by protein sequence and molecular cloning analyses (56, 57) and the human *FCGR2B* gene was then isolated by cross species hybridization. Human *FCGR2B* has similar structure to human *FCGR2A*, being comprised of eight exons. The two major forms of FcγRIIB—FcγRIIB1 and FcγRIIB2 (**Figure 1**)—arise from mRNA splicing which results in the inclusion or exclusion of the C1 exon sequence in FcγRIIB1 and FcγRIIB2 isoforms, respectively (3, 4). The inclusion of the C1 exon sequence in the FcγRIIB1 results in tethering to the membrane of B cells, whereas its absence from FcγRIIB2 allows rapid internalization of the receptor in myeloid cells. Both forms contain the Immunoreceptor Tyrosine-based Inhibitory Motif (ITIM) in their cytoplasmic tails. The extracellular domains are 95% identical to the two domains of FcγRIIA and almost completely identical to the FcγRIIC (3, 8, 17). Although the focus of this review is the human FcγRII, it should be noted that mouse FcγRIIB comprises three splice variants FcγRIIB1, FcγRIIB1′, and FcγRIIB2, with the predicated amino acid sequences of the latter two corresponding to the human FcγRIIB1 and FcγRIIB2 variants. Any functional differences between the two mouse FcγRIIB1 and FcγRIIB1′ forms are unknown (58). There are also amino acid sequence differences between human FcγRIIB1 and mouse FcγRIIB1/1′ and the functional consequences of these are also unknown.

Cellular Expression

As indicated in "General Comments" above, the analysis of expression of human FcγRIIB protein has been historically difficult because of the extremely high sequence conservation of the extracellular domains of FcγRIIB, FcγRIIA, and FcγRIIC and lack of specific monoclonal antibody probes. The high degree of DNA sequence conservation has also confounded analysis. Much of the early literature has relied on either PCRs or interpretation of data using antibodies that are cross-reactive with, or specific for, FcγRIIA or a combination of these methods and reagents. The relatively recent development of such FcγRIIA/C and FcγRIIB specific antibodies (59–61) has now helped to clarify expression patterns, but there are still differences reported between groups using these reagents. Some caution should still be exercised in analysis of the historic literature. Furthermore, cell expression patterns of FcγRIIB in mouse myeloid derived cells is substantially different to human FcγRIIB, thus additional caution is advised in interpreting the data. Nonetheless, it is clear that FcγRIIB (FcγRIIB1) is highly expressed by B cells, and its mRNA has also been identified at lower levels on monocytes (**Table 1**) (62). The levels of FcγRIIB expression are influenced by cytokine exposure. Cytokines such as IL-10, IL-6, and dexamethasone increase expression of FcγRIIB, while TNF-α, C5a and IFN-γ inhibit expression (18–20).

FcγRIIB (FcγRIIB2) is highly expressed on basophils and at low levels on monocytes (63). Expression on other granulocytes is somewhat complex and controversial. The differences in reported expression of FcγRIIB on mast cells may reflect technological limitations or differences in tissue origin of the cells under investigation. Intestinal and cord blood derived mast cells have been reported as expressing FcγRIIB on the basis of mRNA expression (64). In one study using human leukocyte reconstituted mice and a FcγRIIB specific polyclonal antibody, FcγRIIB protein was detected (65). However, skin mast cells lack FcγRIIB surface expression (66) and using a FcγRIIB specific mAb, peripheral blood derived mast cells do not express FcγRIIB (A. Chenoweth personal communication). Neutrophils either lack (60) or express very low levels of FcγRIIB (59), and the

FcγRIIB-specific mAb 2B6 does not usually stain NK cells (60). However, in that proportion (∼20%) of the population where FcγRIIC is expressed, NK staining by FcγRIIB antibodies might be expected as FcγRIIC EC domain is identical to FcγRIIB. A further complication is that FcγRIIC CNV affects control elements of the *FCGR2B* gene permitting FcγRIIB expression in NK cells (67) (see FcγRIIC below).

One of the more interesting features of FcγRIIB is its presence on non-leukocyte cells including airway smooth muscle (68) and liver sinusoidal endothelial cells (69). Its abundance in liver, in the mouse, accounting for three quarters of the total body expression, appears to provide a large sink for the removal in IgG immune complexes, which has been exploited in therapeutic monoclonal antibodies whose Fc portions have been engineered for high affinity binding to FcγRIIB (70, 71). This appears to be a "stand alone" function of FcγRIIB where small immune complexes are internalized without risk of pro-inflammatory activation.

FcγRIIB Modulation of Immunity

FcγRIIB was the first immune "checkpoint" defined (72), with mouse studies showing a pivotal role in controlling autoreactive germinal center B cell activation and survival in mice with dysfunction resulting in loss of tolerance and autoimmunity (73, 74). Mice with humanized immune systems reconstituted with stems cells homozygous for the dysfunctional FcγRIIB Thr[232] allele develop autoantibodies with specificities characteristic of lupus and human rheumatoid arthritis (75). This critical action of its ITIM in controlling the ITAM activation pathway is extensively reviewed elsewhere (25, 76). The ratio of activating vs. inhibitory receptors is a key factor in determining the cellular threshold for cell activation and resulting immune response (18, 77). An ITIM, consensus amino acid sequence YXXL (where X represents any amino acid), is found in the cytoplasmic domains of both FcγRIIB1 and FcγRIIB2. The co-engagement of FcγRIIB with an activating type receptor such as FcγRIIA or the B cell antigen receptor (25) modulates their ITAM-mediated activation signal. FcγRIIB expression on innate effector cells modulates cell activation mediated by activating FcγRs, including dendritic cell maturation and antigen presentation. FcγRIIB also regulates signaling from varied innate cell receptors including TLRs and complement receptors, reviewed in Bournazos et al. (34) and Espeli et al. (78).

Much of the detail in understanding of the ITIM:ITAM system of immune cell modulation has been derived from FcγRIIB1 ITIM-mediated regulation of the B cell receptor (BCR) signaling in mouse B cells. Conventional FcγRIIB-mediated inhibition requires ligand-dependant co-engagement/aggregation of ITAM-containing receptors (79, 80). The FcγRIIB ITIM modulation targets the two major ITAM driven pathways—ITAM tyrosine phosphorylation, and the generation of phospholipid mediators, e.g., Phosphatidylinositol (3,4,5)-trisphosphate (PIP3). Briefly, src kinases such as Lyn kinase, which participate in the phosphorylation of the ITAM of the ligand-clustered activating receptors, also phosphorylate the FcγRIIB ITIM of the co-aggregated inhibitory receptor. Notably, FcγRIIB1 has been reported to be phosphorylated by Lyn and Blk, whereas FcγRIIB2 solely by Blk (81).

The phosphorylated-ITIM of FcγRIIB recruits the inositol phosphatases SHIP1 and SHIP2, as is extensively reviewed in Getahun and Cambier (25). The preferential recruitment of SHIP, over SHP1 and SHP2, to the phosphorylated FcγRIIB cytoplasmic domain is determined by the SHIP SH2 domain's affinity for the pITIM (82). Notably studies of SHIP recruitment to the cytoplasmic domain of mouse FcγRIIB1 found phosphorylation of Tyr^{326}, outside the ITIM, bound the SH2 domain of the adaptor Grb2 which bridged and stabilized the FcγRIIB:SHIP complex (83). Human FcγRIIB lacks an equivalent tyrosine, and has a small adjacent deletion. It fails to recruit Grb2 but still recruits SHIP1 that modulates BCR-induced Ca mobilization (84). SHIP dephosphorylates phosphatidylinositol species, with the predominant *in vivo* substrate being phosphatidylinositol 3,4,5-trisphosphate and ultimately recruits p62 Dok to form a highly active membrane localized enzymatic complex. This inhibits the Ras activation pathway, decreases MAP kinase activation and reduced PLCγ function leads to less activation of PKC. SHIP-dependent ITIM inhibition of the MAP kinase pathway, together with the anti-apoptotic kinase Akt can thereby affect cellular proliferation and survival (25).

The same mechanisms defined for BCR regulation are applicable to human and mouse myeloid cells, where many observations have been confirmed, particularly for FcγRIIB2 regulation of FcεRI (25, 76). Overall FcγRIIB1 and FcγRIIB2 signaling pathways are similar, however their principal functional difference lies in their localization in the cell membrane. The C1 insertion (85) of FcγRIIB1 prolongs membrane retention, whereas FcγRIIB2 is rapidly internalized. The equivalent C1* sequence in FcγRIIA3 also alters membrane localization (see above).

An ITIM independent mechanism of B cell regulation by FcγRIIB has been reported wherein FcγRIIB, by binding antigen bound IgG, co-aggregates with the BCR and prevents the membrane organization of BCR and CD19 (86, 87). In another mode of regulation of the adaptive humoral response, FcγRIIB has been reported to be expressed on plasma cells and binding IgG immune complexes and trigger apoptosis (88). Studies have also identified other mechanisms of FcgRIIB modulation of the IgE receptor and the BCR the existence of which in human cells has not been determined. Mouse bone marrow derived mast cells, which differ phenotypically from human mast cells, showed an unconventional FcγRIIB ITIM-dependent regulation of the high affinity IgE receptor, FcεRI, where intracellular mediated co-aggregation of FcεRI with FcγRIIB occurs independently of the FcγRIIB ectodomain binding to antigen complexed IgG (89).

Cellular Responses

The specific effects of FcγRIIB signaling are dependent on the context of the co-engaged activating receptors and the cell type. In B cells, FcγRIIB1 inhibition of the BCR is a critical immune checkpoint for regulating antibody production (25, 90). The powerful nature of this immune checkpoint is evident from studies in clinical, genetic, and animal models that show that altering the balance between ITIM modulation and

ITAM activation is central to the pathogenesis and severity of disease (91).

As humoral immune responses develop, circulating antigen:antibody complexes simultaneously engage the antigen-specific BCR via the antigen of the complex and FcγRIIB via the Fc region, thereby modulating antigen receptor signaling. In FcγRIIB1, the C1 insertion impairs endocytosis, increasing the interaction time between FcγRIIB1, and the BCR. The C1 insert, irrespective of its position in the cytoplasmic tail, tethers the receptor to the cytoskeleton and so prevents the receptor localizing to coated pits and so disrupting endocytosis (92, 93). A di-leucine motif within the FcγRIIB ITIM sequence is also required for endocytosis (93, 94). Thus, the C1 insert confers cytoskeletal tethering and membrane retention which counter other cytoplasmic tail sequences including the di-leucine residues that would otherwise promote endocytosis.

FcγRIIB2 has also been studied in B cells in experimental systems where it also co-engages the BCR and regulates its function. FcγRIIB2 lacks the cytoplasmic C1 insertion and is rapidly internalized. A rare Tyr^{235}Asp polymorphism occurs within the unique membrane-tethering 19-amino acid insertion of FcγRIIB1. FcγRIIB1-Asp^{235} binding of mouse IgG1 was slightly lower in comparison to the Tyr^{235} variant of FcγRIIB1, as was mIgG1 anti-CD3 induced T cell mitogenesis (95, 96). FcγRIIB1-Asp^{235} retained the capacity to form caps and was effective in down-regulating increases in calcium upon cross-linking by serum IgG (95).

This prolonged surface expression of actively signaling FcγRIIB1 may also be important for the elimination by apoptosis of self-reactive B cells during somatic hyper-mutation (97). Thus, FcγRIIB1 constrains the selective antigen specificity of the humoral immune system and directs the B cell production toward an appropriate antibody repertoire.

FcγRIIB is upregulated after antigen stimulation via immune complexes on follicular DCs (FDCs) (98). FDCs retain immune complexes and recycle them periodically to their plasma membrane, a process believed to be important in development of B cell immune cell memory (99). The presentation of immune complexes by activated FDCs expressing FcγRIIB provides antigens to B cells in a highly immunogenic form by multimerising the antigens, thus extensively crosslinking multiple BCRs, minimizing B cell FcγRIIB ITIM-mediated inhibition and providing co-stimulatory signals (100).

The functional response of a cell that expresses both ITAM-bearing receptors and FcγRIIB can be altered by their expression levels. Basophils express activatory FcεRI and FcγRIIA, as well as FcγRIIB, which can inhibit IgE-induced responses (101, 102). This balance can be altered by IL-3 which upregulates expression of both FcγR, but more strongly enhances FcγRIIB2 expression (101). Under normal physiologic conditions it is believed that FcγRIIA co-aggregation may, by providing activated Lyn, aid FcγRIIB inhibitory function (102).

Monocyte-derived dendritic cells (moDCs) that were treated with IFNγ to upregulate their activating FcγRs (FcγRI and FcγRIIA) had increased IgG-mediated cellular maturation, while moDCs treated with anti-inflammatory concentrations of soluble monomeric IgG (IVIg) to increase FcγRIIB expression had decreased cellular maturation (18). Similarly, monocytes with increased expression of activating FcγRs over FcγRIIB as induced by IFNγ or TNFα had enhanced IgG-triggered cytokine production, while monocytes with enhanced FcγRIIB expression by IL-4 and IL-10 prevented IgG-triggered cytokine production (103). Furthermore, FcγRIIB$^{-/-}$ mouse macrophages developed robust inflammatory responses after exposure to subthreshold concentrations of immune complexes that failed to induce responses in FcγRIIB-expressing cells, demonstrating a role of FcγRIIB in setting a "threshold" for cellular activation (104).

PROPERTIES OF FcγRIIC

Molecular Structure

The expression of the membrane *FCGR2C* is complex. It is subject to a polymorphism (Gln^{13}STOP) wherein ~80% of the population do not express functional FcγRIIC proteins and also CNV, which in turn impacts expression of the *FCGR2B* gene as described above (67, 105). The *FCGR2C* gene arose by recombination between *FCGR2B* and *FCGR2A*. The functional transmembrane FcγRIIC protein encoded by this gene is an activating receptor wherein the extracellular domains are derived from and are identical to FcγRIIB (exons 1–4), but the transmembrane and cytoplasmic tail are derived from the activating type ITAM-containing FcγRIIA (exons 5–8).

Multiple mRNA splice variants of FcγRIIC have been identified (**Figure 1**), though their physiology is unclear. Interestingly, some FcγRIIC-Gln^{13} individuals still lack FcγRIIC expression due to alternative splicing that gives rise to multiple non-functional forms (67). Additionally, the *FCGR2C* locus shows CNV, which may contribute to variation in gene expression, at the transcript and/or protein level, also impacting other FcγRII expression and function (67, 106).

Expression and Cellular Responses

In individuals expressing the activatory FcγRIIC, it has been most extensively studied on NK cells (**Table 1**). NK cells expressing FcγRIIC had increased levels of ADCC upon receptor cross-linking, causing mediator release and lysis of target cells (67, 105–108). Although not extensively studied, it appears that FcγRIIC is also expressed on CD19+ B Cells. Its co-ligation with the BCR caused enhanced BCR signaling and B cell function, relative to FcγRIIB ITIM-dependent negative regulation in the absence of FcγRIIC. This FcγRIIC expression on B cells is associated with systemic lupus erythematosus (SLE) in humans, possibly related to the altered or unbalanced ITAM/ITIM signaling (108).

Interestingly, multiple other SNPs, 114945036, rs138747765, and rs78603008, have been significantly associated with FcγRIIA or FcγRIIC mRNA expression in B cells in European populations (109). However, protein expression data is not yet available.

STRUCTURAL BASIS OF FcγRII INTERACTION WITH IgG

Human FcγRs have distinct binding specificities and affinities for the four IgG subclasses (2). The determination of affinity and IgG subclass specificity has relied on a wide range of methods

TABLE 3 | Relative binding of human IgG by FcγR expressed on the cell surface.

Human FcγR	Human IgG Subclass			
	IgG1	IgG2	IgG3	IgG4
FcγRIIA His^{131}	+++	++	++++	−
FcγRIIA Arg^{131}	++	±	++++	±
FcγRIIB	+	−	+++	+
FcγRIIC	+	−	+++	+

mostly based on the binding of immune complexes to cell-expressed FcγR. More sensitive methods have used recombinant ectodomains and monomeric IgG using highly sensitive cell free systems such as SPR (5, 6, 110). A survey of the literature on the measurement of specificity and affinity of these receptors shows some variation in the methods used and the values calculated. Even the application of more sophisticated methods such as SPR show some degree of variation from group to group. Notwithstanding the variations and limitation in analyses of the interactions, it is clear that the FcγRII family (FcγRIIA, FcγRIIB, and FcγRIIC), are sensors of immune complexes and as such, interact poorly with uncomplexed monomeric IgG (1 μM affinity) but avidly bind immune complexes (5, 6, 15, 110).

There is general agreement that all FcγRII, indeed all FcγR, bind human IgG1 and IgG3 but there are significant differences in the interaction with IgG2 and IgG4 (**Table 3**). The allelic His^{131} form of human FcγRIIA is the only receptor which avidly binds human IgG2 complexes, while FcγRIIA-Arg^{131} binds IgG2 poorly (**Table 3**). However, it is possible that under circumstances of high local concentrations of opsonizing antibodies that binding interactions occur with FcγRIIA-Arg^{131} though whether there is a functional outcome is unknown (6, 111).

In contrast, FcγRIIB binds IgG4 but not IgG2 and moreover, binds IgG1 and IgG3 an approximately 10-fold lower affinity than the activating FcγRIIA. This is consistent with its powerful physiological inhibitory function as IgG binding affinities equal to or higher than the activating receptors might otherwise prevent pro-inflammatory responses that are necessary in resisting infection. Not surprisingly, FcγRIIC has the same IgG binding properties at FcγRIIB (6).

Other factors that affect interactions between IgG and the FcγRII are the size of the IgG immune complex (112), the distribution of epitopes (111, 113), the geometry of the Fc in the complex, and receptor localization in membrane domains (114) which may also influence the avidity of immune complex binding. The state of the cell expressing the receptor (115) can also influence interaction with IgG. FcγRIIA function may be modified by "inside-out signaling" whereby external stimuli such as granulocyte-macrophage colony-stimulating factor (GM-CSF), IL-5, and IL-3 in eosinophils (116) and N-formylmethionyl-leucyl-phenylalanine (fLMP) in neutrophils increase receptor avidity (117). The mechanism for this FcγRIIA "activation" is unknown but could involve receptor dimer forms (5, 115, 117, 118). This inside-out signaling has also been identified for the high affinity IgG receptor, FcγRI,

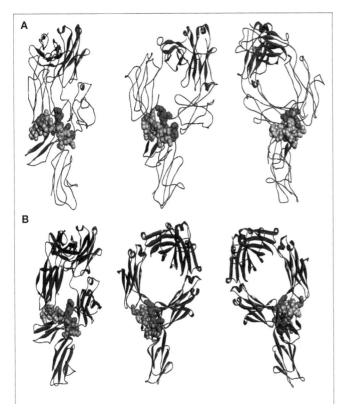

FIGURE 2 | The interaction of IgG-Fc with FcγRIIA and FcγRIIB is similar. The perspectives shown are of two ectodomains of the **(A)** FcγRIIA [adapted from 3RY6 (61)] and **(B)** FcγRIIB [adapted from 3WJJ (123)] (shown in dark blue) in complex with IgG-Fc (shown in gray). The structural components of the receptor contributing to IgG binding are the two tryptophan residues that form the Trp sandwich (red), the BC loop (green), the C'E strand (yellow), and the FG loop (purple), with the "high/low resonder" polymorphic residue His[131]Arg highlighted (orange).

where it is associated with cytoskeletal-dependent clustering of receptors (119).

X-ray crystallographic structural data is available for all FcγR but only in complex with the native or mutated IgG1 (61, 120–122). It is clear that the interaction of FcγRIIA and FcγRIIB with IgG1 is asymmetric. The "bent" FcγR extracellular region of one FcγR molecule inserting between, and making contacts with, both IgG1 H-chain Fcs, as is also the case with other FcγR (**Figure 2**) (2, 124). The key conclusion from these studies is that the principal contact regions of the FcγRIIA and FcγRIIB are similar and occur predominantly within the second domain BC loop, C strand, C'E loop, and the FG loop, with a contribution of the interdomain linker. The BC loop and the interdomain linker provide the two critical tryptophan residues, conserved in all FcγR, that sandwich the Pro[331] of the IgG1 CH2 FG loop.

The lower hinge of IgG has a dominant role in determining the specificity of FcγR interactions. In the case of IgG1, the lower hinge residues, Pro[233]Leu[234]Leu[235]Gly[236]Gly[237], of both H-chains form extensive contacts with FcγRIIA (61). Interestingly, this region is quite different in IgG2 (Pro,Val,Ala,Gly) and suggests that the IgG2 interaction with FcγRIIA may be quite distinct at the atomic level but as yet

no structure of IgG2 in complex with FcγRIIA is known. Nonetheless, the IgG1:FcγRIIA complex structure suggests that the preferential IgG2 binding by FcγRIIA-H[131] over FcγRIIA-R[131]–the "high/low responder" polymorphism (125)—may be explained structurally by the smaller histidine side chain more readily accommodating interaction with the Fc adjacent to the lower hinge compared to the longer arginine side chain (61).

The structural basis for the effect of the rare Gln[127]Lys polymorphism that also affects IgG2 binding is interesting (126). The Lys[127] does not appear to make contact with the IgG1 Fc and sits adjacent to the binding region, so that the effect on Fc binding is presumably indirect. This indicates a possible selective pressure for IgG2 binding by this receptor (126).

ROLES OF FcγRII IN HEALTH AND DISEASE

The balance between activation and inhibitory signaling is important in the control of healthy antibody dependant responses and disturbance to this balance can have adverse, but in some cases positive, consequences to health.

Genetic polymorphism studies of human *FCGR2* genes have helped to establish roles of FcγRII proteins in several autoimmune diseases and in resistance or susceptibility to infectious diseases (**Table 4**). *In vivo* mechanistic studies in experimental animal models, including transgenic and gene replacement systems, have also been helpful in establishing specific protective or deleterious roles of FcγRII in infectious disease, inflammation, autoimmunity, and cancer and have been reviewed extensively elsewhere (139–143).

Infection

The *in vivo* roles of the FcγRII receptor family in humans have been derived by extrapolation of animal studies and by genetic studies of human populations. The FcγRIIA high/low-responder polymorphism influences susceptibility to infections, as FcγRIIA-Arg[131] has poor IgG2 binding (144, 145). Individuals expressing FcγRIIA-His[131] are more resistant to infection by *Streptococcus pneumonia, Haemophilus influenza,* and *Neisseria meningitides*. This is potentially due to more avid binding of IgG2 by FcγRIIA-His[131] over FcγRIIA-Arg[131], consequently resulting in more efficient effector responses such as uptake by phagocytes, induction of degranulation and elastase release by granulocytes *in vivo* (144, 146, 147).

FcγRs do not function in isolation under physiological conditions *in vivo* and it is notable that co-operation between Toll-like receptors (TLRs) and FcγRs is an important feature of effective pathogen elimination (148). TLRs are often co-expressed with FcγRIIA and co-engagement results in enhanced functional responses of these individual receptors, e.g., enhanced TNFα, IL-23, and IL-1β release by DCs (35, 149, 150).

The role of FcγR in HIV is complex and apparently conflicting data may reflect different aspects of HIV infection and clinical outcomes. In a small study of immunocompetent patients who had undergone successful and early antiretroviral treatment, who expressed FcγRIIA-His[131], and had a IgG2 response

TABLE 4 | Function or clinical association of polymorphic residues of FcγRII.

Receptor	Polymorphism	Function/clinical association	Reference
FcγRIIA	Gln27Trp (rs9427397, rs9427398)	Impaired calcium mobilization and MAP kinase phosphorylation; associated with CVID	(127)
	Gln127Lys	Gln[127] interferes with the interaction of adjacent receptor residues with IgG2	(126)
	His131Arg (rs1801274)	His[131] able to bind IgG2; both forms associated with autoimmune disease; allograft rejection and mAb cancer treatment outcomes	(128, 129)
	c.7421871A>G	Permits alternative splicing of the C1* exon resulting in expression of "hyperactive" FcγRIIA3. Risk factor for IVIg anaphylaxis.	(11, 12)
	Hypomethylation	Increased susceptibility genes for Kawasaki disease and IVIg resistance	(130)
FcγRIIB	Promoter haplotype (rs3219018, rs34701572)	Deregulated FcγRIIB expression may contribute to pathogenesis	(59, 131)
	Ile232Thr (rs1050501)	Thr[232] allele does not partition to lipid rafts and is associated with impaired regulation of ITAM signaling, predisposing to SLE but protective for malaria	(132–137)
	Tyr235Asp	Asp[235] has reduced binding, internalization and signaling	(95, 96)
FcγRIIC	Gln13stop	Commonly referred to as the ORF/Stop polymorphism, determines functional expression of receptor, may contribute to autoimmune disease	(105, 106)
	Gln57stop (rs1801274)	Unknown mechanism, associated with autoimmune disease and vaccine efficacy for HIV	(106, 138)

to a gp120 vaccine regime, there was a partial control of viral replication during interruption of anti-retroviral therapy (151). However, analysis of the Vax004 gp120 vaccine trial found no evidence of association of FcγRIIA polymorphism with protection against HIV infection, although this was an unsuccessful vaccine trial overall (152). HIV studies have emphasized the protective role of NK cell FcγRIIIA in antibody dependent cellular cytotoxicity. However, recent studies have found a potent role for FcγRIIA in the protective functions of macrophages and neutrophils, which are abundant effectors at the mucosal sites of HIV acquisition (153). HIV co-infections generate an even more complex clinical picture. FcγRIIA-His[131] homozygous individuals are more susceptible to developing AIDs-related pneumonia, and have an increased risk of placental malaria in HIV-infected women (154) and other perinatal infections (155, 156).

While few resting CD4 T cells express FcγRIIA, these cells are highly relevant to HIV research. Resting CD4 T cells latently infected with HIV are an important target in strategies to eliminate HIV in anti-retroviral therapy (ART) patients, as these quiescent cells provide safe harbor for "silent" virus that, upon reactivation, causes viral recrudescence within weeks of treatment interruption. FcγRIIA was reported as a surface marker of this key quiescent population in ART patients (157) but other studies found no enrichment of HIV proviral DNA by sorting CD4 T cells based on FcγRIIA expression (52, 158). Rather than on resting CD4 T cells, FcγRII expression was mostly on activated CD4 cells associated with transcriptionally active virus (159). Furthermore, another study sorted a CD4+ population that apparently expressed FcγRIIB, not FcγRIIA. However, these FcγRIIB+ cells derived from contaminating B cells, occurring as T-B cell doublets, and also from single CD4 T cells, with a punctate staining pattern that included other B cell markers, and was suggestive of trogocytosis rather than intrinsic CD4 T cell expression (52). These studies indicate some

of the technical challenges that can accompany determining FcγR expression.

Though the numbers are small there is suggestive evidence that polymorphism in the FCGR2C locus, in particular FCGR2C-126 C>T SNP was associated with a protective anti-HIV vaccination response. In the RV144 vaccine trial, individuals homozygous for FCGR2C-126C/C had an estimated vaccine efficacy of 15% whereas individuals homozygous for the FCGR2C-126T/T or heterozygous—126 C/T had an estimated vaccine efficacy of 91% (138). Whether this association relates to effector function via a functional FcγRIIC protein or is due to linkage to another effector system encoded in this chromosomal region is uncertain (109).

FcγRs also have an established role in antibody-dependent enhancement (ADE) of dengue virus (DENV) infection. Immune complexes of DENV opsonized with non- or sub-neutralizing levels of antibodies interact with FcγRs on monocytes, macrophages, and dendritic cells, led to increased uptake, viral replication, and more severe infection (160). In keeping with its modulating role, FcγRIIB inhibits ADE in experimental systems (161). Indeed, while FcγRIIA facilitates DENV entry, mutation of the ITAM to an ITIM significantly inhibited ADE, and conversely, replacing the inhibitory motif in FcγRIIB with an ITAM, conferred ADE capacity (162).

The hypo-functional FcγRIIB-Thr[232] variant is enriched in populations from malaria endemic areas. This suggests that reduced FcγRIIB modulation of responses and a consequential enhancement of B cell and inflammatory cell activation confers a survival advantage in these populations (132, 163). Indeed, enhanced activatory FcR responses including increased phagocytic capacity and TNF production by innate cells and enhanced B cell responses is evident by elevated malaria specific antibody titers (164).

Interestingly, the FcγRIIB-Thr[232] polymorphism has been shown to confer increased phagocytosis of antibody opsonized bacteria by monocyte-derived macrophages (132). Models suggest FcγRIIB is integral for the balance between efficient pathogen clearance and the prevention of the cytokine-mediated effects of sepsis (163). In geographic areas where there is less infectious disease pressure, FcγRIIB-Thr[232] is associated with susceptibility to autoimmunity.

FcγR in Autoimmunity

Imbalance between inhibitory and activatory FcγR functions predisposes individuals to pro-inflammatory autoimmune disease. FcγRIIA activation induces the production of pro-inflammatory cytokines, including IFN and TNFα, which are active in the promotion of inflammation, systemic lupus erythematosus (SLE), Kawasaki disease (KD), Grave's disease, and Rheumatoid Arthritis (RA) (35, 165–167).

The FcγRIIA-His[131] allelic form is associated with other autoimmune diseases, including Guillain-Barré syndrome, ulcerative colitis and KD, possibly due to increased inflammatory cell activation via IgG2 (168–170).The FcγRIIA-Arg[131] allelic form is associated with susceptibility to SLE, angina pectoris, acute coronary syndrome (ACS), myasthenia gravis, and RA (171–174). This may be related to the impaired ability of FcγRIIA-Arg[131] to process and recycle IgG2, causing the release of pro-inflammatory cytokines, aggravating disease (175, 176).

Other FcγRIIA polymorphisms, although less well characterized, are associated with inflammatory diseases. Recently a glutamine/tryptophan polymorphism at position 27 (Gln[27]Trp) has been identified, where homozygous individuals were over represented in CVID (127). No difference in expression was observed and FcγRIIA-Trp[27] had modest impairment of calcium mobilization and MAP kinase phosphorylation *in vitro* (127).

Epigenetic modifications of *FCGR2A* such as hypomethylation have also been described in CVID patients, particularly at the promoter CpG site cg24422489 (130, 169). This increased susceptibility for KD and resistance to Ig replacement therapy, with significant hypomethylation of FcγRIIA in patients with acute KD and coronary artery lesions (130, 169, 177).

The recently described rare intronic A>G SNP that controls expression of the splice variant FcγRIIA3 occurs in <1% of healthy subjects (11, 12). However, it is associated with KD, immune thrombocytopenia (ITP), and CVID (11). Furthermore, severe adverse reactions in response to immunoglobulin replacement therapy occurred in patients expressing FcγRIIA3 and neutrophil activation (mediator and elastase release) was enhanced. Increased signaling by FcγRIIA3 was due to its altered membrane localization and longer membrane retention time (11, 12). Thus, increased inflammatory responses toward therapeutic IgG may paradoxically diminish the utility of the major treatment regime in this subset of CVID patients.

Polymorphism and CNV of activatory FcγRIIC is associated with increased severity of RA and ITP (106, 178). This has been attributed to expression variance in these individuals causing an imbalance between activatory and inhibitory signals.

Since the inhibitory FcγRIIB forms modulate the activation of B cells and innate effector cells, decreased expression of the FcγRIIB leads to dysregulated antibody function and increased antibody-dependant inflammatory cell responses and thus increased susceptibility to autoimmune diseases. Polymorphisms in the *FCGR2B* promoter or transmembrane domain of FcγRIIB influence receptor expression and signaling potency and are associated with susceptibility to autoimmune diseases including SLE, Goodpasture's disease, ITP, and RA (133–135, 156, 179, 180). Multiple polymorphisms in the promoter region of *FCGR2B* have been identified. The promoter haplotype *FCGR2B*−386G>C SNP in combination with *FCGR2B*-120T>A SNP (*FCGR2B*-386C +−120A) enhances promoter activity and transcription, however this enhanced haplotype has low prevalence (59, 131). *FCGR2B*-343G>C SNP is enriched in European American SLE patients and homozygous expression of *FCGR2B*-343C is linked to SLE susceptibility (131, 179). This is due to decreased AP1 transcription complex binding, which causes decreased FcγRIIB expression on B cells and macrophages and altered antigen clearance (179).

The frequency of the transmembrane polymorphism FcγRIIB-Thr[232]Ile differs among different ethnic populations, with FcγRIIB-Thr[232] associated with SLE in Asian but not African American or European populations (134). FcγRIIB-Thr[232] shows reduced lateral mobility in the membrane which impairs its ability to inhibit the co-localization of BCR and CD19 microclusters and consequent B cell activation (181). This causes increased B cell and myeloid cell activation (133, 136, 137), which elevates B cell (antibody) responses and heightens IgG-dependant pro-inflammatory responses, resulting in autoimmunity.

Cancer

The roles of FcγR in cancer relate largely to the harnessing of antibody-dependant effector functions such as ADCC or ADCP by therapeutic mAbs during the treatment [reviewed in (2, 139)]. However, it also appears that mAb therapy may also have long term therapeutic benefits. Studies on DCs indicate that FcγRIIA activation is necessary and sufficient to induce a strong T cell anti-tumor cellular immunity inducing long term anti-tumor vaccine-like or "vaccinal effects" in humanized mice (48). Engagement of FcγRIIA induced DC maturation and up-regulation of costimulatory molecules, priming them for optimal antigen presentation and cross-presentation, thus stimulating long-term anti-tumor T cell memory (48).

Conversely, the inhibitory role of FcγRIIB may be disadvantageous to antibody-based therapies and other immune stimulating therapies. Thus, blocking inhibitory function of FcγRIIB on effector cells or antigen presenting cells such as DCs might be a strategy to enhance anti-tumor immune responses during immunotherapy (18, 182, 183).

HARNESSING OR TARGETING FcγRII FOR ANTIBODY BASED THERAPIES

Monoclonal antibodies are a versatile class of biotherapeutic drugs because of the multifunctional nature of the antibody molecule. IgG-based therapeutic mAbs are effective for the treatment of a variety of diseases due to their high specificity and affinity for their target antigen and, in some cases, their strong induction of FcγR effector functions. Depending on the nature of the disease and molecule, the mAb efficacy may depend on one or more mechanisms of action, ranging from simple antigen neutralization, complement-dependent cytotoxicity, FcγR-dependant cellular effector functions, or inhibition via FcγRIIB. Thus, effective patient responses can be dependent on FcγR based mechanisms, e.g., altered binding due to the FcγRIIA-His^{131}Arg polymorphism, which influence the efficacy of therapeutic mAbs such as rituximab and cetuximab (184, 185).

The efficacy of the anti-EGFR mAb, cetuximab, and subsequent progression free survival was associated with expression of the His^{131} variant of FcγRIIA (185). Patients with the FcγRIIA-His^{131} genotype also responded better to rituximab treatment in non-Hodgkin's lymphoma (184). Conversely, FcγRIIB expression on lymphoma cells is a risk factor for anti-CD20 rituximab therapy failure due to FcγRIIB internalizing the CD20:rituximab complex and thereby reducing exposure of the opsonized lymphoma cell to the immune effector systems (186).

Inhibition of activatory FcγR could block early development of inflammatory disease. This has been explored experimentally in humanized mouse models of RA, using antibody fragments (or small molecules) designed to bind human FcγRIIA to inhibit disease (29, 187). Synthetic FcR mimetics have also been used to block the function of FcγRIIA in vitro (188) and the modulation of FcγRIIA and FcγRIIB function in humans (189).

FcγRIIB is a powerful modulator of ITAM-dependent receptors such as the BCR or high affinity FcεRI. Strategies to harness this powerful inhibitory capacity are being developed by engineering mAb Fc regions with enhanced and/or selective engagement with FcγRIIB. Such strategies rely on the co-engagement of FcγRIIB with the mAb-targeted activating receptor. This engineering of therapeutic mAbs with increased affinity to FcγRIIB has diverse clinical applications. Indeed, anti-CD19 binds the BCR complex and the engineered Fc co-engages FcγRIIB with increased affinity, suppressing B cell activation without B cell depletion (190, 191). This novel approach to treat autoimmune disease demonstrates the importance of understanding FcγR biology and interactions with IgG in order to optimally exploit antibody functions for specific therapies.

Another example is the anti-IgE, omalizumab, an effective treatment for allergic asthma by neutralizing IgE binding to FcεRI. Mutations introduced in XmAb7195, an omalizumab "equivalent" antibody, enhanced affinity for FcγRIIB. Like omalizumab, XmAb7195 binds to and neutralizes circulating IgE (71). However, its enhanced Fc interaction with FcγRIIB may also promote co-aggregation of FcγRIIB with the BCR of IgE+ B cells, and may suppress activation of the BCR, diminishing allergic antibody production. In addition, data from mouse studies suggest that the XmAb7195:IgE complexes are rapidly removed from the circulation via FcγRIIB expressed in the liver endothelium (71).

FcγR Targeted Therapies

In some autoimmune diseases, auto-antibodies activate inflammatory cell effector functions against self-antigens leading to tissue destruction. One strategy used to ameliorate this destructive pathogenesis is the use of soluble FcγRs, which compete for auto-antibody binding with cell-based FcγRs thereby preventing induction of the cell-based effector functions (1, 9). Pre-clinical studies have demonstrated that the use of these soluble FcγRs suppresses the Arthus reaction, collagen-induced arthritis, and SLE (192, 193). A soluble recombinant form of FcγRIIB, named SM101, is a potential treatment for the treatment of ITP and SLE and has progressed into clinical trials (194, 195).

Small chemical entities (SCEs) specific for FcγRIIA have also been reported to inhibit immune complex-induced responses including platelet activation and aggregation, and TNF secretion by macrophages in vitro (187). Furthermore, in vivo testing of these SCEs in FcγRIIA transgenic mice also inhibited the development and stopped the progression of collagen-induced arthritis (CIA) (187). Hence, these SCE FcγRIIA antagonists demonstrated their potential as anti-inflammatory agents for pro-inflammatory immune complex-dependent autoimmune diseases.

CONCLUSIONS

FcγRII receptors and their variants play important roles in the healthy immune response to infection, as well as in the pathologies of autoimmunity and the efficacy of therapeutic mAb treatments in cancer. Our expanding knowledge of these widely expressed FcγR and their signaling pathways may provide insight as to how we can exploit this intricate immunomodulatory system for therapeutic and diagnostic purposes. Harnessing FcR-dependent cellular effector systems through therapeutic mAbs, or by blocking effector functions, is becoming an increasingly useful tool to treat an extensive range of diseases.

AUTHOR CONTRIBUTIONS

JA drafted the manuscript. AC, BW, and PMH provided additional text and all authors reviewed the manuscript.

FUNDING

This work was funded by Australian National Health and Medical Research Council: PMH, JA, AC, and BW supported by NHMRC project grants 1079946, 1067484, and grants-in-aid from the Pendergast Trust and Walkom Trust.

REFERENCES

1. Hogarth PM. Fc receptors are major mediators of antibody based inflammation in autoimmunity. *Curr Opin Immunol.* (2002) 14:798–802. doi: 10.1016/S0952-7915(02)00409-0

2. Hogarth PM, Pietersz GA. Fc receptor-targeted therapies for the treatment of inflammation, cancer and beyond. *Nat Rev Drug Discov.* (2012) 11:311–31. doi: 10.1038/nrd2909

3. Qiu WQ, De Bruin D, Brownstein BH, Pearse R, Ravetch JV. Orgaization of the human and mouse low-affinity FcγR genes: duplication an

recombination. *Science*. (1990) 248:732–5. doi: 10.1126/science. 2139735

4. Brooks DG, Qiu WQ, Luster AD, Ravetch JV. Structure and expression of human IgG FcRII(CD32). Functional heterogeneity is encoded by the alternatively spliced products of multiple genes. *J Exp Med*. (1989) 170:1369–85. doi: 10.1084/jem.170.4.1369

5. Powell MS, Barton PA, Emmanouilidis D, Wines BD, Neumann GM, Peitersz GA, et al. Biochemical analysis and crystallisation of Fc gamma RIIa, the low affinity receptor for Ig. *Immunol Lett G*. (1999) 68:17–23. doi: 10.1016/S0165-2478(99)00025-5

6. Bruhns P, Iannascoli B, England P, Mancardi DA, Fernandez N, Jorieux S, et al. Specificity and affinity of human Fcgamma receptors and their polymorphic variants for human IgG subclasses. *Blood*. (2009) 113:3716–25. doi: 10.1182/blood-2008-09-179754

7. Lu J, Mold C, Du Clos TW, Sun PD. Pentraxins and Fc receptor-mediated immune responses. *Front Immunol*. (2018) 9:2607. doi: 10.3389/fimmu.2018.02607

8. Hibbs ML, Bonadonna L, Scott BM, McKenzie IF, Hogarth PM. Molecular cloning of a human immunoglobulin G Fc receptor. *Proc Natl Acad Sci USA*. (1988) 85:2240–4. doi: 10.1073/pnas.85.7.2240

9. Ierino FL, Hulett MD, McKenzie IF, Hogarth PM. Mapping epitopes of human Fc gamma RII (CDw32) with monoclonal antibodies and recombinant receptors. *J Immunol*. (1993) 150:1794–803.

10. Ierino FL, Powell MS, McKenzie IFC, Hogarth PM. Recombinant soluble human Fc gamma RII: production, characterization, and inhibition of the Arthus reaction. *J Exp Med*. (1993) 178:1617–28. doi: 10.1084/jem.178.5.1617

11. van der Heijden J, Geissler J, van Mirre E, van Deuren MJ, van der Meer W, Salama ATK, et al. A novel splice variant of FcgammaRIIa: a risk factor for anaphylaxis in patients with hypogammaglobulinemia. *J Allergy Clin Immunol*. (2013) 131:1408–16 e5. doi: 10.1016/j.jaci.2013. 02.009

12. Anania JC, Trist HT, Palmer CS, Tan PS, Kouskousis BP, Chenoweth AM, et al. The rare anaphylaxis-associated FcγRIIa3 exhibits distinct characteristics from the canonical FcγRIIa1. *Front Immunol*. (2018) 9:1809. doi: 10.3389/fimmu.2018.01809

13. Amigorena S, Bonnerot C, Drake JR, Choquet D, Hunziker W, Guillet JG, et al. Cytoplasmic domain heterogeneity and functions of IgG Fc receptors in B lymphocytes. *Science*. (1992) 256:1808–12. doi: 10.1126/science.1535455

14. Astier A, de la Salle H, de la Salle C, Bieber T, Esposito-Farese ME, Freund M, et al. Human epidermal Langerhans cells secrete a soluble receptor for IgG (Fc gamma RII/CD32) that inhibits the binding of immune complexes to Fc gamma R+ cells. *J Immunol*. (1994) 152:201–12.

15. Trist HM, Tan PS, Wines BD, Ramsland PA, Orlowski E, Stubbs J, et al. Polymorphisms and interspecies differences of the activating and inhibitory FcgammaRII of Macaca nemestrina influence the binding of human IgG subclasses. *J Immunol*. (2014) 192:792–803. doi: 10.4049/jimmunol.1301554

16. Hogarth PM, Anania JC, Wines BD. The FcgammaR of humans and non-human primates and their interaction with IgG: implications for induction of inflammation, resistance to infection and the use of therapeutic monoclonal antibodies. *Curr Top Microbiol Immunol*. (2014) 382:321–52. doi: 10.1007/978-3-319-07911-0_15

17. Hulett MD, Hogarth PM. Molecular basis of Fc receptor function. *Adv Immunol*. (1994) 57:1–127. doi: 10.1016/S0065-2776(08)60671-9

18. Boruchov AM, Heller G, Veri MC, Bonvini E, Ravetch JV, Young JW. Activating and inhibitory IgG Fc receptors on human DCs mediate opposing functions. *J Clin Invest*. (2005) 115:2914–23. doi: 10.1172/JCI 24772

19. Shushakova N, Skokowa J, Schulman J, Baumann U, Zwirner J, Schmidt RE, et al. C5a anaphylatoxin is a major regulator of activating versus inhibitory FcgammaRs in immune complex-induced lung disease. *J Clin Invest*. (2002) 110:1823–30. doi: 10.1172/JCI16577

20. Guyre PM, Morganelli PM, Miller R. Recombinant immune interferon increases immunoglobulin G Fc receptors on cultured human mononuclear phagocytes. *J Clin Invest*. (1983) 72:393–7. doi: 10.1172/JCI110980

21. te Velde AA, de Waal Malefijt R, Huijbens RJ, de Vries JE, Figdor CG. IL-10 stimulates monocyte Fc gamma R surface expression and cytotoxic activity. Distinct regulation of antibody-dependent cellular cytotoxicity by IFN-gamma, IL-4, and IL-10. *J Immunol*. (1992) 149:4048–52.

22. Engelhardt W, Matzke J, Schmidt RE. Activation-dependent expression of low affinity IgG receptors Fc gamma RII(CD32) and Fc gamma RIII(CD16) in subpopulations of human T lymphocytes. *Immunobiology*. (1995) 192:297–320. doi: 10.1016/S0171-2985(11)80172-5

23. Holgado MP, Sananez I, Raiden S, Geffner JR, Arruvito L. CD32 ligation promotes the activation of CD4(+) T cells. *Front Immunol*. (2018) 9:2814. doi: 10.3389/fimmu.2018.02814

24. Metzger H. Transmembrane signaling: the joy of aggregation. *J Immunol*. (1992) 149:1477–87.

25. Getahun A, Cambier JC. Of ITIMs, ITAMs, and ITAMis: revisiting immunoglobulin Fc receptor signaling. *Immunol Rev*. (2015) 268:66–73. doi: 10.1111/imr.12336

26. Barrow AD, Trowsdale J. You say ITAM and I say ITIM, let's call the whole thing off: the ambiguity of immunoreceptor signalling. *Eur J Immunol*. (2006) 36:1646–53. doi: 10.1002/eji.200636195

27. Mkaddem SB, Murua A, Flament H, Titeca-Beauport D, Bounaix C, Danelli L, et al. Lyn and Fyn function as molecular switches that control immunoreceptors to direct homeostasis or inflammation. *Nat Commun*. (2017) 8:246. doi: 10.1038/s41467-017-00294-0

28. Ganesan LP, Fang H, Marsh CB, Tridandapani S. The protein-tyrosine phosphatase SHP-1 associates with the phosphorylated immunoreceptor tyrosine-based activation motif of Fc gamma RIIa to modulate signaling events in myeloid cells. *J Biol Chem*. (2003) 278:35710–7. doi: 10.1074/jbc.M305078200

29. Ben Mkaddem S, Hayem G, Jonsson F, Rossato E, Boedec E, Boussetta T, et al. Shifting FcgammaRIIA-ITAM from activation to inhibitory configuration ameliorates arthritis. *J Clin Invest*. (2014) 124:3945–59. doi: 10.1172/JCI74572

30. Campbell KS. Suppressing the killer instinct. *Sci Signal*. (2016) 9:fs8. doi: 10.1126/scisignal.aaf6348

31. Kanamaru Y, Pfirsch S, Aloulou M, Vrtovsnik F, Essig M, Loirat C, et al. Inhibitory ITAM signaling by Fc alpha RI-FcR gamma chain controls multiple activating responses and prevents renal inflammation. *J Immunol*. (2008) 180:2669–78. doi: 10.4049/jimmunol.180.4.2669

32. Rossato E, Ben Mkaddem S, Kanamaru Y, Hurtado-Nedelec M, Hayem G, Descatoire V, et al. Reversal of Arthritis by Human Monomeric IgA Through the Receptor-Mediated SH2 Domain-Containing Phosphatase 1 Inhibitory Pathway. *Arthritis Rheumatol*. (2015) 67:1766–77. doi: 10.1002/art. 39142

33. Aloulou M, Ben Mkaddem S, Biarnes-Pelicot M, Boussetta T, Souchet H, Rossato E, et al. IgG1 and IVIg induce inhibitory ITAM signaling through FcgammaRIII controlling inflammatory responses. *Blood*. (2012) 119:3084–96. doi: 10.1182/blood-2011-08-376046

34. Bournazos S, Wang TT, Ravetch JV. The role and function of Fcgamma receptors on myeloid cells. *Microbiol Spectr*. (2016) 4:6. doi: 10.1128/microbiolspec.MCHD-0045-2016

35. Vogelpoel LT, Baeten DL, de Jong EC, den Dunnen J. Control of cytokine production by human fc gamma receptors: implications for pathogen defense and autoimmunity. *Front Immunol*. (2015) 6:79. doi: 10.3389/fimmu.2015.00079

36. Booth JW, Kim MK, Jankowski A, Schreiber AD, Grinstein S. Contrasting requirements for ubiquitylation during Fc receptor-mediated endocytosis and phagocytosis. *EMBO J*. (2002) 21:251–8. doi: 10.1093/emboj/21.3.251

37. Zhang CY, Booth JW. Differences in endocytosis mediated by FcgammaRIIA and FcgammaRIIB2. *Mol Immunol*. (2011) 49:329–37. doi: 10.1016/j.molimm.2011.09.003

38. Indik Z, Kelly C, Chien P, Levinson AI, Schreiber AD. Human Fc gamma RII, in the absence of other Fc gamma receptors, mediates a phagocytic signal. *J Clin Invest*. (1991) 88:1766–71. doi: 10.1172/JCI115496

39. Dai X, Jayapal M, Tay HK, Reghunathan R, Lin G, Too CT, et al. Differential signal transduction, membrane trafficking, and immune effector functions mediated by FcgammaRI versus FcgammaRIIa. *Blood*. (2009) 114:318–27. doi: 10.1182/blood-2008-10-184457

40. Huang ZY, Chien P, Indik ZK, Schreiber AD. Human platelet FcgammaRIIA and phagocytes in immune-complex clearance. *Mol Immunol*. (2011) 48:691–6. doi: 10.1016/j.molimm.2010.11.017

41. Chen K, Nishi H, Travers R, Tsuboi N, Martinod K, Wagner DD, et al. Endocytosis of soluble immune complexes leads to their clearance by

FcgammaRIIIB but induces neutrophil extracellular traps via FcgammaRIIA *in vivo*. *Blood*. (2012) 120:4421–31. doi: 10.1182/blood-2011-12-401133

42. Worth RG, Chien CD, Chien P, Reilly MP, McKenzie SE, Schreiber AD. Platelet FcgammaRIIA binds and internalizes IgG-containing complexes. *Exp Hematol*. (2006) 34:1490–5. doi: 10.1016/j.exphem.2006.06.015

43. Richards JO, Karki S, Lazar GA, Chen H, Dang W, Desjarlais JR. Optimization of antibody binding to FcgammaRIIa enhances macrophage phagocytosis of tumor cells. *Mol Cancer Ther*. (2008) 7:2517–27. doi: 10.1158/1535-7163.MCT-08-0201

44. Sallusto F, Lanzavecchia A. Efficient presentation of soluble antigen by cultured human dendritic cells is maintained by granulocyte/macrophage colony-stimulating factor plus interleukin 4 and downregulated by tumor necrosis factor alpha. *J Exp Med*. (1994) 179:1109–18. doi: 10.1084/jem.179.4.1109

45. Wallace PK, Tsang KY, Goldstein J, Correale P, Jarry TM, Schlom J, et al. Exogenous antigen targeted to FcgammaRI on myeloid cells is presented in association with MHC class I. *J Immunol Methods*. (2001) 248:183–94. doi: 10.1016/S0022-1759(00)00351-3

46. Platzer B, Stout M, Fiebiger E. Antigen cross-presentation of immune complexes. *Front Immunol*. (2014) 5:140. doi: 10.3389/fimmu.2014.00140

47. Amigorena S. Fc gamma receptors and cross-presentation in dendritic cells. *J Exp Med*. (2002) 195:F1–3. doi: 10.1084/jem.20011925

48. DiLillo DJ, Ravetch JV. Differential Fc-receptor engagement drives an anti-tumor vaccinal effect. *Cell*. (2015) 161:1035–45. doi: 10.1016/j.cell.2015.04.016

49. Graziano RF, Fanger MW. Fc gamma RI and Fc gamma RII on monocytes and granulocytes are cytotoxic trigger molecules for tumor cells. *J Immunol*. (1987) 139:3536–41.

50. Krutmann J, Kirnbauer R, Kock A, Schwarz T, Schopf E, May LT, et al. Cross-linking Fc receptors on monocytes triggers IL-6 production. Role in anti-CD3-induced T cell activation. *J Immunol*. (1990) 145:1337–42.

51. Simms HH, Gaither TA, Fries LF, Frank MM. Monokines released during short-term Fc gamma receptor phagocytosis up-regulate polymorphonuclear leukocytes and monocyte-phagocytic function. *J Immunol*. (1991) 147:265–72.

52. Osuna CE, Lim SY, Kublin JL, Apps R, Chen E, Mota TM, et al. Evidence that CD32a does not mark the HIV-1 latent reservoir. *Nature*. (2018) 561:E20–8. doi: 10.1038/s41586-018-0495-2

53. Chauhan AK. Human CD4(+) T-cells: a role for low-affinity Fc receptors. *Front Immunol*. (2016) 7:215. doi: 10.3389/fimmu.2016.00215

54. Canobbio I, Stefanini L, Guidetti GF, Balduini C, Torti M. A new role for FcgammaRIIA in the potentiation of human platelet activation induced by weak stimulation. *Cell Signal*. (2006) 18:861–70. doi: 10.1016/j.cellsig.2005.07.014

55. Gardiner EE, Karunakaran D, Arthur JF, Mu FT, Powell MS, Baker RI, et al. Dual ITAM-mediated proteolytic pathways for irreversible inactivation of platelet receptors: de-ITAM-izing FcgammaRIIa. *Blood*. (2008) 111:165–74. doi: 10.1182/blood-2007-04-086983

56. Hibbs ML, Walker ID, Kirszbaum L, Pietersz GA, Deacon NJ, Chambers GW, et al. The murine Fc receptor for immunoglobulin: purification, partial amino acid sequence, and isolation of cDNA clones. *Proc Natl Acad Sci USA*. (1986) 83:6980–4. doi: 10.1073/pnas.83.18.6980

57. Lewis VA, Koch T, Plutner H, Mellman I. A complementary DNA clone for a macrophage-lymphocyte Fc receptor. *Nature*. (1986) 324:372–5. doi: 10.1038/324372a0

58. Latour S, Fridman WH, Daeron M. Identification, molecular cloning, biologic properties, and tissue distribution of a novel isoform of murine low-affinity IgG receptor homologous to human Fc gamma RIIB1. *J Immunol*. (1996) 157:189–97.

59. Su K, Yang H, Li X, Li X, Gibson AW, Cafardi JM, et al. Expression profile of FcgammaRIIb on leukocytes and its dysregulation in systemic lupus erythematosus. *J Immunol*. (2007) 178:3272–80. doi: 10.4049/jimmunol.178.5.3272

60. Veri MC, Gorlatov S, Li H, Burke S, Johnson S, Stavenhagen J, et al. Monoclonal antibodies capable of discriminating the human inhibitory Fcgamma-receptor IIB (CD32B) from the activating Fcgamma-receptor IIA (CD32A): biochemical, biological and functional characterization. *Immunology*. (2007) 121:392–404. doi: 10.1111/j.1365-2567.2007.02588.x

61. Ramsland PA, Farrugia W, Bradford TM, Sardjono CT, Esparon S, Trist HM, et al. Structural basis for Fc gammaRIIa recognition of human IgG and formation of inflammatory signaling complexes. *J Immunol*. (2011) 187:3208–17. doi: 10.4049/jimmunol.1101467

62. Joshi T, Ganesan LP, Cao X, Tridandapani S. Molecular analysis of expression and function of hFcgammaRIIbl and b2 isoforms in myeloid cells. *Mol Immunol*. (2006) 43:839–50. doi: 10.1016/j.molimm.2005.06.037

63. Tsang MW, Nagelkerke SQ, Bultink IE, Geissler J, Tanck MW, Tacke CE, et al. Fc-gamma receptor polymorphisms differentially influence susceptibility to systemic lupus erythematosus and lupus nephritis. *Rheumatology*. (2016) 55:939–48. doi: 10.1093/rheumatology/kev433

64. Sellge G, Barkowsky M, Kramer S, Gebhardt T, Sander LE, Lorentz A, et al. Interferon-gamma regulates growth and controls Fcgamma receptor expression and activation in human intestinal mast cells. *BMC Immunol*. (2014) 15:27. doi: 10.1186/1471-2172-15-27

65. Burton OT, Epp A, Fanny ME, Miller SJ, Stranks AJ, Teague JE, et al. Tissue-specific expression of the low-affinity IgG receptor, FcgammaRIIb, on human mast cells. *Front Immunol*. (2018) 9:1244. doi: 10.3389/fimmu.2018.01244

66. Zhao W, Kepley CL, Morel PA, Okumoto LM, Fukuoka Y, Schwartz LB. Fc gamma RIIa, not Fc gamma RIIb, is constitutively and functionally expressed on skin-derived human mast cells. *J Immunol*. (2006) 177:694–701. doi: 10.4049/jimmunol.177.1.694

67. van der Heijden J, Breunis WB, Geissler J, de Boer M, van den Berg TK, Kuijpers TW. Phenotypic variation in IgG receptors by nonclassical FCGR2C alleles. *J Immunol*. (2012) 188:1318–24. doi: 10.4049/jimmunol.1003945

68. Xia YC, Schuliga M, Shepherd M, Powell M, Harris T, Langenbach SY, Tan PS, et al. Functional expression of IgG-Fc receptors in human airway smooth muscle cells. *Am J Respir Cell Mol Biol*. (2011) 44:665–72. doi: 10.1165/rcmb.2009-0371OC

69. Ganesan LP, Kim J, Wu Y, Mohanty S, Phillips GS, Birmingham DJ, et al. FcgammaRIIb on liver sinusoidal endothelium clears small immune complexes. *J Immunol*. (2012) 189:4981–8. doi: 10.4049/jimmunol.1202017

70. Iwayanagi Y, Igawa T, Maeda A, Haraya K, Wada NA, Shibahara N, et al. Inhibitory FcgammaRIIb-mediated soluble antigen clearance from plasma by a pH-dependent antigen-binding antibody and its enhancement by Fc engineering. *J Immunol*. (2015) 195:3198–205. doi: 10.4049/jimmunol.1401470

71. Chu SY, Horton HM, Pong E, Leung IW, Chen H, Nguyen DH, et al. Reduction of total IgE by targeted coengagement of IgE B-cell receptor and FcgammaRIIb with Fc-engineered antibody. *J Allergy Clin Immunol*. (2012) 129:1102–15. doi: 10.1016/j.jaci.2011.11.029

72. Phillips NE, Parker DC. Fc-dependent inhibition of mouse B cell activation by whole anti-mu antibodies. *J Immunol*. (1983) 130:602–6.

73. Tiller T, Kofer J, Kreschel C, Busse CE, Riebel S, Wickert S, et al. Development of self-reactive germinal center B cells and plasma cells in autoimmune Fc gammaRIIB-deficient mice. *J Exp Med*. (2010) 207:2767–78. doi: 10.1084/jem.20100171

74. Nimmerjahn F, Ravetch JV. Fcgamma receptors as regulators of immune responses. *Nat Rev Immunol*. (2008) 8:34–47. doi: 10.1038/nri2206

75. Baerenwaldt A, Lux A, Danzer H, Spriewald BM, Ullrich E, Heidkamp G, et al. Fcgamma receptor IIB (FcgammaRIIB) maintains humoral tolerance in the human immune system *in vivo*. *Proc Natl Acad Sci USA*. (2011) 108:18772–7. doi: 10.1073/pnas.1111810108

76. Daeron M, Lesourne R. Negative signaling in Fc receptor complexes. *Adv Immunol*. (2006) 89:39–86. doi: 10.1016/S0065-2776(05)89002-9

77. Liu Y, Masuda E, Blank MC, Kirou KA, Gao X, Park MS, et al. Cytokine-mediated regulation of activating and inhibitory Fc gamma receptors in human monocytes. *J Leukoc Biol*. (2005) 77:767–76. doi: 10.1189/jlb.0904532

78. Espeli M, Smith KG, Clatworthy MR. FcgammaRIIB and autoimmunity. *Immunol Rev*. (2016) 269:194–211. doi: 10.1111/imr.12368

79. Hunter S, Indik ZK, Kim MK, Cauley MD, Park JG, Schreiber AD. Inhibition of Fcgamma receptor-mediated phagocytosis by a nonphagocytic Fcgamma receptor. *Blood*. (1998) 91:1762–8.

80. Malbec O, Fong DC, Turner M, Tybulewicz VL, Cambier JC, Fridman WH, et al. Fc epsilon receptor I-associated lyn-dependent phosphorylation of Fc gamma RIIB during negative regulation of mast cell activation. *J Immunol*. (1998) 160:1647–58.

81. Bewarder N, Weinrich V, Budde P, Hartmann D, Flaswinkel H, Reth M, et al. *In vivo* and *in vitro* specificity of protein tyrosine kinases for immunoglobulin G receptor (FcgammaRII) phosphorylation. *Mol Cell Biol.* (1996) 16:4735–43. doi: 10.1128/MCB.16.9.4735

82. Lesourne R, Bruhns P, Fridman WH, Daeron M. Insufficient phosphorylation prevents fc gamma RIIB from recruiting the SH2 domain-containing protein-tyrosine phosphatase SHP-1. *J Biol Chem.* (2001) 276:6327–36. doi: 10.1074/jbc.M006537200

83. Isnardi I, Lesourne R, Bruhns P, Fridman WH, Cambier JC, Daeron M. Two distinct tyrosine-based motifs enable the inhibitory receptor FcgammaRIIB to cooperatively recruit the inositol phosphatases SHIP1/2 and the adapters Grb2/Grap. *J Biol Chem.* (2004) 279:51931–8. doi: 10.1074/jbc.M410261200

84. Isnardi I, Bruhns P, Bismuth G, Fridman WH, Daeron M. The SH2 domain-containing inositol 5-phosphatase SHIP1 is recruited to the intracytoplasmic domain of human FcgammaRIIB and is mandatory for negative regulation of B cell activation. *Immunol Lett.* (2006) 104:156–65. doi: 10.1016/j.imlet.2005.11.027

85. Aman MJ, Tosello-Trampont AC, Ravichandran K. Fc gamma RIIB1/SHIP-mediated inhibitory signaling in B cells involves lipid rafts. *J Biol Chem.* (2001) 276:46371–8. doi: 10.1074/jbc.M104069200

86. Fong DC, Brauweiler A, Minskoff SA, Bruhns P, Tamir I, Mellman I, et al. Mutational analysis reveals multiple distinct sites within Fc gamma receptor IIB that function in inhibitory signaling. *J Immunol.* (2000) 165:4453–62. doi: 10.4049/jimmunol.165.8.4453

87. Wang J, Li Z, Xu L, Yang H, Liu W. Transmembrane domain dependent inhibitory function of FcgammaRII. *Protein Cell B.* (2018) 9:1004–12. doi: 10.1007/s13238-018-0509-8

88. Xiang Z, Cutler AJ, Brownlie RJ, Fairfax K, Lawlor KE, Severinson E, et al. FcgammaRIIb controls bone marrow plasma cell persistence and apoptosis. *Nat Immunol.* (2007) 8:419–29. doi: 10.1038/ni1440

89. Gast M, Preisinger C, Nimmerjahn F, Huber M. IgG-independent Co-aggregation of FcepsilonRI and FcgammaRIIB Results in LYN-and SHIP1-dependent tyrosine phosphorylation of FcgammaRIIB in murine bone marrow-derived mast cells. *Front Immunol.* (2018) 9:1937. doi: 10.3389/fimmu.2018.01937

90. Lehmann B, Schwab I, Bohm S, Lux A, Biburger M, Nimmerjahn F. FcgammaRIIB: a modulator of cell activation and humoral tolerance. *Expert Rev Clin Immunol.* (2012) 8:243–54. doi: 10.1586/eci.12.5

91. Malbec O, Daeron M. The mast cell IgG receptors and their roles in tissue inflammation. *Immunol Rev.* (2007) 217:206–21. doi: 10.1111/j.1600-065X.2007.00510.x

92. Miettinen HM, Matter K, Hunziker W, Rose JK, Mellman I. Fc receptor endocytosis is controlled by a cytoplasmic domain determinant that actively prevents coated pit localization. *J Cell Biol.* (1992) 116:875–88. doi: 10.1083/jcb.116.4.875

93. Budde P, Bewarder N, Weinrich V, Schulzeck O, Frey J. Tyrosine-containing sequence motifs of the human immunoglobulin G receptors FcRIIb1 and FcRIIb2 essential for endocytosis and regulation of calcium flux in B cells. *J Biol Chem.* (1994) 269:30636–44.

94. Hunziker W, Fumey C. A di-leucine motif mediates endocytosis and basolateral sorting of macrophage IgG Fc receptors in MDCK cells. *EMBO J.* (1994) 13:2963–9. doi: 10.1002/j.1460-2075.1994.tb06594.x

95. Van Den Herik-Oudijk JG, Westerdaal NA, Henriquez NV, Capel PJ, Van De Winkel IE. Functional analysis of human Fc gamma RII (CD32) isoforms expressed in B lymphocytes. *J Immunol.* (1994) 152:574–85.

96. Warmerdam PA van den Herik-Oudijk IE, Parren PW, Westerdaal NA, van de Winkel JG, Capel PJ. Interaction of a human Fc gamma RIIb1 (CD32) isoform with murine and human IgG subclasses. *Int Immunol.* (1993) 5:239–47. doi: 10.1093/intimm/5.3.239

97. Pearse RN, Kawabe T, Bolland S, Guinamard R, Kurosaki T, Ravetch JV. SHIP recruitment attenuates Fc gamma RIIB-induced B cell apoptosis. *Immunity.* (1999) 10:753–60. doi: 10.1016/S1074-7613(00)80074-6

98. Fakher M, Wu J, Qin D, Szakal A, Tew J. Follicular dendritic cell accessory activity crosses MHC and species barriers. *Eur J Immunol.* (2001) 31:176–85. doi: 10.1002/1521-4141(200101)31:1<176::AID-IMMU176>3.0.CO;2-H

99. Sukumar S, El Shikh ME, Tew JG, Szakal AK. Ultrastructural study of highly enriched follicular dendritic cells reveals their morphology and the periodicity of immune complex binding. *Cell Tissue Res.* (2008) 332:89–99. doi: 10.1007/s00441-007-0566-4

100. El Shikh ME, El Sayed RM, Sukumar S, Szakal AK, Tew JG. Activation of B cells by antigens on follicular dendritic cells. *Trends Immunol.* (2010) 31:205–11. doi: 10.1016/j.it.2010.03.002

101. Cassard L, Jonsson F, Arnaud S, Daeron M. Fcgamma receptors inhibit mouse and human basophil activation. *J Immunol.* (2012) 189:2995–3006. doi: 10.4049/jimmunol.1200968

102. Cady CT, Powell MS, Harbeck RJ, Giclas PC, Murphy JR, Katial RK, et al. IgG antibodies produced during subcutaneous allergen immunotherapy mediate inhibition of basophil activation via a mechanism involving both FcgammaRIIA and FcgammaRII. *Immunol Lett B.* (2010) 130:57–65. doi: 10.1016/j.imlet.2009.12.001

103. Wijngaarden S, van de Winkel JG, Jacobs KM, Bijlsma JW, Lafeber FP, van Roon JA. A shift in the balance of inhibitory and activating Fcgamma receptors on monocytes toward the inhibitory Fcgamma receptor IIb is associated with prevention of monocyte activation in rheumatoid arthritis. *Arthritis Rheum.* (2004) 50:3878–87. doi: 10.1002/art.20672

104. Clynes R, Maizes JS, Guinamard R, Ono M, Takai T, Ravetch JV. Modulation of immune complex-induced inflammation *in vivo* by the coordinate expression of activation and inhibitory Fc receptors. *J Exp Med.* (1999) 189:179–85. doi: 10.1084/jem.189.1.179

105. Metes D, Ernst LK, Chambers WH, Sulica A, Herberman RB, Morel PA. Expression of functional CD32 molecules on human NK cells is determined by an allelic polymorphism of the FcgammaRIIC gene. *Blood.* (1998) 91:2369–80.

106. Breunis WB, van Mirre E, Bruin M, Geissler J, de Boer M, Peters M, et al. Copy number variation of the activating FCGR2C gene predisposes to idiopathic thrombocytopenic purpura. *Blood.* (2008) 111:1029–38. doi: 10.1182/blood-2007-03-079913

107. Ernst LK, Metes D, Herberman RB, Morel PA. Allelic polymorphisms in the FcgammaRIIC gene can influence its function on normal human natural killer cells. *J Mol Med.* (2002) 80:248–57. doi: 10.1007/s00109-001-0294-2

108. Li X, Wu J, Ptacek T, Redden DT, Brown EE, Alarcon GS, et al. Allelic-dependent expression of an activating Fc receptor on B cells enhances humoral immune responses. *Sci Transl Med.* (2013) 5:216ra175. doi: 10.1126/scitranslmed.3007097

109. Peng X, Li SS, Gilbert PB, Geraghty DE, Katze MG. FCGR2C Polymorphisms associated with HIV-1 vaccine protection are linked to altered gene expression of Fc-gamma receptors in human B cells. *PLoS ONE.* (2016) 11:e0152425. doi: 10.1371/journal.pone.0152425

110. Warncke M, Calzascia T, Coulot M, Balke N, Touil R, Kolbinger F, et al. Different adaptations of IgG effector function in human and nonhuman primates and implications for therapeutic antibody treatment. *J Immunol.* (2012) 188:4405–11. doi: 10.4049/jimmunol.1200090

111. Wines BD, Vanderven HA, Esparon SE, Kristensen AB, Kent SJ, Hogarth PM. Dimeric FcgammaR ectodomains as probes of the Fc receptor function of anti-influenza virus Ig. *J Immunol G.* (2016) 197:1507–16. doi: 10.4049/jimmunol.1502551

112. Lux A, Yu X, Scanlan CN, Nimmerjahn F. Impact of immune complex size and glycosylation on IgG binding to human FcgammaRs. *J Immunol.* (2013) 190:4315–23. doi: 10.4049/jimmunol.1200501

113. Wines BD, Tan CW, Duncan E, McRae S, Baker RI, Andrews RK, et al. Dimeric FcgammaR ectodomains detect pathogenic anti-platelet factor 4-heparin antibodies in heparin-induced thrombobocytopenia. *J Thromb Haemost.* (2018) 16:2520–25. doi: 10.1111/jth.14306

114. Bournazos S, Hart SP, Chamberlain LH, Glennie MJ, Dransfield I. Association of FcgammaRIIa (CD32a) with lipid rafts regulates ligand binding activity. *J Immunol.* (2009) 182:8026–36. doi: 10.4049/jimmunol.0900107

115. Kanters D, ten Hove W, Luijk B, van Aalst C, Schweizer RC, Lammers JW, et al. Expression of activated Fc gamma RII discriminates between multiple granulocyte-priming phenotypes in peripheral blood of allergic asthmatic subjects. *J Allergy Clin Immunol.* (2007) 120:1073–81. doi: 10.1016/j.jaci.2007.06.021

116. Graziano RF, Looney RJ, Shen L, Fanger MW. Fc gamma R-mediated killing by eosinophils. *J Immunol.* (1989) 142:230–5.

117. Nagarajan S, Venkiteswaran K, Anderson M, Sayed U, Zhu C, Selvaraj P. Cell-specific, activation-dependent regulation of neutrophil CD32A ligand-binding function. *Blood.* (2000) 95:1069–77.

118. Maxwell KF, Powell MS, Hulett MD, Barton PA, McKenzie IF, Garrett TP, et al. Crystal structure of the human leukocyte Fc receptor, Fc gammaRIIa. *Nat Struct Biol.* (1999) 6:437–42. doi: 10.1038/8241

119. Brandsma AM, Schwartz SL, Wester MJ, Valley CC, Blezer GL A, Vidarsson G, et al. Mechanisms of inside-out signaling of the high-affinity IgG receptor FcgammaR. *Sci Signal I.* (2018) 11:540. doi: 10.1126/scisignal.aaq0891

120. Lu J, Sun PD. Structural mechanism of high affinity FcgammaRI recognition of immunoglobulin. *Immunol Rev G.* (2015) 268:192–200. doi: 10.1111/imr.12346

121. Radaev S, Sun P. Recognition of immunoglobulins by Fcgamma receptors. *Mol Immunol.* (2002) 38:1073–83. doi: 10.1016/S0161-5890(02)00036-6

122. Sondermann P, Oosthuizen V. X-ray crystallographic studies of IgG-Fc gamma receptor interactions. *Biochem Soc Trans.* (2002) 30:481–6. doi: 10.1042/bst0300481

123. Mimoto F, Igawa T, Kuramochi T, Katada H, Kadono S, Kamikawa T, et al. Novel asymmetrically engineered antibody Fc variant with superior FcgammaR binding affinity and specificity compared with afucosylated Fc variant. *MAbs.* (2013) 5:229–36. doi: 10.4161/mabs.23452

124. Caaveiro JM, Kiyoshi M, Tsumoto K. Structural analysis of Fc/FcgammaR complexes: a blueprint for antibody design. *Immunol Rev.* (2015) 268:201–21. doi: 10.1111/imr.12365

125. Warnerdanm OAM, van de Winkel J, Gosselin EJ, Capel JG. Molecular basis for a polymorphism of human Fc gamma receptor II (CD32). *J Exp Med.* (1990) 172:19–25. doi: 10.1084/jem.172.1.19

126. Norris CF, Pricop L, Millard SS, Taylor SM, Surrey S, Schwartz E, et al. A naturally occurring mutation in Fc gamma RIIA: a Q to K127 change confers unique IgG binding properties to the R131 allelic form of the receptor. *Blood.* (1998) 91:656–62.

127. Flinsenberg TW, Janssen WJ, Herczenik E, Boross P, Nederend M, Jongeneel LH, et al. A novel FcgammaRIIa Q27W gene variant is associated with common variable immune deficiency through defective FcgammaRIIa downstream signaling. *Clin Immunol.* (2014) 155:108–17. doi: 10.1016/j.clim.2014.09.006

128. Warmerdam PA van de Winkel JG, Vlug A, Westerdaal NA, Capel PJ. A single amino acid in the second Ig-like domain of the human Fc gamma receptor II is critical for human IgG2 binding. *J Immunol.* (1991) 147:1338–43.

129. Parren PW, Warmerdam PA, Boeije LC, Arts J, Westerdaal NA, Vlug A, et al. On the interaction of IgG subclasses with the low affinity Fc gamma RIIa (CD32) on human monocytes, neutrophils, and platelets. Analysis of a functional polymorphism to human IgG2. *J Clin Invest.* (1992) 90:1537–46. doi: 10.1172/JCI116022

130. Kuo HC, Hsu YW, Wu MS, Woon PY, Wong HS, Tsai LJ, et al. FCGR2A promoter methylation and risks for intravenous immunoglobulin treatment responses in kawasaki disease. *Mediators Inflamm.* (2015) 2015:564625. doi: 10.1155/2015/564625

131. Su K, Wu J, Edberg JC, Li X, Ferguson P, Cooper GS, et al. A promoter haplotype of the immunoreceptor tyrosine-based inhibitory motif-bearing FcgammaRIIb alters receptor expression and associates with autoimmunity. I. Regulatory FCGR2B polymorphisms and their association with systemic lupus erythematosus. *J Immunol.* (2004) 172:7186–91. doi: 10.4049/jimmunol.172.11.7186

132. Willcocks LC, Carr EJ, Niederer HA, Rayner TF, Williams TN, Yang W, et al. A defunctioning polymorphism in FCGR2B is associated with protection against malaria but susceptibility to systemic lupus erythematosus. *Proc Natl Acad Sci USA.* (2010) 107:7881–5. doi: 10.1073/pnas.0915133107

133. Floto RA, Clatworthy MR, Heilbronn KR, Rosner DR, MacAry PA, Rankin A, et al. Loss of function of a lupus-associated FcgammaRIIb polymorphism through exclusion from lipid rafts. *Nat Med.* (2005) 11:1056–8. doi: 10.1038/nm1288

134. Kyogoku C, Dijstelbloem HM, Tsuchiya N, Hatta Y, Kato H, Yamaguchi A, et al. Fcgamma receptor gene polymorphisms in Japanese patients with systemic lupus erythematosus: contribution of FCGR2B to genetic susceptibility. *Arthritis Rheum.* (2002) 46:1242–54. doi: 10.1002/art.10257

135. Li X, Wu J, Carter RH, Edberg JC, Su K, Cooper GS, et al. A novel polymorphism in the Fcgamma receptor IIB (CD32B) transmembrane region alters receptor signaling. *Arthritis Rheum.* (2003) 48:3242–52. doi: 10.1002/art.11313

136. Kono H, Kyogoku C, Suzuki T, Tsuchiya N, Honda H, Yamamoto K, et al. FcgammaRIIB Ile232Thr transmembrane polymorphism associated with human systemic lupus erythematosus decreases affinity to lipid rafts and attenuates inhibitory effects on B cell receptor signaling. *Hum Mol Genet.* (2005) 14:2881–92. doi: 10.1093/hmg/ddi320

137. Xu L, Xia M, Guo J, Sun X, Li H, Xu C, et al. Impairment on the lateral mobility induced by structural changes underlies the functional deficiency of the lupus-associated polymorphism FcgammaRIIB-T232. *J Exp Med.* (2016) 213:2707–27. doi: 10.1084/jem.20160528

138. Li SS, Gilbert PB, Tomaras GD, Kijak G, Ferrari G, Thomas R, et al. FCGR2C polymorphisms associate with HIV-1 vaccine protection in RV144 trial. *J Clin Invest.* (2014) 124:3879–90. doi: 10.1172/JCI75539

139. Kaifu T, Nakamura A. Polymorphisms of immunoglobulin receptors and the effects on clinical outcome in cancer immunotherapy and other immune diseases: a general review. *Int Immunol.* (2017) 29:319–325. doi: 10.1093/intimm/dxx041

140. Li X, Gibson AW, Kimberly RP. Human FcR polymorphism and disease. *Curr Top Microbiol Immunol.* (2014) 382:275–302. doi: 10.1007/978-3-319-07911-0_13

141. Li X, Kimberly RP. Targeting the Fc receptor in autoimmune disease. *Expert Opin Ther Targets.* (2014) 18:335–50. doi: 10.1517/14728222.2014.877891

142. Nakamura A, Kubo T, Takai T. Fc receptor targeting in the treatment of allergy, autoimmune diseases and cancer. *Adv Exp Med Biol.* (2008) 640:220–33. doi: 10.1007/978-0-387-09789-3_17

143. Willcocks LC, Smith KG, Clatworthy MR. Low-affinity Fcgamma receptors, autoimmunity and infection. *Expert Rev Mol Med.* (2009) 11:e24. doi: 10.1017/s1462399409001161

144. Rodriguez ME, van der Pol WL, Sanders LA, van de Winkel JG. Crucial role of FcgammaRIIa (CD32) in assessment of functional anti-Streptococcus pneumoniae antibody activity in human sera. *J Infect Dis.* (1999) 179:423–33. doi: 10.1086/314603

145. Yuan FF, Wong M, Pererva N, Keating J, Davis AR, Bryant JA, et al. FcgammaRIIA polymorphisms in Streptococcus pneumoniae infection. *Immunol Cell Biol.* (2003) 81:192–5. doi: 10.1046/j.1440-1711.2003.01158.x

146. Pathan N, Faust SN, Levin M. Pathophysiology of meningococcal meningitis and septicaemia. *Arch Dis Child.* (2003) 88:601–7. doi: 10.1136/adc.88.7.601

147. Nicu EA, Van der Velden U, Everts V, Van Winkelhoff AJ, Roos D, Loos BG. Hyper-reactive PMNs in FcgammaRIIa 131 H/H genotype periodontitis patients. *J Clin Periodontol.* (2007) 34:938–45. doi: 10.1111/j.1600-051X.2007.01136.x

148. van Egmond M, Vidarsson G, Bakema JE. Cross-talk between pathogen recognizing Toll-like receptors and immunoglobulin Fc receptors in immunity. *Immunol Rev.* (2015) 268:311–27. doi: 10.1111/imr.12333

149. Wenink MH, Santegoets KC, Roelofs MF, Huijbens R, Koenen HJ, van Beek R, et al. The inhibitory Fc gamma IIb receptor dampens TLR4-mediated immune responses and is selectively up-regulated on dendritic cells from rheumatoid arthritis patients with quiescent disease. *J Immunol.* (2009) 183:4509–20. doi: 10.4049/jimmunol.0900153

150. Bakema JE, Tuk CW, van Vliet SJ, Bruijns SC, Vos JB, Letsiou S, et al. Antibody-opsonized bacteria evoke an inflammatory dendritic cell phenotype and polyfunctional Th cells by cross-talk between TLRs and FcRs. *J Immunol.* (2015) 194:1856–66. doi: 10.4049/jimmunol.1303126

151. French MA, Tanaskovic S, Law MG, Lim A, Fernandez S, Ward LD, et al. Vaccine-induced IgG2 anti-HIV p24 is associated with control of HIV in patients with a 'high-affinity' FcgammaRIIa genotype. *AIDS.* (2010) 24:1983–90. doi: 10.1097/QAD.0b013e32833c1ce0

152. Forthal DN, Gabriel EE, Wang A, Landucci G, Phan TB. Association of Fcgamma receptor IIIa genotype with the rate of HIV infection after gp120 vaccination. *Blood.* (2012) 120:2836–42. doi: 10.1182/blood-2012-05-431361

153. Sips M, Krykbaeva M, Diefenbach TJ, Ghebremichael M, Bowman BA, Dugast AS, et al. Fc receptor-mediated phagocytosis in tissues as a potent mechanism for preventive and therapeutic HIV vaccine strategies. *Mucosal Immunol.* (2016) 9:1584–95. doi: 10.1038/mi.2016.12

154. Brouwer KC, Lal AA, Mirel LB, Otieno J, Ayisi J, Van Eijk AM, et al. Polymorphism of Fc receptor IIa for immunoglobulin G is associated with placental malaria in HIV-1-positive women in western Kenya. *J Infect Dis.* (2004) 190:1192–8. doi: 10.1086/422850

155. Groux H, Gysin J. Opsonization as an effector mechanism in human protection against asexual blood stages of Plasmodium falciparum: functional role of IgG subclasses. *Res Immunol.* (1990) 141:529–42. doi: 10.1016/0923-2494(90)90021-P

156. Brouwer KC, Lal RB, Mirel LB, Yang C, van Eijk AM, Ayisi J, et al. Polymorphism of Fc receptor IIa for IgG in infants is associated with susceptibility to perinatal HIV-1 infection. *AIDS.* (2004) 18:1187–94. doi: 10.1097/00002030-200405210-00012

157. Descours B, Petitjean G, Lopez-Zaragoza JL, Bruel T, Raffel R, Psomas C, et al. CD32a is a marker of a CD4 T-cell HIV reservoir harbouring replication-competent proviruses. *Nature.* (2017) 543:564–7. doi: 10.1038/nature21710

158. Perez L, Anderson J, Chipman J, Thorkelson A, Chun TW, Moir S, et al. Conflicting evidence for HIV enrichment in CD32(+) CD4 T cells. *Nature.* (2018) 561:E9–16. doi: 10.1038/s41586-018-0493-4

159. Abdel-Mohsen M, Kuri-Cervantes L, Grau-Exposito J, Spivak AM, Nell RA, Tomescu C, et al. CD32 is expressed on cells with transcriptionally active HIV but does not enrich for HIV DNA in resting T cells. *Sci Transl Med.* (2018) 10:437. doi: 10.1126/scitranslmed.aar6759

160. Gan ES, Ting DH, Chan KR. The mechanistic role of antibodies to dengue virus in protection and disease pathogenesis. *Expert Rev Anti Infect Ther.* (2017) 15:111–9. doi: 10.1080/14787210.2017.1254550

161. Chan KR, Zhang SL, Tan HC, Chan YK, Chow A, Lim AP, et al. Ligation of Fc gamma receptor IIB inhibits antibody-dependent enhancement of dengue virus infection. *Proc Natl Acad Sci USA.* (2011) 108:12479–84. doi: 10.1073/pnas.1106568108

162. Boonnak K, Slike BM, Donofrio GC, Marovich MA. Human FcgammaRII cytoplasmic domains differentially influence antibody-mediated dengue virus infection. *J Immunol.* (2013) 190:5659–65. doi: 10.4049/jimmunol.1203052

163. Clatworthy MR, Smith KG. FcgammaRIIb balances efficient pathogen clearance and the cytokine-mediated consequences of sepsis. *J Exp Med.* (2004) 199:717–23. doi: 10.1084/jem.20032197

164. Brownlie RJ, Lawlor KE, Niederer HA, Cutler AJ, Xiang Z, Clatworthy MR, et al. Distinct cell-specific control of autoimmunity and infection by FcgammaRIIb. *J Exp Med.* (2008) 205:883–95. doi: 10.1084/jem.20072565

165. Bave U, Magnusson M, Eloranta ML, Perers A, Alm GV, Ronnblom L. Fc gamma RIIa is expressed on natural IFN-alpha-producing cells (plasmacytoid dendritic cells) and is required for the IFN-alpha production induced by apoptotic cells combined with lupus Ig. *J Immunol G.* (2003) 171:3296–302. doi: 10.4049/jimmunol.171.6.3296

166. Yu X, Lazarus AH. Targeting FcgammaRs to treat antibody-dependent autoimmunity. *Autoimmun Rev.* (2016) 15:510–2. doi: 10.1016/j.autrev.2016.02.006

167. Smith KG, Clatworthy MR. FcgammaRIIB in autoimmunity and infection: evolutionary and therapeutic implications. *Nat Rev Immunol.* (2010) 10:328–43. doi: 10.1038/nri2762

168. van der Pol WL, van den Berg LH, Scheepers RH van der Bom JG, van Doorn PA, van Koningsveld R, et al. IgG receptor IIa alleles determine susceptibility and severity of Guillain-Barre syndrome. *Neurology.* (2000) 54:1661–5. doi: 10.1212/WNL.54.8.1661

169. Khor CC, Davila S, Breunis WB, Lee YC, Shimizu C, Wright VJ, et al. Genome-wide association study identifies FCGR2A as a susceptibility locus for Kawasaki disease. *Nat Genet.* (2011) 43:1241–6. doi: 10.1038/ng.981

170. Asano K, Matsushita T, Umeno J, Hosono N, Takahashi A, Kawaguchi T, et al. A genome-wide association study identifies three new susceptibility loci for ulcerative colitis in the Japanese population. *Nat Genet.* (2009) 41:1325–9. doi: 10.1038/ng.482

171. Raaz D, Herrmann M, Ekici AB, Klinghammer L, Lausen B, Voll RE, et al. FcgammaRIIa genotype is associated with acute coronary syndromes as first manifestation of coronary artery disease. *Atherosclerosis.* (2009) 205:512–6. doi: 10.1016/j.atherosclerosis.2009.01.013

172. Karassa FB, Bijl M, Davies KA, Kallenberg CG, Khamashta MA, Manger K, et al. Role of the Fcgamma receptor IIA polymorphism in the antiphospholipid syndrome: an international meta-analysis. *Arthritis Rheum.* (2003) 48:1930–8. doi: 10.1002/art.11059

173. Raaz-Schrauder D, Ekici AB, Munoz LE, Klinghammer L, Voll RE, Leusen JH et al. Patients with unstable angina pectoris show an increased frequency of the Fc gamma RIIa R131 allele. *Autoimmunity.* (2012) 45:556–64. doi: 10.3109/08916934.2012.682665

174. van der Pol WL, Jansen MD, Kuks JB, de Baets M, Leppers-van de Straat, Wokke JH, et al. Association of the Fc gamma receptor IIA-R/R131 genotype with myasthenia gravis in Dutch patients. *J Neuroimmunol.* (2003) 144:143–7. doi: 10.1016/j.jneuroim.2003.08.043

175. Mathsson L, Lampa J, Mullazehi M, Ronnelid J. Immune complexes from rheumatoid arthritis synovial fluid induce FcgammaRIIa dependent and rheumatoid factor correlated production of tumour necrosis factor-alpha by peripheral blood mononuclear cells. *Arthritis Res Ther.* (2006) 8:R64. doi: 10.1186/ar1926

176. Ronnelid J, Tejde A, Mathsson L, Nilsson-Ekdahl K, Nilsson B. Immune complexes from SLE sera induce IL10 production from normal peripheral blood mononuclear cells by an FcgammaRII dependent mechanism: implications for a possible vicious cycle maintaining B cell hyperactivity in SLE. *Ann Rheum Dis.* (2003) 62:37–42. doi: 10.1136/ard.62.1.37

177. Chang LS, Lo MH, Li SC, Yang MY, Hsieh KS, Kuo HC. The effect of FcgammaRIIA and FcgammaRIIB on coronary artery lesion formation and intravenous immunoglobulin treatment responses in children with Kawasaki disease. *Oncotarget.* (2017) 8:2044–52. doi: 10.18632/oncotarget.13489

178. Stewart-Akers AM, Cunningham A, Wasko MC, Morel PA. Fc gamma R expression on NK cells influences disease severity in rheumatoid arthritis. *Genes Immun.* (2004) 5:521–9. doi: 10.1038/sj.gene.6364121

179. Blank MC, Stefanescu RN, Masuda E, Marti F, King PD, Redecha PB, et al. Decreased transcription of the human FCGR2B gene mediated by the−343 G/C promoter polymorphism and association with systemic lupus erythematosus. *Hum Genet.* (2005) 117:220–7. doi: 10.1007/s00439-005-1302-3

180. Radstake TR, Franke B, Wenink MH, Nabbe KC, Coenen MJ, Welsing P, et al. The functional variant of the inhibitory Fcgamma receptor IIb (CD32B) is associated with the rate of radiologic joint damage and dendritic cell function in rheumatoid arthritis. *Arthritis Rheum.* (2006) 54:3828–37. doi: 10.1002/art.22275

181. Xu L, Li G, Wang J, Fan Y, Wan Z, Zhang S, et al. Through an ITIM-independent mechanism the FcgammaRIIB blocks B cell activation by disrupting the colocalized microclustering of the B cell receptor and CD19. *J Immunol.* (2014) 192:5179–91. doi: 10.4049/jimmunol.1400101

182. Cassard L, Cohen-Solal JF, Fournier EM, Camilleri-Broet S, Spatz A, Chouaib S, et al. Selective expression of inhibitory Fcgamma receptor by metastatic melanoma impairs tumor susceptibility to IgG-dependent cellular response. *Int J Cancer.* (2008) 123:2832–9. doi: 10.1002/ijc.23870

183. Gul N, van Egmond M. Antibody-dependent phagocytosis of tumor cells by macrophages: a potent effector mechanism of monoclonal antibody therapy of cancer. *Cancer Res.* (2015) 75:5008–13. doi: 10.1158/0008-5472.CAN-15-1330

184. Weng WK, Levy R. Two immunoglobulin G fragment C receptor polymorphisms independently predict response to rituximab in patients with follicular lymphoma. *J Clin Oncol.* (2003) 21:3940–7. doi: 10.1200/JCO.2003.05.013

185. Bibeau F, Lopez-Crapez E, Di Fiore F, Thezenas S, Ychou M, Blanchard F, et al. Impact of Fc{gamma}RIIa-Fc{gamma}RIIIa polymorphisms and KRAS mutations on the clinical outcome of patients with metastatic colorectal cancer treated with cetuximab plus irinotecan. *J Clin Oncol.* (2009) 27:1122–9. doi: 10.1200/JCO.2008.18.0463

186. Vaughan AT, Chan CH, Klein C, Glennie MJ, Beers SA, Cragg MS. Activatory and inhibitory Fcgamma receptors augment rituximab-mediated internalization of CD20 independent of signaling via the cytoplasmic domain. *J Biol Chem.* (2015) 290:5424–37. doi: 10.1074/jbc.M114.593806

187. Pietersz GA, Mottram PL van de Velde NC, Sardjono CT, Esparon S, Ramsland PA, et al. Inhibition of destructive autoimmune arthritis in

FcgammaRIIa transgenic mice by small chemical entities. *Immunol Cell Biol.* (2009) 87:3–12. doi: 10.1038/icb.2008.82

188. Boonyarattanakalin S, Martin SE, Sun Q, Peterson BR. A synthetic mimic of human Fc receptors: defined chemical modification of cell surfaces enables efficient endocytic uptake of human immunoglobulin-G. *J Am Chem Soc.* (2006) 128:11463–70. doi: 10.1021/ja062377w

189. Belostocki K, Park MS, Redecha PB, Masuda E, Salmon JE, Pricop L. FcgammaRIIa is a target for modulation by TNFalpha in human neutrophils. *Clin Immunol.* (2005) 117:78–86. doi: 10.1016/j.clim.2005.07.001

190. Chu SY, Yeter K, Kotha R, Pong E, Miranda Y, Phung S, et al. Suppression of rheumatoid arthritis B cells by XmAb5871, an anti-CD19 antibody that coengages B cell antigen receptor complex and Fcgamma receptor IIb inhibitory receptor. *Arthritis Rheumatol.* (2014) 66:1153–64. doi: 10.1002/art.38334

191. Horton HM, Chu SY, Ortiz EC, Pong E, Cemerski S, Leung IW, et al. Antibody-mediated coengagement of FcgammaRIIb and B cell receptor complex suppresses humoral immunity in systemic lupus erythematosus. *J Immunol.* (2011) 186:4223–33. doi: 10.4049/jimmunol.1003412

192. Ellsworth JL, Hamacher N, Harder B, Bannink K, Bukowski TR, Byrnes-Blake K, et al. Recombinant soluble human FcgammaR1A (CD64A) reduces inflammation in murine collagen-induced arthritis. *J Immunol.* (2009) 182:7272–9. doi: 10.4049/jimmunol.0803497

193. Magnusson SE, Andren M, Nilsson KE, Sondermann P, Jacob U, Kleinau S. Amelioration of collagen-induced arthritis by human recombinant soluble FcgammaRIIb. *Clin Immunol.* (2008) 127:225–33. doi: 10.1016/j.clim.2008.02.002

194. Konstaninova TS, Leonidovna IV, Hellmann A, Kyrcz-Krzemien S, Tillmanns S, Sondermann P, et al. Interim results from a phase Ib/IIa clinical trial with the soluble Fc-gamma IIb receptor SM101 for the treatment of primary immune thrombocytopenia. *Blood.* (2012) 120:3388.

195. Tillmanns S, Kolligs C, D'Cruz DP, Doria A, Hachulla E, Voll RE, et al. SM101, a novel recombinant, soluble, human FcgIIB receptor, in the treatment of systemic lupus erythematosus: results of a doubleblind, placebo-controlled multicenter study. *Am Coll Rheumatol.* (2014) 66:S1238.

7

Inside-Out Control of Fc-Receptors

*Leo Koenderman**

Department of Respiratory Medicine and Laboratory of Translational Immunology, University Medical Center Utrecht, Utrecht, Netherlands

Correspondence:
Leo Koenderman
l.koenderman@umcutrecht.nl

Receptors recognizing the Fc-part of immunoglobulins (FcR) are important in the engagement of phagocytes with opsonized micro-organisms, but they also play a major role in the pathogenesis of chronic inflammatory diseases. Different FcRs are specifically recognizing and binding the different classes of immunoglobulins, transmitting different signals into the cell. The function of IgG (FcγR's) and IgA (FcαR) recognizing receptors is controlled by cellular signals evoked by activation of heterologous receptors in a process generally referred to as inside-out control. This concept is clearly described for the regulation of integrin receptors. Inside-out control can be achieved at different levels by modulation of: (i) receptor affinity, (ii) receptor avidity/valency, (iii) interaction with signaling chains, (iv) interaction with other receptors and (v) localization in functionally different membrane domains. The inside-out control of FcRs is an interesting target for novel therapy by therapeutical antibodies as it can potentiate or decrease the functionality of the response to the antibodies depending on the mechanisms of the diseases they are applied for.

Keywords: inside-out control, immunoglobulins, priming, activation, phagocytes, Fc-receptors

INTRODUCTION

Immunoglobulins have evolved during evolution as a link between the antigen-specific adaptive immunity and the molecular pattern driven innate immune system. These molecules contain an antigen-specific variable region brought about by gene rearrangement in B-cells. The underlying mechanisms for this rearrangement has been reviewed elsewhere (1). For the purpose of this review it suffices to say that this variable part enables specific binding to antigens beyond the common patterns recognized by the innate immune system. After the antibody binds the antigen via the variable regions, the constant region of the immunoglobulins denoted as Fc part can be recognized by other immune cells and facilitate the immune response (2–4).

The Fc-part of immunoglobulins is relevant at three different levels. First of all the Fc-part determines the human (sub)class of the immunoglobulin: IgA (IgA1 and IgA2), IgD, IgE, IgG (IgG1, IgG2a, IgG2b, IgG3, and IgG4) and IgM. During gene rearrangement the B-cell determines, guided by cytokines in its environment, which (sub)class of immunoglobulin is later produced by the respective plasma cells. The second level is the propensity of some classes of immunoglobulins to activate and fixate complement, which greatly enhances the recognition of antigens through recognition of C3b and C3bi by complement receptors (CR1/CD35 and CR3/CD11b) on phagocytic cells. The binding of immunoglobulins and complement fragments to antigens is generally referred to as opsonization.

Finally, the third level by which the Fc-part of immunoglobulins is important, is the recognition by specific Fc-receptors. These Fc receptors are mainly expressed by effector cells of the innate immune response [for excellent reviews see (2–7)].

Every class of immunoglobulins has specific receptors that can recognize these subclass specific Fc portions. These receptors are indicated by Greek letters: FcγR for IgG, FcαR for IgA, FcεR for IgE, FcδR of IgD and FcμR for IgM. Apart from these receptors also the neonatal FcR (FcRn) is expressed by stromal cells and is involved in transfer of immunoglobulins from blood to the tissue (8). Some of the immunoglobulins have more receptors with various affinities for the different subclasses as IgG comes in 5 subclasses (IgG1, IgG2a, IgG2b, IgG3, and IgG4) and IgA in two (IgA1 and IgA2). The situation with IgA is even more complex as the molecules are found as both monomers and dimers, and on mucosal surfaces as dimers with a J-chain and secretory component. The latter form of IgA is referred to as secretory IgA, which can still be recognized by FcαR (2, 3). However, additional receptors for the secretory component can modify the binding characteristics of secretory IgA (9).

The FcRs are under tight control as the immune system should evoke a balanced response to invading micro-organisms as well as to signals that can lead to aberrant activation of the immune system such as seen in chronic inflammatory disease including autoimmune disorders (10). Too much activation leads to collateral damage to the host tissue, whereas too little activation can lead to infections. The control of the function of the FcRs is the subject of this review.

FC-RECEPTOR FUNCTIONING IN THE INNATE IMMUNE RESPONSE

The best known function of FcRs is their role in phagocytosis and killing of opsonized targets. Phagocytosis refers to the process of specialized cells of the immune system that can engulf and take up targets into intracellular organelles called phagosomes (11). These phagosomes are closed and do not have any link with the extracellular milieu. In these organelles the cells can induce a very hostile environment by which the phagocytosed target is killed. This is mediated by multiple processes: fusion of granules filled with cytotoxic proteins, enzymes and peptides, production of toxic oxygen intermediates by a membrane bound NADPH-oxidase, and a lowering of the pH in the phagosome (12).

The fusion of the granules with the phagosome is often referred to as degranulation. This fusion of the phagosome with the granules leads to the formation of so-called phagolysosomes in which the actual killing of microbes takes place. Degranulation is not only into these phagolysomes, but occurs also by fusion of the granules with the plasma membrane. Then the cytotoxic components are liberated into the extracellular space, where they are involved in killing of the targets outside the cell. It will be clear that this extracellular process comes with a cost: damage to the healthy host tissues (13). This process of extracellular killing is also employed by eosinophils and macrophages killing large multicellular targets such as helminths; targets several times larger than the immune cells. Patnode et al. (14) describe clear swarming behavior of eosinophils interacting with helminths that leads to a "together we are strong" type of killing. There is a clear synergism in killing mediated by degranulation and the activation

of the NADPH-oxidase; the other major mechanism involved in killing of micro-organisms by phagocytes (15).

It will be clear from the above that FcRs are very important in the interaction of the host with pathogens. This review will focus on two classes of FcRs as these are important in phagocytosis and killing of micro-organisms: FcγR and FcαR. Six genes encode FcγR's in humans: FcγRI (CD64), FcγRIIA (CD32A), FcγRIIB (CD32B), FcγRIIC (CD32C), FcγRIIIA (CD16A), and FcγRIIIB (CD16B) (4). These receptors are expressed by various immune cells in different combinations and have different affinities for the different IgG subclasses (4). There are several IgA receptors: FcαRI (CD89), transferrin-receptor-1 (CD71), asialoglycoprotein-receptor (ASGPR/), Fcα/μR, FcRL4, and DC-SIGN/SIGNR1 (2). However, the best studied in the context of immune function and phagocytosis is FcαRI (CD89) and, therefore, we will focus on this IgA-receptor in this review.

Signal Transduction

Signal transduction of FcRs has been studied in detail and reviewed by Bournazos et al. (16). In short, broadly three modules of signaling are found for these receptors: (1) Direct signaling by the receptor itself (CD32s), (2) Via an accessory common FcRγ-chain (CD64 and CD16A and CD89), and (3) indeterminate signaling because of the absence of an intracellular tail [Glycosylphosphatidylinisotol (GPI) anchored CD16B].

Direct Signaling

Direct signaling by CD32 is mediated by immunoreceptor tyrosine-based activation motif (ITAM/CD32A and CD32C) (17) and by immunoreceptor tyrosine-based inhibitory motif (ITIM/CD32B) (18). These motifs determine whether the receptors are activating or inhibitory. It is important to emphasize that signaling starts by cross-linking of the receptor leading to activation of phosphatases such as SHP and SHIP, and members of the src-family of tyrosine kinases (19–21). This leads to phosphorylation of the important tyrosine residues in the ITAM/ITIM motifs from where various signaling cascades are initiated. Phosphorylation of ITAMs lead to activation of the cells (22), whereas phosphorylation of ITIMs lead to cell inhibition (23). The mechanisms involved in the control of CD32B have been excellently reviewed by Getahun and Cambier (24).

Signaling via an Accessory Common FcRγ-Chain

Signaling via an accessory common FcRγ-chain is also mediated by ITAM motifs present in the γ-chain. Here the main signaling is not mediated by the intracellular tail of the FcR itself, but by the FcRγ-chain that is associated with the receptor. This mode of action is found for CD16A, CD64, and CD89. Similar signals are initiated compared to direct signaling from the receptor (25–27).

Indeterminate Signaling

Indeterminate signaling seems to be the characteristic of CD16B expressed at high levels on human neutrophils. This receptor lacks both an intra-cellular portion and a transmembrane domain as it linked with the membrane with a GPI-linkage (28). However, it is likely too simple to consider this receptor as signaling dead. Various studies indicate that cross-linking CD16B evokes signaling characterized by e.g., changes in intracellular free Ca^{2+} ($[Ca^{2+}]_i$) (29). The general idea is that cross-linking leads to an engagement with other receptors that in turn activate a signaling cascade. The identity of such a receptor in CD16B signaling remains to be defined, but studies indicate that integrins and integrin associated proteins might be candidates(30). Such mechanism *in trans* can also be part of signaling through the other signaling FcRs (30, 31). This paradigm will be discussed in more detail later in the review.

Most of the IgG and IgA receptors exhibit a low or intermediate affinity for their monovalent ligands with an exception for FcγRI/CD64 that has a high affinity for monomeric IgG. The low affinity receptors do not bind to monomeric ligand or this binding is so low affinity that it is difficult to determine *in vivo* (32). The consequence of this low affinity is that these receptors only bind to multivalent ligand such as found in immune complexes as well as Ig coated surfaces such as found on opsonized micro-organisms(3). This in contrast to FcγRI that is always bound to IgG, but that interestingly does not lead to appreciable signaling (33).

An additional mode of control of FcRs is the multimerisation of the receptor into clusters at the cell membrane by which their valency increases (34). Modulation of this valency is a means by which the cell can facilitate the interaction with Ig-coated surface.

THE CONCEPT OF INSIDE-OUT CONTROL

The Concept of Inside-Out Control Identified in Integrin Function

The concept of inside-out control of immune receptors was first put forward for the function of integrins (35). It basically refers to an increase in receptor affinity, valency and/or function induced by intracellular signals initiated by heterologous stimuli. A very clear example is the finding that a mutation of the Kindlin-3 gene in patients with leukocyte adhesion deficiency III leads to a complete block in the functionality of β2 chain containing integrins LFA-1, Mac-1 and p150.95 (36). The genes and expression of these receptors are normal, but functionality is lacking leading to a clinical phenotype reminiscent of LAD1 where the β2-chain (CD18) gene is mutated and expression of the CD18 integrins is absent (37). A similar situation is found for the fibrinogen receptor (αIIb/β3) that is dysfunctional in these Kindlin-3 deficient patients. The molecular mechanisms underlying inside-out control of integrins is excellently reviewed by the group of Ginsberg et al. (35, 38).

Inside-Out Control of FcR

Next to integrins various studies show that also FcγR's and FcαR are subjected to inside-out control (39–43). In contrast to integrins where a consensus is present that this mechanism is important, this concept has not yet been generally accepted for FcR function. The main problem with the latter receptors is that many immune cells express multiple FcRs for the same ligand Ig which makes the study of individual receptors difficult. The studies that have focused on inside-out control of specific FcRs have either been performed with cells endogenously expressing only a single Fc-receptor or cell models dependent on cytokines exogenously expressing single Fc-receptors (39–42, 44).

FcγRII

An excellent cell to study the inside-out control of FcγRIIA is the human eosinophil. This cell isolated from the blood of healthy control only expresses this FcγR. Early work showed that eosinophils carefully isolated in a non-primed fashion hardly bind beads coated with human IgG while they clearly express FcγRII as visualized in FACS based assays (42). Short term pre-incubation with cytokines such as IL-5 and GM-CSF or chemotaxins such as platelet-activating factor (PAF) lead to clear binding of the cells to these Ig-coated particles, whereas the expression of the receptor on the cell surface was unaltered. This model also allowed the manipulation with different pharmacological inhibitors to find out which signaling models are important in this inside-out control (44). These experiments identified that the MEK-MAP-kinase based signaling in these cells is important as MEK inhibitors clearly block the interaction of pre-activated eosinophils with Ig-coated particles (44). These findings basically imply that different cytokines differentially engaging different signaling pathways can steer the inside-out control of FcγRII: those that engage MEK-MAPK such as IL-5 steer the function of FcγRII, whereas those that more engage PI-3K and p38 such as IL-4 more activate FcαR [see below and (44)]. Similar experiments are very difficult to perform with neutrophils because of the high co-expression of FcγRIII (CD16B). It should be emphasized that Huizinga et al. have shown that FcγRII is also the main signaling IgG-receptor in neutrophils (45) and most likely controlled by a similar signaling module as operational for FcαR (42). However, direct experimental proof is lacking. Interestingly, Aleman et al. (46) described the importance of FcγRIIIB in netosis of neutrophils supporting the concept of FcγRIIIB as a signaling receptor.

FcαRI

This receptor is expressed by multiple immune cells including eosinophils. It is, however, important to mention that FcαRI on eosinophils is heavily glycosylated and behaves differently in SDS-PAGE gels when compared with the receptor present in e.g., neutrophils (47). Comparable with serum-IgG coated beads, only (cytokine) primed eosinophils interact with IgA-coated beads (44). However, for FcαR mediated interaction between IgA-coated targets and primed eosinophils the PI-3-kinase signaling pathway is important. This has important consequences as cytokines such as IL-4 that primarily engage this pathway without apparent activation of the MAP-kinase pathway only induce binding of eosinophils with IgA coated targets and not IgG coated targets (44). Interaction with IgG coated beads is not sensitive for (cytokine) priming, likely because FcγRIIIB that is highly expressed by neutrophils can facilitate the interaction with IgG coated beads.

These findings have consequences *in vivo* as differential priming with different mediators at different times and places will determine whether innate immune cells will engage with opsonized particles. It is important to emphasize that eosinophils isolated from patients with allergic diseases exhibit a primed phenotype with respect to binding to IgG and IgA coated beads (48). This implies that these cells have engaged with Th2 driven cytokines and other mediators leading to long term priming of the cells as the primed phenotype persisted during the whole isolation procedure *ex vivo*. Thus, the FcRs retain their primed phenotype for a long time *in vitro*. The situation *in vivo* is less clear as the group of Chilvers et al. put forward the hypothesis that part of the primed phenotype of granulocytes associated with primed FcRs deprimes in the lung *in vivo* (49, 50). This concept, however, has been tested for neutrophils but not for eosinophils. The expression of multiple FcRs on neutrophils precludes a simple testing of the hypothesis that depriming leads to deactivated FcRs on granulocytes.

The mechanisms underlying inside-out control are multiple, complex and cross-interacting. They can be at the level of the receptor itself, associated signaling partner molecules, clustering of homologous and heterologous receptors allowing activation in *trans* and last but not least changes in organization of plasma membrane specialized areas such as lipid rafts and caps.

The functionality of FcRs expressed on the plasma membrane can be accomplished at different levels: (1) changes in valency (multiple receptors are engaged by multivalent ligands on opsonized surfaces (see **Figure 1**), and (2) changes in affinity of single receptors for their ligands.

The valency of receptors is very important as the consensus in the field is that cross-linking of receptors by multiple ligands on the opsonized surface is the main trigger for activation through FcRs (34). It is generally believed that tyrosine kinases binding the one FcR cross-phosphorylate tyrosine residues in ITAM's/ITIM's of the adjacent FcRs. This then initiates the signaling cascades leading to the activation of the downstream functions. So these receptors have to come together in order to be able to signal. Cross-linking by itself seems to be sufficient for signaling as artificial cross-linking by receptor antibodies leads to phosphorylation of the receptors and induction of signaling (29, 51). However, artificial cross-linking does not completely recapitulate the activation induced by natural ligand. This is nicely illustrated by the finding that cross-linking of FcγRIIIB (CD16B) that does not have any intracellular tail leads to changes in intracellular free Ca^{2+} ($[Ca^{2+}]_i$) whereas no signaling motif is present in this receptor. Although it might be that cross-linking of FcγRIIIB engages FcγRIIA through the Fc-portion of the CD16 antibody. In addition, such changes in $[Ca^{2+}]_i$ are not necessarily induced by natural ligand in the form of immune complexes (45) or serum-opsonized particles (52). Thus, caution should be taken to apply artificial cross-linking of the receptor as surrogate for FcR signaling. It is also difficult to test the hypothesis that an increase in valency (receptor clustering) is sufficient for FcR signaling as it is difficult to accomplish this without additionally affecting the receptor affinity for its ligand.

The affinity of low-affinity receptors for their ligands is difficult to determine as monomeric ligand does not bind with sufficient affinity even after inside-out activation. This makes sense as the immune system ideally does not want to interact with monomeric Ig's in blood and mucosal tissues. Therefore, it is very difficult to study valency and affinity of FcRs as two

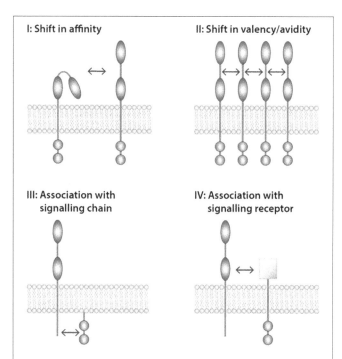

FIGURE 1 | Levels of inside-out control of FcRs . Inside-out control can be accomplished at four levels. The first level is modulation of affinity of single receptors opening up the binding domain(s) of the immunoglobulin domains (illustrated by ➴) facilitating the activation of the receptor which in turn signals through signaling motifs (illustrated by ●) present in the receptor. The second level is induction of lateral movement of the receptor increasing the valency of the receptor. The third level is the interaction with signaling chains such as FcRγ-chain that transmit the signal-tranduction pathways. The fourth level is the trans-activation through an associated heterologous signaling receptor (illustrated by ■).

independent mechanisms and, therefore, the functionality of FcR in the remainder of this review is the resultant of both increased valency and affinity.

THE IMPORTANCE OF THE INTRACELLULAR TAIL OF FcRs IN INSIDE-OUT CONTROL

In order for inside-out control to be affecting the functionality of FcRs these signals should converge at the intracellular tail of the FcRs such as also found for integrins (38). This concept is studied in more molecular detail for two FcRs: FcαRI (CD89) and FcγRI (CD64) (39–41, 53, 54).

The Importance of Serine263 in the Intracellular Tail of FcαRI

Initial studies indicated that several kinases, PI-3-kinase, MAP kinase and p38 were critically involved in the activation of the functionality of FcαRI (40, 41, 48). This was found both in primary cells (leukocytes) as well as cell lines ectopically expressing this receptor. Inhibitors of these kinases modulated the activation FcαRI even in the absence of the accessory common Fcγ-chain. This implies that phosphorylation is involved in the direct control of the functionality of FcαRI. However, there were no clear consensus motifs present in the intracellular tail that are preferentially phosphorylated by any of these kinases. In depth analysis of the receptor led to the conclusion that FcαRI expressed in resting cells was constitutively phosphorylated and thus that kinase activity was already found in the cytosol of resting cells (41). This led to the concept that FcαRI is actively suppressed in its function by constitutive phosphorylation of the receptor. By studying FcαRI receptor mutants transfected into cytokine-dependent Ba/F3 cells it was found that a serine residue at the 263 position in the intracellular tail is essential for the functionality of FcαRI in the context of binding to IgA-coated beads. Mutation of the serine residue to alanine led to a constitutively active receptor supporting the concept that an active kinase is important in keeping the receptor in a non-functional state. This hypothesis was supported by the finding that the S>D mutation, introducing a negative charge at the 263 position, lead to a non-functional receptor as if it was constitutively phosphorylated (41).

Ten Broeke et al. recently provided evidence that the identity of this constitutively active kinase is glycogen synthase kinase-3 (GSK-3) (43), a kinase that is constitutively active in resting cells such as leukocytes and its activity is inhibited by phosphorylation (43). Interestingly, such phosphorylation can be mediated by cytokine-induced activation of the PI-3K and protein kinase-Cζ (PKCζ) -axis (43). This leads to a model were the function of FcαRI is actively suppressed by phosphorylation by GSK-3 in unactivated cells. Cytokine-induced activation of PI-3K followed by activation of PKCζ leads to phosphorylation and inactivation of GSK-3. This in turn leads to dephosphorylation and activation of FcαRI. It is still unclear at which level the control of dephosphorylating of the receptor is achieved. It might be that a constitutive active phosphatase dephosphorylates the receptor or that such enzyme is actively controlled by inside out signals such as found for FcγRI (39). Unfortunately, a similar concept has not been developed in any detail for the inside-out control of FcγRII.

Mechanism of Inside-Out Control of FcγRI (CD64) Functionality: The Tail and Importance of Phosphatase Activity

The situation is different with FcγRI as this is a high affinity receptor able to bind to monomeric IgG. The general idea is that this receptor is always occupied by ligand under conditions such as found in the plasma. Nonetheless, several indications in studies by the group of Leusen et al. (55) provided evidence that this receptor irrespective of bound monomeric IgG can still bind to immune complexes. Only this latter binding is sensitive for inside-out control. The receptor ectopically expressed in hematopoietic cell lines is sensitive for inside-out signaling. The concept arising from this study is that the phosphatase PP2A is the driving enzyme involved in dephosphorylating the receptor and thereby activating its functionality (39). Here again the phosphorylated receptor has a low functionality and dephosphorylation leads to activation. The underlying

mechanisms are not yet completely understood, but recently Brandsma et al. have described that inside-out control of FcγRI is at least in part mediated by lateral movement of the receptor in the membrane (54). It is tempting to speculate that this modulation of movement will be important for the control of valency of this receptor.

The Intracellular Tail and the Inside-Out Control of FcγRII (CD32)

The importance of the intracellular tail of FcγRII comes from experiments in cell lines showing that ectopically expressing tail-less version of FcγRIIA/B is accompanied by a blunted signaling response (17). To test the hypothesis that the tail of FcγRIIA is also important in phagocytes Clark et al. (56) transduced neutrophils with a cell permeant peptide encompassing the intracellular tail of FcγRIIA. They could show that this peptide decreased Ca^{2+} signaling as well as formation of phagolysosomes in human neutrophils.

It is clear that the intracellular tails of FcγRIIA/B, FcγRIIIA, and FcαRI are important for signaling. However, tail-less mutants co-expressed with other receptors such as integrins are still able to transmit signals indicating the intimate cross-talk between these receptors and alternative signaling chains (57).

INSIDE-OUT CONTROL AND RECEPTOR INTERACTIONS

The view that only valency and affinity are important for the inside-out function of Fc-receptors is too simple. The complexity of the ligands (uni/multi valent, fixed complement etc.), immune complexes and opsonized microbes, is very relevant. Here additional proteins and other ligands are present/expressed that can bind to a multitude of additional receptors on innate effector cells e.g., integrins, Toll-like receptors, glucan receptors, complement receptors etc. It is to be expected that differential inside-control mechanisms will control some if not all of these receptors. It will be clear that the net result of all these interactions will lead to a very complex situation that is difficult to understand from the view of individual receptor function.

FcγR/FcγR Cross-Talk

Most innate effector cells express multiple FcRs and most multiple FcγR's. Monocytes and macrophages express FcγRI, FcγRII, and FcγRIII, neutrophils FcγRIIA and FcγRIIIB. Eosinophils only express FcγRIIA and maybe FcγRIIB/C. Cross-talk between FcγRII and FcγRIIIA/B has been suggested by various experiments. Co-crosslinking of FcγRIIA and FcγRIIIB leads to a clear activation of neutrophils characterized by changes in $[Ca^{2+}]_I$ and downstream functions (29). On NK-cells FcγRIIA and FcγRIIIA cross-modulate their functions (58). It is tempting to speculate that subtle changes in inside-out control of these individual receptors will influence the end result of co-activation.

FcR-Integrin Cross-Talk

Several studies have shown that the interaction of primary cells expressing both integrin receptors and FcRs with opsonized targets is characterized by a clear cross-talk (30, 59–61). Again this is best shown in cells that express relatively little different FcRs to exclude interference of above mentioned FcγR/FcγR interactions. Again eosinophils are an interesting cell model as they only express FcγRIIA as activating FcγR. It has clearly been shown that a synergism is present when a surface is expressing integrin ligands such C3bi (ligand of Mac-1/CR3) together with Ig's. Van der Bruggen et al. have shown that yeast opsonized with both ligands is superior when compared with yeast only coated with Ig's or complement (60). However, a trivial explanation might be that the affinity/avidity of the opsonin receptors might be higher when both ligands are present.

Ortiz-Stern et al. have described the importance of cross-linking of FcγRIIIB on neutrophils in modulation of β1-integrins whereas cross-linking of FcγRIIA and FcγRIIIb both lead to activation of β2-integrins (62). More of this type of cross-talk between FcRs and integrins has been reviewed by this group (59). Relevant for this concept is the finding that a genetic polymorphism in the FcγRIIIb gene affects the interaction of this receptor with FcγRIIA and Mac-1/CR3 (CD11b/CD18) (63).

FcR-TLR Cross-Talk

Apart from functional interactions between opsonin and integrin receptors, the function of FcRs is also modulated by multiple other receptors. An important class are the pattern recognition receptors such as toll-like receptors. These receptors can engage with FcR signaling by physical interaction as well as through signaling after ligand binding (64). Indeed, co-immunoprecipitation studies in murine neutrophils have shown that TLR4 (LPS-receptor) physically interacts with FcγRIII upon binding to its ligand LPS (64). It is good to emphasize that there are marked differences in FcRs and Toll-like receptors between mouse and man (4, 65).

For cross-talk between FcR and TLR both receptors do not need to physically interact as the main signaling pathways induced by TLR activation, NFκb, MAP-kinases and PI-3 kinase, are important in inside-out control of FcγRIIA and FcαRI. More of these interactions between FcR and TLR have been excellently reviewed recently (66).

Inside Control of FcRs by Other Receptors or Signaling Molecules

Apart from TLR's there is a whole range of cytokine/chemokine receptors and glucan receptors that all have in common that they engage in signaling pathways important for inside-out control of FcRs. It will be clear that these signals control the interaction between innate effector cells and their targets. This mechanism has been known for a long time and was generally referred to as priming: a process that does not induce a certain cell function by itself but greatly enhances this response to a (heterologous) agonist (67). Particularly, cytotoxic responses are sensitive for such priming responses that act as "safety locks" to prevent aspecific activation of inflammatory cells. Part of such a priming response is mediated by the interaction of FcRs with function modulating membrane proteins.

Not many membrane receptors/chains other than FcR-γchain, additional FcRs or integrins have been described to be involved in the functionality of FcRs. The correct expression of FcRs is

dependent on the presence of β-2 (CD18) integrins. Kindzelskii et al. have described the aberrant capping responses of membrane proteins including FcγRIII and the urokinase receptor in patients with leukocyte adhesion deficiency I (LADI) (68). The data imply that a physical cross talk between integrins and FcRs is part of the correct functioning of FcRs (57). The reverse has not been published.

Next to these aforementioned binding partners periplakin has been implicated in the regulation of function of FcγRI (69). The authors described that periplakin was important in receptor recycling as well as ligand affinity. Periplakin has also been implicated in the control of G-protein coupled receptors, which might important for the signaling of FcR in trans (70) (see below).

INSIDE-OUT CONTROL AND GLYCOSYLATION OF FC-RECEPTORS AND IMMUNOGLOBULINS

In recent years another concept of inside-out control has emerged. It turned out that differences in glycosylation of Fc-receptors has a major impact on their functionality as has recently been reviewed by Hayes et al. (71). This mode of control is nicely illustrated by Patel et al. (72) showing that the function of FcγRIIIA on NK-cells is dependent on its glycan composition. This implies that post-translational processing of FcR is of importance for their functionality on the cell membrane (73). It is not only the glycosylation of FcRs that is important, but also the glycosylation of the different Ig's as large differences are found between the functionality of certain Ig's depending on their N-glycan content (74, 75). Interestingly, also anti-inflammatory characteristics of IgG can be attributed to differences in glycosylation (76). In conclusion, by affecting glycosylation of both FcRs as well as Ig's immune cells can steer the immune response. This has major consequences for designing therapeutical antibodies (77).

INSIDE-OUT CONTROL AND SIGNALING IN *TRANS*

As mentioned before FcRs can signal through their intracellular tail and/or through an accessory FcRγ chain constitutively associated with the receptor. A third mechanism is activation in trans through heterologous receptors associated with the FcRs only after (pre)activation. This concept of signaling in *trans* has been identified many years ago for signaling through G-protein coupled receptors directly activating growth factor receptors such as the EGF receptor (78). This mode of transactivation between receptors seems important for FcRs. Several interesting interactions have been published.

FcRs and Other FcRs

Most of the data regarding transactivation of FcRs to other FcRs is indirect. Nevertheless, several lines of evidence show that co-crosslinking of different FcRs leads to differences in signaling. Vossebeld et al. showed that co-crosslinking FcγRII and FcγRIII lead to more mobilization of intracellular free Ca²⁺

(29). This study also implied a function for FcγRIII as this PI-linked protein was still able to modulate signaling through FcγRIIA. Other studies have shown that cross-linked FcRs lead to differences in the activation of the MAPkinase signaling pathways (20, 79). Interestingly, co-crosslinking of FcRs leads to differential of adhesive phenotypes dependent on the type of FcR and their polymorphisms (80). This mechanism might be important in the fine tuning of responses of leukocytes with different immune complexes. A next level of complexity comes from studies showing functional antagonistic behavior of FcγRIIA and FcγRIIIB (81). These authors provided evidence that immune complexes that are endocytosed by FcγRIIIB are cleared that is considered as anti-inflammatory whilst this process mediated by FcγRIIA leads to Netosis that is considered to be pro-inflammatory. These studies imply that subtle changes brought about by inside out signaling determines the type of the immune response.

FcRs and Integrins

Most data on FcR signaling in *trans* is through integrins. Many studies imply that FcRs pair with different integrins upon activation with immune complexes or by crosslinking of the receptors by anti-receptor antibodies. However, these experiments in primary cells that cannot be genetically manipulated are difficult to interpret in terms of receptor specific signaling as there will be interplay between these receptors, and other modulating membrane receptors where it is basically impossible to determine which signal originates from which signaling chain. To circumvent these "chicken and the egg" issues experiments have been performed in cell lines ectopically expressing FcRs and integrins. Poo et al. have described the physical interaction between FcγRIII and Mac-1 (CD11b) in fibroblasts (82). A similar finding described the interaction between FcγRII and Mac-1 (57). This latter interaction is important for FcγRII mediated phagocytosis. Indirect experiments show that these interactions are also important in the response of neutrophils with opsonized particles (83). The concept that Mac-1 can transduce signals for other Mac-1 binding partners has been described before (84).

The Interaction Between FcRs and G-Protein Coupled Receptors (GPCR)

The interaction between FcRs and G-protein coupled receptors (GPCR) can cross regulate their functions. It has been established that the function of FcγRII on eosinophils is upregulated by priming evoked by agonists of GPCR (67). However, it is uncertain whether a physical interaction between FcγRII and GPCR is necessary or that the activated GPCR activates the receptor by cytosolic signaling. Relevant is, however, that periplakin that regulates the functionality of FcγRI (CD64) can also bind GPCR's (70) supporting a potential bridging role of periplakin between FcRs and GPCR's. Such functions have been amply described in the control of integrins, which has been recently reviewed by Ye et al. (38).

FcRs With Other Proteins

FcRs with other proteins have been described but one should be aware of the fact that the intimate interaction between integrins and FcRs might preclude the identification of other binding partners: in multimolecular complexes these proteins such as integrin associated protein (85) or thrombospondin (86) might bind to integrins rather than the associated FcR.

INSIDE-OUT CONTROL, MEMBRANE DOMAINS, AND LATERAL MOVEMENT

Up to now the functionality of FcRs has been described as if the receptors are free flowing in the plane of the plasma membrane. This is, however, a too simple view as the membrane is organized in domains with different fluidities. Best studied are the micro domains rich in cholesterol also referred to as lipid rafts (87). But other specialized domains such as found in the lamellipodium (88) and uropods (89) are also characterized as being enriched in important receptors and signaling molecules. Receptors can therefore be localized at different membrane compartments that are relatively slowly interacting. Not much is known regarding the distribution of FcRs in these different domains, but recent studies support the importance of lateral mobility of FcRs in the plain of the membrane and the importance of co-localization in these domains (54). In addition, Ten Broeke et al. provided evidence that dephosphorylation of FcαRI and functional activation of the receptor is associated with enhanced lateral movement of the receptor and possibly an increase in valency of the receptor (43). Moreover, data of Yang et al. implied that cross-linking of FcγRIIIb (CD16b) leads to lipid raft mediated activation of SHP2 (51).

INSIDE-OUT CONTROL AND THE HIGH AFFINITY RECEPTOR FOR IGE, FCεRI

The main emphasis in this review was inside-out control of IgG and IgA receptors as this process was best described in this context. However, several studies clearly indicate that also the function of FcεRI is controlled by inside-out signals. This control has been excellently reviewed by Kraft and Kinet (90). Important for this review is the requirement of expression of the tetraspanin CD63 for optimal functionality of FcεRI on mast cells (91). As CD63 is expressed in granules this finding links degranulation with an optimal function of FcεRI. Several other processes are involved in the control of FcεRI by either activating (92) or inhibiting the receptor (93). These processes are now seen as therapeutic targets in allergic diseases (6).

THE IMPLICATIONS OF INSIDE-OUT CONTROL IN CLINICAL APPLICATIONS OF HUMANIZED ANTIBODIES

The implications of FcR inside-out control for the treatment of patients with clinical humanized antibodies are just emerging. The approach will obviously depend on the requirement of effector cells in such therapy and the FcR that they express. Treatment with blocking antibodies directed against single molecules (such as cytokines, complement fragments, and chemokines) might not be directly affected by inside-out control of FcRs as these receptors do not have an obvious role here. However, FcRs play a role in clearance of these target-antibody complexes as the majority is cleared by endocytosis and will subsequently be degraded in the lysosomal compartment (53). This may indicate that therapeutic antibodies might be more rapidly cleared in patients with inflammatory diseases that are characterized by the presence of priming mediators in the peripheral blood or tissue (94). Under these conditions inhibition of inside-out control might be a therapeutic target as it might preserve therapeutic doses of these antibodies allowing lower dosing of the antibodies.

The situation with several antibodies might be more complex. Particularly, those antibodies blocking the function of cellular receptors are of interest. On the one hand, one might want to inhibit inside-out control for preservation of sufficient therapeutical concentrations (see above) on the other inside-out activation might be beneficial for the clinical effect. The idea behind this conception is the following. Anti-receptor antibodies or antibodies directed against cell bound cytokines not only block these molecules, but they might also enable the cell expressing these proteins to be killed (95). This is mediated by antibody or complement dependent cytotoxicity: ADCC or CDC, respectively. Binding of antibodies and/or complement to cells leads to opsonization. Phagocytic receptors are particularly directed against multivalent ligands such as a surface covered with antibodies or complement. The phagocytes will then activate the same armamentarium normally employed for the killing of micro-organisms. The result is a cytotoxic response toward the opsonized cell instead of micro-organism. As both complement receptors such as complement receptor 3 (CR3/Mac-1/CD11b) and FcRs such as FcγRIIA (CD32) and FcαRI (CD89) are very sensitive for inside-out activation it will be clear that this activation is very important for the clinical action (53, 84). Not much is known regarding these issues in humans *in vivo* some studies now imply that ADCC is often important for the clinical effect of therapeutic antibodies (96, 97). A clear example is the anti-IL5R antibody, Benralizumab, which functions through ADCC (95) of IL5Rα+ cells [eosinophils,

basophils and possibly ILC2 (98)]. The concept of inside-out activation of the ADCC under these conditions has not been applied to these clinical studies.

The overall conclusion whether or not inside-out control should be considered in augmenting the therapeutic is likely to be dependent on the mode(s) of action of the therapeutic antibodies. It is, however, clear that this complexity should be considered gaining optimal therapeutic effectiveness of current and new antibodies.

CONCLUSION

Inside-out control of FcRs as well as integrins functions as a safety lock preventing collateral damage evoked by innate immune effector cells. Here a clear cross-talk is present between the adaptive immune response producing priming mediators and the innate immune system that adapt to these signals. Part of the priming mediators liberated during inflammation leads to inside-out control of FcRs potentiating these receptors. This very complex mechanism is based on modulation of valency of the receptors, their affinity, their interaction with other signaling chains and receptors and their localization in specialized membrane areas such as lipid rafts. The many levels of control will make it possible to fine tune the inside out control with therapeutic molecules only affecting part of this process. This will allow stratified therapy such that the therapeutic effect is maximal while the normal function of phagocytes is preserved.

AUTHOR CONTRIBUTIONS

The author confirms being the sole contributor of this work and has approved it for publication.

FUNDING

This work was supported by Universitair Medisch Centrum Utrecht.

ACKNOWLEDGMENTS

Dr. N. Vrisekoop is thanked for critically reading the manuscript.

REFERENCES

1. Nussenzweig MC. Immune receptor editing: revise and select. *Cell.* (1998) 95:875–8. doi: 10.1016/S0092-8674(00)81711-0
2. Mkaddem SB, Christou I, Rossato E, Berthelot L, Lehuen A, Monteiro RC. IgA, IgA receptors, and their anti-inflammatory properties. *Curr Top Microbiol Immunol.* (2014) 382:221–35. doi: 10.1007/978-3-319-07911-0_10
3. Monteiro RC, Van De Winkel JGJ. IgA Fc receptors. *Annu Rev Immunol.* (2003) 21:177–204. doi: 10.1146/annurev.immunol.21.120601.141011
4. Ravetch J, Bolland S. IgG Fc receptor. *Annu Rev Immunol.* (2001) 19:275–90. doi: 10.1146/annurev.immunol.19.1.275
5. Hargreaves CE, Rose-Zerilli MJJ, Machado LR, Iriyama C, Hollox EJ, Cragg MS, et al. Fcγ receptors: genetic variation, function, and disease. *Immunol Rev.* (2015) 268:6–24. doi: 10.1111/imr.12341

6. MacGlashan Jr DW. IgE-dependent signaling as a therapeutic target for allergies. *Trends Pharmacol Sci.* (2012) 33:502–9. doi: 10.1016/j.tips.2012.06.002
7. Monteiro RC. Role of IgA and IgA fc receptors in inflammation. *J Clin Immunol.* (2010) 30:1–9. doi: 10.1007/s10875-009-9338-0
8. Roopenian DC, Akilesh S. FcRn: the neonatal Fc receptor comes of age. *Nat Rev Immunol.* (2007) 7:715–25. doi: 10.1038/nri2155
9. Lamkhioued B, Gounni AS, Gruart V, Pierce A, Capron A, Capron M. Human eosinophils express a receptor for secretory component. Role in secretory IgA-dependent activation. *Eur J Immunol.* (1995) 25:117–25. doi: 10.1002/eji.1830250121
10. Karsten CM, Köhl J. The immunoglobulin, IgG Fc receptor and complement triangle in autoimmune diseases. *Immunobiology.* (2012) 217:1067–79. doi: 10.1016/j.imbio.2012.07.015

11. Gordon S. Phagocytosis: an immunobiologic process. *Immunity*. (2016) 44:463–75. doi: 10.1016/j.immuni.2016.02.026

12. Segal AW. How neutrophils kill microbes. *Annu Rev Immunol*. (2005) 23:197–223. doi: 10.1146/annurev.immunol.23.021704.115653

13. Bardoel BW, Kenny EF, Sollberger G, Zychlinsky A. The balancing act of neutrophils. *Cell Host Microbe*. (2014) 15:526–36. doi: 10.1016/j.chom.2014.04.011

14. Patnode ML, Bando JK, Krummel MF, Locksley RM, Rosen SD. Leukotriene B₄ amplifies eosinophil accumulation in response to nematodes. *J Exp Med*. (2014) 211:1281–8. doi: 10.1084/jem.20132336

15. Yazdanbakhsh M, Tai PC, Spry CJ, Gleich GJ, Roos D. Synergism between eosinophil cationic protein and oxygen metabolites in killing of schistosomula of *Schistosoma mansoni*. *J Immunol*. (1987) 138:3443–7.

16. Bournazos S, Wang TT, Dahan R, Maamary J, Ravetch JV. Signaling by antibodies: recent progress. *Annu Rev Immunol*. (2017) 35:285–311. doi: 10.1146/annurev-immunol-051116-052433

17. Van den Herik-Oudijk IE, Capel PJA, van der Bruggen T, Van den Winkel JGJ. Identification of signaling motifs within human FcγRIIa and FcγRIIb isoforms. *Blood*. (1995) 85:2202–11.

18. Roghanian A, Stopforth RJ, Dahal LN, Cragg MS. New revelations from an old receptor: immunoregulatory functions of the inhibitory Fc gamma receptor, FcγRIIB (CD32B). *J Leukoc Biol*. (2018) 103:1077–88. doi: 10.1002/JLB.2MIR0917-354R

19. Huang Z, Hunter S, Kim M-K, Indik ZK, Schreiber AD. The effect of phosphatases SHP-1 and SHIP-1 on signaling by the ITIM- and ITAM-containing Fcγ receptors FcγRIIB and FcγRIIA. *J Leukoc Biol*. (2003) 73:823–9. doi: 10.1189/jlb.0902454

20. Rollet-Labelle E, Gilbert C, Naccache PH. Modulation of human neutrophil responses to CD32 cross-linking by serine/threonine phosphatase inhibitors: cross-talk between serine/threonine and tyrosine phosphorylation. *J Immunol*. (2000) 164:1020–8. doi: 10.4049/jimmunol.164.2.1020

21. Sato K, Ochi A. Superclustering of B cell receptor and Fc gamma RIIB1 activates Src homology 2-containing protein tyrosine phosphatase-1. *J Immunol*. (1998) 161:2716–22.

22. Underhill DM, Goodridge HS. The many faces of ITAMs. *Trends Immunol*. (2007) 28:66–73. doi: 10.1016/j.it.2006.12.004

23. Verbrugge A, Meyaard L. Signaling by ITIM-bearing receptors. *Curr Immunol Rev*. (2005) 1:201–12. doi: 10.2174/1573395054065160

24. Getahun A, Cambier JC. Of ITIMs, ITAMs, and ITAMis: revisiting immunoglobulin Fc receptor signaling. *Immunol Rev*. (2015) 268:66–73. doi: 10.1111/imr.12336

25. Morton HC, Van Den Herik-Oudijk IE, Vossebeld P, Snijders A, Verhoeven AJ, Capel PJA, et al. Functional association between the human myeloid immunoglobulin A Fc receptor (CD89) and FcR gamma chain: molecular basis for CD89/FcR gamma chain association. *J Biol Chem*. (1995) 270:29781–7. doi: 10.1074/jbc.270.50.29781

26. Van Vugt MJ, Heijnen IA, Capel PJ, Park SY, Ra C, Saito T, et al. FcR gamma-chain is essential for both surface expression and function of human Fc gamma RI (CD64) *in vivo*. *Blood*. (1996) 87:3593–99.

27. Wirthmueller BU, Kurosaki T, Murakami MS, Ravetch JV, Wirthmueller U. Signal transduction by Fc gamma RIII (CD16) is mediated through the gamma chain. *J Exp Med*. (1992) 175:1381–90. doi: 10.1084/jem.175.5.1381

28. Huizinga TW, van der Schoot CE, Jost C, Klaassen R, Kleijer M, von dem Borne AE, et al. The PI-linked Fc gamma RIII is released on stimulation of neutrophils. *Nature*. (1988) 333:667–9. doi: 10.1038/333667a0

29. Vossebeld PJM, Kessler J, Von dem Borne AEGK, Roos D, Verhoeven AJ. Heterotypic FcγR clusters evoke a synergistic Ca2+response in human neutrophils. *J Biol Chem*. (1995) 270:10671–9. doi: 10.1074/jbc.270.18.10671

30. Petty HR, Worth RG, Todd RF. Interactions of integrins with their partner proteins in leukocyte membranes. *Immunol Res*. (2002) 25:75–95. doi: 10.1385/IR:25:1:75

31. Reumaux D, Kuijpers TW, Hordijk PL, Duthilleul P, Roos D. Involvement of Fcγ receptors and β2 integrins in neutrophil activation by anti-proteinase-3 or anti-myeloperoxidase antibodies. *Clin Exp Immunol*. (2003) 134:344–50. doi: 10.1046/j.1365-2249.2003.02280.x

32. van de Winkel JG, van Ommen R, Huizinga TW, de Raad MA, Tuijnman WB, Groenen PJ, et al. Proteolysis induces increased binding affinity of the monocyte type II FcR for human IgG. *J Immunol*. (1989) 143:571–8.

33. Hulett MD, Hogarth PM. The second and third extracellular domains of FcγRI (CD64) confer the unique high affinity binding of IgG2a. *Mol Immunol*. (1998) 35:989–96. doi: 10.1016/S0161-5890(98)00069-8

34. Ortiz DF, Lansing JC, Rutitzky L, Kurtagic E, Prod'homme T, Choudhury A, et al. Elucidating the interplay between IgG-Fc valency and FcγR activation for the design of immune complex inhibitors. *Sci Transl Med*. (2016) 8:365ra158. doi: 10.1126/scitranslmed.aaf9418

35. Faull RJ, Ginsberg MH. Inside-out signaling through integrins. *J Am Soc Nephrol*. (1996) 7:1091–7.

36. Kuijpers TW, Van De Vijver E, Weterman MAJ, De Boer M, Tool ATJ, Van Den Berg TK, et al. LAD-1/variant syndrome is caused by mutations in FERMT3. *Blood*. (2009) 113:4740–6. doi: 10.1182/blood-2008-10-182154

37. Springer TA. Inherited deficiency of the Mac-1, LFA-1, p150,95 glycoprotein family and its molecular basis. *J Exp Med*. (1984) 160:1901–18. doi: 10.1084/jem.160.6.1901

38. Ye F, Kim C, Ginsberg MH. Molecular mechanism of inside-out integrin regulation. *J Thromb Haemost*. (2011) 9:20–5. doi: 10.1111/j.1538-7836.2011.04355.x

39. Bakema JE, Bakker A, de Haij S, Honing H, Bracke M, Koenderman L, et al. Inside-out regulation of Fc RI (CD89) depends on PP2A. *J Immunol*. (2008) 181:4080–8. doi: 10.4049/jimmunol.181.6.4080

40. Bracke M, Nijhuis E, Lammers JJ, Coffer PJ, Koenderman L. A critical role for PI 3-kinase in cytokine-induced Fc alpha -receptor activation. *Blood*. (2000) 95:2037–43.

41. Bracke M, Lammers JWJ, Coffer PJ, Koenderman L. Cytokine-induced inside-out activation of FcαR (CD89) is mediated by a single serine residue (S263) in the intracellular domain of the receptor. *Blood*. (2001) 97:3478–83. doi: 10.1182/blood.V97.11.3478

42. Koenderman L, Hermans SW, Capel PJ, van de Winkel JG. Granulocyte-macrophage colony-stimulating factor induces sequential activation and deactivation of binding via a low-affinity IgG Fc receptor, hFc gamma RII, on human eosinophils. *Blood*. (1993) 81:2413–9.

43. ten Broeke T, Honing H, Brandsma A, Jacobino S, Bakema J, Kanters D, et al. FcalphaRI dynamics are regulated by GSK-3 and PKCzeta during cytokine mediated inside-out signaling. *Front Immunol*. (2018) 9:3191. doi: 10.3389/fimmu.2018.03191

44. Bracke M, Coffer PJ, Lammers JW, Koenderman L. Analysis of signal transduction pathways regulating cytokine-mediated Fc receptor activation on human eosinophils. *J Immunol*. (1998) 161:6768–74.

45. Huizinga TW, van Kemenade F, Koenderman L, Dolman KM, von dem Borne AE, Tetteroo PA, et al. The 40-kDa Fc gamma receptor (FcRII) on human neutrophils is essential for the IgG-induced respiratory burst and IgG-induced phagocytosis. *J Immunol*. (1989) 142:2365–9.

46. Alemán OR, Mora N, Cortes-Vieyra R, Uribe-Querol E, Rosales C. Differential use of human neutrophil Fc γ receptors for inducing neutrophil extracellular trap formation. *J Immunol Res*. (2016) 2016:1–17.·doi: 10.1155/2016/2908034

47. Monteiro RC, Hostoffer RW, Cooper MD, Bonner JR, Gartland GL, Kubagawa H. Definition of immunoglobulin A receptors on eosinophils and their enhanced expression in allergic individuals. *J Clin Invest*. (1993) 92:1681–5. doi: 10.1172/JCI116754

48. Bracke M, van De Graaf E, Lammers JW, Coffer PJ, Koenderman L. In vivo priming of FcalphaR functioning on eosinophils of allergic asthmatics. *J Leukoc Biol*. (2000b) 68:655–61. doi: 10.1189/jlb.68.5.655

49. Kitchen E, Rossi A, Condliffe A, Haslett C, Chilvers E. Demonstration of reversible priming of human neutrophils using platelet- activating factor. *Blood*. (1996) 88:4330–7.

50. Summers C, Chilvers ER, Michael Peters A. Mathematical modeling supports the presence of neutrophil depriming in vivo. *Phys Rep*. (2014) 2:e00241. doi: 10.1002/phy2.241

51. Yang H, Jiang H, Song Y, Chen DJ, Shen XJ, Chen JH. Neutrophil CD16b crosslinking induces lipid raft-mediated activation of SHP-2 and affects cytokine expression and retarded neutrophil apoptosis. *Exp Cell Res*. (2018) 362:121–31. doi: 10.1016/j.yexcr.2017.11.009

52. Koenderman L, Tool ATJ, HooyBrink B, Roos D, Hansen CA, Williamson JR, et al. Adherence of human neutrophils changes Ca2+signaling during activation with opsonized particles. *FEBS Lett*. (1990) 270:49–52. doi: 10.1016/0014-5793(90)81232-D

53. Brandsma AM, Jacobino SR, Meyer S, ten Broeke T, Leusen JHW. Fc receptor inside-out signaling and possible impact on antibody therapy. *Immunol Rev.* (2015) 268:74–87. doi: 10.1111/imr.12332

54. Brandsma AM, Schwartz SL, Wester MJ, Valley CC, Blezer GLA, Vidarsson G, et al. Mechanisms of inside-out signaling of the high-affinity IgG receptor FcγRI. *Sci Signal.* (2018) 11:eaaq0891. doi: 10.1126/scisignal.aaq0891

55. Van Der Poel CE, Karssemeijer RA, Boross P, Van Der Linden JA, Blokland M, Van De Winkel JGJ, et al. Cytokine-induced immune complex binding to the high-affinity IgG receptor, FcγRI, in the presence of monomeric IgG. *Blood.* (2010) 116:5327–33. doi: 10.1182/blood-2010-04-280214

56. Clark AJ, Petty HR. A cell permeant peptide containing the cytoplasmic tail sequence of Fc receptor type IIA reduces calcium signaling and phagolysosome formation in neutrophils. *Cell Immunol.* (2010) 261:153–8. doi: 10.1016/j.cellimm.2009.12.002

57. Worth RG, Mayo-Bond L, van de Winkel JG, Todd 3rd RF, Petty HR. CR3 (alphaM beta2; CD11b/CD18) restores IgG-dependent phagocytosis in transfectants expressing a phagocytosis-defective Fc gammaRIIA (CD32) tail-minus mutant. *J Immunol.* (1996) 157:5660–5.

58. Arase N, Arase H, Park SY, Ohno H. Association with FcR gamma is essential for activation signal through NKR-P1 (CD161) in Natural Killer (NK) cells and NK1.1 + T Cells. *J Exp Med.* (1997) 186:1957–63. doi: 10.1084/jem.186.12.1957

59. Ortiz-Stern A, Rosales C. Cross-talk between Fc receptors and integrins. *Immunol Lett.* (2003) 90:137–43. doi: 10.1016/j.imlet.2003.08.004

60. van der Bruggen T, Kok PT, Raaijmakers JA, Lammers JW, Koenderman L. Cooperation between Fc gamma receptor II and complement receptor type 3 during activation of platelet-activating factor release by cytokine-primed human eosinophils. *J Immunol.* (1994) 153:2729–35.

61. Worth RG, Kim M-K, Kindzelskii AL, Petty HR, Schreiber AD. Signal sequence within FcRIIA controls calcium wave propagation patterns: apparent role in phagolysosome fusion. *Proc Natl Acad Sci USA.* (2003) 100:4533–8. doi: 10.1073/pnas.0836650100

62. Ortiz-Stern A, Rosales C. FcγRIIIB stimulation promotes β1 integrin activation in human neutrophils. *J Leukoc Biol.* (2005) 77:787–99. doi: 10.1189/jlb.0504310

63. Urbaczek AC, Toller-Kawahisa JE, Fonseca LM, Costa PI, Faria CMQG, Azzolini AECS, et al. Influence of FcγRIIIb polymorphism on its ability to cooperate with FcγRIIa and CR3 in mediating the oxidative burst of human neutrophils. *Hum Immunol.* (2014) 75:785–90. doi: 10.1016/j.humimm.2014.05.011

64. Rittirsch D, Flierl MA, Day DE, Nadeau BA, Zetoune FS, Sarma JV, et al. Cross-talk between TLR4 and FcγReceptorIII (CD16) pathways. *PLoS Pathog.* (2009) 5:e1000464. doi: 10.1371/journal.ppat.1000464

65. Rehli M. Of mice and men: species variations of toll-like receptor expression. *Trends Immunol.* (2002) 23:375–8. doi: 10.1016/S1471-4906(02)02259-7

66. van Egmond M, Vidarsson G, Bakema JE. Cross-talk between pathogen recognizing toll-like receptors and immunoglobulin Fc receptors in immunity. *Immunol Rev.* (2015) 268:311–27. doi: 10.1111/imr.12333

67. Coffer PJ, Koenderman L. Granulocyte signal transduction and priming: cause without effect? *Immunol Lett.* (1997) 57:27–31. doi: 10.1016/S0165-2478(97)00067-9

68. Kindzelskii AL, Xue W, Todd 3rd RF, Boxer LA, Petty HR. Aberrant capping of membrane proteins on neutrophils from patients with leukocyte adhesion deficiency. *Blood.* (1994) 83:1650–5.

69. Beekman JM, Bakema JE, van de Winkel JGJ, Leusen JHW. Direct interaction between FcgammaRI (CD64) and periplakin controls receptor endocytosis and ligand binding capacity. *Proc Natl Acad Sci USA.* (2004) 101:10392–7. doi: 10.1073/pnas.0401217101

70. Milligan G, Murdoch H, Kellett E, White JH, Feng GJ. Interactions between G-protein-coupled receptors and periplakin: a selective means to regulate G-protein activation. *Biochem Soc Trans.* (2004) 32:878–80. doi: 10.1042/BST0320878

71. Hayes JM, Wormald MR, Rudd PM, Davey GP. Fc gamma receptors: glycobiology and therapeutic prospects. *J Inflamm Res.* (2016) 9:209–19. doi: 10.2147/JIR.S121233

72. Patel KR, Roberts JT, Subedi GP, Barb AW. Restricted processing of CD16a/Fc receptor IIIa N-glycans from primary human NK cells impacts structure and function. *J Biol Chem.* (2018) 293:3477–89. doi: 10.1074/jbc.RA117.001207

73. Oliva KD, Cavanaugh JM, Cobb BA. Antibody receptors steal the sweet spotlight. *J Biol Chem.* (2018) 293:3490–1. doi: 10.1074/jbc.H118.001955

74. Dekkers G, Rispens T, Vidarsson G. Novel concepts of altered immunoglobulin G galactosylation in autoimmune diseases. *Front Immunol.* (2018) 9:553. doi: 10.3389/fimmu.2018.00553

75. Quast I, Peschke B, Lünemann JD. Regulation of antibody effector functions through IgG Fc N-glycosylation. *Cell Mol Life Sci.* (2017) 74:837–47. doi: 10.1007/s00018-016-2366-z

76. Nimmerjahn F, Böhm S, Kao D. Sweet and sour: the role of glycosylation for the anti-inflammatory activity of immunoglobulin G. *Curr Top Microbiol Immunol.* (2014) 382:393–417. doi: 10.1007/978-3-319-07911-0_18

77. Jennewein MF, Alter G. The immunoregulatory roles of antibody glycosylation. *Trends Immunol.* (2017) 38:358–72. doi: 10.1016/j.it.2017.02.004

78. Voisin L, Foisy S, Giasson E, Lambert C, Moreau P, Meloche S. EGF receptor transactivation is obligatory for protein synthesis stimulation by G protein-coupled receptors. *Am J Physiol Physiol.* (2002) 283:C446–55. doi: 10.1152/ajpcell.00261.2001

79. Sánchez-Mejorada G, Rosales C. Signal transduction by immunoglobulin Fc receptors. *J Leukoc Biol.* (1998) 63:521–33. doi: 10.1002/jlb.63.5.521

80. Jakus Z, Berton G, Ligeti E, Lowell CA, Mocsai A. Responses of neutrophils to anti-integrin antibodies depends on costimulation through low affinity Fc Rs: full activation requires both integrin and nonintegrin signals. *J Immunol.* (2004) 173:2068–77. doi: 10.4049/jimmunol.173.3.2068

81. Chen K, Nishi H, Travers R, Tsuboi N, Martinod K, Wagner DD, et al. Endocytosis of soluble immune complexes leads to their clearance by FcγRIIIB but induces neutrophil extracellular traps via FcγRIIA *in vivo*. *Blood.* (2012) 120:4421–31. doi: 10.1182/blood-2011-12-401133

82. Poo H, Krauss JC, Mayo-Bond L, Todd RF, Petty HR. Interaction of Fcγ receptor type IIIB with complement receptor type 3 in fibroblast transfectants: evidence from lateral diffusion and resonance energy transfer studies. *J Mol Biol.* (1995) 247:597–603. doi: 10.1016/S0022-2836(05)80141-X

83. Koenderman L, Van Der Bruggen T, Kok PT, Raaijmakers JA, Lammers JW. *Cooperation Between Fc Gamma Receptor II and Complement Receptor Type 3 During Activation of Platelet-Activating factor release by cytokine-primed human eosinophils.* (2018). Available online at: http://www.jimmunol.org/content/153/6/2729

84. Van Spriel AB, Leusen JHW, Van Egmond M, Dijkman HBPM, Assmann KJM, Mayadas TN, et al. Mac-1 (CD11b/CD18) is essential for Fc receptor-mediated neutrophil cytotoxicity and immunologic synapse formation. *Blood.* (2001) 97:2478–86. doi: 10.1182/blood.V97.8.2478

85. Schwartz MA, Brown EJ, Fazeli B. A 50-kDa integrin-associated protein is required for integrin-regulated calcium entry in endothelial cells. *J Biol Chem.* (1993) 268:19931–4.

86. Chung J, Gao AG, Frazier WA. Thrombospondin acts via integrin-associated protein to activate the platelet integrin alpha(IIb)beta3. *J Biol Chem.* (1997) 272:14740–6. doi: 10.1074/jbc.272.23.14740

87. Lingwood D, Simons K. Lipid rafts as a membrane-organizing principle. *Science.* (2010) 327:46–50. doi: 10.1126/science.1174621

88. Swaney KF, Huang C-H, Devreotes PN. Eukaryotic chemotaxis: a network of signaling pathways controls motility, directional sensing, and polarity. *Annu Rev Biophys.* (2010) 39:265–89. doi: 10.1146/annurev.biophys.093008.131228

89. Hind LE, Vincent WJB, Huttenlocher A. Leading from the back: the role of the uropod in neutrophil polarization and migration. *Dev Cell.* (2016) 38:161–9. doi: 10.1016/j.devcel.2016.06.031

90. Kraft S, Kinet JP. New developments in FcεRI regulation, function and inhibition. *Nat Rev Immunol.* (2007) 7:365–78. doi: 10.1038/nri2072

91. Kraft S, Jouvin M-H, Kulkarni N, Kissing S, Morgan ES, Dvorak AM, et al. The tetraspanin CD63 is required for efficient IgE-mediated mast cell degranulation and anaphylaxis. *J Immunol.* (2013) 191:2871–8. doi: 10.4049/jimmunol.1202323

92. Kuehn HS, Beaven MA, Ma HT, Kim MS, Metcalfe DD, Gilfillan AM. Synergistic activation of phospholipases Cγ and Cβ: A novel mechanism for PI3K-independent enhancement of FcεRI-induced mast cell mediator release. *Cell Signal.* (2008) 20:625–36. doi: 10.1016/j.cellsig.2007.11.016

93. Sabato V, Verweij MM, Bridts CH, Levi-Schaffer F, Gibbs BF, De Clerck LS, et al. CD300a is expressed on human basophils and seems to inhibit

IgE/FcεRI-dependent anaphylactic degranulation. *Cytom Part B Clin Cytom.* (2012) 82:132–8. doi: 10.1002/cyto.b.21003

94. Mukherjee M, Lim HF, Thomas S, Miller D, Kjarsgaard M, Tan B, et al. Airway autoimmune responses in severe eosinophilic asthma following low-dose Mepolizumab therapy. *Allergy Asthma Clin Immunol.* (2017) 13:2. doi: 10.1186/s13223-016-0174-5

95. Ghazi A, Trikha A, Calhoun WJ. Benralizumab – a humanized mAb to IL-5Rα with enhanced antibody-dependent cell-mediated cytotoxicity – a novel approach for the treatment of asthma. *Expert Opin Biol Ther.* (2012) 12:113–8. doi: 10.1517/14712598.2012.642359

96. Choudary KB. Monoclonal antibodies with ADCC and CDC enhancement for therapy. *Int J Pharma Bio Sci.* (2013) 4:B588–99.

97. Strohl WR. Current progress in innovative engineered antibodies. *Protein Cell.* (2018) 9:86–120. doi: 10.1007/s13238-017-0457-8

98. Smith SG, Chen R, Kjarsgaard M, Huang C, Oliveria JP, O'Byrne PM, et al. Increased numbers of activated group 2 innate lymphoid cells in the airways of patients with severe asthma and persistent airway eosinophilia. *J Allergy Clin Immunol.* (2016) 137:75–86.e8. doi: 10.1016/j.jaci.2015.05.037

8

Antibody Epitope Specificity for dsDNA Phosphate Backbone is an Intrinsic Property of the Heavy Chain Variable Germline Gene Segment used

Tatjana Srdic-Rajic[1], Heinz Kohler[2], Vladimir Jurisic[3] and Radmila Metlas[4*]

[1] Department of Experimental Pharmacology, National Cancer Research Center, Belgrade, Serbia, [2] Department of Microbiology and Immunology, University of Kentucky, Lexington, KY, United States, [3] Faculties of Medicinal Science, University of Kragujevac, Kragujevac, Serbia, [4] Vinča Institute of Nuclear Science, University of Belgrade, Belgrade, Serbia

*Correspondence:
Radmila Metlas
metlas.r@sbb.rs

Analysis of protein sequences by the informational spectrum method (ISM) enables characterization of their specificity according to encoded information represented with defined frequency (F). Our previous data showed that F(0.367) is characteristic for variable heavy chain (VH) domains (a combination of variable (V), diversity (D) and joining (J) gene segments) of the anti-phosphocholine (PC) T15 antibodies and mostly dependent on the CDR2 region, a site for PC phosphate group binding. Because the T15 dsDNA-reactive U4 mutant also encodes F(0.367), we hypothesized that the same frequency may also be characteristic for anti-DNA antibodies. Data obtained from an analysis of 60 spontaneously produced anti-DNA antibody VH domain sequences supported our hypothesis only for antibodies, which use V gene segment in germline configuration, such as S57(VH31), MRL-DNA22, and VH11, members of the VH1 (J558) and VH7 (S107) gene families. The important finding is that out of seven V gene segments used by spontaneous anti-DNA antibodies, F(0.367) is only expressed by the germline configuration of these three V gene segments. The data suggest that antibody specificity for the phosphate group moiety delineated as F(0.367) is the intrinsic property of the V germline gene segments used, whereas paratope/epitope interaction with antigens bearing this epitope, such as PC or dsDNA, requires corresponding antibody VH conformation that is susceptible to somatic mutation(s).

Keywords: anti-DNA antibodies, anti-PC antibodies, VH germline genes, Characterization of antibody specificity by ISM, dsDNA reactive antibodies

INTRODUCTION

Natural autoantibodies, mainly IgM whose heavy chains are encoded by unmutated VDJ genes, play a role in immune system homeostasis, provide the first line of defense against infections, and may play a role in autoimmune disease as somatically mutated IgG autoantibodies (1, 2). The highly diverse CDR3 loops are assumed as the key determinant of specificity in antigen recognition, but in nonsomatically mutated antibodies, binding sites may consist of germline-encoded CDR1 and CDR2 sequences dominating in a number of contacts, whereas light chains play a subsidiary role to heavy chains (3, 4). It was also suggested that in contrast to antigen specificity determined by CDR3 (5), germline-encoded CDR1 and CDR2 sequences accommodate binding to a number of different unrelated antigens (6). The analyses also showed that despite the potential to generate almost unlimited variability, the CDR regions exhibit a small number of core main chain conformations termed "canonical structures" (7). In particular, a limited repertoire of the main chain adopted conformations dependent on the loop length and a few key conserved residues at defined positions (8) has been assigned to CDR1 and CDR2 regions (9).

One of the best studied primary antibody responses to phosphocholine (PC) is T15 antibody expressing heavy and light chain products of the T15(V1) and Vk22 germline genes in mice (10–13). It is of interest that in ontogeny, T15 predominant clonotypes appear about 1 week after birth (14), whereas PC-specific responses or precursors were detected as early as 1 day after birth (15). An important finding is that the heavy chains of T15 and other PC binding proteins bearing M603 and M167 idiotypic determinants are derived from a single germline T15(V1) gene segment and three light chains, i.e., T15 (VK22), M603 (VK8), and M167 (VK24) (13, 16, 17).

Crystallography studies of the anti-PC binding antibody provide evidence for the PC contact residues, revealing that favorable interaction of the choline moiety is with CDR1 Glu-35, whereas specific interactions occur between the phosphate group and charged groups such as CDR2 Arg-52 that produce a large favorable electrostatic interaction and Lys-54 that helps neutralize the PC negative charge (18, 19). The data obtained from mutagenesis experiments conferred importance of CDR2 Arg-52 as a site for interaction with the PC phosphate group (20), whereas interaction with the carrier involves different sites (21). The role of CDR2 H52-H56 motif in nucleic acid binding was also demonstrated by analyses of monoclonal autoantibodies derived from lupus-prone mice (22).

On the other hand, T15 CDR2 sequence VH50-60 region, a part of the self-binding domain (homophilicity), enhances antibody potency (23). The CDR2 of T15 antibody, according to our view, may also have an immunoregulatory role in the ontogeny of natural Tregs and consequently in the control of T15 and some anti-DNA antibody diversification (24).

Anti-DNA antibodies recognize a considerable number of different epitopes, and their exact nature is only partially known (25). Anti-dsDNA antibodies may react with linear and conformational determinants exposed on the double helix of DNA and cross-react with different antigens (26). For example, a similar arrangement of phosphate groups in the DNA sugar-phosphate backbone and phospholipids may explain cross-reactivity (27).

Sequence analysis of anti-dsDNA antibodies from autoimmune mice revealed a high frequency of mutations and the presence of basic amino acids in the CDRs, such as Arg and Lys and polar Asn with the potential to interact with structures within dsDNA (28–31) or, when gained during

affinity maturation, be critical for CDR3 region interaction with histone-DNA complex (32–34). This complex according to a hapten-carrier-like model, may initiate production of both anti-dsDNA and other anti-nucleosome antibodies [reviewed in (35)].

In prior studies, we have shown that antibody VH domains of anti-PC T15 and T15 dsDNA binding somatic mutant, U4 (13), encode characteristic sequence information represented with F(0.367) (36). In this report, we extended this finding by showing that F(0.367) is also expressed by several anti-DNA antibody VH domains that use V germline or somatically mutated S57(VH31), MRL-DNA22, and VH11 gene segments of the VH1 (J558) and VH7 (S107) gene families, as well as that protein sequences of these germline genes in addition to T15(V1) encode an intrinsic epitope specificity represented by F(0.367). Obtained data suggests that as long as the frequency is expressed by an antibody VH domain (a) the corresponding conformation for paratope/epitope interaction might be preserved despite somatic mutations and (b) because of somatic mutation(s), interaction with another antigen bearing the same epitope might be achieved and vice versa, loss of the characteristic frequency may cause achievement of a new epitope specificity.

METHOD

The sequence analysis was performed by applying the informational spectrum method (ISM). The physicomathematical basis of ISM was described in detail elsewhere (37), and here, we will only point the basic steps involved by the method. According to the ISM approach, also denoted as resonant recognition model (RRM) (38), protein sequences are transformed into signals by assignment of numerical values of each amino acid. These values correspond to electron–ion interaction potential (39) determining electronic properties of amino acids that are responsible for their intermolecular interactions (40–43). The signal obtained is decomposed in periodical function by Fourier transformation. The result is a series of frequencies and their amplitudes (the informational spectrum, IS). Detailed steps (43) that precede obtaining the IS by the ISM are explained in the **Supplementary Information**. The obtained frequencies correspond to the distribution of structural motifs with defined physicochemical characteristics determining the biological function of the sequence. When comparing proteins that share the same biological function, the technique allows detection of code/frequency pairs in IS, which are specific for their common biological properties. This common information is represented by characteristic peaks in the cross-spectrum (CIS) of proteins. The method is insensitive to the location of the motifs and, thus, does not require the previous alignment of the sequence. A measure of similarity for each peak is a signal-to-noise ratio (S/N), which represents a ratio between signal intensity at one particular IS frequency and the mean value of the whole spectrum which depends on the number of the sequences used in the analysis.

Abbreviations: CDR, Hypervariable region; CIS, Cross-spectral analysis; EIIP, Electron-ion interaction potential; ISM, Informational spectrum method; IS, Informational spectrum; RRM, Resonant recognition model; S/N, Signal-to-noise ratio; VH, Variable heavy chain.

RESULTS

Our previous data showed that VH domain of the anti-PC T15 idiotype antibody that uses an unmutated copy of the V germline gene T15(V1) (16, 17), as well as anti-PC binding antibodies of different idiotypes, encode information represented with F(0.367) in short F(0.37) (36). We also showed that F(0.37), is independent of a single substitution-glutamic acid to alanine, at position 35 in the T15 antibody CDR1 region, causing reactivity acquisition for dsDNA (13) but depends on mutations in CDR2 region (36). In this report, seven V germline gene amino acid sequences used by spontaneous anti-DNA antibodies (31) were analyzed; of which, only three showed F(0.367) in individual spectra such as S57(VH31) (30), MRL-DNA22 (44) germline gene segments members of the VH1(J558) gene family, and VH11 (45) member of the VH7(S107) gene family. The CIS of the T15(V1), S57(VH31), MRL-DNA22, and VH11 V germline gene segment amino acid sequences is presented in **Figure 1A**, revealing a peak at F(0.367). The T15(V1) V germline gene segment from the VH7(S107) gene family is introduced because VH domains of antibodies that express F(0.367), as we have shown previously (36), use this V gene segment in germline configuration (13, 16, 17). The CIS of the four V germline gene segments used by anti-DNA antibodies (31), such as BWDNA16, 2F2, BWDNA7, and VH283, which do not express F(0.367) is presented in **Supplementary Table 1**, revealing that characteristic peak is not at F(0.367).

In this report, the analysis was performed on 60 spontaneous anti-DNA VH domain sequences (31); of which, 20 are encoded by the V gene segments that express F(0.367). However, F(0.367) expression is limited, because only six antibody VH domains retained this characteristic (30%). Thus, we found that F(0.367) is expressed by IgG 74.c2 out of three individually analyzed VH domains of anti-DNA antibodies that use VH11 V gene segment or by IgG 17s-c2 out of nine analyzed anti-DNA antibodies that use S57(VH31) as well as IgG 17s.83, IgG 17s-c3, IgM 111.185, and IgM 165.27 out of eight analyzed VH domains encoded by MRL-DNA22 V gene segment. The CIS of the VH domains of these antibodies is shown in **Figure 1B** revealing a dominant peak at F(0.367). It might be concluded that some anti-DNA antibodies encoded by these V gene segments have lost F(0.367) as the result of somatic mutations.

In **Figure 1C**, CIS of VH domains for 54 anti-DNA VH domains is shown which, in an individual spectrum, does not express F(0.367) and thus do not encode epitope specificity for phosphate groups of dsDNA backbone. It should be emphasized that a peak at F(0.023) with dominant S/N value is detected for the V gene segments (**Figure 1A**), whereas it is a unique peak in the CIS (**Figure 1C**) obtained for anti-DNA VH domains, whose individual sequences do not express F(0.367) a feature relevant for the specificity here analyzed. An analysis of antibodies reactive with ssDNA, Z-DNA, and chromatin further confirms the connection between F(0.367) expression and antibody specificity for the phosphate group of B DNA backbone as shown in **Supplementary Figures 1B–D**.

It is of interest to note that comparison of the V gene segments and VH domain contribution to S/N value for the peak at F(0.367) revealed an insignificant CDR3 region contribution (**Table 1**).

We further made an attempt to determine peptide position in the V gene segment sequences mostly contributing to the F(0.367) expression. The data obtained showed that for T15(V1), VH11(VH7), S57[VH31(VH1)], and MRL-DNA22(VH1) V germline gene segments, these peptides involve residues at positions 35–66, 36–67, 46–65, and 46–77, respectively. The most important finding is that selected peptides include CDR2 regions that are abundant in basic residues (**Table 2**), indicating an CDR2 role in both F(0.367) expression and interaction with an antigenic determinant shared by the PC hapten and dsDNA.

The data obtained from the VH domains analysis of two preimmune natural polyreactive autoantibodies, E7 and D23 (46), which react with antigens such as DNA, myosin, actin, tubulin, spectrin, and trinitrophenol, revealed that F(0.367) was not expressed (**Figure 1D**), meaning that epitope specificity of these antibodies differs from dsDNA-reactive anti-DNA antibodies here analyzed. The CDR2 regions of these autoantibodies are in germline configuration and with a reduced number of basic residues.

DISCUSSION

Previously, using ISM for protein sequence analysis (37), we showed that antibody VH domains of T15 PC binding antibody and U4 dsDNA binding antibody encode information determining sequence specificity represented with characteristic frequency F(0.367), in short F(0.37) (36). We also showed that this frequency is dependent on the type of residues in the CDR2 region and insensitive to a residue substitution in CDR1 (36) of the T15 U4 mutant (13). In this report, we extend these findings by showing that F(0.367) is not only expressed by VH domains of T15 and some spontaneous anti-DNA antibodies from autoimmune mice but is found to be also intrinsic for the V germline gene segments used by these antibodies.

It has been shown that anti-PC binding antibody VH encoded by T15(V1) V gene segment of the VH7(S107) germline gene family (13, 16, 17) form strong interactions between the PC phosphate group and charged residues in the CDR2 region, such as Arg-52 and Lys-54, whereas CDR1 region Glu-35 is involved in choline binding (17, 18). Therefore, F(0.367) expressed by antibodies such as T15, T15 somatic mutant U4, and some anti-DNA antibodies may characterize epitope specificity, that is, specificity for phosphate groups present on different antigens such as PC hapten and dsDNA. Furthermore, the data presented showed that expression of the S/N$_{F(0.367)}$ mostly depends on antibody V gene segments, and thus, a contribution of the CDR3 regions is insignificant (**Table 1**). It should be emphasized that IgG V gene segments of anti-DNA antibodies expressing F(0.367) can be close to germline configuration such as antibodies 74.c2 and 17s.83 encoded by the V gene segment VH11 of the VH7 (S107) gene family and MRL-DNA22 of the gene family VH1 (J558), respectively (31), suggesting that some mutations are tolerable as they do not affect the specificity delineated by the F(0.367). However, they differed in CDR3 regions (31), and their

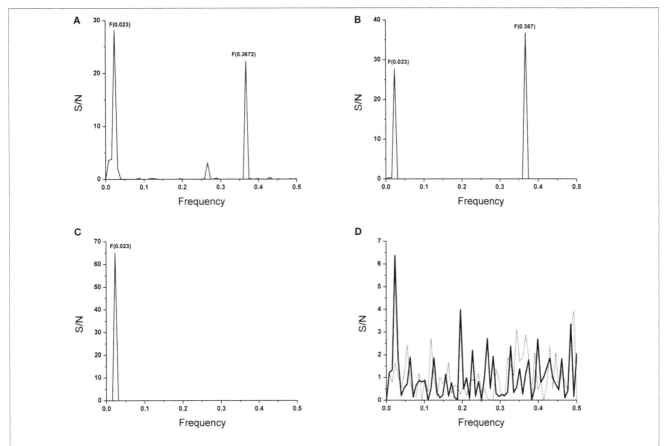

FIGURE 1 | ISM analysis of the V germline genes and antibody VH domain protein sequences. The CIS of the V germline genes segments of VH1, VH11, S57(VH31) and MRL-DNA22 which shows characteristic F(0.367) relevant for the biological activity here followed and activity irrelevant F(0.023) **(A)**. The CIS of the VH domains of antibodies 74.c2 encoded by the V gene segment VH11, a member of the VH7 (S107) gene family, 17s-c2 encoded by the V gene segment S57(VH31) and 17s.83, 17s-c3, 111.185 and 165.27 encoded by V gene segment MRL-DNA22 of the VH1 (J558) gene family **(B)**. CIS of all anti-DNA antibodies which in individual spectrum does not express F(0.367) **(C)**. The IS of the preimmune natural polyreactive autoantibodies which use V gene segments from VH2 (Q52) gene family such as D23 VH domain (___) and superimposed IS of the E7 VH domain (......) **(D)**. The abscissa represents the frequencies from the Fourier transform of the sequence of electron-ion interaction potential (EIIP). The lowest frequency is 0.0 and the highest is 0.5. The ordinate represents the signal to noise ratio (S/N) corresponding to each frequency component in the informational spectrum (IS).

TABLE 1 | Contribution of antibody VH domains and corresponding V gene segments to $S/N_{F(0.367)}$.

Antibodies	Antibody isotype	V germline gene segment used	VH gene family	$S/N_{F(0.367)}$	
				Domains	V gene segments
T15	IgG	T15(V1)	VH7 (S107)*	3.727	3.544
U4	IgG	T15(V1)	VH7 (S107)*	3.950	3.821
74.c2	IgG	VH11	VH7 (S107)*	5.622	5.304
17s-c2	IgG	S57(VH31)	VH1 (J558)*	4.148	4.008
17s.83	IgG	DNA22	VH1 (J558)*	3.789	3.383
17s-c3	IgG	DNA22	VH1 (J558)*	4.434	3.944
111.185	IgM	DNA22	VH1 (J558)*	3.963	3.623
165.27	IgM	DNA22	VH1 (J558)*	3.731	3.259

*Old nomenclature for VH gene families is given in parenthesis.

contribution to F(0.367) expression is insignificant (**Table 1**), whereas IgM 111.185 (MRL-DNA22) anti-DNA antibody (31) retains V gene segment in germline configuration. The data presented may be in accord with the idea that V germline gene segments prone to bind a dsDNA epitope should be less dependent on CDR3 regions (48).

Anti-dsDNA antibodies derived from autoimmune mouse models revealed that they have undergone somatic mutations suggesting their role in achievement of the corresponding conformation. Thus, an important finding obtained from sequence analysis showed the presence of basic amino acids Arg, Lys, and His and, perhaps, the uncharged Asn in CDRs (28–31),

TABLE 2 | Sequence alignment for CDR2 regions of the V gene segments.

V gene segments	Germline configuration	Antibody	CDR2 region amino acid sequence
			(abc)
MRL-DNA22	+		N I Y P G S S S T N Y N E **K** F **K** S
MRL-DNA22		111.185	– – – – – – – – – – – – – – – – –
MRL-DNA22		165.27	– – – – – – – – – – – – – – – – –
MRL-DNA22		17s.83	N – – – – – I I – **H** F N – **K** – **K** N
MRL-DNA22		17s-c3	E – – – **R** – G N I Y Y N – **K** – **K** G
			(abc)
S57(VH31)	+		W I Y S G S G N T **K** Y N E **K** F **K** D
S57(VH31)		17s-c2	– – – P – – – N – **K** – N – **K** – **K** –
VH11	+		L I **R** N **K** A N G Y T T E Y S A S V **K** G
VH11		74-c2	– – **R** N **K** – N D – – – – – – – – – **K** –
			(a b c)
T15(V1)	+		A S **R** N **K** A N D Y T T E Y S A S V **K** G
T15(V1)		T15	– – **R** N **K** – N – – – – – – – – – **K** –
T15(V1)		U4	– – **R** N **K** – N – – – – – – – – – **K** –
VH1210.7	+		Y I S Y S G S T Y Y N P S L **K** S
VH1210.7		E7	– – – – – – – – – – – – – – – –
VH101	+		V I W S G G S T D Y N A A F I S
VH101		D23	– – – – – – – – – – – – – – – – –

The CDR2 region sequences (aa 50-65) for V germline genes and epitope specific anti-DNA antibodies shown in the single letter code were taken from Tillman et al. (31). Origin of these V germline gene sequences are: S57(VH31) (30), MRL-DNA22 (44), VH11 (45). Sequences for T15(V1), as well as E7 and D23 antibodies are taken from Diamond and Scharff (13), Crews et al. (16), Rudikoff et al. (17), and Baccala et al. (46) respectively. Within the compared antibody V gene segments dashes indicate identity with the reference germline gene sequences, while basic residues are shown in bold. Numbering is according to Kabat et al. (47).

whereas Arg in the CDR3 has an important contribution in DNA specificity for DNA-histone complexes (32–34). However, cationic amino acids were not necessary for immune deposit formation (49). Thus, another goal of this study was to examine the role of the CDR2 regions in F(0.367) expression and in particular the content of basic residues in the CDR2 regions of V germline genes used by anti-DNA antibodies. The data obtained showed that peptides within sequences mostly contributing to F(0.367) expression cover residues at position 35–66 for T15(V1), 36–67 for VH11, 46–65 for S57(VH31), and 46–77 for MRL-DNA22. It should be emphasized that these peptide sequences include the CDR2 region enriched in basic residues of T15(V1), VH11, S57(VH31), and MRL-DNA22 germline genes and are also present in CDR2 regions of antibody VH domains (**Table 2**). It can be seen that type and positions of the basic residues for CDR2 of the T15(V1) and VH11 V germline gene segments and anti-DNA antibody V gene segments are the same and S57(VH31) differs slightly. The MRL-DNA22 anti-DNA IgM isotypes are close to germline configuration, whereas IgG differs in the type and position of basic residues (**Table 2**). The CDR2 regions of natural polyreactive autoantibodies are in germline configuration and have one or two basic residues, confirming that both the number and position in CDR2 regions are important for antibody epitope specificity.

The findings presented indicate that antibody specificity for an antigenic determinant (epitope) in the context of different antigens might be identified by the ISM approach (37).

The method applied made a possible correlation between primary antibody structure and specificity delineated by a characteristic frequency.

The main conclusion is that antibody VH domain sequences can encode ability expressed as characteristic frequency, to interact with non-protein structures of various molecules after achievement of the corresponding conformation by somatic mutations.

AUTHOR CONTRIBUTIONS

TS-R and RM developed the study design, analyzed the data and wrote the paper. HK and VJ revised the paper.

FUNDING

This work was supported by a grant from the Ministry of Education, Science and Technological Development of the Republic of Serbia (Grant No. 1 75056).

ACKNOWLEDGMENTS

The authors express their gratitude to Dr V. Veljkovic for useful consultation.

REFERENCES

1. Nguyen TT, Baumgarth N. Natural IgM and the development of B cell-mediated Autoimmune diseases. *Crit Rev Immunol* (2016) 36:163–77.doi: 10.1615/CritRevImmunol.2016018175

2. Holodick NE, Rodríguez-Zhurbenko N, Hernández AM. Defining natural antibodies. *Front Immunol.* (2017) 26:872. doi: 10.3389/fimmu.2017.00872

3. Ohno S, Mori N, Matsunaga T. Antigen-binding specificities of antibodies are primarily determined by seven residues of VH. *Proc Natl Acad Sci USA.* (1985) 82:2945–9.

4. Liang Z, Chang S, Youn MS, Mohan C. Molecular hallmarks of anti-chromatin antibodies associated with the lupus susceptibility locus, Sle1. *Mol Immunol.* (2009) 46:2671–81. doi: 10.1016/j.molimm.2008.12.034

5. Xu J, Davis M: Diversity in the CDR3 region of VH is sufficient for most antibody specificities. *Immunity* (2000) 13:37–45. doi: 10.1002/jmr.2592

6. Willis JR, Briney BS, DeLuca SL, Crowe JE Jr., Meiler J. Human germline antibody gene segments encode polyspecific antibodies. *PLoS Comput Biol.* (2013) 9:e1003045. doi: 10.1371/journal.pcbi.1003045

7. Chothia C, Lesk A. Canonical structures for the hypervariable regions o immunoglobulins. *J Mol Biol.* (1987) 196:901–17.

8. Al-Lazikani B, Lesk AM, Chothia C. Standard conformations for the canonical structures of immunoglobulins. *J Mol Biol.* (1997) 273:927–48. doi: 10.1006/jmbi.1997.1354

9. Chothia C, Lesk AM, Gherardi E, Tomlinson IM, Walter G, Marks JD, et al. Structural repertoire of the human VH segments. *J Mol Biol.* (1992) 227:799–817.

10. Köhler H. The response to phosphorylcholine. Dissecting an immune response. *Trans Rev.* (1975) 27:24–56.

11. Lieberman RM, Potter EB, Mushinski W, Humphrey Jr, Rudikoff S. Genetics of a new IgVH(T15 idiotype) marker in the mouse regulating natural antibody to phosphorylcholine. *J Exp Med* (1974) 139:983–1001.

12. Claflin JL, Lieberman R, Davie JM. Clonal nature of the immune response to phosphorylcholine. I. Specificity, class, and idiotype of phosphorylcholine-binding receptors on lymphoid cells. *J Exp Med.* (1974) 139:58–73.

13. Diamond B, Scharff MD. Somatic mutation of the T15 heavy chain gives rise to an antibody with autoantibody specificity. *Proc Natl Acad Sci USA.* (1984) 81:5841–4.

14. Sigal NH, Pickard AR, Metcalf ES, Gearhart PJ, Klinman NR. Expression of phosphorylcholine-specific B cells during murine development. *J Exp Med.* (1977) 146:933–48.

15. Fung J, Kohler H. Late clonal selection and expansion of the TEPC-15 germ-line specificity. *J Exp Med.* (1980) 152:1262–73.

16. Crews S, Griffin J, Huang H, Calame K, Hood L. A single VH gene segment encodes the immune response to phosphorylcholine: somatic mutation is correlated with the class of the antibody. *Cell* (1981) 25:59–66.

17. Rudikoff S, Potter M. Size differences among immunoglobulin heavy chains from phosphorylcholine-binding proteins. *Proa Natl Acad Sci USA.* (1976) 73:2109–12.

18. Segal DM, Padlan EA, Cohen GH, Rudikoff S, Potter M, Davies DR. The three dimensional structure of a phosphorylcholine-binding mouse immunoglobulin Fab and the nature of the antigen binding site. *Proc Natl Acad Sci USA.* (1974) 71:4298–302.

19. Padlan EA, Davies DR, Rudikoff S, Potter M. Structural basis for the specificity of phosphorylcholine-binding immunoglobulins. *Immunochemistry* (1976) 13:945–9.

20. Chen C, Roberts VA, Rittenberg MB. Generation and analysis of random point mutations in an antibody CDR2 sequence: many mutated antibodies lose their ability to bind antigen. *J Exp Med.* (1992) 176:855–66.

21. Andres CM, Maddalena A, Hudak S, Young NM, Claflin JL. Anti-phosphocholine hybridoma antibodies. II. Functional analysis of binding sites within three antibody families. *J Exp Med.* (1981) 154:1584–98.

22. Chang S, Yang L, Moon YM, Cho YG, Min SY, Kim TJ, et al. Anti-nuclear antibody reactivity in lupus may be partly hard-wired into the primary b-cell repertoire. *Mol Immunol.* (2009) 46:3420–6. doi: 10.1016/j.molimm.2009.07.014

23. Kohler H, Bayry J, Kaveri SV. The homophilic domain – an immunological archetype. *Front Immunol.* (2016) 7:106–11. doi: 10.3389/fimmu.2016.00106

24. Metlas R, Srdic-Rajic T, Kohler H. Cooperation of intrathymic T15 idiotype-bearing B and complementary T cells in ontogeny of natural Treg cells involved in establishment of T15 clonal dominance. *Immunol Lett.* (2018) 200:52–4. doi: 10.1016/j.imlet.2018.07.002

25. Isenberg DA, Ehrenstein MR, Longhurst C, Kalsi JK. The origin, sequence, structure, and consequences of developing anti-DNA antibodies. A human perspective. *Arthritis Rheum.* (1994) 37:169–80.

26. Jang YJ, Stollar BD. Anti-DNA antibodies: aspects of structure and pathogenicity. *Cell Mol Life Sci.* (2003) 60:309–20.

27. Lafer EM, Rauch J, Andrzejewski JR, Mudd D, Furie B, Furie B, et al. Polyspecific monoclonal lupus autoantibodies reactive with both polynucleotides and phospholipids. *J Exp Med.* (1981) 153:897–909.

28. Radic MZ, Weigert M. Genetic and structural evidence for antigen selection of anti-DNA antibodies. *Annu Rev Immunol.* (1994) 12:487–520.

29. Eilat D, Webster DM, Rees AR: V region sequences of antiDNA and anti-RNA autoantibodies from NZB/NZW F1 mice. *J Immunol.* (1988) 141:1745–53.

30. Shlomchik M, Mascelli M, Shan H, Radic MZ, Pisetsky D, Marshak-Rothstein A, et al. Anti- DNA antibodies from autoimmune mice arise by clonal expansion and somatic mutation. *J Exp Med.* (1990) 171:265–92.

31. Tillman DM, Jou NT, Hill RJ, Marion TN. Both IgM and IgG anti-DNA antibodies are the products of clonally selective B cell stimulation in (NZB x NZW)F1 mice. *J Exp Med.* (1992) 176: 761–779.

32. Detanico T, Guo W, Wysocki LJ. Predominant role for activation-induced cytidine deaminase in generating IgG anti-nucleosomal antibodies of murine SLE. *J Autoimmun.* (2015) 58:67–77. doi: 10.1016/j.jaut.2015.01.006

33. Guth AM, Zhang X, Smith D, Detanico T, Wysocki LJ. Chromatin specificity of anti-doublestranded DNA antibodies and a role for Arg residues in the third complementarity-determining region of the heavy chain. *J Immunol.* (2003) 171:6260–6. doi: 10.4049/jimmunol.171.11.6260

34. Li Z, Schettino EW, Padlan EA, Ikematsu H, Casali P. Structure function analysis of a lupus anti-DNA autoantibody: central role of the heavy chain complementarity-determining region 3 Arg in binding of double- and single-stranded DNA. *Eur J Immunol.* (2000) 30:2015–26.doi: 10.1002/1521-4141(200007)30:7<2015::AID-IMMU2015>3.0.CO;2-5

35. Rekvig OP. The anti-DNA antibody: origin and impact, dogmas and controversies. *Nat Rev Rheumatol.* (2015) 11:530–40. doi: 10.1038/nrrheum.2015.69

36. Srdic-Rajic T, Kekovic G, Davidovic DM, Metlas R. Phosphocholine-binding antibody activities are hierarchically encoded in the sequence of the heavy-chain variable region: dominance of self-association activity in the T15 idiotype. *Int Immunol* (2013) 25:345–52. doi: 10.1093/intimm/dxs156

37. Veljkovic V, Cosić I, Dimitrijević B, Lalović D. Is it possible to analyze DNA and protein sequences by the method of digital signal processing? *IEEE Trans BME* (1985) 32:337-41.

38. Cosic I. Macromolecular bioactivity: is it Resonant Interaction between Molecules? – Theory and Applications. *IEEE Trans BME* (1994) 41:1101–14.

39. Veljkovic V, Slavic I. Simple general-model pseudopotential. *Phys Rev Let.* (1972) 29:105–6.

40. Veljkovic V. *Theoretical Approach to Preselection of Cancerogens and Chemical Carcinogenesis.* New York, NY: Gordon and Breach (1980).

41. Veljkovic V, Cosic I. A Novel Method of Protein Analysis for Prediction of Biological Function: Application to Tumor Toxins. *Cancer Biochem. Biophys* (1987) 9:139–48.

42. Veljkovic V, Metlas R. Identification of nanopeptide from HTLV3., LAV and ARV-2 envelope gp120 determining binding to T4 cell surface protein. *Cancer Biochem Biophys.* (1988) 10:91–106.

43. Veljkovic N, Glisic S, Prljic J, Perovic V, Botta M, Veljkovic V. Discovery of new therapeutic targets by the informational spectrum method. *Curr Protein Pep Sci.* (2008) 9:493–506. doi: 10.2174/138920308785915245

44. Kofler, R, Strohal R, Balderas RS, Johnson ME, Noonan DJ, Duchosal MA, et al. Immunoglobulin k light chain variable region complex organization and immunoglobulin genesencoding anti-DNA autoantibodies in lupus mice. *J Clin Invest.* (1988) 82:852–60.

45. Clarke SH, Claflin JL, Rudikoff S. Polymorphisms in immunoglobulin heavy chains suggesting gene conversion. *Proc Natl Acad Sci USA.* (1982) 79:3280–4.

46. Baccala R, Quang TV, Gilbert M, Ternynck T, Avrameas S. Two murine natural polyreactive autoantibodies are encoded by nonmutated germ-line genes. *Proc Natl Acad Sci USA.* (1989) 86: 4624–8

47. Kabat EA, Wu TT, Reid-Miller M, Perry HM, Gottesman KS. *Sequences of Proteins of Immunological Interest.* Bethesda, MD: U.S. Government Printing Office (1987).

48. Maranhão AQ, Costa MBW, Guedes L, Moraes-Vieira PM, Raiol T, Brigido MM. A mouse variable gene fragment binds to DNA independently of the BCR context: a possible role for immature B-cell repertoire establishment. *PLoS ONE* (2013) 8:e72625. doi: 10.1371/journal.pone.00 72625

49. Katz MS, Foster MH, Madaio MP. Independently derived murine glomerular immune deposit-forming anti-DNA antibodies are encoded by near-identical VH gene sequences. *J Clin Invest.* (1993) 91:402–8.

9

Multiple Variables at the Leukocyte Cell Surface Impact Fc γ Receptor-Dependent Mechanisms

Kashyap R. Patel, Jacob T. Roberts and Adam W. Barb *

Roy J. Carver Department of Biochemistry, Biophysics, and Molecular Biology, Iowa State University, Ames, IA, United States

*Correspondence:
Adam W. Barb
abarb@iastate.edu

Fc γ receptors (FcγR) expressed on the surface of human leukocytes bind clusters of immunoglobulin G (IgG) to induce a variety of responses. Many therapeutic antibodies and vaccine-elicited antibodies prevent or treat infectious diseases, cancers and autoimmune disorders by binding FcγRs, thus there is a need to fully define the variables that impact antibody-induced mechanisms to properly evaluate candidate therapies and design new intervention strategies. A multitude of factors influence the IgG-FcγR interaction; one well-described factor is the differential affinity of the six distinct FcγRs for the four human IgG subclasses. However, there are several other recently described factors that may prove more relevant for disease treatment. This review covers recent reports of several aspects found at the leukocyte membrane or outside the cell that contribute to the cell-based response to antibody-coated targets. One major focus is recent reports covering post-translational modification of the FcγRs, including asparagine-linked glycosylation. This review also covers the organization of FcγRs at the cell surface, and properties of the immune complex. Recent technical advances provide high-resolution measurements of these often-overlooked variables in leukocyte function and immune system activation.

Keywords: antibody, IgG, N-glycosylation, post-translation modification, ADCC—antibody dependent cellular cytotoxicity, immune complex, ADCP—antibody dependent cellular phagocytosis

INTRODUCTION: THE IMPORTANCE OF MODULATING THE Fc-FcγR INTERACTION

Immunoglobulin G (IgG) is the most thoroughly studied and well characterized molecule of the humoral immune response. IgG activates the immune system through cell-bound Fc γ Receptors (FcγRs; **Figure 1**). The IgG fragment antigen-binding (Fab) domains confer specificity and affinity toward an antigen while the distinct hinge and fragment crystallizable (Fc) domain of the four IgG subclasses (IgG1-4) provide the structural basis for specificity and affinity to bind FcγRs (1). The six structurally distinct members of the classical human FcγRs (FcγRI or CD64, FcγRIIa/CD32a, FcγRIIb/CD32b, FcγRIIc/CD32c, FcγRIIIa/CD16a, and FcγRIIIb/CD16b) are expressed on leukocytes of both the myeloid and lymphoid lineage (**Figure 2**). This group of proteins can be divided into two types: activating receptors (CD64, CD32a, CD32c, CD16a, and CD16b) that lead to cell activation through immunoreceptor tyrosine-based activation motifs (ITAM) on cytosolic tails or on co-receptor molecules, and an inhibitory receptor (CD32b) that signals through immunoreceptor tyrosine-based inhibitory motifs (ITIM) (2–4). Only CD32s contain ITAM or ITIM domains, and the other receptors must associate with an ITAM-containing

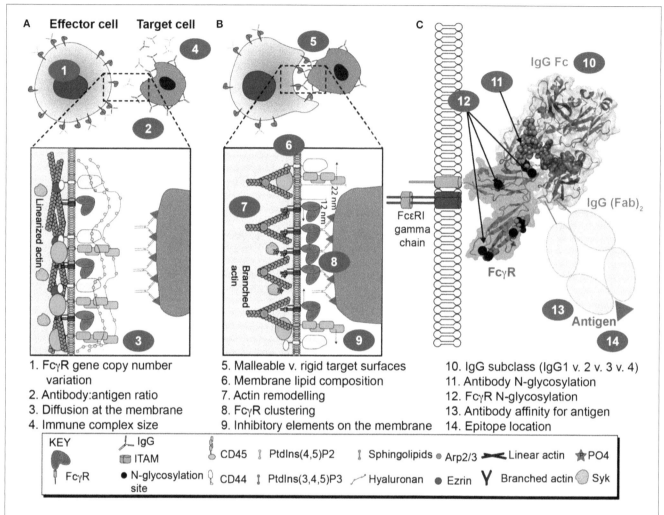

FIGURE 1 | Multiple variables affect FcγR-mediated immune function. **(A)** cellular variables influencing FcγR activity that are present before the effector cell engages a target cell. **(B)** cellular variables influencing FcγR-mediated activity while the effector cell is engaged with a target cell. **(C)** molecular variables associated with the FcγRs, antibody, and antigen.

adaptor protein (FcεRI γ chain or CD3 ζ chain) (3, 5) (**Figure 2**). In either situation, the ratio of activating to inhibiting signals determines the outcome of an immune response (6).

Receptor clustering is essential for FcγR signaling. Circulating IgG coats an antigen to form an oligomeric complex, positioning the Fc portions of the IgG molecules away from the target surface and exposed to interact with FcγRs. The antibody-coated target is also referred to as an immune complex. The multiple IgG molecules of the immune complex provide an opportunity for multivalent interactions with FcγR-expressing leukocytes and must compete with non-complexed serum antibodies occupying the FcγRs that will, in turn, cluster FcγRs on the cell surface (7, 8). Depending on the receptors engaged, the clustering of the extracellular domains triggers phosphorylation of tyrosine in the ITAMs or ITIMs, which subsequently recruits signaling molecules that promote a cellular response (9). The types of FcγR-mediated effector cell responses are diverse and include, but are not limited to, antibody-dependent cellular cytotoxicity

(ADCC), antibody-dependent cellular phagocytosis (ADCP), release of cytokines and antigen uptake for presentation (10–14). FcγRs are critical for maintaining immune system homeostasis as well as preventing pathogenic infections and they play a major role in inflammatory diseases and autoimmune disorders (9, 13, 15–17). The combination of distinct antagonistic and synergistic factors contribute to a considerable functional diversity within this group of antibody receptors. Here we will discuss multiple factors which influence the antibody:FcγR interaction and modify the immune response (**Figure 1**).

RECEPTOR PRESENTATION AT THE CELL SURFACE

FcγRs are predominately expressed on cells originating from hematopoietic progenitor stem cells including dendritic cells, neutrophils, basophils, eosinophils, macrophages, monocytes,

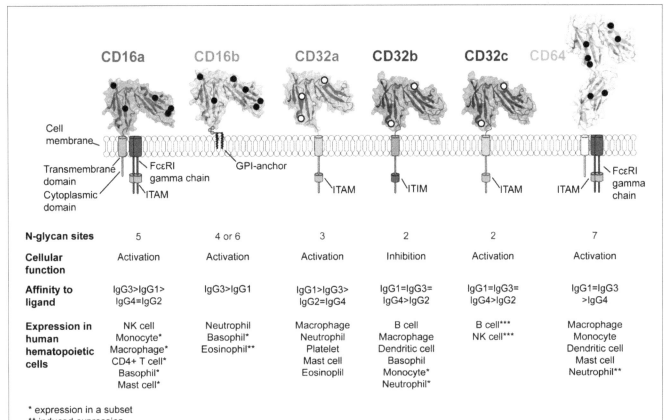

	CD16a	CD16b	CD32a	CD32b	CD32c	CD64
N-glycan sites	5	4 or 6	3	2	2	7
Cellular function	Activation	Activation	Activation	Inhibition	Activation	Activation
Affinity to ligand	IgG3>IgG1>IgG4=IgG2	IgG3>IgG1	IgG1>IgG3>IgG2=IgG4	IgG1=IgG3=IgG4>IgG2	IgG1=IgG3=IgG4>IgG2	IgG1=IgG3>IgG4
Expression in human hematopoietic cells	NK cell Monocyte* Macrophage* CD4+ T cell* Basophil* Mast cell*	Neutrophil Basophil* Eosinophil**	Macrophage Neutrophil Platelet Mast cell Eosinoplil	B cell Macrophage Dendritic cell Basophil Monocyte* Neutrophil*	B cell*** NK cell***	Macrophage Monocyte Dendritic cell Mast cell Neutrophil**

* expression in a subset
** induced expression
*** expressed in a subset of cells

FIGURE 2 | Structures and properties of the human Fc γ receptors. Five receptors are expressed in the majority of the population with CD32c expressed only in a small subset. The ribbon diagrams show the structures of the extracellular antibody-binding domains as determined by x-ray crystallography; overlayed black or white circles indicate the sites of N-glycosylation.

mast cells, NK cells, B cells, a subset of T cells, and platelets as well as non-hematopoietic cell types such as syncytiotrophoblasts at various levels (18–20). FcγR expression varies depending on cell lineage; not surprisingly gene copy number is also implicated in disease. These factors can greatly influence the dynamic ability of the immune system to respond to the diverse repertoire of foreign invaders. Thus, variable surface expression by different immune cell types influences how the immune system responds to a foreign invader. This section will cover the cellular expression of FcγRs and immune modulation of expression through downregulation and induction.

Five activating FcγRs are expressed in humans (**Figure 2**). The highest affinity, CD64, is expressed on monocytes, dendritic cells and macrophages (11), mast cells (21), and neutrophils following IFN-γ exposure (22, 23). The low affinity CD32a is expressed on mast cells, neutrophils, macrophages, eosinophils, and platelets (24). CD32c is expressed by 7–15% of individuals on NK cells and B cells and results from a gene mutation (4). The high/moderate affinity CD16a is expressed predominantly on NK cells, a subset of monocytes, mast cells, basophils, macrophages and is inducible in CD4+ T-cells (25, 26). The low/moderate affinity CD16b is found only in humans and expressed predominantly on

neutrophils (27), a subset of basophils (28) and has inducible expression on eosinophils (29, 30). CD32b is the sole inhibitory receptor and is expressed on basophils, B cells, macrophages, dendritic cells, a subset of monocytes and neutrophils (24). Interestingly, CD32b is also expressed in non-hematopoietic cells, including the endothelium of various organs (31).

Variability in Receptor Amount

Gene duplications in individuals lead to copy number variation (CNV) of some FcγRs in the population. Surprisingly, only CD16a, CD16b, and CD32c of the FcγRs exhibited CNV in a sample population of 600 subjects (32). CNVs have been correlated to autoimmune disorders as well as variations in surface expression levels. CNV of CD16b is correlated to surface expression on neutrophils and implicated in SLE susceptibility (33, 34), as well as other autoimmune disorders (35, 36). Furthermore, CD16a CNV appears to be functionally significant since increased surface expression positively correlated with increasing CD16a gene number (ranging from one to three copies) (32, 35). A CD16a indel has been shown to increase surface expression as well (37).

FcγR amount at the cell surface varies by cell type and receptor identity (**Figure 2**). On neutrophils, there are an estimated 100,000–300,000 surface exposed CD16b molecules and 10,000–40,000 CD32a molecules (38, 39). The predominant monocyte subtype at roughly 80% of the pool, "classical" monocytes, does not express CD16a. "Non-classical" monocytes express CD16a at a level of roughly 10,000 CD16a molecules per cell but upon differentiation into macrophages express 40,000 CD16a molecules per cell while CD32 remained the same at ~10,000 molecules per cell (40). Another study found macrophages express 5–10 fold higher CD64, CD32a, and CD32b while CD16a expression was comparable to non-classical monocytes. M2c macrophages expressed overall higher levels of FcγRs than M1 macrophages with the following order of expression: CD32a, CD32b > CD64 > CD16a (41). A high number of CD16a molecules are expressed on CD16+ NK cells (100,000-250,000) (42).

Expression levels also vary based on the cell status. Following activation, innate immune cells can induce expression of FcγRs (23, 25, 29, 30, 35). There is also evidence of receptor downregulation upon activation. Downregulation mechanisms include both decreases in expression as well as shedding FcγR from the cell surface following metalloproteinase cleavage. CD32a is shed from Langerhans cells and also expressed as a soluble form (43). CD32b is shed upon activation of B-cells (44). CD16a and CD16b are likewise shed upon activation of NK cells and neutrophils at a known cleavage site by the metalloprotease ADAM17 (45–48). Intriguingly, sCD16b is relatively abundant in serum (~5 nM) (49) and levels vary based on the immune state of the individual (50). Surprisingly, CD64 is the only human FcγR in which a soluble, serum-borne form has not been reported. This may be explained by the presence of a third extracellular CD64 domain in place of the cleavage site found in CD32s and CD16s (**Figure 2**).

Soluble FcγR forms modulate immune responses. Soluble CD16b binds myeloid cells, NK cells, subsets of T cells, B cells, and monocytes through complement receptor 3 (CR3 or Mac-1 or αM β2, comprised of CD11b/CD18) and complement receptor 4 (CR4 or αx β2, comprised of CD11c/CD18). These interactions cause the release of IL6 and IL8 by monocytes and indicate a potential role for soluble CD16b in inflammation (51). Shedding of CD16a from NK cells allows disengagement of the immune synapse from the target cell and the subsequent ability to kill again. One study demonstrated that repeated engagement by CD16a depleted perforin, however, shedding of CD16a allowed perforin replenishment upon subsequent activation by another activating receptor, Natural killer group 2 member D (NKG2D), which recognizes ligands not normally expressed on healthy tissue (52). Thus, it appears that the act of shedding of CD16 can allow disengagement of the foreign particle which would be crucial for the immune cell's survival and preservation of potential future cytolytic activity. Though shed receptors are proinflammatory and recruit immune cells as discussed above, a complete picture of the mechanisms of regulating surface expression upon immune activation is not currently available.

Receptor Clustering at the Membrane Is Required for Effector Function

The correct presentation of FcγRs on the cell membrane is essential for proper immune cell function. ADCC can destroy virally infected cells and cancer cells, and is thus a target for monoclonal antibody (mAb) therapies (53). ADCP is also an important mechanism in mAb therapy targeting malignant cells (14). ADCC and ADCP are dependent on the ability of low to moderate affinity FcγRs to cluster on fluid plasma membranes for activation to occur (54) (**Figure 1**). Equally important is the regulation of these receptors when no activation signal is present.

Proper activation of FcγRs following Fc engagement by macrophages requires clustering of FcγRs and the displacement of inhibitory receptors. In one study utilizing murine RAW 264.7 cells, segregation of CD45, a phosphatase responsible for dephosphorylating ITAMs, is dependent on antigen distance from the target membrane (55) (**Figure 1**). It appears that if the antibody is >10 nm from the target surface, there is a substantially impaired ADCP response. This phenomenon is due to the location of the epitope; epitopes closer to the surface exclude the inhibitory CD45 molecule (which stands ~22 nm tall vs. FcγR-IgG complex = 11.5 nm) from the immune synapse. Interestingly, a follow-up study that focused on FDA-approved mAbs found the targets were small surface proteins (<10 nm in height) suggesting there may be a requirement for mAb epitopes to be located close to the surface for therapeutic efficacy. CD45 was also excluded from the immune synapse in activated human T cells (56). Another study concerning inhibitory module segregation on human macrophages demonstrates CD64, but not CD32a, and inhibitory signal regulating protein α (SIRPα), in conjunction with CD47 (a receptor that inhibits macrophage phagocytosis), are clustered on quiescent cells but upon activation segregate in a process regulated by spleen tyrosine kinase (SYK)-dependent actin cytoskeleton reorganization (57). Recently, FcγR diffusion has been shown to be inhibited by the CD44 transmembrane protein which is immobilized by linearized actin filaments via ezrin/radixen/moesin (ERM) and binds hyaluronan in the glycocalyx (58). This study used primary human macrophages as well as murine cell lines and murine models, utilizing single particle tracking found CD44 and hyaluronan decreased the diffusion rate of FcγRs, while also sterically blocking the binding of FcγRs to immune complexes (**Figure 1**).

Receptor clustering overwhelms constitutive inhibition as described previously, allowing phosphorylation of the ITAM. ITAMs are phosphorylated via SYK, Src family kinase (SFKs) or ζ-chain-associated protein kinase 70 (ZAP-70) for downstream activation of phosphoinositide-3-kinase (PI3K), NF-κB, extracellular signal regulated kinase (ERK), phosphatidyl inositol 4-phosphate 5-kinase γ (PIP5Kγ), GTPases and other SRC-family kinases (53, 54, 59, 60). Along with FcγR clustering, actin polymerization and depolymerization is equally important for phagocytosis in RAW 264.7 macrophages by creating lammellipodium/pseudopods. These protrusions are controlled by Rac GTPase and lipid composition (54, 59) (**Figure 1**). Clustering has also been observed on the plasma membrane of murine derived macrophages using total internal reflection microscopy (TIRF) of a lipid bilayer supporting IgG (61). The FcγR microcluster appears on the macrophage pseudopod edge and is subsequently transported to a synapse-like structure thereby recruiting SYK and production of PtdIns(3–5)P3 coordinated with lamellar actin polymerization. Another study on quiescent human macrophages found lateral diffusion of FcγRs is regulated by tonic activity of SYK causing actin cytoskeleton organization to increase the likelihood of FcγRs to be pre-clustered upon finding a pathogen (62).This study further described differential FcγR mobility upon activation. FcγRs at the periphery of the actin-rich pseudopod were more mobile than those already immobilized by binding of IgG-rich regions. The authors explained that this mobility difference is controlled by SYK-mediated regulation of the actin-cytoskeleton which would increase the likelihood of FcγRs to engage more IgG molecules at the leading edge of the lamellipodium/pseudopod and not waste time diffusing into already IgG-dependent, FcγR-immobilized, actin-rich rich regions of plasma membrane. Mobility of FcγRs was described earlier to be decreased at the trailing end of polarized macrophages by CD44 that was bound to linear actin and connected to hyaluronan (58). It was also found in this study that on the leading edge of polarized macrophages, the side that encounters opsonized material, Arp2/3-driven actin branching predominates, initiated by phosphotidlyinosotide (3–5)-trisphosphate production, and increased FcγR mobility allowing for more efficient clustering at the immune synapse. When Arp2/3-driven actin branching predominates, it was found CD44 is more mobile allowing greater FcγR mobility (**Figure 1**).

In the human NK92 cell line, transduced to express CD16a, a study showed β2 integrins mediate the dynamics of FcγR receptor microclusters in a protein-tyrosine kinase 2 (Pyk2)-dependent manner, controlling the rate of target cell destruction by ADCC (63). β2 integrins bind ICAM-1 on the target cell allowing adhesion and signal transduction through Pyk2 for actin remodeling and the subsequent enhancement of FcγR mobility. Furthermore, sites of granule release are surrounded by clusters of CD16a and release points are devoid of actin. Human NK cell lytic granules also converge at the surface in a dynein and integrin-signal dependent manner which aids spatial targeting of the weaponized molecules to limit off-target damage (64). Surprisingly, CD16a is essential for ADCC of human CD16+ monocytes and upon CD16a engagement, β2 integrins are activated along with TNFα secretion thereby indicating that non-classical monocytes (CD16+) are the sole monocyte class capable of ADCC (65).

During the early stages of phagocytosis by RAW 264.7 cells, direct contact between FcγRs and IgG is increased by greater IgG density on particles, and increased IgG density results in an increased level of early signals. However, late stage signals are "all or nothing," not concentration dependent, and regulated by PI3K concentration in the phagocytic membranes (66). In this study, low IgG density decreased the amount of opsonized particles but not the rate of phagosome formation and low IgG density particles that did result in phagocytosis recruited the same amounts of late stage signaling molecules (PIP3, Protein

kinase C ε type, p85 subunit) and actin. Overall it appears that FcγRs control the initial binding process essential for scanning the foreign particle and initial activation by binding IgG and later stages of commitment to destruction of the particle are controlled by both IgG density and membrane lipid composition.

On murine and human macrophages, receptor clustering upon activation is consistent with a change in the heterogeneity of the membrane lipid composition to a highly ordered phagosomal membrane that is heavily enriched in sphingolipids and ceramide but lacking cholesterol (67) (**Figure 1**). The authors state that lipid remodeling mediates F-actin remodeling and the biophysical characteristics of the phagosomal membrane are essential for phagocytosis. On human B cells, a polymorphism of the inhibitory receptor CD32b (Ile232Thr) located in the middle of the transmembrane domain, is described to decrease inhibitory function (68). This mutation was shown to result in aberrant localization to a sphingolipid and cholesterol rich region in contrast to the Ile232 wild-type. Aberrant localization is not surprising considering the introduction of a polar residue into the transmembrane domain (69). Furthermore, the ability of CD32b to inhibit B cell receptor (BCR)-mediated PIP3 production, AKT, phospholipase C-γ-2 (PLCγ2) activation and calcium mobilization was impaired in cells expressing the CD32b Thr232 allotype as compared to Ile232. The authors indicate the FcγR locus was associated with SLE and this polymorphism may promote disease. Thus, it appears lipid composition is important for FcγR-mediated mechanisms.

The unique construction of CD16b indicates the potential for a different activation mechanism for neutrophils. Neutrophils predominantly express CD16b with 10-fold less CD32a. CD32a signal transduction is well described and thought to be the canonical FcγR signal transduction via phosphorylation of ITAMs and subsequent SYK recruitment (70). However, CD16b contains a GPI anchor and does not have a polypeptide transmembrane domain nor is it known to associate with a signaling coreceptor, therefore, it is unclear how CD16b promotes signaling in neutrophils (**Figure 2**). CD16b plays a role in the initial binding of immune complexes in concert with β2 integrins (71). Currently there are conflicting studies suggesting that CD16b can transduce a signal on its own (70, 72, 73), or it transduces a signal by acting with CD32a (74). A recent study found CD16b cross-linking increased IL-10 and TNFα expression, phosphorylated SHP-2 in a lipid-raft mediated manner and inhibited apoptosis in neutrophils. Lipid composition certainly may be an important part of CD16b signal transduction in mechanisms similar to those discussed previously for macrophage phagocytosis and CD32b on B-cells, however the role of lipids in neutrophil activation is not understood (75–81). Interestingly proteinase 3 (PR3), CD16b, cytochrome b558, and NADPH oxidase co-immunoprecipitate on lipid rafts and PR3 and CD16b colocalize in confocal imaging suggesting these may interact in a lipid raft (75). Other findings suggest CD16b signals in conjunction with CR3 via lectin-like interactions (82), leading to neutrophil respiratory bursts (72). The function of GPI-linked CD16b remains undefined despite the high abundance of CD16b in the body and critical roles in mAb therapies (83).

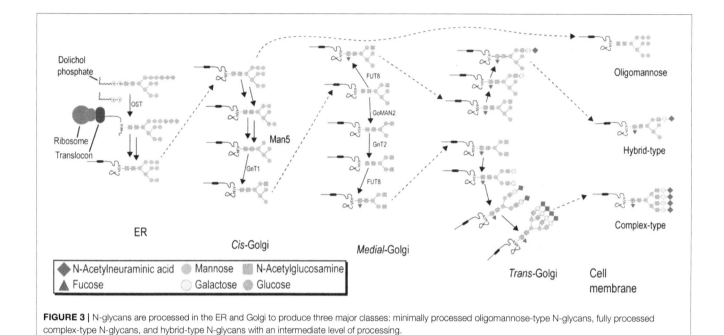

FIGURE 3 | N-glycans are processed in the ER and Golgi to produce three major classes: minimally processed oligomannose-type N-glycans, fully processed complex-type N-glycans, and hybrid-type N-glycans with an intermediate level of processing.

The Type of FcγR Membrane Anchor Impacts Activation

There are clear differences between the signaling and antibody-binding affinity of soluble and membrane-anchored FcγR forms. However, less is known about the effects of the specific FcγR membrane anchors on affinity and cell activation. All FcγRs are localized to the membrane by a transmembrane polypeptide moiety or a glycosylphosphatidylinositol (GPI) moiety (CD16b only) (**Figure 2**). A micropipette adhesion assay demonstrated CD16a attached to microspheres via a GPI anchor bound roughly 5-fold tighter to IgG1-coated red blood cells (RBCs) than CD16a tethered by a transmembrane domain (84, 85). Interestingly, it also appears IgG1-coated spheres treated with phosphoinositide phospholipase C (PIPLC) to remove the diacylglycerol moiety bound to GPI-linked CD16a with 12-fold less affinity. These authors observed a 60-fold decrease when the GPI-anchor was completely removed. A CD16b-GPI construct showed 2-fold decrease of affinity upon PIPLC treatment and an 11-fold decrease following removal of the GPI-anchor. The authors hypothesized that enhancement of binding affinity associated with the GPI anchor may be due to an allosteric effect on CD16, changing the structure to bind IgG more effectively; such an allosteric mechanism was observed with other GPI-anchored proteins (80). Further studies will be required to fully elucidate how the GPI-anchor affects CD16b and how specific aspects of the membrane anchor confers distinct properties *in vivo*.

POST-TRANSLATIONAL MODIFICATION OF THE ANTIBODY AND RECEPTOR

Asparagine-linked (N-) glycosylation is one of the most common protein modifications performed by the eukaryotic cell and is a substantial modification of all FcγRs [**Figure 2**;

for a thorough review of N-glycan processing, see (86)].It is important to note, however, the resulting glycans processed in the ER and Golgi can be grouped into three distinct forms: (1) minimally-processed oligomannose type N-glycans, (2) intermediate processed hybrid-type N-glycans with processing on one of the two core mannose branches, and (3) highly-processed complex-type N-glycans with extensively modified branches (**Figure 3**).

Several variables introduce a significant degree of heterogeneity into the N-glycan present at any single site on a glycoprotein, ranging from substrate availability, protein anchor type, to accessibility of N-glycan site, potentially creating a vast diversity of protein forms and functions (87–90). This heterogeneity also renders glycoproteins challenging targets for *in vitro* studies to characterize structure. Minimally-processed hybrid and oligomannose type N-glycans are not expected at the cell surface because these forms harbor terminal mannose residues that may bind to the mannose receptor and elicit an immune response (91, 92). Though many previous glycomics studies report high levels of oligomannose N-glycans recovered from primary cells, the abundance of these under-processed forms is likely due to cell lysis and recovery of unprocessed glycans from the ER. If under-processed forms are present on the cell surface, these must be protected from binding to the mannose receptor. Therefore, highly processed complex-type N-glycans are expected as the predominant species at the cell surface.

The functional impact of N-glycosylation at the conserved asparagine 297 residues in IgG1 is well established. IgG1 glycosylation at Asn-297 is essential for the IgG-FcγR interaction (93). The N-glycosylation profile of serum IgG changes due to multiple factors, including age, gender, infection, pregnancy, and disease (94–97). The variation in IgG1 Fc glycoforms is known to change antibody affinity toward the

FcγRs (98), and this fact has also been leveraged to develop glycoengineered mAbs and anti-inflammatory glycoforms of intravenous immunoglobulin (IVIG) (99, 100). The wealth of knowledge regarding IgG glycoforms is due in large part to protein abundance and ease of obtaining samples. However, little is known about the glycosylation of FcγRs on immune cells.

FcγRs are heavily glycosylated molecules, containing two to seven N-glycans (**Figure 2**). The extent of FcγR modification was evident as early as 1988 as certain FcγRs from native tissue migrated much slower in SDS-PAGE gels than expected based on the polypeptide mass alone. Furthermore, the migration rate increased after treatment to specifically remove N-glycans (101, 102). There is a prominent gap in knowledge about the impact of FcγR N-glycosylation on immune function largely due to limited studies of the native FcγRs purified from primary leukocytes. However, it is known that CD16a expressed by NK cells had a distinct N-glycosylation profile when compared CD16a expressed by cultured monocytes, though this determination was made using lectin binding (103) and surface CD16a on the NK cell and monocyte displayed differential antibody-binding affinity that was attributed to differences in cell-specific CD16a N-glycosylation (104).

Even though native glycoforms of all FcγRs are not known, the effect of N-glycosylation on binding affinity has been well characterized *in vitro* using protein expressed with mammalian cells. Aglycosylated, recombinant, soluble (s)FcγRs bind IgG1 Fc at different affinities than glycosylated forms, thus the IgG-FcγR interaction is sensitive to receptor N-glycosylation (105–107). Recent studies reported substantial differences in affinity for sFcγRs expressed in recombinant systems (106, 108–110), N-glycosylation profiles of NK cell CD16a and soluble CD16b from serum revealed surprising heterogeneity and substantial differences from recombinantly-expressed protein (109, 111).

Specific CD16a Glycoforms Bind Antibody With High Affinity Comparable to CD64

The analysis of N-glycan composition from FcγRs provides a characteristic profile of a protein (112). Glycomics analysis of CD16a on circulating NK cells from three healthy donors revealed a surprising abundance of under-processed forms (~45% hybrid and oligomannose-type N-glycans). CD16a is N-glycosylated at five sites (**Figure 2**). The remainder of the N-glycans were primarily complex type, biantennary N-glycan structures with a high degree of sialylation (78%) and fucosylation (89%) (109). The under-processed forms do not likely originate from unprocessed CD16a in the ER because all of the observed hybrid forms were sialylated, a modification that occurs in the late Golgi compartments (113) (**Figure 3**). Moreover, the presence of oligomannose type N-glycans on CD16a from almost all recombinant sources suggests that restricted processing is a conserved feature (108–110). N-glycans at Asn38 and Asn74 were not observed using this glycomics approach to study NK cell CD16a; perhaps these large glycans ionize too poorly to be observed in a derivatized form, but robust

ionization of the peptide provides measurable signals for CD16b N38 and N74 glycopeptides (111).

Recombinant expression has thus far failed to generate CD16 with glycan profiles matching those measured for CD16a or CD16b from primary cells. CD16a is the most heavily studied FcγR due to its role in ADCC and the associated therapeutic applications. Glycomics characterization of soluble extracellular domain of CD16a (sCD16a) from HEK293, NS0, and CHO cell lines showed stark differences when compared to CD16a from NK cells, including a high abundance (over 90% compared to 55% in NK cells) of biantennary and triantennary complex type N-glycans with low levels of sialylation (108–110). Moreover, each recombinant system has the potential to synthesize unique N-glycan structures that are not commonly found on native human proteins, such as LacDiNAc (GlcNAc-GalNAc) from HEK293 cells, α-Gal epitopes (αGal-βGal-βGlcNAc), terminal N-acetylglycolylneuraminic acid in NS0 cells and only α-2,3 linked sialic acids in CHO cells (106, 114). These terminal modifications can potentially alter the binding affinity to IgG in an unexpected and undesirable manner.

Differences between native and recombinant CD16a processing render studies of binding affinity using recombinant material suboptimal, however, these materials still represent the best option for many *in vitro* studies. Furthermore, binding affinity measurements have utilized the soluble extracellular FcγR domains due to challenges associated with extracting full-length material from the membrane. Tethering CD16a to the membrane changes the N-glycosylation, likely due to differential localization within the Golgi (88, 109). Unfortunately, the N-glycosylation profile of full-length CD16a (frCD16a) expressed with HEK293 cells revealed an N-glycan profile unlike that found on NK cells (109). N-glycans from frCD16a showed less under-processed oligomannose and hybrid types (27% in frCD16a and 45% in NK cell CD16a) and the complex-type N-glycans were highly branched. Thus, cell-type specific glycosylation accounts for the dissimilar N-glycan profile on CD16a from primary and recombinant sources and impacts binding affinity measurement, as discussed below.

Recombinant FcγRs are valuable to characterize the role of N-glycosylation on IgG binding affinity, despite clear differences in N-glycan processing when compared to endogenous material. One recent study reported a 40-fold increase in affinity toward afucosylated IgG1-Fc (G0 form) when complex type N-glycans on CD16a were replaced with Man_5 N-glycans (110). This gain revealed that CD16a can bind with an affinity comparable to CD64, the "high affinity FcγR." A comparable study demonstrated that higher amounts of larger sialylated complex type N-glycans on CD16a expressed in CHO cells correlated with lower affinity for Rituximab (108).

Of five CD16a N-glycans, only two appear essential for high affinity interactions. Mutating the protein to eliminate N-glycan addition with N45Q and N162Q substitutions reduced the affinity for IgG1-Fc (109, 115–117). However, the reported influence of N-glycan composition was primarily driven by the N-glycan at N162: only the N162Q mutation abolished the affinity gain due to Man_5 N-glycans on CD16a (110). These observations are in agreement with the fact that glycans at N45 and N162 form interactions with the CD16a polypeptide and influence protein structure (118) and glycans at these two sites showed the greatest restriction in N-glycan processing using the HEK293 and CHO systems (119). Thus, cell-type specific CD16a N-glycosylation patterns influence affinity for IgG1 and a range of potential affinities are accessible purely through modifying N-glycan processing.

N-glycosylation of CD16b

CD16b is a highly similar paralogue of CD16a and only found in humans (97% sequence homology of the extracellular antibody-binding domain). However, two common CD16b alleles encode either four (NA1) or six (NA2) N-glycosylation sites (120, 121) (**Figure 2**). Considerable site-specific diversity in N-glycan structures was present on sCD16b obtained from 2l of pooled human serum (111). Serum sCD16b is generated by ADAM17 cleavage of cell surface CD16b upon neutrophil activation (48). Thus, sCD16b were likely membrane bound when the N-glycans were being processed. The N-glycans at each site had unique profiles ranging from smaller oligomannose type N-glycans at N45 to large complex type N-glycans with extensive elongation, sialylation, and fucosylation at N38 and N74, unlike sCD16b expressed in recombinant systems (106, 114, 122). Additionally, allele specific (NA1 and NA2) N-glycosylation profile at N162 and N45 of donor matched serum and neutrophil CD16b confirmed the observations of CD16b from pooled serum, revealing moderate variability in the abundance of the most prominent glycoforms (123). The profile of sCD16b from serum was distinct from CD16a expressed by NK cells that displayed a greater level of under-processed N-glycans (109, 111). The presence of oligomannose type N-glycans only at N45 strongly suggests under-processing of N-glycan is restricted to a single site on the protein with as many as six N-glycosylation sites (111).

The stark differences in the glycosylation profile of sCD16b from serum compared to recombinant sCD16b further emphasized the importance of cell type specific N-glycosylation. Glycomics analysis of CD16b from HEK293, NS0 and BHK revealed mainly multiantennary complex type N-glycans with a high degree of sialylation and fucosylation (106, 114, 122). The N-glycosylation profile of recombinant sCD16a and sCD16b are comparable as most of the N-glycosylation sites are shared (124). There was a minimal difference (2-fold increase) in affinity when sCD16b-Man5 binding to IgG1-Fc (G0F form) was compared to sCD16b with complex-type N-glycans (110). This was surprising considering that the extracellular antibody binding domains of CD16a and CD16b (NA2) differ at only four amino acid residues. Moreover, both CD16s are functionally distinct because CD16a-complex type has a 15-fold greater affinity for IgG-Fc than CD16b-complex type (110). The affinity and sensitivity to glycan composition for CD16b was improved to that of CD16a by mutating a single residue, Asp129, to Gly based on the CD16a sequence (124). The authors demonstrate with x-ray crystallography and molecular dynamics simulations that Asp129 buckles the CD16b backbone upon binding IgG1 Fc. Thus, buckling shifts a nearby residue, Arg155, which makes a different contact with the N162-glycan that is not observed in CD16a.

N-glycosylation of CD32

The N-glycosylation profiles of sCD32a and sCD32b expressed with recombinant systems were highly comparable (106, 108, 114). There are two to three N-glycosylation sites on CD32: CD32a (3), CD32b (2), and CD32c (2; 32b and 32c have identical extracellular domains) (**Figure 2**). Glycomics analysis of CD32a and CD32b expressed in HEK293, NS0, and CHO displayed predominantly biantennary and triantennary complex type N-glycan structures with a low degree of sialylation and varying levels of fucose (106, 108, 110, 114). Binding affinity between sCD32a and sCD32b was comparable and neither appeared sensitive to N-glycan composition as sCD32(a or b)-Man5 and sCD32(a or b)-complex type bound IgG1 Fc with similar affinities (106, 110). CD32a polymorphisms (R131 or H131) cause differences in binding to IgG subtypes, potentially changing the sensitivity of immune complexes to phagocytosis by neutrophils and monocytes (121, 125). However, N-glycan analysis on the receptor expressed in CHO cells showed no substantial difference in glycosylation pattern between the two CD32a allotypes (108). The site-specific N glycosylation profile and native N-glycosylation profile for any CD32 is not currently available.

N-glycosylation of CD64 Also Impacts Binding Affinity

The high affinity FcγR, CD64, is distinct from other FcγRs because it contains an additional extracellular domain (126). Moreover, CD64 can potentially receive N-glycosylation modification at seven sites in its extracellular domain (**Figure 2**). A comparative glycomics analysis of the sCD64 expressed in HEK293, NS0, and CHO cell lines showed biantennary and multi-antennary complex type N-glycans with varying degrees of sialylation and fucosylation as the most abundant glycoforms (106, 108, 114). A distinct feature which was conserved across sCD64 expressed in all three cell lines was the higher abundance of oligomannose structures when compared to recombinant CD16 or CD32. It was speculated that the presence of Man5 forms (the most abundant oligomannose N-glycan in these cell types) conferred a stabilizing effect toward IgG1 binding since the higher abundance of Man5 forms (14.4% in NS0 and 5.2% in CHO) correlated with an increase in binding affinity to Rituximab (108). According to the authors, the increased affinity was due to the lack of core fucose on the Man5 structure which can potentially prevent steric hindrance effects similar to that observed in fucosylated N-glycan on IgG1 (115, 127). The authors also observed that the presence of large sialylated complex type N-glycans on CD64 correlated with reduced binding affinity for Rituximab, indicating that these glycans destabilized the interaction (108). Even though N-glycan composition on CD64 can affect IgG1 affinity, the N-glycosylation profile of native CD64 and the composition of N-glycans at each site remains unknown.

N-glycosylation processing depends on the amino acid sequence and secondary structures which affect the exposure of substrate monosaccharide residues to the glycan processing enzymes (**Figure 3**). Presence of both the under-processed and highly-processed (tetraantennary sialylated) N-glycan structures on NK cell CD16a and recombinant sCD64 suggests site-specific glycan modification. Oligomannose structures at specific sites on sCD16a have been implicated in modulating IgG affinity; similarly, specific sites on CD64 can be involved in modulating CD64-IgG1 affinity (108, 110). Thus, a thorough analysis of site-specific N-glycosylation analysis of recombinant and endogenous FcγRs from all expressing tissues is required to fully elucidate the role of N-glycosylation pattern at specific sites in affinity modulation.

HOW MULTIVALENCY IMPACTS IgG-FcγR INTERACTIONS

Investigating factors that contribute to the monovalent affinity of IgG-FcγRs interaction revealed clear differences in the affinity of antibody subclasses for certain receptors, however, multivalent avidity likely determines the *in vivo* immunological response initiated by these interactions. High IgG concentrations in the serum of ~10 mg/ml provide monomeric antibody to the receptors at a concentration of ~67 μM, vastly exceeding the K_D of IgG1 for all human receptors (7). Thus, surface-borne FcγRs are occupied on cells circulating in the peripheral compartment and multivalent interactions must compete with monomeric IgG to cluster receptors (7, 8). Receptor cross-linking and clustering on the effector cell surface is essential for signal transduction through FcγRs, thus multivalent immune complexes or opsonized targets are the functionally appropriate ligands for the receptors (**Figure 1**) (54, 128). Distinct FcγRs are engaged depending on the responding cell type, the IgG subclass, the antibody concentration on the opsonized target, and the size of immune complex (**Figures 1, 2**) (129, 130). Furthermore, the differential binding of immune complexes has therapeutic as well as pathogenic properties, especially during infection and autoimmune disease but not all aspects are well-defined (9, 15). Therefore, defining the critical factors associated with immune complex recognition is required to fully understand the antibody-mediated immune response.

Immune Complex Size Determines Effector Function

The importance of interactions between multiple monovalent ligands and multiple receptors is well known, however, the study of multivalent interactions remains challenging. Early attempts to generate multivalent immune complexes through heat aggregation of IgG produced aggregates with varied valency, immunogenicity and ill-defined sizes (131, 132). Technological advances in recent years produced immune complexes of defined size and valency which accurately represent those generated *in vivo* (130). Functional interrogation using defined immune complex revealed that immune complex size contributes to interactions with FcγRs.

Immune Complex Size Affects Binding

The concentration of antigen-specific antibody in the serum and likewise immune complex size is expected to change during an immune response, and size-associated changes in the immune response are well described (130, 133). Nimmerjahn and coworkers used well-defined immune complexes formed by all four IgG subclasses binding to FcγRs expressed on a CHO cell surface to systematically determine that there was a clear size-dependent gain in binding by IgG2 and IgG4 immune complexes and the size of an immune complex can overcome IgG glycan truncation, a modification that destroys the monovalent interaction (134). Moreover, the binding patterns were comparable to experiments using primary leukocytes that increased cytokine secretion in response to larger immune complexes. These data led to a mathematical model that describes effects of valency and IgG subclass on *in vivo* function (135). The differential binding due to a change in the size of immune complex can potentially lead to substantial changes in cell signaling and recent technical advances provide a means to quantitate signaling with cell-based assays (136).

Role of Immune Complex Size in Autoimmune Disorders

The formation of immune complexes with soluble self-antigen is implicated in the pathophysiology of several autoimmune diseases (137). IVIG is a frequent treatment for a variety of autoimmune disorders, but the exact mechanism of action is not known (138). Even though there is a well-documented role of CD32b in decreasing an immune response triggered by autoantibody immune complexes in murine model of immune thrombocytopenia (ITP) (139), a recent study demonstrated that engaging the inhibitory CD32b alone is not responsible for the decrease in phagocytosis of RBC opsonized by autoantibody in human ITP patients. Instead, the direct engagement of IgG by CD64 and CD32a caused the decrease in phagocytosis (140). Surprisingly, though IVIG dimers and multimers are not necessary for therapeutic efficacy in murine models for ITP, small IVIG oligomers provided more potent inhibition of phagocytosis, indicating a role of IVIG immune complexes in blocking pathogenic immune complexes from binding to activating FcγRs (141). Consistent with this observation, immune complexes formed with the anti-citrullinated protein antibodies isolated from rheumatoid arthritis patients bound preferentially to activating and not inhibiting FcγRs expressed on CHO cells (142). Moreover, CD64 on activated neutrophils and CD32a on macrophages were recognized as receptors for the autoantibody immune complex, eliciting the secretion of pro-inflammatory cytokines. These observations formed the basis for developing engineered multivalent immune complexes as therapeutic options.

Considerations Regarding Immune Complex Size in Therapeutic Development

Multivalent synthetic immune complexes show promise and may prove useful in the clinic. For example, a trivalent IgG-Fc construct inhibited autoantibody-mediated FcγR-dependent cellular responses in primary human cells and autoimmune murine models (143). Likewise, an engineered hexameric-Fc construct bound to primary differentiated human macrophages and triggered internalization, colocalizing with the activating FcγRs and elicited a decrease in the phagocytosis of antiCD20-coated human B cells and platelets in a murine ITP model (144). The hexameric Fc construct did not trigger internalization of CD32b and exhibited a much shorter serum half-life in animal models than IgG1, however, the inhibition was effective for several days after the initial injection, suggesting a potential for clinical use. In contrast to the approach of preventing the internalization of pathogenic immune complex to block phagocytosis of healthy cells or activating a pro-inflammatory response, a designed bispecific antibody formed larger complexes that neutralized soluble antigens, leading to rapid clearance from serum of a murine model (145). Thus, studies of multivalent IgG-FcγR interactions provide guidance for the development of effective therapeutic options. However, there are multiple antibody and antigen associated factors which govern the antigenicity of immune complexes that must be considered when designing antibodies with defined FcγR-dependent functions.

Features of the Antibody and Antigen That Impact Antigenicity of the Immune Complex *in vivo*
The Ratio of Antibody to Antigen
Antibody concentration relative to antigen changes throughout the progression of an immune response against an infectious pathogen. Considering influenza infection as an example, the B-cell response can take up to 7–14 days to produce antibodies (146). Generally, the antigen-specific antibody titers increased by up to 10.2-fold, depending on the patient, vastly changing the antibody to antigen ratio and the antibody production can be sustained or subside depending on clearance of the organism.

A minimal threshold of antibody density must be surpassed to elicit an immune response during encounters between an opsonized target and effector cell, typically seen during pathogenic infection (147, 148). Antibody concentrations that exceed the threshold lead to an increase in phagocytic activity, as demonstrated by primary mouse bone marrow derived macrophages phagocytosing opsonized sheep erythrocytes. Moreover, at relatively high concentrations of IgG, a valency dependent induction of IL-10 production was seen (148). Similarly, infection with *Cryptococcus neoformans* in mice could be cleared using a specific ratio of antibody to antigen, ratios with excessive antibody led to a detrimental host response mainly due to a reduction in pro-inflammatory cytokines secretion in organs associated with the infection (149). Apart from changes in cytokine secretion potential, larger immune complexes formed with high concentrations of neutralizing antibody against dengue virus actually inhibited antibody-dependent enhancement by binding to the inhibitory receptor CD32b on phagocytic monocytes (150). Thus, relative antibody concentration can modulate immune response in an FcγR-dependent manner by altering the size and concentration of immune complexes; this effect may be similar to the therapeutic benefit of IVIG in autoimmune conditions.

Concentration of the Immune Complex
Immune complex concentration likewise impacts viral infection. Apart from the traditional view of Fab-mediated neutralizing activity, Fc dependent effector functions are becoming increasingly recognized in protection against viral infection (16, 17, 151). Classical FcγR-dependent protective mechanisms such as ADCC and ADCP, as well as antibody dependent enhancement of infection, are influenced by the size of the immune complex and IgG subtype coating the viral particle (17, 152). The production of a high concentration of immune complexes are common during chronic viral infection in mice (153). However, high concentrations do not always lead to favorable outcomes. A high concentration of immune complex blocked FcγRs on primary murine macrophages and dendritic cells, negatively impacting viral clearance, and other FcγR-related activity (153). These phenomena were independent of CD32b and reversed once the immune complex concentration was reduced. Thus, the role of FcγRs during pathogen infection is complex and varied but there is a clear dependence of cellular response based on immune complex size and concentration, similar to that observed in autoimmune disease discussed above.

Affinity of the Antibody for Antigen
At a fixed antibody concentration, the affinity of the antibody toward the antigen can determine how many Fcs are displayed on the immune complex and are available to interact with FcγRs (154). A recent study showed that at saturating concentrations, antibodies with high affinity for antigen elicited a weaker ADCC response compared to antibodies with lower affinity (K_D = 0.8 nM and 72 nM, respectively) (155). The observed difference in the immune response was attributed to the higher proportion of monovalent antigen binding displayed by the lower affinity antibody, recruiting a larger number of antibodies to the cell surface and increasing the number of Fcs available to the leukocyte. A notable feature of this observation is the initial IgG response often produces antibodies with antigen-binding affinities similar to the lower affinity antibody in this study. Antibody concentration and antibody-antigen affinity are not the only factors affecting immunogenicity of immune complex. A comparative analysis of three anti-TNFα antibodies with a range of affinities (K_D = 0.18–5.1 nM) showed that the size and composition of the immune complex was determined by the properties associated with epitope location and binding energetics (156).

Epitope and Antigen Location
Location of the epitope influences the immune response. Neutralizing antibodies targeting the stalk region of the influenza hemagglutinin protein induced FcγR-dependent cytotoxicity while antibodies binding the head domain did not (12). A comparable analysis of anti-Ebola antibodies showed that binding to the most membrane distal portion of viral surface glycoprotein elicited the highest ADCP and antibody-dependent neutrophil phagocytosis (ADNP) compared to antibodies that bound to the membrane proximal regions (157). Even though epitope location on the antigen is not directly implicated in changes in immune complex size in these studies, it is likely

that the epitope location causes changes in immune complex properties since three different monoclonal antibodies against different epitopes on sCD154 and TNFα also formed different immune complexes (156, 158). In other cases, the height of the antigen from the target surface affected phagocytosis in a valency-independent manner (55). Antigens which are <10 nm from target surface promoted phagocytosis when compared to antigens further away from the surface because close contact between target and effector cell surface was necessary to exclude effector cell the inhibitory CD45 from the immune synapse following FcγRs clustering (as noted above). Additionally, antibodies binding West Nile virus epitopes that are normally buried can form immune complexes, given sufficient incubation time, though these immune complexes are smaller and led to lower neutralization levels (154). Thus, location of the epitope can affect the immune response but the effect of epitope location on immune complex size is not fully understood.

The location of the antigen (soluble or cell bound) affects FcγR clustering and the subsequent immune response. A soluble antigen may form relatively smaller immune complexes which are endocytosed but a cell surface antigen forms a relatively larger opsonized target that is more likely phagocytized as determined using mouse bone marrow-derived macrophages (133). Both mechanisms, triggered through FcγRs, are distinct and induce different signaling and subsequent immune responses (128, 159). In one example, small soluble immune made with soluble CD154 would be expected to be endocytosed, and CD154 tethered to a T cell membrane led to the formation of very large complexes at the cell surface (158). Surprisingly, the specific monoclonal antibody greatly influenced the immune complex structure. It is also known that opsonized targets can exhibit lateral diffusion on the leukocyte surface which also affects the multivalent interaction with FcγRs (160).

Malleable vs. Rigid Target Surfaces

In addition to size and shape, deformability of the target also impacts activation. The phagocytosis of opsonized polyacrylamide beads tuned to exhibit different rigidity established that phagocytosis of ridged particles was preferred over relatively more deformable particles by mouse bone marrow-derived macrophages (161). A related study demonstrated that murine macrophage RAW264.7 cells phagocytosed emulsion droplets at a lower IgG concentration when compared to solid particles (162). It was speculated that the attachment of IgG on the surface of rigid particles prevents the lateral diffusion of opsonizing antibodies, while lateral diffusion was observed in opsonized emulsion droplet. Thus, the location of the antigen, which facilitated higher cell surface FcγRs interaction at lower antibody concentrations, can affect recognition of the complex.

IgG-Subclass Impact Immune Response

FcγR binding is also affected by IgG subclass. Specificity of a specific IgG subclass binding to a FcγR is largely studied in context of a monovalent interaction (23), however, immune complexes and opsonized target cells are the natural ligands. Additionally, specific IgG subclasses are related to various

disorders indicating immune complex composition is important (1, 152, 163). Therefore, studying these interactions in a multivalent form is required to accurately determine their binding properties and the subsequent immune response. The observation that immune complexes of certain IgG subclasses only bind at higher concentrations indicates that IgG subclass is also a variable which can affect the immune response (164).

The Fcs of different IgG subclasses have distinct amino acid residues and hinge regions which can affect binding to the FcγRs, despite a high degree of sequence conservation (**Figure 2**) (1). A systematic analysis of multivalent binding for the four human IgG subclasses to the cell surface FcγRs revealed the IgG2 and IgG4 subclasses, which showed minimal affinity in a monovalent interaction, bound as immune complexes to FcγRs expressed on CHO cells at higher concentrations (164). This study also demonstrated that allotype variants of FcγRs had different binding properties toward immune complexes generated by different IgG subtypes. CD16a V158 bound IgG3 immune complexes with high affinity while CD16a F158 bound more weakly and CD32a H131 had a higher affinity to IgG2 immune complex compared to CD32a R131. Another report showed that the CD32a H131 variant bound to IgG1, IgG2, and IgG3 with higher affinity than CD32a R131. This observation may explain why the CD32a R131 allotype is associated with greater susceptibility to bacterial infections and autoimmune disorders (163). Thus, the wide range of binding affinities displayed by FcγRs toward IgG subclass specific immune complexes can impact clinical outcome.

The use of different IgG subclasses in designed immune complexes can also impact potential therapeutic use. Incubation of a hexameric IgG1 Fc construct, discussed above as an inhibitor of phagocytosis, elicited the release of higher cytokine levels in whole blood when compared to PBMCs, likely due to CD16b engagement on neutrophils (not present in PBMCs) (165). Furthermore, the hexameric IgG1 Fc construct also triggered release of cytokines from platelets through a CD32a-dependent interaction. However, a hexameric IgG4 Fc construct did not promote the release of cytokines from neutrophils or platelets. This result is consistent with the reduced affinity of IgG4 for CD16b and CD32a when compared with IgG1, highlighting the potential utility of specific FcγR interactions.

SUMMARY

The multitude of factors influencing the immune system each affects a wide range of responses. This review covers a relatively limited collection of variables that contribute to an FcγR-dependent immune response (**Figure 1**). There appear to be few inviolable laws governing this aspect of the immune system, and every newly discovered variable introduce a new handle to tune the immune response, at least *in vitro*. It is well known that different monoclonal antibodies to a single target elicit different responses, in many cases through the mechanisms described here. If any lessons are to be learned, it is that each antibody must be thoroughly evaluated using systems that recapitulate as closely as possible endogenous immune system components.

One striking example of this tenet is the observation that the efficacy of a hexameric IgG1 Fc increased when neutrophils and platelets were incorporated in an *in-vitro* assay with PBMCs (165). Moreover, soluble complement components can also bind the immune complex to affect the immune response as reported in few studies described above (130, 148, 149). Laboratory studies often focus on immune complexes formed by monoclonal antibodies, but that is likely not the case *in vivo* with a polyclonal immune response to vaccines or infection; one study demonstrated that a mixture of disease neutralizing and disease enhancing antibodies against *Bacillus anthracis* formed immune complexes that elicited a protective immune response (166). Thus, these observations highlight the complex yet important features associated with studying FcγRs function *in vivo*.

Animal models have, and will continue to have, an important role in studies designed to understand human FcγRs in immune function. Despite the differences in FcγR cellular expression patterns and minor differences in binding affinities to human IgG subclass, animal (mainly murine and non-human primate) models have sufficiently recapitulated human FcγR biology to be used for studying FcγR function and test therapeutic molecules (167–173). A recent study determined that the mouse FcγRIV and the human equivalent to human CD16a both share the conserved N-glycosylation site at N162 which mediates tight binding to afucosylated mouse IgG similar to observations in human system, and human IgG binds mouse FcγRs with similar affinity patterns as human FcγRs demonstrating conservation of certain functional features of human FcγR biology in mouse model (170, 174). Furthermore, several studies mentioned in this review have employed murine autoimmune models, humanized models, cell lines or primary cells to test efficacy of engineered antibody products and delineate mechanistic aspects of the FcγRs dependent cellular response, demonstrating that these models are indispensable for understanding human FcγR biology (61, 66, 139, 141, 143, 162). The two successful strategies to attain humanized FcγR mouse models eliminate the influence of mouse FcγRs in studying human FcγR function

in these models and can uncover novel role of FcγRs in autoimmune disorders, infection and cancer immunity (175, 176). However, important yet undefined FcγR variables including post-translational modification including glycosylation as well as copy number variation and interaction with coexpressed membrane proteins likely vary in animal models. It is likely that organism diversity in these key variables likewise differentially impacts immune function, comparable to the diversity attributed to protein coding regions and gene variability between species.

It is worth highlighting the role of post translation modification of the FcγRs as another critical variable that is overlooked due to the historical inability to resolve differences in the glycosylation of endogenous material. One future challenge will be matching the level of detail known regarding serum IgG glycosylation with studies of functionally-relevant FcγR modifications as these have the potential to exert an enormous influence on the immune response. Differential gene expression profiles of the glycan modifying enzymes are present in monocytes, dendritic cells, and macrophages, suggesting the potential for the functionally-relevant differentiation and maturation specific N-glycosylation modifications (177). A complete understanding of the immune response will require the definition of these recently discovered variables, with the likelihood that more variables will emerge.

AUTHOR CONTRIBUTIONS

All authors listed have made a substantial, direct and intellectual contribution to the work, and approved it for publication.

ACKNOWLEDGMENTS

This material is based upon work supported by the National Institutes of Health under Award No. R01 GM115489 (NIGMS) and by the Roy J. Carver Department of Biochemistry, Biophysics & Molecular Biology at Iowa State University.

REFERENCES

1. Vidarsson G, Dekkers G, Rispens T. IgG subclasses and allotypes: from structure to effector functions. *Front Immunol.* (2014) 5:520. doi: 10.3389/fimmu.2014.00520

2. Bolland S, and Ravetch JV. Inhibitory Pathways triggered by ITIM-containing receptors. *Adv Immunol.* (1999) 72:149–77. doi: 10.1016/S0065-2776(08)60019-X

3. Isakov N. Immunoreceptor tyrosine-based activation motif (ITAM), a unique module linking antigen and Fc receptors to their signaling cascades. *J Leukocyte Biol.* (1997) 61:6–16. doi: 10.1002/jlb.61.1.6

4. Li X, Wu J, Ptacek T, Redden DT, Brown EE, Alarcón GS, et al. Allelic-dependent expression of an activating Fc receptor on B cells enhances humoral immune responses. *Sci Transl Med.* (2013) 5:216ra175. doi: 10.1126/scitranslmed.3007097

5. Turner M, Schweighoffer E, Colucci F, Di Santo JP, Tybulewicz VL. Tyrosine kinase SYK: essential functions for immunoreceptor signalling. *Immunol Today* (2000) 21:148–54. doi: 10.1016/S0167-5699(99)01574-1

6. Nimmerjahn F, Ravetch JV. Fcγ receptors: old friends and new family members. *Immunity* (2006) 24:19–28. doi: 10.1016/j.immuni.2005.11.010

7. Kelton JG, Singer J, Rodger C, Gauldie J, Horsewood P, Dent P. The concentration of IgG in the serum is a major determinant of Fc-dependent reticuloendothelial function. *Blood* (1985) 66:490–5.

8. Mirre E, van Teeling JL, Meer JWM, Bleeker WK, Hack CE. Monomeric IgG in intravenous Ig preparations is a functional antagonist of FcγRII and FcγRIIIb. *J Immunol.* (2004) 173:332–9. doi: 10.4049/jimmunol.173 .1.332

9. Li X, Kimberly RP. Targeting the Fc receptor in autoimmune disease. *Exp Opin Ther Targets* (2014) 18:335–50. doi: 10.1517/14728222.2014.877891

10. Boross P, van Montfoort N, Stapels DAC, van der Poel CE, Bertens C, Meeldijk J, et al. FcRγ-chain ITAM signaling is critically required for cross-presentation of soluble antibody-antigen complexes by dendritic cells. *J Immunol.* (2014) 193:5506–14. doi: 10.4049/jimmunol.1302012

11. Daëron M. Fc Receptor biology. *Ann Rev Immunol.* (1997) 15:203–34. doi: 10.1146/annurev.immunol.15.1.203

12. DiLillo DJ, Tan GS, Palese P, Ravetch JV. Broadly neutralizing hemagglutinin stalk–specific antibodies require FcγR interactions for protection against influenza virus *in vivo*. *Nat Med.* (2014) 20:143–51. doi: 10.1038/nm.3443

13. Vogelpoel LTC, Baeten DLP, de Jong EC, den Dunnen J. Control of cytokine production by human fc gamma receptors: implications

for pathogen defense and autoimmunity. *Front Immunol.* (2015) 6:79. doi: 10.3389/fimmu.2015.00079

14. Weiskopf K, Weissman IL. Macrophages are critical effectors of antibody therapies for cancer. *MAbs* (2015) 7:303–10. doi: 10.1080/19420862.2015.1011450

15. Bournazos S, DiLillo DJ, Ravetch JV. The role of Fc–FcγR interactions in IgG-mediated microbial neutralization. *J Exp Med.* (2015) 212:1361–9. doi: 10.1084/jem.20151267

16. Chan KR, Ong EZ, Mok DZ, Ooi EE. Fc receptors and their influence on efficacy of therapeutic antibodies for treatment of viral diseases. *Exp Rev Anti Infect Ther.* (2015) 13:1351–60. doi: 10.1586/14787210.2015.1079127

17. Lu LL, Suscovich TJ, Fortune SM, Alter G. Beyond binding: antibody effector functions in infectious diseases. *Nat Rev Immunol.* (2018) 18:46–61. doi: 10.1038/nri.2017.106

18. Lyden TW, Robinson JM, Tridandapani S, Teillaud JL, Garber SA, Osborne JM, et al. The Fc receptor for IgG expressed in the villus endothelium of human placenta is Fc gamma RIIb2. *J Immunol.* (2001) 166:3882–9. doi: 10.4049/jimmunol.166.6.3882

19. Simister NE, Story CM, Chen H-L, Hunt JS. An IgG-transporting Fc receptor expressed in the syncytiotrophoblast of human placenta. *Eur J Immunol.* (1996) 26:1527–31. doi: 10.1002/eji.1830260718

20. Wainwright SD, Holmes CH. Distribution of Fc gamma receptors on trophoblast during human placental development: an immunohistochemical and immunoblotting study. *Immunology* (1993) 80:343–51.

21. Okayama Y, Kirshenbaum AS, Metcalfe DD. Expression of a functional high-affinity IgG receptor, FcγRI, on human mast cells: up-regulation by IFN-γ. *J Immunol.* (2000) 164:4332–9. doi: 10.4049/jimmunol.164.8.4332

22. Cassatella MA, Flynn RM, Amezaga MA, Bazzoni F, Vicentini F, Trinchieri G. Interferon gamma induces in human neutrophils and macrophages expression of the mRNA for the high affinity receptor for monomeric IgG (Fc gamma R-I or CD64). *Biochem Biophys Res Commun.* (1990) 170:582–8. doi: 10.1016/0006-291X(90)92131-I

23. Ravetch JV, Kinet JP. Fc receptors. *Annu Rev Immunol.* (1991) 9:457–92. doi: 10.1146/annurev.iy.09.040191.002325

24. Rosales C. Fcγ receptor heterogeneity in leukocyte functional responses. *Front Immunol.* (2017) 8:280. doi: 10.3389/fimmu.2017.00280

25. Chauhan AK, Chen C, Moore TL, DiPaolo RJ. Induced expression of FcγRIIIa (CD16a) on CD4+ T cells triggers generation of IFN-γhigh subset. *J Biol Chem.* (2015) 290:5127–40. doi: 10.1074/jbc.M114.599266

26. Ravetch JV, Bolland S. IgG Fc Receptors. *Annu Rev Immunol.* (2001) 19:275–90. doi: 10.1146/annurev.immunol.19.1.275

27. Ravetch JV, Perussia B. Alternative membrane forms of Fc gamma RIII(CD16) on human natural killer cells and neutrophils. Cell type-specific expression of two genes that differ in single nucleotide substitutions. *J Exp Med.* (1989) 170:481–97. doi: 10.1084/jem.170.2.481

28. Meknache N, Jönsson F, Laurent J, Guinnepain M-T, Daëron M. Human basophils express the glycosylphosphatidylinositol-anchored low-affinity igg receptor FcγRIIIB (CD16B). *J Immunol.* (2009) 182:2542–50. doi: 10.4049/jimmunol.0801665

29. Davoine F, Lavigne S, Chakir J, Ferland C, Boulay M-È, Laviolette M. Expression of FcγRIII (CD16) on human peripheral blood eosinophils increases in allergic conditions. *J Allergy Clin Immunol.* (2002) 109:463–9. doi: 10.1067/mai.2002.121952

30. Zhu X, Hamann KJ, Muñoz NM, Rubio N, Mayer D, Hernrreiter A, et al. Intracellular Expression of FcγRIII (CD16) and its mobilization by chemoattractants in human eosinophils. *J Immunol.* (1998) 161:2574–9.

31. Anderson CL, Ganesan LP, Robinson JM. The biology of the classical Fcγ receptors in non-hematopoietic cells. *Immunol Rev.* (2015) 268:236–40. doi: 10.1111/imr.12335

32. Breunis WB, van Mirre E, Geissler J, Laddach N, Wolbink G, van der Schoot E, et al. Copy number variation at the FCGR locus includes FCGR3A, FCGR2C and FCGR3B but not FCGR2A and FCGR2B. *Hum Mutat.* (2009) 30:E640–50. doi: 10.1002/humu.20997

33. Morris DL, Roberts AL, Witherden AS, Tarzi R, Barros P, Whittaker JC, et al. Evidence for both copy number and allelic (NA1/NA2) risk at the FCGR3B locus in systemic lupus erythematosus. *Eur J Hum Genet.* (2010) 18:1027–31. doi: 10.1038/ejhg.2010.56

34. Niederer HA, Clatworthy MR, Willcocks LC, Smith KGC. FcγRIIB, FcγRIIIB, and systemic lupus erythematosus. *Ann N Y Acad Sci.* (2010) 1183:69–88. doi: 10.1111/j.1749-6632.2009.05132.x

35. Franke L, Bannoudi H, Jansen DTSL, Kok K, Trynka G, Diogo D, et al. Association analysis of copy numbers of FC-gamma receptor genes for rheumatoid arthritis and other immune-mediated phenotypes. *Eur J Hum Genet.* (2016) 24:263–70. doi: 10.1038/ejhg.2015.95

36. Martorana D, Bonatti F, Alberici F, Gioffredi A, Reina M, Urban ML, et al. Fcγ-receptor 3B (FCGR3B) copy number variations in patients with eosinophilic granulomatosis with polyangiitis. *J Allergy Clin Immunol.* (2016) 137:1597–9.e8. doi: 10.1016/j.jaci.2015.09.053

37. Lassaunière R, Shalekoff S, Tiemessen CT. A novel FCGR3A intragenic haplotype is associated with increased FcγRIIIa/CD16a cell surface density and population differences. *Hum Immunol.* (2013) 74:627–34. doi: 10.1016/j.humimm.2013.01.020

38. Huizinga TW, Kerst M, Nuyens JH, Vlug A, Borne AE, Roos D, et al. Binding characteristics of dimeric IgG subclass complexes to human neutrophils. *J Immunol.* (1989) 142:2359–64.

39. Huizinga TW, Roos D, von dem Borne, AE. Neutrophil Fc-gamma receptors: a two-way bridge in the immune system. *Blood* (1990) 75:1211–4.

40. Clarkson SB, Ory PA. CD16. Developmentally regulated IgG Fc receptors on cultured human monocytes. *J Exp Med.* (1988) 167:408–20. doi: 10.1084/jem.167.2.408

41. Herter S, Birk MC, Klein C, Gerdes C, Umana P, Bacac M. Glycoengineering of therapeutic antibodies enhances monocyte/macrophage-mediated phagocytosis and cytotoxicity. *J Immunol.* (2014) 192:2252–60. doi: 10.4049/jimmunol.1301249

42. Perussia B, Acuto O, Terhorst C, Faust J, Lazarus R, Fanning V, et al. Human natural killer cells analyzed by B73.1, a monoclonal antibody blocking Fc receptor functions. II. Studies of B73.1 antibody-antigen interaction on the lymphocyte membrane. *J Immunol.* (1983) 130:2142–8.

43. de La Salle C, Esposito-Farese M-E, Bieber T, Moncuit J, Morales M, Wollenberg A, et al. Release of soluble FcγRII/CD32 molecules by human langerhans cells: a subtle balance between shedding and secretion? *J Invest Dermatol.* (1992) 99:S15–7. doi: 10.1111/1523-1747.ep12668250

44. Sármay G, Rozsnyay Z, Gergely J. Fcγ RII expression and release on resting and activated human B lymphocytes. *Molecul Immunol.* (1990) 27:1195–200. doi: 10.1016/0161-5890(90)90022-R

45. Huizinga TWJ, van der Schoot CE, Jost C, Klaassen R, Kleijer M, von dem Borne AEGK, et al. The Pi-linked receptor FcRIII is released on stimulation of neutrophils. *Nature* (1988) 333:667–9. doi: 10.1038/333667a0

46. Jing Y, Ni Z, Wu J, Higgins L, Markowski TW, Kaufman DS, et al. Identification of an ADAM17 cleavage region in human CD16 (FcγRIII) and the engineering of a non-cleavable version of the receptor in NK cells. *PLoS ONE* (2015) 10:e0121788. doi: 10.1371/journal.pone.0121788

47. Middelhoven P, Ager A, Roos D, Verhoeven A. Involvement of a metalloprotease in the shedding of human neutrophil FcγRIIIB. *FEBS Lett.* (1997) 414:14–8. doi: 10.1016/S0014-5793(97)00959-9

48. Galon J, Moldovan I, Galinha A, Provost-Marloie MA, Kaudewitz H, Roman-Roman S, et al. Identification of the cleavage site involved in production of plasma soluble Fc gamma receptor type III (CD16). *Eur J Immunol.* (1998) 28:2101–7. doi: 10.1002/(SICI)1521-4141(199807)28:07<2101::AID-IMMU2101>3.0.CO;2-W

49. Huizinga TW, de Haas M, Kleijer M, Nuijens JH, Roos D, Borne AE. Soluble Fc gamma receptor III in human plasma originates from release by neutrophils. *J Clin Invest.* (1990) 86:416–23. doi: 10.1172/JCI114727

50. Teillaud JL, Bouchard C, Astier A, Teillaud C, Tartour E, Michon J, et al. Natural and recombinant soluble low-affinity FcγR: detection, purification, and functional activities. *ImmunoMethods* (1994) 4:48–64. doi: 10.1006/immu.1994.1007

51. Galon J, Gauchat JF, Mazières N, Spagnoli R, Storkus W, Lötze M, et al. Soluble Fcgamma receptor type III (FcgammaRIII, CD16) triggers cell activation through interaction with complement receptors. *J Immunol.* (1996) 157:1184–92.

52. Srpan K, Ambrose A, Karampatzakis A, Saeed M, Cartwright ANR, Guldevall K, et al. Shedding of CD16 disassembles the NK cell immune synapse and boosts serial engagement of target cells. *J Cell Biol.* (2018) 217:3267–83. doi: 10.1083/jcb.201712085

53. Wang W, Erbe AK, Hank JA, Morris ZS, Sondel PM. NK cell-mediated antibody-dependent cellular cytotoxicity in cancer immunotherapy. *Front Immunol.* (2015) 6:368. doi: 10.3389/fimmu.2015.00368

54. Goodridge HS, Underhill DM, Touret N. Mechanisms of Fc receptor and dectin-1 activation for phagocytosis. *Traffic* (2012) 13:1062–71. doi: 10.1111/j.1600-0854.2012.01382.x

55. Bakalar MH, Joffe AM, Schmid EM, Son S, Podolski M, Fletcher DA. Size-dependent segregation controls macrophage phagocytosis of antibody-opsonized targets. *Cell* (2018) 174:131–42.e13. doi: 10.1016/j.cell.2018.05.059

56. Chang VT, Fernandes RA, Ganzinger KA, Lee SF, Siebold C, et al. Initiation of T cell signaling by CD45 segregation at "close contacts." *Nat Immunol.* (2016) 17:574–82. doi: 10.1038/ni.3392

57. Lopes FB, Balint S, Valvo S, Felce JH, Hessel EM, Dustin ML, et al. Membrane nanoclusters of FcgammaRI segregate from inhibitory SIRPalpha upon activation of human macrophages. *J Cell Biol.* (2017) 216:1123–41. doi: 10.1083/jcb.201608094

58. Freeman SA, Vega A, Riedl M, Collins RF, Ostrowski PP, Woods EC, et al. Transmembrane pickets connect cyto- and pericellular skeletons forming barriers to receptor engagement. *Cell* (2018) 172:305–17.e10. doi: 10.1016/j.cell.2017.12.023

59. Flannagan RS, Harrison RE, Yip CM, Jaqaman K, Grinstein S. Dynamic macrophage "probing" is required for the efficient capture of phagocytic targets. *J Cell Biol.* (2010) 191:1205–18. doi: 10.1083/jcb.201007056

60. Mao YS, Yamaga M, Zhu X, Wei Y, Sun H-Q, Wang J, et al. Essential and unique roles of PIP5K-γ and -α in Fcγ receptor-mediated phagocytosis. *J Cell Biol.* (2009) 184:281–96. doi: 10.1083/jcb.200806121

61. Lin J, Kurilova S, Scott BL, Bosworth E, Iverson BE, Bailey EM, et al. TIRF imaging of Fc gamma receptor microclusters dynamics and signaling on macrophages during frustrated phagocytosis. *In BMC Immunol.* (2016) 17:5. doi: 10.1186/s12865-016-0143-2

62. Jaumouillé V, Farkash Y, Jaqaman K, Das R, Lowell CA, Grinstein S. Actin cytoskeleton reorganization by Syk regulates Fcγ receptor responsiveness by increasing its lateral mobility and clustering. *Dev Cell* (2014) 29:534–46. doi: 10.1016/j.devcel.2014.04.031

63. Steblyanko M, Anikeeva N, Campbell KS, Keen JH, Sykulev Y. Integrins influence the size and dynamics of signaling microclusters in a Pyk2-dependent manner. *J Biol Chem.* (2015) 290:11833–42. doi: 10.1074/jbc.M114.614719

64. Hsu HT, Mace EM, Carisey AF, Viswanath DI, Christakou AE, Wiklund M., et al. NK cells converge lytic granules to promote cytotoxicity and prevent bystander killing. *J Cell Biol.* (2016) 215:875–89. doi: 10.1083/jcb.201604136

65. Yeap WH, Wong KL, Shimasaki N, Teo ECY, Quek JKS, Yong HX, et al. CD16 is indispensable for antibody-dependent cellular cytotoxicity by human monocytes. *Sci Rep.* (2016) 6:srep34310. doi: 10.1038/srep34310

66. Zhang Y, Hoppe AD, Swanson JA. Coordination of Fc receptor signaling regulates cellular commitment to phagocytosis. *Proc Natl Acad Sci USA.* (2010) 107:19332–7. doi: 10.1073/pnas.1008248107

67. Magenau A, Benzing C, Proschogo N, Don AS, Hejazi L, Karunakaran D, et al. Phagocytosis of IgG-coated polystyrene beads by macrophages induces and requires high membrane order. *Traffic* (2011) 12:1730–43. doi: 10.1111/j.1600-0854.2011.01272.x

68. Kono H, Kyogoku C, Suzuki T, Tsuchiya N, Honda H, Yamamoto K, et al. FcgammaRIIB Ile232Thr transmembrane polymorphism associated with human systemic lupus erythematosus decreases affinity to lipid rafts and attenuates inhibitory effects on B cell receptor signaling. *Hum Mol Genet.* (2005) 14:2881–92. doi: 10.1093/hmg/ddi320

69. Scheiffele P, Roth MG, Simons K. Interaction of influenza virus haemagglutinin with sphingolipid-cholesterol membrane domains via its transmembrane domain. *EMBO J.* (1997) 16:5501–8. doi: 10.1093/emboj/16.18.5501

70. García-García E, Nieto-Castañeda G, Ruiz-Saldaña M, Mora N, Rosales C. FcgammaRIIA and FcgammaRIIIB mediate nuclear factor activation through separate signaling pathways in human neutrophils. *J Immunol.* (2009) 182:4547–56. doi: 10.4049/jimmunol.0801468

71. Coxon A, Cullere X, Knight S, Sethi S, Wakelin MW, Stavrakis G, et al. FcγRIII mediates neutrophil recruitment to immune complexes: a mechanism for neutrophil accumulation in immune-mediated inflammation. *Immunity* (2001) 14:693–704. doi: 10.1016/S1074-7613(01)00150-9

72. Zhou MJ, Brown EJ. CR3 (Mac-1, alpha M beta 2, CD11b/CD18) and Fc gamma RIII cooperate in generation of a neutrophil respiratory burst: requirement for Fc gamma RIII and tyrosine phosphorylation. *J Cell Biol.* (1994) 125:1407–16. doi: 10.1083/jcb.125.6.1407

73. Zhou M, Lublin DM, Link DC, Brown EJ. Distinct tyrosine kinase activation and triton X-100 insolubility upon FcγRII or FcγRIIIB ligation in human polymorphonuclear leukocytes. Implications for immune complex activation of the respiratory burst. *J Biol Chem.* (1995) 270:13553–60. doi: 10.1074/jbc.270.22.13553

74. Anderson CL, Shen L, Eicher DM, Wewers MD, Gill JK. Phagocytosis mediated by three distinct Fc gamma receptor classes on human leukocytes. *J Exp Med.* (1990) 171:1333–45. doi: 10.1084/jem.171.4.1333

75. David A, Fridlich R, Aviram I. The presence of membrane Proteinase 3 in neutrophil lipid rafts and its colocalization with FcgammaRIIIb and cytochrome b558. *Exp Cell Res.* (2005) 308:156–65. doi: 10.1016/j.yexcr.2005.03.034

76. Fernandes MJG, Rollet-Labelle E, Paré, G, Marois S, Tremblay ML, Teillaud JL, et al. CD16b associates with high-density, detergent-resistant membranes in human neutrophils. *Biochem J.* (2006) 393:351–9. doi: 10.1042/BJ20050129

77. Green JM, Schreiber AD, Brown EJ. Role for a glycan phosphoinositol anchor in Fcγ receptor synergy. *J Cell Biol.* (1997) 139:1209–17. doi: 10.1083/jcb.139.5.1209

78. Marois L, Paré G, Vaillancourt M, Rollet-Labelle E, Naccache PH. Fc gammaRIIIb triggers raft-dependent calcium influx in IgG-mediated responses in human neutrophils. *J Biol Chem.* (2011) 286:3509–19. doi: 10.1074/jbc.M110.169516

79. Munro S. Lipid rafts: elusive or illusive? *Cell* (2003) 115:377–88. doi: 10.1016/S0092-8674(03)00882-1

80. Paulick MG, Bertozzi CR. The glycosylphosphatidylinositol anchor: a complex membrane-anchoring structure for proteins. *Biochemistry* (2008) 47:6991–7000. doi: 10.1021/bi8006324

81. Yang H, Jiang H, Song Y, Chen DJ, Shen XJ, Chen JH. Neutrophil CD16b crosslinking induces lipid raft-mediated activation of SHP-2 and affects cytokine expression and retarded neutrophil apoptosis. *Exp Cell Res.* (2018) 362:121–31. doi: 10.1016/j.yexcr.2017.11.009

82. Zhou M, Todd RF, van de Winkel JG, Petty HR. Cocapping of the leukoadhesin molecules complement receptor type 3 and lymphocyte function-associated antigen-1 with Fc gamma receptor III on human neutrophils. Possible role of lectin-like interactions. *J Immunol.* (1993) 150:3030–41.

83. Golay J, Roit FD, Bologna L, Ferrara C, Leusen JH, Rambaldi A, et al. Glycoengineered CD20 antibody obinutuzumab activates neutrophils and mediates phagocytosis through CD16B more efficiently than rituximab. *Blood* (2013) 122:3482–91. doi: 10.1182/blood-2013-05-504043

84. Chesla SE, Li P, Nagarajan S, Selvaraj P, Zhu C. The membrane anchor influences ligand binding two-dimensional kinetic rates and three-dimensional affinity of FcγRIII (CD16). *J Biol Chem.* (2000) 275:10235–46. doi: 10.1074/jbc.275.14.10235

85. Jiang N, Chen W, Jothikumar P, Patel JM, Shashidharamurthy R, Selvaraj P, et al. Effects of anchor structure and glycosylation of Fcγ receptor III on ligand binding affinity. *Mol Biol Cell* (2016) 27:3449–58. doi: 10.1091/mbc.e16-06-0470

86. Moremen KW, Tiemeyer M, Nairn AV. Vertebrate protein glycosylation: diversity, synthesis and function. *Nat Rev Molecul Cell Biol.* (2012) 13:448–62. doi: 10.1038/nrm3383

87. Hirschberg CB, Robbins PW, Abeijon C. Transporters of nucleotide sugars, ATP, and nucleotide sulfate in the endoplasmic reticulum and Golgi apparatus. *Annu Rev Biochem.* (1998) 67:49–69. doi: 10.1146/annurev.biochem.67.1.49

88. Wheeler SF, Rudd PM, Davis SJ, Dwek RA, Harvey DJ. Comparison of the N-linked glycans from soluble and GPI-anchored CD59 expressed in CHO cells. *Glycobiology* (2002) 12:261–71. doi: 10.1093/glycob/12.4.261

89. Thaysen-Andersen M, Packer NH. Site-specific glycoproteomics confirms that protein structure dictates formation of N-glycan type, core fucosylation

and branching. *Glycobiology* (2012) 22:1440–52. doi: 10.1093/glycob/cws110

90. Varki A. Biological roles of glycans. *Glycobiology* (2017) 27:3–49. doi: 10.1093/glycob/cww086

91. Chui D, Sellakumar G, Green R, Sutton-Smith M, McQuistan T, Marek K, et al. Genetic remodeling of protein glycosylation *in vivo* induces autoimmune disease. *Proc Natl Acad Sci USA.* (2001) 98:1142–7. doi: 10.1073/pnas.98.3.1142

92. Lee SJ, Evers S, Roeder D, Parlow AF, Risteli J, Risteli L, et al. Mannose receptor-mediated regulation of serum glycoprotein homeostasis. *Science* (2002) 295:1898–901. doi: 10.1126/science.1069540

93. Subedi GP, Barb AW. The structural role of antibody N-glycosylation in receptor interactions. *Structure* (2015) 23:1573–83. doi: 10.1016/j.str.2015.06.015

94. Chen G, Wang Y, Qiu L, Qin X, Liu H, Wang X, et al. Human IgG Fc-glycosylation profiling reveals associations with age, sex, female sex hormones and thyroid cancer. *J Proteom.* (2012) 75:2824–34. doi: 10.1016/j.jprot.2012.02.001

95. Dekkers G, Rispens T, Vidarsson G. Novel concepts of altered immunoglobulin G galactosylation in autoimmune diseases. *Front Immunol.* (2018) 9:553. doi: 10.3389/fimmu.2018.00553

96. Gardinassi LG, Dotz V, Hipgrave Ederveen A, de Almeida RP, Nery Costa CH, Costa DL, et al. Clinical severity of visceral leishmaniasis is associated with changes in immunoglobulin g fc N-glycosylation. *MBio* (2014) 5:e01844. doi: 10.1128/mBio.01844-14

97. Yu X, Wang Y, Kristic J, Dong J, Chu X, Ge S, et al. Profiling IgG N-glycans as potential biomarker of chronological and biological ages: a community-based study in a Han Chinese population. *Medicine* (2016) 95:e4112. doi: 10.1097/MD.0000000000004112

98. Subedi GP, Barb AW. The immunoglobulin G1 N-glycan composition affects binding to each low affinity Fc γ receptor. *MAbs* (2016) 8:1512–24. doi: 10.1080/19420862.2016.1218586

99. Bruggeman CW, Dekkers G, Visser R, Goes NWM, van den Berg TK, Rispens T, et al. IgG glyco-engineering to improve IVIg potency. *Front Immunol.* (2018) 9:2442. doi: 10.3389/fimmu.2018.02442

100. Li T, DiLillo DJ, Bournazos S, Giddens JP, Ravetch JV, Wang L-X. Modulating IgG effector function by Fc glycan engineering. *Proc Natl Acad Sci USA.* (2017) 114:3485–90. doi: 10.1073/pnas.1702173114

101. Fleit HB, Kuhnle M. Biochemical characterization of an Fc gamma receptor purified from human neutrophils. *J Immunol.* (1988) 140:3120–5.

102. Lanier LL, Ruitenberg JJ, Phillips JH. Functional and biochemical analysis of CD16 antigen on natural killer cells and granulocytes. *J Immunol.* (1988) 141:3478–85.

103. Edberg JC, Barinsky M, Redecha PB, Salmon JE, Kimberly RP. Fc gamma RIII expressed on cultured monocytes is a N-glycosylated transmembrane protein distinct from Fc gamma RIII expressed on natural killer cells. *J Immunol.* (1990) 144:4729–34.

104. Edberg JC, Kimberly RP. Cell type-specific glycoforms of Fc gamma RIIIa (CD16): differential ligand binding. *J Immunol.* (1997) 159:3849–57.

105. Galon J, Robertson MW, Galinha A, Maziéres N, Spagnoli R, Fridman W-H, et al. Affinity of the interaction between Fcgamma receptor type III (FcγRIII) and monomeric human IgG subclasses. Role of FcγRIII glycosylation. *Eur J Immunol.* (1997) 27:1928–32. doi: 10.1002/eji.1830270816

106. Hayes JM, Frostell A, Cosgrave EF, Struwe WB, Potter O, Davey GP, et al. Fc gamma receptor glycosylation modulates the binding of IgG glycoforms: a requirement for stable antibody interactions. *J Proteome Res.* (2014) 13:5471–85. doi: 10.1021/pr500414q

107. Jung ST, Kang TH, Georgiou G. Efficient expression and purification of human aglycosylated Fcγ receptors in Escherichia coli. *Biotechnol Bioeng.* (2010) 107:21–30. doi: 10.1002/bit.22785

108. Hayes JM, Frostell A, Karlsson R, Müller S, Martín SM, Pauers M, et al. Identification of Fc gamma receptor glycoforms that produce differential binding kinetics for rituximab. *Mol Cell Proteom.* (2017) 16:1770–88. doi: 10.1074/mcp.M117.066944

109. Patel KR, Roberts JT, Subedi GP, and Barb AW. Restricted processing of CD16a/Fc γ receptor IIIa N-glycans from primary human NK cells impacts structure and function. *J Biol Chem.* (2018) 293:3477–89. doi: 10.1074/jbc.RA117.001207

110. Subedi GP, Barb AW. CD16a with oligomannose-type N-glycans is the only "low affinity" Fc γ receptor that binds the IgG crystallizable fragment with high affinity *in vitro*. *J Biol Chem.* (2018) 293:16842–50. doi: 10.1074/jbc.RA118.004998

111. Yagi H, Takakura D, Roumenina LT, Fridman WH, Sautes-Fridman C, Kawasaki N, et al. Site-specific N-glycosylation analysis of soluble Fcgamma receptor IIIb in human serum. *Sci Rep.* (2018) 8:2719. doi: 10.1038/s41598-018-21145-y

112. Ruhaak LR, Xu G, Li Q, Goonatilleke E, Lebrilla CB. Mass spectrometry approaches to glycomic and glycoproteomic analyses. *Chem Rev.* (2018) 118:7886–930. doi: 10.1021/acs.chemrev.7b00732

113. Qian R, Chen C, Colley KJ. Location and mechanism of α2,6-Sialyltransferase dimer formation role of cysteine residues in enzyme dimerization, localization, activity, and processing. *J Biol Chem.* (2001) 276:28641–9. doi: 10.1074/jbc.M103664200

114. Cosgrave EF, Struwe WB, Hayes JM, Harvey DJ, Wormald MR, Rudd PM. N-linked glycan structures of the human Fcgamma receptors produced in NS0 cells. *J Proteome Res.* (2013) 12:3721–37. doi: 10.1021/pr400344h

115. Falconer DJ, Subedi GP, Marcella AM, Barb AW. Antibody Fucosylation lowers the FcγRIIIa/CD16a affinity by limiting the conformations sampled by the N162-Glycan. *ACS Chem Biol.* (2018) 13:2179–89. doi: 10.1021/acschembio.8b00342

116. Ferrara C, Stuart F, Sondermann P, Brunker P, Umana P. The carbohydrate at FcgammaRIIIa Asn-162. An element required for high affinity binding to non-fucosylated IgG glycoforms. *J Biol Chem.* (2006) 281:5032–6. doi: 10.1074/jbc.M510171200

117. Shibata-Koyama M, Iida S, Okazaki A, Mori K, Kitajima-Miyama K, Saitou S, et al. The N-linked oligosaccharide at FcγRIIIa Asn-45: an inhibitory element for high FcγRIIIa binding affinity to IgG glycoforms lacking core fucosylation. *Glycobiology* (2009) 19:126–34. doi: 10.1093/glycob/cwn110

118. Subedi GP, Falconer DJ, Barb AW. Carbohydrate-polypeptide contacts in the antibody receptor CD16A identified through solution NMR spectroscopy. *Biochemistry* (2017) 56:3174–7. doi: 10.1021/acs.biochem.7b00392

119. Zeck A, Pohlentz G, Schlothauer T, Peter-Katalinić J, Regula JT. Cell type-specific and site directed N-glycosylation pattern of FcγRIIIa. *J Proteome Res.* (2011) 10:3031–9. doi: 10.1021/pr1012653

120. Ory PA, Goldstein IM, Kwoh EE, Clarkson SB. Characterization of polymorphic forms of Fc receptor III on human neutrophils. *J Clin Invest.* (1989) 83:1676–81. doi: 10.1172/JCI114067

121. Salmon JE, Edberg JC, Brogle NL, Kimberly RP. Allelic polymorphisms of human Fc gamma receptor IIA and Fc gamma receptor IIIB. Independent mechanisms for differences in human phagocyte function. *J Clin Invest.* (1992) 89:1274–81. doi: 10.1172/JCI115712

122. Takahashi N, Cohen-Solal J, Galinha A, Fridman WH, Sautes-Fridman C, Kato K. N-glycosylation profile of recombinant human soluble Fcgamma receptor III. *Glycobiology* (2002) 12:507–15. doi: 10.1093/glycob/cwf063

123. Washburn N, Meccariello R, Duffner J, Getchell K, Holte K, Prod'homme T, et al. Characterization of endogenous human FcγRIII by mass spectrometry reveals site, allele and sequence specific glycosylation. *Molecul Cell Proteom.* (2018) 17:mcp.RA118.001142. doi: 10.1074/mcp.RA118.001142

124. Roberts JT, Barb AW. A single amino acid distorts the Fc γ receptor IIIb / CD16b structure upon binding immunoglobulin G1 and reduces affinity relative to CD16a. *J Biol Chem.* (2018) 293:19899–908. doi: 10.1074/jbc.RA118.005273

125. Parren PW, Warmerdam PA, Boeije LC, Arts J, Westerdaal NA, Vlug A, et al. On the interaction of IgG subclasses with the low affinity Fc gamma RIIa (CD32) on human monocytes, neutrophils, and platelets. Analysis of a functional polymorphism to human IgG2. *J Clin Invest.* (1992) 90:1537–46. doi: 10.1172/JCI116022

126. Harrison PT, Allen JM. High affinity IgG binding by FcgammaRI (CD64) is modulated by two distinct IgSF domains and the transmembrane domain of the receptor. *Protein Eng.* (1998) 11:225–32. doi: 10.1093/protein/11.3.225

127. Shields RL, Lai J, Keck R, O'Connell LY, Hong K, Meng YG, et al. Lack of fucose on human IgG1 N-linked oligosaccharide improves binding to human Fcgamma RIII and antibody-dependent cellular toxicity. *J Biol Chem.* (2002) 277:26733–40. doi: 10.1074/jbc.M202069200

128. Huang Z-Y, Barreda DR, Worth RG, Indik ZK, Kim M-K, Chien P, et al. Differential kinase requirements in human and mouse Fc-gamma receptor phagocytosis and endocytosis. *J Leukoc Biol.* (2006) 80:1553–62. doi: 10.1189/jlb.0106019

129. Chen K, Nishi H, Travers R, Tsuboi N, Martinod K, Wagner DD, et al. Endocytosis of soluble immune complexes leads to their clearance by FcγRIIIB but induces neutrophil extracellular traps via FcγRIIA *in vivo*. *Blood* (2012) 120:4421–31. doi: 10.1182/blood-2011-12-401133

130. Voice JK, Lachmann PJ. Neutrophil Fc gamma and complement receptors involved in binding soluble IgG immune complexes and in specific granule release induced by soluble IgG immune complexes. *Eur J Immunol.* (1997) 27:2514–23. doi: 10.1002/eji.1830271008

131. Ostreiko KK, Tumanova IA, Sykulev YK. Production and characterization of heat-aggregated IgG complexes with pre-determined molecular masses: light-scattering study. *Immunol Lett.* (1987) 15:311–6. doi: 10.1016/0165-2478(87)90134-9

132. St Clair JB, Detanico T, Aviszus K, Kirchenbaum GA, Christie M, Carpenter JF, et al. Immunogenicity of Isogenic IgG in aggregates and immune complexes. *PLoS ONE* (2017) 12:e0170556. doi: 10.1371/journal.pone.0170556

133. Koval M, Preiter K, Adles C, Stahl PD, Steinberg TH. Size of IgG-opsonized particles determines macrophage response during internalization. *Exp Cell Res.* (1998) 242:265–73. doi: 10.1006/excr.1998.4110

134. Lux A, Yu X, Scanlan CN, Nimmerjahn F. Impact of immune complex size and glycosylation on IgG binding to human FcgammaRs. *J Immunol.* (2013) 190:4315–23. doi: 10.4049/jimmunol.1200501

135. Robinett RA, Guan N, Lux A, Biburger M, Nimmerjahn F, Meyer AS. Dissecting FcgammaR regulation through a multivalent binding model. *Cell Syst.* (2018) 7:41–8.e5. doi: 10.1016/j.cels.2018.05.018

136. Stopforth RJ, Oldham RJ, Tutt AL, Duriez P, Chan HTC, Binkowski BF, et al. Detection of experimental and clinical immune complexes by measuring SHIP-1 recruitment to the inhibitory FcγRIIB. *J Immunol.* (2018) 200:1937–50. doi: 10.4049/jimmunol.1700832

137. Suurmond J, Diamond B. Autoantibodies in systemic autoimmune diseases: specificity and pathogenicity. *J Clin Invest.* (2015) 125:2194–202. doi: 10.1172/JCI78084

138. Zuercher AW, Spirig R, Baz Morelli A, Käsermann F. IVIG in autoimmune disease - Potential next generation biologics. *Autoimmun Rev.* (2016) 15:781–5. doi: 10.1016/j.autrev.2016.03.018

139. Samuelsson A, Towers TL, Ravetch JV. Anti-inflammatory activity of IVIG mediated through the inhibitory Fc receptor. *Science* (2001) 291:484–6. doi: 10.1126/science.291.5503.484

140. Nagelkerke SQ, Dekkers G, Kustiawan I, van de Bovenkamp FS, Geissler J, Plomp R, et al. Inhibition of FcgammaR-mediated phagocytosis by IVIg is independent of IgG-Fc sialylation and FcgammaRIIb in human macrophages. *Blood* (2014) 124:3709–18. doi: 10.1182/blood-2014-05-576835

141. Tremblay T, Paré I, Bazin R. Immunoglobulin G dimers and immune complexes are dispensable for the therapeutic efficacy of intravenous immune globulin in murine immune thrombocytopenia. *Transfusion* (2013) 53:261–9. doi: 10.1111/j.1537-2995.2012.03725.x

142. Kempers AC, Nejadnik MR, Rombouts Y, Ioan-Facsinay A, van Oosterhout M, Jiskoot W, et al. Fc gamma receptor binding profile of anti-citrullinated protein antibodies in immune complexes suggests a role for FcgammaRI in the pathogenesis of synovial inflammation. *Clin Exp Rheumatol.* (2018) 36:284–93.

143. Ortiz DF, Lansing JC, Rutitzky L, Kurtagic E, Prod'homme T, Choudhury A, et al. Elucidating the interplay between IgG-Fc valency and FcγR activation for the design of immune complex inhibitors. *Sci Transl Med.* (2016) 8:365ra158. doi: 10.1126/scitranslmed.aaf9418

144. Qureshi OS, Rowley TF, Junker F, Peters SJ, Crilly S, Compson J, et al. Multivalent Fc γ -receptor engagement by a hexameric Fc-fusion protein triggers Fc γ -receptor internalisation and modulation of Fc γ -receptor functions. *Sci Rep.* (2017) 7:17049. doi: 10.1038/s41598-017-17255-8

145. Kasturirangan S, Rainey GJ, Xu L, Wang X, Portnoff A, Chen T, et al. Targeted Fcγ receptor (FcγR)-mediated clearance by a biparatopic bispecific antibody. *J Biol Chem.* (2017) 292:4361–70. doi: 10.1074/jbc.M116.770628

146. Freeman G, Perera RAPM, Ngan E, Fang VJ, Cauchemez S, Ip DKM, et al. Quantifying homologous and heterologous antibody titer rises after influenza virus infection. *Epidemiol Infect.* (2016) 144:2306–16. doi: 10.1017/S0950268816000583

147. Bachmann MF, Kalinke U, Althage A, Freer G, Burkhart C, Roost H-P, et al. The role of antibody concentration and avidity in antiviral protection. *Science* (1997) 276:2024–7. doi: 10.1126/science.276.5321.2024

148. Gallo P, Goncalves R, Mosser DM. The influence of IgG density and macrophage Fc (gamma) receptor cross-linking on phagocytosis and IL-10 production. *Immunol Lett.* (2010) 133:70–7. doi: 10.1016/j.imlet.2010.07.004

149. Taborda CP, Rivera J, Zaragoza O, Casadevall A. More is not necessarily better: prozone-like effects in passive immunization with IgG. *J Immunol.* (2003) 170:3621–30. doi: 10.4049/jimmunol.170.7.3621

150. Chan KR, Zhang SL-X, Tan HC, Chan YK, Chow A, Lim APC, et al. Ligation of Fc gamma receptor IIB inhibits antibody-dependent enhancement of dengue virus infection. *Proc Natl Acad Sci USA.* (2011) 108:12479–84. doi: 10.1073/pnas.1106568108

151. Corey L, Gilbert PB, Tomaras GD, Haynes BF, Pantaleo G, Fauci AS. Immune correlates of vaccine protection against HIV-1 acquisition. *Sci Transl Med.* (2015) 7:310rv7. doi: 10.1126/scitranslmed.aac7732

152. Ferrante A, Beard LJ, Feldman RG. IgG subclass distribution of antibodies to bacterial and viral antigens. *Pediatr Infec Dis J.* (1990) 9:516. doi: 10.1097/00006454-199008001-00004

153. Yamada DH, Elsaesser H, Lux A, Timmerman JM, Morrison SL, de la Torre JC, et al. Suppression of Fcgamma-receptor-mediated antibody effector function during persistent viral infection. *Immunity* (2015) 42:379–90. doi: 10.1016/j.immuni.2015.01.005

154. Dowd KA, Jost CA, Durbin AP, Whitehead SS, Pierson TC. A dynamic landscape for antibody binding modulates antibody-mediated neutralization of west nile virus. *PLoS Pathog.* (2011) 7:e1002111. doi: 10.1371/journal.ppat.1002111

155. Mazor Y, Yang C, Borrok MJ, Ayriss J, Aherne K, Wu H, et al. Enhancement of immune effector functions by modulating IgG's intrinsic affinity for target antigen. *PLoS ONE* (2016) 11:e0157788. doi: 10.1371/journal.pone.0157788

156. Kim MS, Lee SH, Song MY, Yoo TH, Lee BK, Kim YS. Comparative analyses of complex formation and binding sites between human tumor necrosis factor-alpha and its three antagonists elucidate their different neutralizing mechanisms. *J Mol Biol.* (2007) 374:1374–88. doi: 10.1016/j.jmb.2007.10.034

157. Saphire EO, Schendel SL, Fusco ML, Gangavarapu K, Gunn BM, Wec AZ, et al. Systematic analysis of monoclonal antibodies against Ebola virus GP defines features that contribute to protection. *Cell* (2018) 174:938–52.e13. doi: 10.1016/j.cell.2018.07.033

158. Ferrant JL, Wilson CA, Benjamin CD, Hess DM, Hsu Y-M, Karpusas M, et al. Variation in the ordered structure of complexes between CD154 and anti-CD154 monoclonal antibodies. *Molecul Immunol.* (2002) 39:77–84. doi: 10.1016/S0161-5890(02)00045-7

159. Booth JW, Kim M-K, Jankowski A, Schreiber AD, Grinstein S. Contrasting requirements for ubiquitylation during Fc receptor-mediated endocytosis and phagocytosis. *EMBO J.* (2002) 21:251–8. doi: 10.1093/emboj/21.3.251

160. Cherry RJ. Rotational and lateral diffusion of membrane proteins. *Biochim Biophys Acta* (1979) 559:289–327. doi: 10.1016/0304-4157(79)90009-1

161. Beningo KA, Wang YL. Fc-receptor-mediated phagocytosis is regulated by mechanical properties of the target. *J Cell Sci.* (2002) 115:849–56.

162. Ben M'Barek K, Molino D, Quignard S, Plamont MA, Chen Y, Chavrier P, et al. Phagocytosis of immunoglobulin-coated emulsion droplets. *Biomaterials* (2015) 51:270–7. doi: 10.1016/j.biomaterials.2015.02.030

163. Shashidharamurthy R, Zhang F, Amano A, Kamat A, Panchanathan R, Ezekwudo D, et al. Dynamics of the interaction of human IgG subtype immune-complexes with cells expressing R and H allelic forms of a low affinity Fc gamma receptor CD32A. *J Immunol.* (2009) 183:8216–24. doi: 10.4049/jimmunol.0902550

164. Bruhns P, Iannascoli B, England P, Mancardi DA, Fernandez N, Jorieux S, et al. Specificity and affinity of human Fcγ receptors and their polymorphic variants for human IgG subclasses. *Blood* (2009) 113:3716–25. doi: 10.1182/blood-2008-09-179754

165. Rowley TF, Peters SJ, Aylott M, Griffin R, Davies NL, Healy LJ, et al. Engineered hexavalent Fc proteins with enhanced Fc-gamma receptor avidity

provide insights into immune-complex interactions. *Commun Biol.* (2018) 1:146. doi: 10.1038/s42003-018-0149-9

166. Chow S-K, Smith C, MacCarthy T, Pohl MA, Bergman A, Casadevall A. Disease-enhancing antibodies improve the efficacy of bacterial toxin-neutralizing antibodies. *Cell Host Microbe* (2013) 13:417–28. doi: 10.1016/j.chom.2013.03.001

167. Bruhns P. Properties of mouse and human IgG receptors and their contribution to disease models. *Blood* (2012) 119:5640–9. doi: 10.1182/blood-2012-01-380121

168. Chan YN, Boesch AW, Osei-Owusu NY, Emileh A, Crowley AR, Cocklin SL, et al. IgG Binding characteristics of rhesus macaque FcγR. *J Immunol.* (2016) 197:2936–47. doi: 10.4049/jimmunol.1502252

169. Chenoweth AM, Trist HM, Tan P-S, Wines BD, Hogarth PM. The high-affinity receptor for IgG, FcγRI, of humans and non-human primates. *Immunol Rev.* (2015) 268:175–91. doi: 10.1111/imr.12366

170. Dekkers G, Bentlage AEH, Stegmann TC, Howie HL, Lissenberg-Thunnissen S, Zimring J, et al. Affinity of human IgG subclasses to mouse Fc gamma receptors. *MAbs* (2017) 9:767–73. doi: 10.1080/19420862.2017.1323159

171. Derebe MG, Nanjunda RK, Gilliland GL, Lacy ER, Chiu ML. Human IgG subclass cross-species reactivity to mouse and cynomolgus monkey Fcγ receptors. *Immunol Lett.* (2018) 197:1–8. doi: 10.1016/j.imlet.2018.02.006

172. Gillis C, Gouel-Chéron A, Jönsson F, Bruhns P. Contribution of human FcγRs to disease with evidence from human polymorphisms and transgenic animal studies. *Front Immunol.* 5:254. doi: 10.3389/fimmu.2014.00254

173. Hogarth PM, Anania JC, Wines BD. The FcγR of humans and non-human primates and their interaction with IgG: implications for induction of inflammation, resistance to infection and the use of therapeutic monoclonal antibodies. *Curr Top Microbiol Immunol.* (2014) 382:321–52. doi: 10.1007/978-3-319-07911-0_15

174. Dekkers G, Bentlage AEH, Plomp R, Visser R, Koeleman CAM, Beentjes A, et al. Conserved FcγR- glycan discriminates between fucosylated and afucosylated IgG in humans and mice. *Mol Immunol.* (2018) 94:54–60. doi: 10.1016/j.molimm.2017.12.006

175. Lux A, Seeling M, Baerenwaldt A, Lehmann B, Schwab I, Repp R., et al. A humanized mouse identifies the bone marrow as a niche with low therapeutic IgG activity. *Cell Rep.* (2014) 7:236–48. doi: 10.1016/j.celrep.2014.02.041

176. Smith P, DiLillo DJ, Bournazos S, Li F, Ravetch JV. Mouse model recapitulating human Fcγ receptor structural and functional diversity. *Proc Natl Acad Sci USA.* (2012) 109:6181–6. doi: 10.1073/pnas.1203954109

177. Trottein F, Schaffer L, Ivanov S, Paget C, Vendeville C, Groux-Degroote S, et al. Glycosyltransferase and sulfotransferase gene expression profiles in human monocytes, dendritic cells and macrophages. *Glycoconj J.* (2009) 26:1259–74. doi: 10.1007/s10719-009-9244-y

10

Targeting the Antibody Checkpoints to Enhance Cancer Immunotherapy–Focus on FcγRIIB

Ingrid Teige, Linda Mårtensson and Björn L. Frendéus*

BioInvent, Lund, Sweden

*Correspondence:
Björn L. Frendéus
bjorn.frendeus@bioinvent.com

Immunotherapy with therapeutic antibodies has increased survival for patients with hematologic and solid cancers. Still, a significant fraction of patients fails to respond to therapy or acquire resistance. Understanding and overcoming mechanisms of resistance to antibody drugs, and in particular those common to antibody drugs as a class, is therefore highly warranted and holds promise to improve response rates, duration of response and potentially overall survival. Activating and inhibitory Fc gamma receptors (FcγR) are known to coordinately regulate therapeutic activity of tumor direct-targeting antibodies. Similar, but also divergent, roles for FcγRs in controlling efficacy of immune modulatory antibodies e.g., checkpoint inhibitors have been indicated from mouse studies, and were recently implicated in contributing to efficacy in the human clinical setting. Here we discuss evidence and mechanisms by which Fc gamma receptors–the "antibody checkpoints"–regulate antibody-induced antitumor immunity. We further discuss how targeted blockade of the sole known inhibitory antibody checkpoint FcγRIIB may help overcome resistance and boost activity of clinically validated and emerging antibodies in cancer immunotherapy.

Keywords: therapeutic antibody, antibody checkpoint, fc gamma receptor, cancer immunotherapy, drug resistance, tumor microenvironment

INTRODUCTION

Monoclonal antibody-based therapies have revolutionized cancer treatment improving survival for patients with hematologic and solid cancers. The clinically most successful antibodies exert antitumor activity either by targeting tumor cells directly (direct-targeting antibodies) (1–4), or by targeting and activating immune cells that seek up and kill cancer cells in the tumor microenvironment (immune checkpoint antibodies) (5–13).

While both types of mAb are highly potent with cancer curative potential a significant fraction of patients fail to respond or develop resistance to treatment (14–17). An improved understanding of mechanisms underlying resistance, and in particular those common to antibody drugs as a class–including direct-targeting and immune checkpoint antibodies–is needed for rational development of drugs that could help boost efficacy, and prevent or overcome antibody drug resistance. Given the broad use of antibodies in cancer treatment, such drugs would have the potential to fundamentally improve cancer survival.

FcγR Regulation of Antibody-Induced Immunity–"The Antibody Checkpoints"

The Fc receptors (FcR) are the only receptors of the immune system known to regulate the activity of antibodies as a class (18). FcRs orchestrate antibody-induced effector cell responses and immunity through low affinity, high avidity interactions with aggregated antibody Fc-domains of antibody-coated cells or immune complexes, generated following antibody Fv-binding to target receptors. Because Fc domains are conserved between antibodies of a given subclass e.g., IgA, IgE, IgM, or IgG$_1$, IgG$_2$, IgG$_3$ or IgG$_4$, FcRs regulate antibody-induced immune responses irrespective of antigen specificity. For this same reason FcRs regulate immune responses induced both by endogenously generated antibodies (e.g., antibodies mounted in response to infection or underlying inflammatory or autoimmune disease) and recombinantly produced therapeutic monoclonal antibodies (18, 19). Of particular relevance for cancer immunotherapy the Fc gamma receptors (FcγR) are known to regulate the activity of Immunoglobulin G type of antibodies (20), the group to which all antibodies approved for cancer therapy belong.

The family of FcγRs share several characteristics with the T cell immune checkpoints in how they regulate effector cell activation and immune responses (**Figure 1**). Recent work by ourselves and others, reviewed in detail below, demonstrate a critical role for this receptor family as concerted regulators of antibody-induced innate and adaptive immunity. Consequently, the FcγRs are therapeutically important immune checkpoints, and since they control immune activity of IgG antibodies as a class, we propose to refer to them as "antibody checkpoints." We will herein use antibody checkpoint and FcγR interchangeably.

Antibody and T Cell Checkpoints–Similarities and Differences

Like the T cell checkpoints the Fc gamma receptors (FcγR) fall into either of two functionally distinct groups, which coordinately regulate immune effector cell activation and ensuing immune responses (**Figure 1**). Activating FcγR, like co-stimulatory T cell checkpoints, promote effector cell activation, and immunity. In contrast, inhibitory FcγR, like the T cell co-inhibitory checkpoints, block cellular activation and down-modulate immune responses. Adding to complexity, antibody checkpoints may–similar to the T cell checkpoints–promote checkpoint receptor extrinsic signaling by facilitating cross-linking and signaling of ligand receptors (21, 22). In case of the antibody checkpoints, this would equate to FcγR-mediated cross-linking of antibody Fv-targeted receptors (**Figure 2**). Depending on ligand receptor function, such signaling may be activating or inhibitory, as has been described for agonistic CD40 and agonistic Fas antibodies, respectively (23–27). FcγR extrinsic signaling may, or may not, contribute to therapeutic efficacy.

The activating and the inhibitory FcγR receptors transmit their signals into FcγR-bearing immune cell via immunoreceptor tyrosine-based activation motifs (ITAM), and immunoreceptor tyrosine-based inhibitory motifs (ITIM), respectively. Specifically, how target cell-bound antibodies modulate immune

cell activation is determined by their relative engagement of activating and inhibitory Fcγ receptors. This in turn is determined by the size of the FcγR-engaging immune complex, i.e., the number of antibodies coated onto a target cell (determined by cellular expression levels of antibody targeted receptor), availability of activating and inhibitory Fcγ receptors, and antibody isotype. Different antibody isotypes bind with different affinity to activating and inhibitory Fcγ receptors, resulting in different activating: inhibitory (A:I) ratios, and differential ability to mediate e.g., activating FcγR-dependent target cell deletion (28) or inhibitory FcγR-dependent agonism (23, 24).

As in the T cell checkpoint family, there are several activating antibody checkpoints that individually, and collectively, positively regulate antibody-induced cell activation. In humans, the activating FcγR's are: FcγRI (CD64), FcγRIIa (CD32a), FcγRIIc (CD32c), and FcγRIIIa (CD16a) (29, 30). The GPI-linked FcγRIIIb lacks an intracellular signaling domain and ITAM motifs, but is nevertheless often considered an activating FcγR, since it has been shown to promote neutrophil activation and effector cell mediated target cell killing in response to challenge with antibody-coated target cells (31, 32). The activating mouse FcγRs are: FcγRI, FcγRIII, and FcγRIV (28, 30, 33).

Most Fc gamma receptors bind monomeric IgG with low to intermediate (μM) affinity [as reviewed in detail elsewhere (28, 29, 33)]. Immune complex formation allows for high-avidity binding of multimerized IgG Fc's to the low-affinity FcγRs, which are cross-linked, leading to FcγR-expressing cell activation. In contrast, free circulating IgG has too low affinity to promote stable Fc:FcγR binding, and cannot promote FcγR-cross-linking, or cell activation. How high affinity FcγRs e.g., FcγRI and mouse FcγRIV, which may bind monomeric uncomplexed IgG, sense and trigger activation in response to immune complexes and antibody-coated cells remains a subject of debate. It is however clear that the high affinity FcγRs may critically contribute to therapeutic antibody efficacy and pathology (33, 34).

Multiple isoforms and allelic variants of the individual FcγRs are known, and the affinities of the clinically most significant variants for different human IgG subclasses have been described (29). Of particular significance for cancer immunotherapy, two isoforms of the low and intermediary affinity antibody checkpoints FcγRIIa (H131R) and FcγRIIIa (V158F), which bind IgG and antibody-coated target cells with higher affinity and avidity, have been associated with improved survival of diverse cancer patients in response to antibody-based cancer immunotherapy (35–39). These, and additional polymorphisms of low and intermediary affinity activating and inhibitory FcγRs, which alter affinity for IgG, or modulate FcγR expression levels, are further associated with susceptibility to antibody-mediated chronic inflammatory and autoimmune disease (40). Of further functional consequence, there is extensive gene copy number variation in high and low affinity loci that affect expression levels of individual FcγRs (41–43).

The antibody checkpoints differ from the T cell checkpoints in notable and critical aspects, which have important consequences for the type of immune response induced, and for design

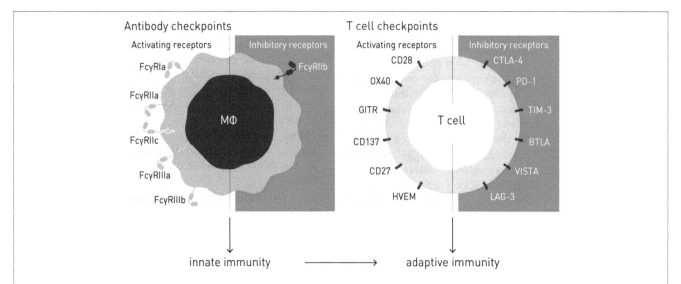

FIGURE 1 | Antibody and T cell checkpoints. Both T cell and antibody checkpoints comprise activating (co-stimulatory) and inhibitory receptors. However, antibody checkpoints are co- expressed only on innate immune cells e.g., macrophages and dendritic cells, and comprise only a single inhibitory member (FcγRIIB).

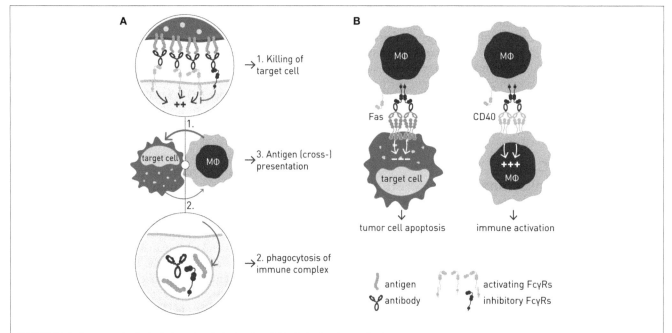

FIGURE 2 | Antibody checkpoint intrinsic and extrinsic signaling. **(A)** Intrinsic signaling. Antibody checkpoints relay aggregated antibody Fc-induced signals into effector cells (MΦ) in a concerted manner through ITAM containing activating (aFcγR) and ITIM-containing inhibitory (iFcγR) Fc gamma receptors. FcγR-expressing cell responses include phagocytosis, immune complex endocytosis, and antigen presentation. **(B)** Extrinsic signaling. Antibody checkpoints promote clustering and signaling induced by antibody targeted receptors in an antibody Fv and Fc co-dependent manner. Cellular responses are determined by the antibody-targeted receptor's function e.g., macrophage co-stimulation or tumor cell apoptosis.

of drugs aimed at harnessing and enhancing FcγR-mediated immunity (**Figure 1**).

Firstly, in contrast to the T cell checkpoints the Fc gamma receptors are not generally expressed on T cells, but principally on cells of the innate immune system, and in a restricted manner on B cells (FcγRIIb) and NK cells (FcγRIIIa and FcγRIIc, the latter in ∼20% of caucasians) (18, 30, 41). In particular cells specialized in MHC class II-restricted antigen presentation, e.g., macrophages and dendritic cells, express both activating and inhibitory FcγRs, enabling fine-tuned regulation of antibody-induced immune responses (28, 44). Consequently, the antibody checkpoints hold the key to unleash antibody-induced immunity first and fore-most through improving innate immune effector mechanisms, e.g., macrophage dependent phagocytosis (ADCP), and dendritic cell mediated antigen presentation, and cross-presentation (45–51). Triggering and enhancing innate immune activation and robust antigen presentation is known to critically contribute to and underlie robust adaptive T cell-mediated antitumor responses, including those induced by antibodies targeting T cell checkpoints (18, 52–54). Modulation of antibody checkpoints therefore has the potential to improve also adaptive antitumor responses, possibly decreasing the threshold of tumor mutational burden for cancers to respond to antibody-mediated cancer immunotherapy (55). Finally, and in stark contrast to the multiple inhibitory T cell checkpoints described, only a single inhibitory antibody checkpoint–Fc gamma receptor IIB–is known (**Figure 1**).

ANTIBODY CHECKPOINTS DETERMINE ANTI-CANCER ANTIBODY EFFICACY

Cancer Cell Direct-Targeting Antibodies

The CD20-specific antibody rituximab was the first antibody to be approved by the FDA for cancer therapy and is arguably the clinically best validated antibody used in cancer immunotherapy. As such rituximab provides a prime example of a tumor cell direct-targeting antibody that has been exhaustively studied from a mechanism-of-action perspective. While multiple mechanisms, including induction of apoptosis and triggering of complement mediated cell lysis, have been proposed to contribute to and underlie rituximab therapeutic activity (56, 57), the strongest preclinical, and clinical evidence point to Fc gamma receptor dependent mechanisms (58–61).

Independent retrospective studies have established a correlation between one or more activating Fc gamma receptors and clinical efficacy in different types of lymphoma. Patients homozygous for high affinity allelic variants of the activating antibody checkpoints FcγRIIIa or FcγRIIa showed improved responses and survival in response to rituximab therapy compared to patients carrying one or more lower affinity alleles (35, 36). Similar links between response and FcγR-dependent mechanisms have been observed for additional cancer cell direct-targeting antibodies e.g., herceptin (anti-Her2) and cetuximab (anti-EGFR) in breast cancer (38) and colorectal patients, respectively (37, 39). These observations have spurred biotech and pharmaceutical companies to engineer antibodies with improved binding to activating antibody checkpoints. Obinutuzumab, a glycoengineered antibody with improved affinity for FcγRIIIa, was approved for clinical use based on increased overall survival in a head-to-head comparison with rituximab in CLL patients (15). Taken together, these observations demonstrate that antibody checkpoints can determine clinical efficacy of cancer cell direct-targeting antibodies.

Consistent with the well-conserved function of activating and inhibitory antibody checkpoints between mouse and man, similar dependencies between activating FcγRs and cancer cell direct-targeting antibodies have been made in mouse cancer experimental models. Further in keeping with common, ITAM-signaling dependent, functions of the several activating antibody

checkpoints, genetic ablation of individual activating FcγRs typically has shown limited effects on *in vivo* therapeutic efficacy compared to ablation of all activatory FcγRs (28, 33, 62).

In stark contrast, genetic deletion of the sole inhibitory antibody checkpoint FcγRIIB fundamentally enhances *in vivo* therapeutic activity of cancer cell direct-targeting antibodies, including those specific for CD20, Her2, and EGFR i.e., clinically validated targets in therapy of hematologic malignancy as well as solid cancer (63). These observations indicate the significant therapeutic potential of targeting the inhibitory antibody checkpoint, and indicate that redundancy needs to be accounted for when seeking to enhance antibody efficacy by modulating activating antibody checkpoints, much as has been observed in targeting of the multiple different T cell checkpoints (6, 14, 64).

Interestingly, and in further support of FcγRIIB being a tractable target in cancer immunotherapy, recent data has demonstrated that this inhibitory antibody checkpoint limits therapeutic antibody efficacy and promotes antibody drug resistance by additional mechanisms distinct from inhibitory signaling in immune effector cells, when expressed on tumor B cells (65) (**Figure 3**). Beers et al. found that FcγRIIB expressed on tumor B cells promoted internalization of rituximab antibody molecules from the tumor B cell surface, increasing antibody consumption and leaving fewer rituximab molecules to engage critical FcγR-dependent effector cell-mediated antitumor activity e.g., ADCP (66). FcγRIIB expression correlated with rituximab internalization across several different lymphoma subtypes studied. Highest and most homogenous expression of FcγRIIB is observed in Chronic Lymphocytic Leukemia (CLL), Mantle cell lymphoma (MCL), and Marginal Zone Lymphoma, although a fraction of Follicular lymphoma (FL) and Diffuse Large B cell Lymphoma show exceptionally high FcγRIIB expression (67, 68). Further consistent with tumor B cell expressed FcγRIIB limiting antibody therapeutic efficacy and promoting antibody resistance, retrospective clinical studies of MCL and FL patients treated with rituximab-containing therapy showed decreased survival of patients with higher FcγRIIB expression on tumor cells (67, 69). Tumor cell expressed FcγRIIB appears to be a general mechanism limiting antibody therapeutic efficacy and promoting antibody drug resistance in the tumor microenvironment. Using a humanized model of treatment refractory B cell leukemia, and the CD52-specific antibody alemtuzumab, Pallasch et al. found that FcγRIIB is highly overexpressed on leukemic tumor cells in such antibody drug-resistant tumor microenvironments, and that shRNA-mediated knock-down of tumor cell FcγRIIB restored responsiveness to therapeutic antibody resulting in animal cure (70). Finally, high expression of FcγRIIB in B cell malignancy may indicate that immunocompetent antibodies to FcγRIIB could have single agent therapeutic activity in this setting (65, 71).

Collectively, these and other observations provided the rationale to develop antagonistic anti-FcγRIIB antibodies that block FcγRIIB-mediated antibody internalization for combination immunotherapy of B cell cancer with direct-targeting antibodies e.g., rituximab (65, 72) (**Figure 3**).

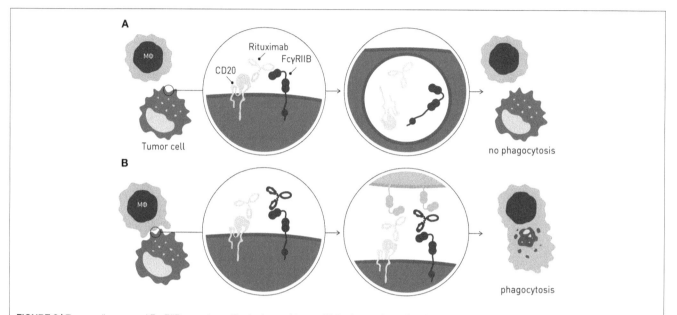

FIGURE 3 | Tumor cell expressed FcγRIIB promotes antibody drug resistance. **(A)** Resistance is mediated by FcγRIIB-mediated removal of antibody molecules from the tumor cell surface through a process of internalization. **(B)** Blocking antibodies to FcγRIIB prevent internalization, leaving greater numbers of therapeutic antibody on the tumor cell surface, promoting immune effector cell-mediated antitumor activity.

Antibodies to Immune Checkpoint Inhibitory Receptors

Antibody targeting of immune inhibitory T cell checkpoints e.g., CTLA-4, PD-1 and PD-L1 has transformed solid cancer therapy shifting focus from cancer cell-direct targeting therapies to immune modulatory drugs, which induce long-term remission and apparent cures albeit in a small fraction of advanced stage cancer patients. Such immune checkpoint-directed therapy has increased overall survival for patients with various cancers, notably including multiple solid cancer types e.g., melanoma, lung, bladder, and head and neck cancer, and are approved by the Food and Drug Administration (14, 73, 74).

While originally thought to act solely via "blocking the brake" on effector T cells (74, 75), recent preclinical and clinical data indicate a critical role for FcγR's in regulating therapeutic efficacy of antibodies to inhibitory T cell checkpoints. Vargas et al. for the first time in human subjects, demonstrated a link between antibody checkpoints, and clinical response to T cell checkpoint targeted antibody therapy (76). Melanoma patients carrying a high affinity allele of the activating FcγRIIIa (V158) showed improved survival in response to treatment with the anti-CTLA-4 antibody ipilimumab compared to patients carrying a lower affinity FcγRIIIa (F158) allele. Interestingly, in the two retrospectively studied cohorts, a prerequisite for response to anti-CTLA-4 antibody therapy was that patients had inflamed tumors i.e., T cells had infiltrated tumors prior to commencing therapy. The observation that antibody checkpoints determine clinical efficacy of ipilimumab was not unexpected, since anti-CTLA-4 antibody therapy in the mouse critically depends on FcγR-mediated deletion of regulatory T cells (77–80), which express CTLA-4 at higher levels compared with effector T

cells in the tumor microenvironment (76). Consistent with co-ordinate regulation of anti-CTLA-4 antibody therapeutic efficacy by the antibody checkpoints, in a FcγR-humanized mouse model antibody variants engineered for enhanced binding to activatory FcγR showed enhanced therapeutic activity (76). In contrast, antibody variants with diminished binding to activating FcγR failed to induce protective immunity against cancer.

So, how about the other clinically validated T cell checkpoints? Do antibody checkpoints regulate the activity also of antibodies targeting the PD-1/PD-L1 axis? Evidence from mouse models suggests that indeed they do. Interestingly, however, these data indicate differential FcγR-regulation for anti-PD-1 and anti-PD-L1 antibodies. Dahan et al. reported that anti-PD-L1 antibodies therapeutic efficacy was enhanced with antibody isotypes that preferentially engage activating over inhibitory antibody checkpoints (81). Conversely, anti-PD-1 antibody variants that did not engage FcγRs showed greatest therapeutic activity, and FcγR-engaging antibodies' activity decreased with increasing A:I ratios. Similarly, Pittet and coworkers found that *in vitro* and *in vivo* efficacy of clinically approved anti-PD-1 antibodies nivolumab and pembrolizumab, and a murine surrogate antibody variant with claimed similar engagement of mouse FcγR compared to these mAb, was compromised by FcγR-engagement (82). Deglycosylation of antibodies with EndoS rendering them incapable of engaging FcγRs, or antibody-mediated FcγR-blockade, significantly improved anti-PD-1 antibody therapeutic activity. This demonstrates that FcγRs negatively regulate anti-PD-1 antibody efficacy. Further studies are needed to dissect the relative importance of activating vs. inhibitory antibody checkpoints in regulating anti-PD-1/PD-L1 antibodies' therapeutic activity.

Antibodies to Immune Checkpoint Co-stimulatory Receptors

The power of treating cancer by engaging patient's own immune defense mechanisms through immunotherapy with antibodies to the co-inhibitory T cell checkpoints, has prompted the question of whether targeting also co-stimulatory immune checkpoints e.g., 4-1BB, OX40, CD40, and GITR can translate into similarly efficacious and perhaps complementary pathways of anti-cancer immunity?

Preclinical and limited clinical data has indicated both single agent activity of antibodies to co-stimulatory immune checkpoints and complementary effects following combination with checkpoint blocking antibodies e.g., anti-PD-1 (83–89). As found for antibodies to the immune inhibitory checkpoints, and as discussed below, efficacy of immune agonist checkpoint antibodies is regulated by the FcγRs (77–79, 89), with some showing preferential engagement of activatory FcγR (i.e., high A:I ratio), and others of inhibitory FcγR (i.e., low A:I ratio), for optimal therapeutic activity (**Table 1**).

So, what is the common denominator determining FcγR-dependency, and preferential engagement of inhibitory vs. activating FcγR for efficacy of individual targets and antibodies? In a recent landmark paper, Beers and co-workers used a multi-pronged approach to study molecular and cellular FcγR-dependent mechanisms underlying therapeutic activity of antibodies to the co-stimulatory immune checkpoint 4-1BB (89). Firstly, the authors used anti-4-1BB antibodies with identical Fv-regions but differing in isotype–therefore targeting the same epitope on 4-1BB but showing preferential engagement of activating (mouse IgG2a, high A:I ratio) or inhibitory (mouse IgG1, low A:I ratio) antibody checkpoints. Second, effects were studied in immunocompetent tumor-bearing animals differing only by FcγR repertoire–expressing only activating, only inhibitory or both activating and inhibitory antibody checkpoints. Using this approach, the authors found that anti-4-1BB antibodies can stimulate anti-tumor immunity by different mechanisms; Boosting of effector CD8+ T cells, or depletion of regulatory T cells (**Figure 4**). Both mechanisms were regulated by antibody interactions with FcγR, but differently so.

Anti-4-1BB antibodies' depletion of intratumoral Treg cells was shown to be dependent on activating FcγR (89). Antibody isotypes with high A:I ratio showed enhanced Treg deletion, and Treg deletion was diminished in animals lacking activating Fc gamma receptors. A similar dependence on activating antibody checkpoints for Treg depletion had previously been demonstrated for antibodies to other immune receptors e.g., GITR, OX40, CD40, CTLA-4, or IL-2R, i.e., independent of specificity for co-stimulatory or inhibitory immune checkpoints (**Table 1**).

Conversely, boosting of CD8+ T cell responses was most pronounced with antibody isotypes of low A:I ratio. The mechanism underlying enhanced CD8+ T cell responses likely involves FcγRIIB-mediated antibody cross-linking, and thereby promoted signaling, of antibody-targeted co-stimulatory 4-1BB receptors on CD8+ T cells. Agonist anti-tumor activity of anti-CD40 antibodies has previously been proposed to rely

on FcγRIIB-mediated antibody cross-linking and promoted signaling in CD40-expressing antigen presenting cells (23, 24) (**Table 1**; **Figure 2B**).

Interestingly, the authors found that concurrent administration of equal doses of high A:I variant (mIgG2a), Treg-depleting, anti-4-1BB antibodies, and low A:I variant (mIgG1), CD8+ T cell boosting, anti-4-1BB antibodies reduced therapeutic efficacy. In contrast, sequential administration of first activating FcγR-optimized antibody to deplete Tregs, followed by inhibitory FcγR-optimized antibody to agonize CD8+ T cells, enhanced therapeutic efficacy compared to single agent treatment. These observations indicated competing mechanisms of high A:I antibody mediated Treg depletion, and low A:I antibody mediated CD8+ T cell boosting. This notion that was corroborated through a series of complementary experiments. In short, although the two studied isotype variant antibodies show preferential binding to activatory (mIgG2a, high A:I ratio) and inhibitory (mIgG1, low A:I ratio) FcγRs, respectively, both antibody variants will co-engage activating and inhibitory FcγRs in vivo, where their "preferred" type (activating or inhibitory) of FcγR on effector cells is limited in numbers, relative to target cell coated antibody Fc's available for FcγR engagement. Therefore, concurrently administered high A:I ratio and low A:I ratio antibodies will compete for binding to available activating and inhibitory FcγR, resulting in a "frustrated system" of suboptimal Treg depletion and suboptimal CD8+ T cell boosting.

Importantly, if translated to human, these findings could have broad implications for cancer immunotherapy. Human IgG1 and IgG4 antibodies–two of the most common isotypes used in cancer immunotherapy–bind human activating and inhibitory FcγRs with rather similar affinity, compared with the more "polar" affinities of mIgG2a and mIgG1 for activating, and inhibitory FcγRs, respectively. Human IgG1 and IgG4 might therefore be expected to be quite sensitive to such competition, which could help explain the poor translation of promising mouse data to the human clinical setting. Further, the findings are likely relevant to other signaling antibody targets, most notably co-stimulatory receptors of the TNF receptor superfamily. Earlier studies had reported decreased efficacy following concurrent treatment with antibodies to OX40 and PD-1, although underlying molecular mechanisms were not studied (88).

Collectively, these observations shed important light on how antibody checkpoints regulate mechanisms common to cancer cell direct-targeting and immune checkpoint targeting antibodies. Therapeutic activity of either type of antibody may rely principally on target cell depletion (e.g., anti-CD20 or anti-IL-2R), cell depletion and block of target receptor signaling (e.g., anti-Her2 or anti-CTLA-4), or strictly on receptor/ligand blockade e.g., anti-PD-1 (**Figure 5**). Thus, classification of antibodies into cancer cell-direct targeting, immune checkpoint blocking, or immune checkpoint agonists, is inadequate and needs revision (98). Instead, careful dissection of individual antibodies' mechanism(s) of action with respect to their ability to block or agonize receptor signaling and/or deplete target cell(s), and their regulation by interactions with

TABLE 1 | Antibody checkpoints determine efficacy and mechanism-of-action of immune modulatory antibodies.

Antibody MoA		Co-stimulatory checkpoints				IL-2R	Co-inhibitory checkpoints		
		GITR	OX40	4-1BB	CD40		CTLA-4	PD-1	PD-L1
High A:I ratio	Effect	Treg depletion			CD40⁺ cell depletion	Treg depletion	Treg depletion	*FcγRs reduce efficacy	TAM depletion?
	FcγR-modulation	aFcγR↑ iFcγR↓	aFcγR↑	aFcγR↑ iFcγR↓	aFcγR↑ iFcγR↓	aFcγR↑ iFcγR↓	aFcγR↑ iFcγR↓		aFcγR↑ iFcγR↓
Low A:I ratio	Effect	Teff costimulation			APC costimul.				
	FcγR-modulation		aFcγR↓ iFcγR↑	aFcγR↓ iFcγR↑	aFcγR↓ iFcγR↑				
FcγR-indep. mAbs	Effect						Block Teff suppression		
	Isotype(s)	rIgG2b	mIgG1	mIgG2a, mIgG1	mIgG1, hIgG1/2/SE/ SELF/V9/V11	rIgG1, mIgG2a	haIgG, hIgG1	mIgG1/2a/ ¹D265A, rIgG1, hIgG4	mIgG1/2a/ ¹D265A
	Clone(s)	DTA-1	OX86	LOB12.0	1C10, 3/23, FGK45, CP-870,893	PC-61	9H10, 4F10, 9D9, ipilimumab	4H2, RPMI-14, nivolumab, pembro	14D8

*Table indicates antibody Mechanism-of-Action (**MoA**) as a function of antibody isotype preferential engagement of activating (**High A:I ratio**) or inhibitory (**Low A:I ratio**) antibody checkpoints. Mechanisms of immune modulatory antibodies to co-stimulatory immune checkpoints, co-inhibitory immune checkpoints or the IL-2R are indicated. **Effect** indicates main cell type and function identified as underlying therapeutic effects of High A:I, and Low A:I variant antibodies, respectively. **FcγR-modulation:** arrows indicate how activatory FcγR (aFcγR) and inhibitory FcγR (iFcγR) positively (↑) or negatively (↓) regulate indicated effect. Bottom two lines indicate antibody isotypes and clones used in referenced studies. **References**: GITR (79), OX40 (90–95), 4-1BB (89), CD40 (23, 24, 96), IL-2R (97), CTLA-4 (76–80), PD-1 (81, 82), PD-L1 (81).*

the antibody checkpoints, will be critical for identification and rational combination of antibodies with complementary non-competing mechanisms-of-action (**Table 1**). As discussed below, such knowledge will additionally pave the way for antibody-checkpoint targeted therapies, e.g., antibody blockade of inhibitory FcγRIIB or Fc-engineering for enhanced affinity to activating FcγR, to help boost efficacy and overcome resistance in the immune suppressed tumor microenvironment.

Targeting the Antibody Checkpoints to Improve Cancer Immunotherapy–Focus on FcγRIIB

The documented role of the antibody checkpoints as master regulators of the clinically most relevant classes of anti-cancer antibodies detailed above, suggests that targeting of this receptor family be an attractive strategy to enhance efficacy and overcome resistance to antibody-based cancer immunotherapy.

While Fc gamma receptor regulation of antibody efficacy is highly functionally conserved between mouse and man, important differences in absolute and relative binding affinities of the species' respective antibody subclasses for their corresponding activating and inhibitory FcγRs have slowed translation into human therapeutic antibody candidates and clinical development. Recent development of FcR-humanized mouse models (99), and highly specific antagonist or agonist antibodies to individual human and mouse activating and inhibitory receptors (30, 65), have now enabled such translation.

Two principal strategies to better harness antibody checkpoint-dependent antitumor immunity have been pursued–Fc engineering or FcγR blockade (**Figure 6**).

Antibody engineering to enhance affinity for activating antibody checkpoints has obtained clinical proof-of-concept through the afucosylated CD20-specific antibody obinutuzumab (15), with additional afucosylated antibodies in late stage clinical development (100). While clinically validated, and elegant in the sense that simple removal of a fucose group of residue N297 in the antibody constant domain results in very significantly enhanced binding to FcγRIIIa (101), this approach has its limitations. Firstly, emerging data indicates that intratumoral macrophages and dendritic cells–critical effectors underlying antibody-induced antitumor immunity (102)–express FcγRIIA and FcγRIIB at highest density (76). Further, FcγRIIA may be the only activating Fc gamma receptor expressed on human dendritic cells, which additionally express FcγRIIB for coordinate regulation of antigen presentation (45). Consequently, harnessing the full potential of antibody checkpoint-regulated anti-cancer immunity is likely to require engagement and enhancement of additional activating FcγRs besides FcγRIIIa, and ideally reduced or no engagement of the inhibitory antibody checkpoint. As discussed below, the great structural similarity between individual activating and inhibitory antibody checkpoint receptors poses significant technical challenges to succeed in engineering of antibodies with such properties. Nevertheless, Fc-engineering by substitution of two or more amino acids has generated antibody molecules with enhanced affinity for both FcγRIIA and FcγRIIIA, albeit with retained or slightly enhanced affinity also for the inhibitory FcγRIIB (103, 104). Whether such molecules will show therapeutically relevant pharmacokinetics or enhanced efficacy remains to be demonstrated in clinical trials.

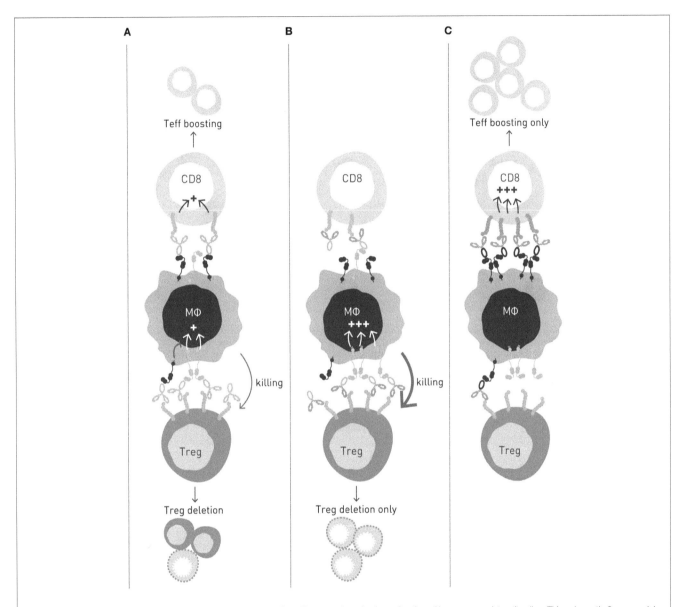

FIGURE 4 | Activating and inhibitory antibody checkpoints determine efficacy and mechanism-of-action of immune agonist antibodies. This schematic figure models **(A)** Antibody engagement of activating and inhibitory FcγRs determine target cell depletion and agonism, respectively. The two mechanism compete when antibody variants (isotype) capable of binding both FcγR are used, resulting in reduced or no therapeutic activity. **(B)** Antibody variants with enhanced binding to activating FcγR (high A:I ratio) show improved depletion of Treg cells, which express higher numbers of receptors compared with effector cells, resulting in immune activation through elimination of suppressor cells. **(C)** Antibody variants with enhanced binding to inhibitory FcγR (low A:I ratio) show improved CD8+ T cell agonism, resulting in immune activation by expansion and boosting of effector cells.

Based on the significant upregulation of the sole inhibitory antibody checkpoint FcγRIIB in the tumor microenvironment (97), and its documented role in conferring resistance to antibody-based therapy in this niche (65, 70, 97), we have pursued antibody-mediated blockade of FcγRIIB as an alternative and complementary approach to Fc-engineering to harness the full potential of antibody checkpoint-regulated immunity. In theory, besides being an apparent critical pan-antibody regulator conferring antibody drug resistance in the tumor microenvironment, targeted blockade of FcγRIIB by a separate antibody has the advantage of enabling

combination therapy and boosted efficacy with multiple existing, clinically validated, antibodies including those engineered for enhanced binding to activating FcγR (65). The strategy does, however, put exquisite requirements on a therapeutic antibody candidate, both from target receptor specificity and function-modulating perspectives. The extracellular, antibody accessible domain, of the inhibitory FcγRIIB is ∼93% homologous with the activating FcγRIIA. Nevertheless, probing of a highly diversified human recombinant antibody library (65), or immunization of mice transgenic for human FcγRIIA (105), generated diverse pools of highly specific

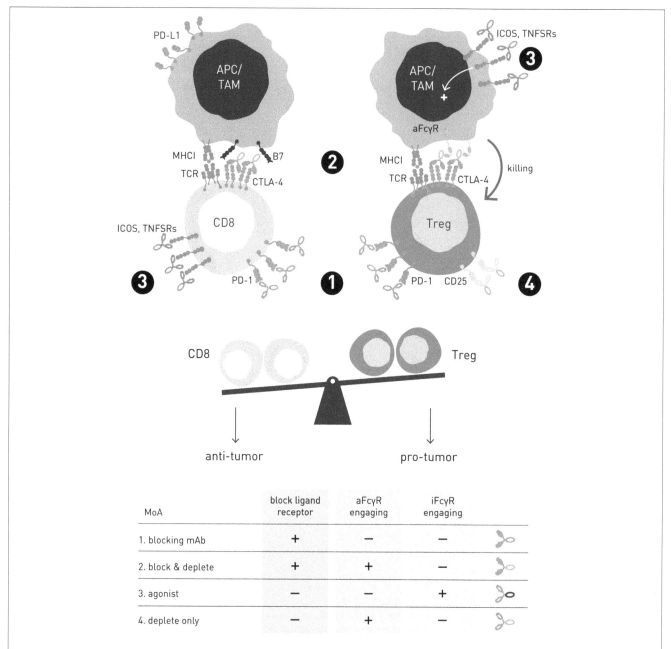

FIGURE 5 | Antibody preferred mechanism-of-action and FcγR-engagement is dependent on target receptor function and expression. This schematic figure models four exemplary antibody MoA's, pertinent to both immune checkpoint and tumor cell direct-targeting antibody types. (1) Blocking mAb. PD-1, a co-inhibitory antibody checkpoint expressed at high and similar levels on intratumoral Treg and Teff cells, is best targeted using a PD-1/PD-L1 blocking Fc-null antibody variant, since FcγR-mediated Teff cell depletion is undesirable (2) Blocking and depleting mAbs. Anti-CTLA-4 is overexpressed on intratumoral Treg compared with Teff, and activatory FcγR-engagement correlates with survival in melanoma patients treated with ipilimumab. Preferred MoA is two-fold: CTLA-4/B7 blockade and Treg depletion through FcγR-dependent mechanisms (3) Agonist mAb Preferred MoA is FcγR-engaging antibody variant, where FcγRs promote receptor cross-linking and signaling. (4) Depletion only mAb. Anti-IL2R antibody preferred MoA is ligand non-blocking and FcγR-dependent (Treg) cell depletion. IL-2R overexpressing Tregs are selectively depleted, while free IL-2 may promote Teff survival and expansion.

antibodies that selectively bound to FcγRIIB, and not to FcγRIIA, and which in a dose-dependent manner blocked immune complex binding to cell surface-expressed FcγRIIB. Functional screening revealed that only a minority of the highly FcγRIIB specific human recombinant antibodies were able to block antibody-induced FcγRIIB inhibitory signaling (65). Remaining candidates either did not block, or agonized, FcγRIIB signaling. The latter category could have therapeutic potential in treatment of chronic inflammatory and autoimmune disease (106).

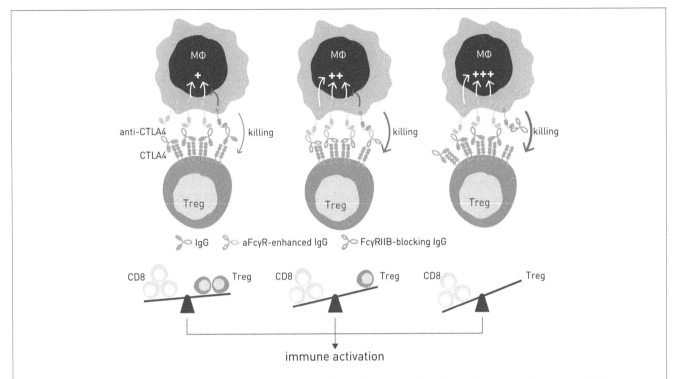

FIGURE 6 | Antibody-induced antitumor immunity can be enhanced by modulation of antibody: FcγR interactions. **Left** panel (no antibody checkpoint modulation). Antibody efficacy is balanced by co-engagement of activating and inhibitory FcγR. **Center** panel (enhanced engagement of activating FcγR). Antibody efficacy is improved through Fc-engineering for enhanced binding to activating FcγR. **Right** panel–Antibody efficacy is enhanced by blockade of the inhibitory FcγRIIB.

Based on observations that FcγRIIB limits antibody efficacy and promotes tumor cell resistance by dual mechanisms in B cell malignancy, acting at the level of both immune effector cells and tumor B cells, we have further characterized the therapeutic potential of antagonistic anti-FcγRIIB antibodies to boost efficacy and overcome resistance to antibody therapy *in vivo* focusing initially on this setting. A lead human antagonistic anti-FcγRIIB IgG1 antibody (6G11 or BI-1206), which showed synergistically enhanced rituximab B cell depletion in FcγRIIB and CD20 humanized mice, and overcame refractoriness of primary leukaemic B cells to anti-CD20-based antibody therapy *in vivo*, is currently in early phase clinical testing (65).

Besides affording efficacy, therapeutic targeting of Fc gamma receptors, whether by blocking antibodies or Fc-engineering, must be safe and associated with therapeutically relevant pharmacokinetics. In addition to its high expression on B cells and certain macrophage/dendritic cells, FcγRIIB has been reported to be highly expressed in mouse and rat liver sinusoidal endothelial cells (LSEC) (107), where they have been implicated in removal of circulating small immune complexes (108). These observations raise potential safety concerns of undesirably cytotoxic activity with therapeutic antibodies targeting FcγRIIB. However, our recent observations of human and mouse liver indicate lower LSEC expression in man (30), and dosing of FcγRIIB humanized mice with therapeutically relevant doses of anti-human FcγRIIB IgG1 antibody 6G11 showed no apparent acute or chronic treatment

related adverse effects (30, 65). Ultimately, the safety and efficacy of targeting FcγRIIB needs to be assessed in human subjects. Two clinical trials are ongoing to evaluate safety and explore efficacy of the BI-1206 antibody as single agent and in combination with rituximab in B cell malignancy (NCT03571568 and NCT02933320). Our ongoing efforts aim at translating observations of FcγRIIB-regulated antitumor immunity to the solid cancer clinical setting.

As noted above FcγRIIB may promote anti-tumor activity by facilitating extrinsic signaling of certain co-stimulatory receptors expressed on tumor or immune cells. A possible strategy to enhance therapeutic activity of such antibodies would therefore be to enhance their affinity for FcγRIIB. In keeping with this, anti-DR5 antibodies carrying the S267E ("SE") mutation, increasing human IgG1 affinity for FcγRIIB several hundred-fold, showed improved tumor regression in mouse models humanized for FcγRIIB (109). Analogously, human IgG2 anti-CD40 antibodies equipped with SE or SE/LF mutated backbones (the latter further increases affinity for FcγRIIB) showed enhanced CD8$^+$ T cell activation, and improved ability to clear tumors, in mice humanized for FcγRs and CD40 (96). However, increasing antibody affinity for FcγRIIB in these two cases improved not only efficacy but also side effects. Increased DR5 agonism of the SE variant anti-DR5 was associated with increased liver enzyme release. SE and SE/LF variant anti-CD40 antibodies increased not only T cell activation and anti-tumor immunity, but also depletion of platelets, which express CD40 (96, 109). Thus, Fc-engineering for enhanced FcγRIIB affinity or selectivity needs close consideration of antibody (Fv-) targeted receptor's cellular distribution and function(s).

CONCLUDING REMARKS

Emerging preclinical and clinical data demonstrate that the activating and inhibitory Fc gamma receptors–the "antibody checkpoints"–control antitumor immunity induced by the clinically most successful antibodies used in cancer immunotherapy. Therapeutics that harness the power of antibody checkpoint-regulated anti-tumor immunity, through Fc-engineering to enhance binding to activating FcγRs, or through blockade of the inhibitory FcγRIIB, have been approved or are in development. If safe and well-tolerated,

these agents hold promise to improve response rates, duration of response, and potentially overall survival for diverse cancer patients.

AUTHOR CONTRIBUTIONS

BF wrote and edited the manuscript and conceived figures. IT helped write the manuscript and conceive figures. LM designed and performed experiments in several of herein reviewed papers, and helped write the current manuscript and helped conceive figures.

ACKNOWLEDGMENTS

We thank Joost Bakker (www.scicomvisuals.com) for help generating schematic figures.

REFERENCES

1. Cheson BD, Leonard JP. Monoclonal antibody therapy for B-cell non-Hodgkin's lymphoma. *N Engl J Med.* (2008) 359:613–26. doi: 10.1056/NEJMra0708875
2. Gradishar WJ. HER2 therapy–an abundance of riches. *N Engl J Med.* (2012) 366:176–8. doi: 10.1056/NEJMe1113641
3. Jonker DJ, O'Callaghan CJ, Karapetis CS, Zalcberg JR, Tu D, Au HJ, et al. Cetuximab for the treatment of colorectal cancer. *N Engl J Med.* (2007) 357:2040–8. doi: 10.1056/NEJMoa071834
4. Lokhorst HM, Plesner T, Laubach JP, Nahi H, Gimsing P, Hansson M, et al. Targeting CD38 with daratumumab monotherapy in multiple myeloma. *N Engl J Med.* (2015) 373:1207–19. doi: 10.1056/NEJMoa1506348
5. Hodi FS, O'Day SJ, McDermott DF, Weber RW, Sosman JA, Haanen JB, et al. Improved survival with ipilimumab in patients with metastatic melanoma. *N Engl J Med.* (2010) 363:711–23. doi: 10.1056/NEJMoa1003466
6. Larkin J, Chiarion-Sileni V, Gonzalez R, Grob JJ, Cowey CL, Lao CD, et al. Combined nivolumab and ipilimumab or monotherapy in untreated melanoma. *N Engl J Med.* (2015) 373:23–34. doi: 10.1056/NEJMoa1504030
7. Brahmer JR, Tykodi SS, Chow LQ, Hwu WJ, Topalian SL, Hwu P, et al. Safety and activity of anti-PD-L1 antibody in patients with advanced cancer. *N Engl J Med.* (2012) 366:2455–65. doi: 10.1056/NEJMoa1200694
8. Topalian SL, Hodi FS, Brahmer JR, Gettinger SN, Smith DC, McDermott DF, et al. Safety, activity, and immune correlates of anti-PD-1 antibody in cancer. *N Engl J Med.* (2012) 366:2443–54. doi: 10.1056/NEJMoa1200690
9. Ribas A, Puzanov I, Dummer R, Schadendorf D, Hamid O, Robert C, et al. Pembrolizumab versus investigator-choice chemotherapy for ipilimumab-refractory melanoma (KEYNOTE-002): a randomised, controlled, phase 2 trial. *Lancet Oncol.* (2015) 16:908–18. doi: 10.1016/S1470-2045(15)00083-2
10. Robert C, Thomas L, Bondarenko I, O'Day S, Weber J, Garbe C, et al. Ipilimumab plus dacarbazine for previously untreated metastatic melanoma. *N Engl J Med.* (2011) 364:2517–26. doi: 10.1056/NEJMoa1104621
11. Robert C, Ribas A, Wolchok JD, Hodi FS, Hamid O, Kefford R, et al. Anti-programmed-death-receptor-1 treatment with pembrolizumab in ipilimumab-refractory advanced melanoma: a randomised dose-comparison cohort of a phase 1 trial. *Lancet.* (2014) 384:1109–17. doi: 10.1016/S0140-6736(14)60958-2
12. Robert C, Long GV, Brady B, Dutriaux C, Maio M, Mortier L, et al. Nivolumab in previously untreated melanoma without BRAF mutation. *N Engl J Med.* (2015) 372:320–30. doi: 10.1056/NEJMoa1412082
13. Weber JS, D'Angelo SP, Minor D, Hodi FS, Gutzmer R, Neyns B, et al. Nivolumab versus chemotherapy in patients with advanced melanoma who progressed after anti-CTLA-4 treatment (CheckMate 037): a randomised, controlled, open-label, phase 3 trial. *Lancet Oncol.* (2015) 16:375–84. doi: 10.1016/S1470-2045(15)70076-8

14. Sharma P, Hu-Lieskovan S, Wargo JA, Ribas A. Primary, adaptive, and acquired resistance to cancer immunotherapy. *Cell.* (2017) 168:707–23. doi: 10.1016/j.cell.2017.01.017
15. Goede V, Fischer K, Busch R, Engelke A, Eichhorst B, Wendtner CM, et al. Obinutuzumab plus chlorambucil in patients with CLL and coexisting conditions. *N Engl J Med.* (2014) 370:1101–10. doi: 10.1056/NEJMoa1313984
16. Baselga J, Cortes J, Kim SB, Im SA, Hegg R, Im YH, et al. Pertuzumab plus trastuzumab plus docetaxel for metastatic breast cancer. *N Engl J Med.* (2012) 366:109–19. doi: 10.1056/NEJMoa1113216
17. Gopal AK, Kahl BS, de Vos S, Wagner-Johnston ND, Schuster SJ, Jurczak WJ, et al. PI3Kdelta inhibition by idelalisib in patients with relapsed indolent lymphoma. *N Engl J Med.* (2014) 370:1008–18. doi: 10.1056/NEJMoa1314583
18. Pincetic A, Bournazos S, DiLillo DJ, Maamary J, Wang TT, Dahan R, et al. Type I and type II Fc receptors regulate innate and adaptive immunity. *Nat Immunol.* (2014) 15:707–16. doi: 10.1038/ni.2939
19. Bournazos S, Woof JM, Hart SP, Dransfield I. Functional and clinical consequences of Fc receptor polymorphic and copy number variants. *Clin Exp Immunol.* (2009) 157:244–54. doi: 10.1111/j.1365-2249.2009.03980.x
20. Nimmerjahn F, Ravetch JV. Fcgamma receptors: old friends and new family members. *Immunity.* (2006) 24:19–28. doi: 10.1016/j.immuni.2005.11.010
21. Carreno BM, Collins M. The B7 family of ligands and its receptors: new pathways for costimulation and inhibition of immune responses. *Annu Rev Immunol.* (2002) 20:29–53. doi: 10.1146/annurev.immunol.20.091101.091806
22. Schildberg FA, Klein SR, Freeman GJ, Sharpe AH. Coinhibitory pathways in the B7-CD28 ligand-receptor family. *Immunity.* (2016) 44:955–72. doi: 10.1016/j.immuni.2016.05.002
23. Li F, Ravetch JV. Inhibitory Fcgamma receptor engagement drives adjuvant and anti-tumor activities of agonistic CD40 antibodies. *Science.* (2011) 333:1030–4. doi: 10.1126/science.1206954
24. White AL, Chan HT, Roghanian A, French RR, Mockridge CI, Tutt AL, et al. Interaction with FcgammaRIIB is critical for the agonistic activity of anti-CD40 monoclonal antibody. *J Immunol.* (2011) 187:1754–63. doi: 10.4049/jimmunol.1101135
25. Xu Y, Szalai AJ, Zhou T, Zinn KR, Chaudhuri TR, Li X, et al. Fc gamma Rs modulate cytotoxicity of anti-Fas antibodies: implications for agonistic antibody-based therapeutics. *J Immunol.* (2003) 171:562–8. doi: 10.4049/jimmunol.171.2.562
26. Wilson NS, Yang B, Yang A, Loeser S, Marsters S, Lawrence D, et al. An Fcgamma receptor-dependent mechanism drives antibody-mediated target-receptor signaling in cancer cells. *Cancer Cell.* (2011) 19:101–13. doi: 10.1016/j.ccr.2010.11.012
27. Deng R, Cassady K, Li X, Yao S, Zhang M, Racine J, et al. B7H1/CD80 interaction augments PD-1-dependent T cell apoptosis

and ameliorates graft-versus-host disease. *J Immunol.* (2015) 194:560–74. doi: 10.4049/jimmunol.1402157

28. Nimmerjahn F, Ravetch JV. Divergent immunoglobulin g subclass activity through selective Fc receptor binding. *Science.* (2005) 310:1510–2. doi: 10.1126/science.1118948

29. Bruhns P, Iannascoli B, England P, Mancardi DA, Fernandez N, Jorieux S, et al. Specificity and affinity of human Fcgamma receptors and their polymorphic variants for human IgG subclasses. *Blood.* (2009) 113:3716–25. doi: 10.1182/blood-2008-09-179754

30. Tutt AL, James S, Laversin SA, Tipton TR, Ashton-Key M, French RR, et al. Development and characterization of monoclonal antibodies specific for mouse and human Fcgamma receptors. *J Immunol.* (2015) 195:5503–16. doi: 10.4049/jimmunol.1402988

31. Kimberly RP, Ahlstrom JW, Click ME, Edberg JC. The glycosyl phosphatidylinositol-linked Fc gamma RIIIPMN mediates transmembrane signaling events distinct from Fc gamma RII. *J Exp Med.* (1990) 171:1239–55. doi: 10.1084/jem.171.4.1239

32. Golay J, Da Roit F, Bologna L, Ferrara C, Leusen JH, Rambaldi A, et al. Glycoengineered CD20 antibody obinutuzumab activates neutrophils and mediates phagocytosis through CD16B more efficiently than rituximab. *Blood.* (2013) 122:3482–91. doi: 10.1182/blood-2013-05-504043

33. Nimmerjahn F, Bruhns P, Horiuchi K, Ravetch JV. FcgammaRIV: a novel FcR with distinct IgG subclass specificity. *Immunity.* (2005) 23:41–51. doi: 10.1016/j.immuni.2005.05.010

34. Mancardi DA, Albanesi M, Jonsson F, Iannascoli B, Van Rooijen N, Kang X, et al. The high-affinity human IgG receptor FcgammaRI (CD64) promotes IgG-mediated inflammation, anaphylaxis, and antitumor immunotherapy. *Blood.* (2013) 121:1563–73. doi: 10.1182/blood-2012-07-442541

35. Cartron G, Dacheux L, Salles G, Solal-Celigny P, Bardos P, Colombat P, et al. Therapeutic activity of humanized anti-CD20 monoclonal antibody and polymorphism in IgG Fc receptor FcgammaRIIIa gene. *Blood.* (2002) 99:754–8. doi: 10.1182/blood.V99.3.754

36. Weng WK, Levy R. Two immunoglobulin G fragment C receptor polymorphisms independently predict response to rituximab in patients with follicular lymphoma. *J Clin Oncol.* (2003) 21:3940–7. doi: 10.1200/JCO.2003.05.013

37. Zhang W, Gordon M, Schultheis AM, Yang DY, Nagashima F, Azuma M, et al. FCΓR2A and FCΓR3A polymorphisms associated with clinical outcome of epidermal growth factor receptor expressing metastatic colorectal cancer patients treated with single-agent cetuximab. *J Clin Oncol.* (2007) 25:3712–8. doi: 10.1200/JCO.2006.08.8021

38. Musolino A, Naldi N, Bortesi B, Pezzuolo D, Capelletti M, Missale G, et al. Immunoglobulin G fragment C receptor polymorphisms and clinical efficacy of trastuzumab-based therapy in patients with HER-2/neu-positive metastatic breast cancer. *J Clin Oncol.* (2008) 26:1789–96. doi: 10.1200/JCO.2007.14.8957

39. Mellor JD, Brown MP, Irving HR, Zalcberg JR, Dobrovic A. A critical review of the role of Fc gamma receptor polymorphisms in the response to monoclonal antibodies in cancer. *J Hematol Oncol.* (2013) 6:1. doi: 10.1186/1756-8722-6-1

40. Gillis C, Gouel-Cheron A, Jonsson F, Bruhns P. Contribution of human FcgammaRs to disease with evidence from human polymorphisms and transgenic animal studies. *Front Immunol.* (2014) 5:254. doi: 10.3389/fimmu.2014.00254

41. van der Heijden J, Breunis WB, Geissler J, de Boer M, van den Berg TK, Kuijpers TW. Phenotypic variation in IgG receptors by nonclassical FCΓR2C alleles. *J Immunol.* (2012) 188:1318–24. doi: 10.4049/jimmunol.1003945

42. Breunis WB, van Mirre E, Geissler J, Laddach N, Wolbink G, van der Schoot E, et al. Copy number variation at the FCΓR locus includes FCΓR3A, FCΓR2C and FCΓR3B but not FCΓR2A and FCΓR2B. *Hum Mutat.* (2009) 30:E640–50. doi: 10.1002/humu.20997

43. Koene HR, Kleijer M, Roos D, de Haas M, Von dem Borne AE. Fc gamma RIIIB gene duplication: evidence for presence and expression of three distinct Fc gamma RIIIB genes in NA(1+,2+)SH(+) individuals. *Blood.* (1998) 91:673–679.

44. Guilliams M, Bruhns P, Saeys Y, Hammad H, Lambrecht BN. The function of Fcgamma receptors in dendritic cells and macrophages. *Nat Rev Immunol.* (2014) 14:94–108. doi: 10.1038/nri3582

45. DiLillo DJ, Ravetch JV. Differential Fc-Receptor engagement drives an anti-tumor vaccinal effect. *Cell.* (2015) 161:1035–45. doi: 10.1016/j.cell.2015.04.016

46. Regnault A, Lankar D, Lacabanne V, Rodriguez A, Thery C, Rescigno M, et al. Fcgamma receptor-mediated induction of dendritic cell maturation and major histocompatibility complex class I-restricted antigen presentation after immune complex internalization. *J Exp Med.* (1999) 189:371–80. doi: 10.1084/jem.189.2.371

47. Kalergis AM, Ravetch JV. Inducing tumor immunity through the selective engagement of activating Fcgamma receptors on dendritic cells. *J Exp Med.* (2002) 195:1653–9. doi: 10.1084/jem.20020338

48. Diaz de Stahl T, Heyman B. IgG2a-mediated enhancement of antibody responses is dependent on FcRgamma+ bone marrow-derived cells. *Scand J Immunol.* (2001) 54:495–500. doi: 10.1046/j.1365-3083.2001.01000.x

49. Dhodapkar KM, Kaufman JL, Ehlers M, Banerjee DK, Bonvini E, Koenig S, et al. Selective blockade of inhibitory Fcgamma receptor enables human dendritic cell maturation with IL-12p70 production and immunity to antibody-coated tumor cells. *Proc Natl Acad Sci USA.* (2005) 102:2910–5. doi: 10.1073/pnas.0500014102

50. Desai DD, Harbers SO, Flores M, Colonna L, Downie MP, Bergtold A, et al. Fc gamma receptor IIB on dendritic cells enforces peripheral tolerance by inhibiting effector T cell responses. *J Immunol.* (2007) 178:6217–26. doi: 10.4049/jimmunol.178.10.6217

51. van Montfoort N, t Hoen PA, Mangsbo SM, Camps MG, Boross P, Melief CJ, et al. Fcgamma receptor IIb strongly regulates Fcgamma receptor-facilitated T cell activation by dendritic cells. *J Immunol.* (2012) 189:92–101. doi: 10.4049/jimmunol.1103703

52. Broz ML, Binnewies M, Boldajipour B, Nelson AE, Pollack JL, Erle DJ, et al. Dissecting the tumor myeloid compartment reveals rare activating antigen-presenting cells critical for T cell immunity. *Cancer Cell.* (2014) 26:638–52. doi: 10.1016/j.ccell.2014.09.007

53. Spranger S, Bao R, Gajewski TF. Melanoma-intrinsic beta-catenin signalling prevents anti-tumour immunity. *Nature.* (2015) 523:231–5. doi: 10.1038/nature14404

54. Salmon H, Idoyaga J, Rahman A, Leboeuf M, Remark R, Jordan S, et al. Expansion and activation of CD103(+) dendritic cell progenitors at the tumor site enhances tumor responses to therapeutic PD-L1 and BRAF inhibition. *Immunity.* (2016) 44:924–38. doi: 10.1016/j.immuni.2016.03.012

55. Alexandrov LB, Nik-Zainal S, Wedge DC, Aparicio SA, Behjati S, Biankin AV, et al. Signatures of mutational processes in human cancer. *Nature.* (2013) 500:415–21. doi: 10.1038/nature12477

56. Maloney DG. Anti-CD20 antibody therapy for B-cell lymphomas. *N Engl J Med.* (2012) 366:2008–16. doi: 10.1056/NEJMct1114348

57. Wang SY, Veeramani S, Racila E, Cagley J, Fritzinger DC, Vogel CW, et al. Depletion of the C3 component of complement enhances the ability of rituximab-coated target cells to activate human NK cells and improves the efficacy of monoclonal antibody therapy in an *in vivo* model. *Blood.* (2009) 114:5322–30. doi: 10.1182/blood-2009-01-200469

58. Biburger M, Aschermann S, Schwab I, Lux A, Albert H, Danzer H, et al. Monocyte subsets responsible for immunoglobulin G-dependent effector functions *in vivo*. *Immunity.* (2011) 35:932–44. doi: 10.1016/j.immuni.2011.11.009

59. Montalvao F, Garcia Z, Celli S, Breart B, Deguine J, Van Rooijen N, et al. The mechanism of anti-CD20-mediated B cell depletion revealed by intravital imaging. *J Clin Invest.* (2013) 123:5098–103. doi: 10.1172/JCI70972

60. Uchida J, Hamaguchi Y, Oliver JA, Ravetch JV, Poe JC, Haas KM, et al. The innate mononuclear phagocyte network depletes B lymphocytes through Fc receptor-dependent mechanisms during anti-CD20 antibody immunotherapy. *J Exp Med.* (2004) 199:1659–69. doi: 10.1084/jem.20040119

61. Biburger M, Lux A, Nimmerjahn F. How immunoglobulin G antibodies kill target cells: revisiting an old paradigm. *Adv Immunol.* (2014) 124:67–94. doi: 10.1016/B978-0-12-800147-9.00003-0

62. Park S, Jiang Z, Mortenson ED, Deng L, Radkevich-Brown O, Yang X, et al. The therapeutic effect of anti-HER2/neu antibody depends

on both innate and adaptive immunity. *Cancer Cell.* (2010) 18:160–70. doi: 10.1016/j.ccr.2010.06.014

63. Clynes RA, Towers TL, Presta LG, Ravetch JV. Inhibitory Fc receptors modulate *in vivo* cytotoxicity against tumor targets. *Nat Med.* (2000) 6:443–6. doi: 10.1038/74704

64. Postow MA, Chesney J, Pavlick AC, Robert C, Grossmann K, McDermott D, et al. Nivolumab and ipilimumab versus ipilimumab in untreated melanoma. *N Engl J Med.* (2015) 372:2006–17. doi: 10.1056/NEJMoa1414428

65. Roghanian A, Teige I, Martensson L, Cox KL, Kovacek M, Ljungars A, et al. Antagonistic human FcgammaRIIB (CD32B) antibodies have anti-tumor activity and overcome resistance to antibody therapy *in vivo. Cancer Cell.* (2015) 27:473–88. doi: 10.1016/j.ccell.2015.03.005

66. Beers SA, French RR, Chan HT, Lim SH, Jarrett TC, Vidal RM, et al. Antigenic modulation limits the efficacy of anti-CD20 antibodies: implications for antibody selection. *Blood.* (2010) 115:5191–201. doi: 10.1182/blood-2010-01-263533

67. Lim SH, Vaughan AT, Ashton-Key M, Williams EL, Dixon SV, Chan HT, et al. Fc gamma receptor IIb on target B cells promotes rituximab internalization and reduces clinical efficacy. *Blood.* (2011) 118:2530–40. doi: 10.1182/blood-2011-01-330357

68. Camilleri-Broet S, Cassard L, Broet P, Delmer A, Le Touneau A, Diebold J, et al. FcgammaRIIB is differentially expressed during B cell maturation and in B-cell lymphomas. *Br J Haematol.* (2004) 124:55–62. doi: 10.1046/j.1365-2141.2003.04737.x

69. Lee CS, Ashton-Key M, Cogliatti S, Rondeau S, Schmitz SF, Ghielmini M, et al. Expression of the inhibitory Fc gamma receptor IIB (FCΓR2B, CD32B) on follicular lymphoma cells lowers the response rate to rituximab monotherapy (SAKK 35/98). *Br J Haematol.* (2015) 168:145–8. doi: 10.1111/bjh.13071

70. Pallasch CP, Leskov I, Braun CJ, Vorholt D, Drake A, Soto-Feliciano YM, et al. Sensitizing protective tumor microenvironments to antibody-mediated therapy. *Cell.* (2014) 156:590–602. doi: 10.1016/j.cell.2013.12.041

71. Rankin CT, Veri MC, Gorlatov S, Tuaillon N, Burke S, Huang L, et al. CD32B, the human inhibitory Fc-gamma receptor IIB, as a target for monoclonal antibody therapy of B-cell lymphoma. *Blood.* (2006) 108:2384–91. doi: 10.1182/blood-2006-05-020602

72. Vaughan AT, Iriyama C, Beers SA, Chan CH, Lim SH, Williams EL, et al. Inhibitory FcgammaRIIb (CD32b) becomes activated by therapeutic mAb in both cis and trans and drives internalization according to antibody specificity. *Blood.* (2014) 123:669–77. doi: 10.1182/blood-2013-04-490821

73. Pardoll DM. The blockade of immune checkpoints in cancer immunotherapy. *Nat Rev Cancer.* (2012) 12:252–64. doi: 10.1038/nrc3239

74. Topalian SL, Drake CG, Pardoll DM. Immune checkpoint blockade: a common denominator approach to cancer therapy. *Cancer Cell.* (2015) 27:450–61. doi: 10.1016/j.ccell.2015.03.001

75. Ostrand-Rosenberg S, Horn LA, Haile ST. The programmed death-1 immune-suppressive pathway: barrier to antitumor immunity. *J Immunol.* (2014) 193:3835–41. doi: 10.4049/jimmunol.1401572

76. Arce Vargas F, Furness AJS, Litchfield K, Joshi K, Rosenthal R, Ghorani E, et al. Fc effector function contributes to the activity of human anti-CTLA-4 antibodies. *Cancer Cell.* (2018) 33:649–663 e644. doi: 10.1016/j.ccell.2018.02.010

77. Selby MJ, Engelhardt JJ, Quigley M, Henning KA, Chen T, Srinivasan M, et al. Anti-CTLA-4 antibodies of IgG2a isotype enhance antitumor activity through reduction of intratumoral regulatory T cells. *Cancer Immunol Res.* (2013) 1:32–42. doi: 10.1158/2326-6066.CIR-13-0013

78. Simpson TR, Li F, Montalvo-Ortiz W, Sepulveda MA, Bergerhoff K, Arce F, et al. Fc-dependent depletion of tumor-infiltrating regulatory T cells co-defines the efficacy of anti-CTLA-4 therapy against melanoma. *J Exp Med.* (2013) 210:1695–710. doi: 10.1084/jem.20130579

79. Bulliard Y, Jolicoeur R, Windman M, Rue SM, Ettenberg S, Knee DA, et al. Activating Fc gamma receptors contribute to the antitumor activities of immunoregulatory receptor-targeting antibodies. *J Exp Med.* (2013) 210:1685–93. doi: 10.1084/jem.20130573

80. Peggs KS, Quezada SA, Chambers CA, Korman AJ, Allison JP. Blockade of CTLA-4 on both effector and regulatory T cell compartments contributes to the antitumor activity of anti-CTLA-4 antibodies. *J Exp Med.* (2009) 206:1717–25. doi: 10.1084/jem.20082492

81. Dahan R, Sega E, Engelhardt J, Selby M, Korman AJ, Ravetch JV. FcgammaRs modulate the anti-tumor activity of antibodies targeting the PD-1/PD-L1 axis. *Cancer Cell.* (2015) 28:285–95. doi: 10.1016/j.ccell.2015.08.004

82. Arlauckas SP, Garris CS, Kohler RH, Kitaoka M, Cuccarese MF, Yang KS, et al. *In vivo* imaging reveals a tumor-associated macrophage-mediated resistance pathway in anti-PD-1 therapy. *Sci Transl Med.* (2017) 9:eaal3604. doi: 10.1126/scitranslmed.aal3604

83. Beatty GL, Chiorean EG, Fishman MP, Saboury B, Teitelbaum UR, Sun W, et al. CD40 agonists alter tumor stroma and show efficacy against pancreatic carcinoma in mice and humans. *Science.* (2011) 331:1612–6. doi: 10.1126/science.1198443

84. Weinberg AD, Rivera MM, Prell R, Morris A, Ramstad T, Vetto JT, et al. Engagement of the OX-40 receptor *in vivo* enhances antitumor immunity. *J Immunol.* (2000) 164:2160–9. doi: 10.4049/jimmunol.164.4.2160

85. Melero I, Shuford WW, Newby SA, Aruffo A, Ledbetter JA, Hellstrom KE, et al. Monoclonal antibodies against the 4-1BB T-cell activation molecule eradicate established tumors. *Nat Med.* (1997) 3:682–5. doi: 10.1038/nm0697-682

86. Guo Z, Wang X, Cheng D, Xia Z, Luan M, Zhang S. PD-1 blockade and OX40 triggering synergistically protects against tumor growth in a murine model of ovarian cancer. *PLoS ONE.* (2014) 9:e89350. doi: 10.1371/journal.pone.0089350

87. Turk MJ, Guevara-Patino JA, Rizzuto GA, Engelhorn ME, Sakaguchi S, Houghton AN. Concomitant tumor immunity to a poorly immunogenic melanoma is prevented by regulatory T cells. *J Exp Med.* (2004) 200:771–82. doi: 10.1084/jem.20041130

88. Messenheimer DJ, Jensen SM, Afentoulis ME, Wegmann KW, Feng Z, Friedman DJ, et al. Timing of PD-1 blockade is critical to effective combination immunotherapy with anti-OX40. *Clin Cancer Res.* (2017) 23:6165–77. doi: 10.1158/1078-0432.CCR-16-2677

89. Buchan SL, Dou L, Remer M, Booth SG, Dunn SN, Lai C, et al. Antibodies to costimulatory receptor 4-1BB enhance anti-tumor immunity via T regulatory cell depletion and promotion of CD8 T cell effector function. *Immunity.* (2018) 49:958–70.e7. doi: 10.1016/j.immuni.2018.09.014

90. Bulliard Y, Jolicoeur R, Zhang J, Dranoff G, Wilson NS, Brogdon JL. OX40 engagement depletes intratumoral Tregs via activating FcgammaRs, leading to antitumor efficacy. *Immunol Cell Biol.* (2014) 92:475–80. doi: 10.1038/icb.2014.26

91. Marabelle A, Kohrt H, Sagiv-Barfi I, Ajami B, Axtell RC, Zhou G, et al. Depleting tumor-specific Tregs at a single site eradicates disseminated tumors. *J Clin Invest.* (2013) 123:2447–63. doi: 10.1172/JCI64859

92. Piconese S, Valzasina B, Colombo MP. OX40 triggering blocks suppression by regulatory T cells and facilitates tumor rejection. *J Exp Med.* (2008) 205:825–39. doi: 10.1084/jem.20071341

93. Kjaergaard J, Tanaka J, Kim JA, Rothchild K, Weinberg A, Shu S. Therapeutic efficacy of OX-40 receptor antibody depends on tumor immunogenicity and anatomic site of tumor growth. *Cancer Res.* (2000) 60:5514–21.

94. Linch SN, Kasiewicz MJ, McNamara MJ, Hilgart-Martiszus IF, Farhad M, Redmond WL. Combination OX40 agonism/CTLA-4 blockade with HER2 vaccination reverses T-cell anergy and promotes survival in tumor-bearing mice. *Proc Natl Acad Sci USA.* (2016) 113:E319–27. doi: 10.1073/pnas.1510518113

95. Gough MJ, Ruby CE, Redmond WL, Dhungel B, Brown A, Weinberg AD. OX40 agonist therapy enhances CD8 infiltration and decreases immune suppression in the tumor. *Cancer Res.* (2008) 68:5206–15. doi: 10.1158/0008-5472.CAN-07-6484

96. Dahan R, Barnhart BC, Li F, Yamniuk AP, Korman AJ, Ravetch JV. Therapeutic activity of agonistic, human anti-CD40 monoclonal antibodies requires selective FcgammaR engagement. *Cancer Cell.* (2016) 29:820–31. doi: 10.1016/j.ccell.2016.05.001

97. Arce Vargas F, Furness AJS, Solomon I, Joshi K, Mekkaoui L, Lesko MH, et al. Fc-Optimized Anti-CD25 depletes tumor-infiltrating regulatory T cells and synergizes with PD-1 blockade to eradicate established tumors. *Immunity.* (2017) 46:577–86. doi: 10.1016/j.immuni.2017.03.013

98. Chen DS, Mellman I. Oncology meets immunology: the cancer-immunity cycle. *Immunity.* (2013) 39:1–10. doi: 10.1016/j.immuni.2013.07.012

99. Smith P, DiLillo DJ, Bournazos S, Li F, Ravetch JV. Mouse model recapitulating human Fcgamma receptor structural and functional diversity. *Proc Natl Acad Sci USA.* (2012) 109:6181–6. doi: 10.1073/pnas.1203954109

100. Pereira NA, Chan KF, Lin PC, Song Z. The "less-is-more" in therapeutic antibodies: Afucosylated anti-cancer antibodies with enhanced antibody-dependent cellular cytotoxicity. *MAbs.* (2018) 10:693–711. doi: 10.1080/19420862.2018.1466767

101. Shields RL, Lai J, Keck R, O'Connell LY, Hong K, Meng YG, et al. Lack of fucose on human IgG1 N-linked oligosaccharide improves binding to human Fcgamma RIII and antibody-dependent cellular toxicity. *J Biol Chem.* (2002) 277:26733–40. doi: 10.1074/jbc.M202069200

102. Engblom C, Pfirschke C, Pittet MJ. The role of myeloid cells in cancer therapies. *Nat Rev Cancer.* (2016) 16:447–62. doi: 10.1038/nrc.2016.54

103. Richards JO, Karki S, Lazar GA, Chen H, Dang W, Desjarlais JR. Optimization of antibody binding to FcgammaRIIa enhances macrophage phagocytosis of tumor cells. *Mol Cancer Ther.* (2008) 7:2517–27. doi: 10.1158/1535-7163.MCT-08-0201

104. Lazar GA, Dang W, Karki S, Vafa O, Peng JS, Hyun L, et al. Engineered antibody Fc variants with enhanced effector function. *Proc Natl Acad Sci USA.* (2006) 103:4005–10. doi: 10.1073/pnas.0508123103

105. Veri MC, Gorlatov S, Li H, Burke S, Johnson S, Stavenhagen J, et al. Monoclonal antibodies capable of discriminating the human inhibitory Fcgamma-receptor IIB (CD32B) from the activating Fcgamma-receptor IIA (CD32A): biochemical, biological and functional characterization. *Immunology.* (2007) 121:392–404. doi: 10.1111/j.1365-2567.2007.02588.x

106. Veri MC, Burke S, Huang L, Li H, Gorlatov S, Tuaillon N, et al. Therapeutic control of B cell activation via recruitment of Fcgamma receptor IIb (CD32B) inhibitory function with a novel bispecific antibody scaffold. *Arthritis Rheum.* (2010) 62:1933–43. doi: 10.1002/art.27477

107. Berntzen G, Andersen JT, Ustgard K, Michaelsen TE, Mousavi SA, Qian JD, et al. Identification of a high affinity FcgammaRIIA-binding peptide that distinguishes FcgammaRIIA from FcgammaRIIB and exploits FcgammaRIIA-mediated phagocytosis and degradation. *J Biol Chem.* (2009) 284:1126–35. doi: 10.1074/jbc.M803584200

108. Ganesan LP, Kim J, Wu Y, Mohanty S, Phillips GS, Birmingham DJ, et al. FcgammaRIIb on liver sinusoidal endothelium clears small immune complexes. *J Immunol.* (2012) 189:4981–8. doi: 10.4049/jimmunol.1202017

109. Li F, Ravetch JV. Apoptotic and antitumor activity of death receptor antibodies require inhibitory Fcgamma receptor engagement. *Proc Natl Acad Sci USA.* (2012) 109:10966–71. doi: 10.1073/pnas.1208698109

11

FcγRIIIb Restricts Antibody-Dependent Destruction of Cancer Cells by Human Neutrophils

Louise W. Treffers[1], Michel van Houdt[1], Christine W. Bruggeman[1], Marieke H. Heineke[2], Xi Wen Zhao[1], Joris van der Heijden[1], Sietse Q. Nagelkerke[1,3], Paul J. J. H. Verkuijlen[1], Judy Geissler[1], Suzanne Lissenberg-Thunnissen[1], Thomas Valerius[4], Matthias Peipp[4], Katka Franke[1], Robin van Bruggen[1], Taco W. Kuijpers[1,3], Marjolein van Egmond[2], Gestur Vidarsson[1], Hanke L. Matlung[1†] and Timo K. van den Berg[1,2*†]

[1] Sanquin Research, and Landsteiner Laboratory, Amsterdam UMC, University of Amsterdam, Amsterdam, Netherlands, [2] Department of Molecular Cell Biology and Immunology, Amsterdam UMC, Amsterdam Infection and Immunity Institute, Vrije Universiteit Amsterdam, Amsterdam, Netherlands, [3] Emma Children's Hospital, Amsterdam UMC, University of Amsterdam, Amsterdam, Netherlands, [4] Division of Stem Cell Transplantation and Immunotherapy, Department of Internal Medicine II, Kiel University, Kiel, Germany

*Correspondence:
Timo K. van den Berg
t.k.vandenberg@sanquin.nl

[†] These authors have contributed equally to this work

The function of the low-affinity IgG-receptor FcγRIIIb (CD16b), which is uniquely and abundantly expressed on human granulocytes, is not clear. Unlike the other Fcγ receptors (FcγR), it is a glycophosphatidyl inositol (GPI) -anchored molecule and does not have intracellular signaling motifs. Nevertheless, FcγRIIIb can cooperate with other FcγR to promote phagocytosis of antibody-opsonized microbes by human neutrophils. Here we have investigated the role of FcγRIIIb during antibody-dependent cellular cytotoxicity (ADCC) by neutrophils toward solid cancer cells coated with either trastuzumab (anti-HER2) or cetuximab (anti-EGFR). Inhibiting FcγRIIIb using CD16-F(ab')$_2$ blocking antibodies resulted in substantially enhanced ADCC. ADCC was completely dependent on FcγRIIa (CD32a) and the enhanced ADCC seen after FcγRIIIb blockade therefore suggested that FcγRIIIb was competing with FcγRIIa for IgG on the opsonized target cells. Interestingly, the function of neutrophil FcγRIIIb as a decoy receptor was further supported by using neutrophils from individuals with different gene copy numbers of FCGR3B causing different levels of surface FcγRIIIb expression. Individuals with one copy of FCGR3B showed higher levels of ADCC compared to those with two or more copies. Finally, we show that therapeutic antibodies intended to improve FcγRIIIa (CD16a)-dependent natural killer (NK) cell ADCC due to the lack of fucosylation on the N-linked glycan at position N297 of the IgG$_1$ heavy chain Fc-region, show decreased ADCC as compared to regularly fucosylated antibodies. Together, these data confirm FcγRIIIb as a negative regulator of neutrophil ADCC toward tumor cells and a potential target for enhancing tumor cell destruction by neutrophils.

Keywords: FcγRIIIb, neutrophil, ADCC, cancer, granulocyte, Fc-receptor, CNV, glycoengineering

INTRODUCTION

Fc-receptors play a vital role in cancer immunotherapy by inducing ADCC and antibody dependent cellular phagocytosis (ADCP). Most cancer targeting therapeutic antibodies currently on the market are of the IgG class, and thus human FcγRs constitute the key receptors for ADCC during cancer immunotherapy (1). The principal FcγR receptor on neutrophils required for mediating ADCC of solid cancer cells appears to be FcγRIIa (2, 3), with ~30–60-thousand copies expressed per cell (4), sometimes in combination with the activating receptor FcγRIIc, present on a minority of about 15–20% of Caucasian individuals (5). The high affinity receptor FcγRI (CD64) is only present on activated neutrophils, but does generally not contribute to ADCC of solid cancer cells even when expressed (3). Both FcγRI and FcγRIIa signal via immunoreceptor tyrosine-based activation motifs (ITAM), encoded in the cytoplasmic tail of the receptors (FcγRIIa) or in the associated γ-chain (FcγRI). Lastly, neutrophils express the highly abundant, 100–200-thousand copies per cell, low affinity receptor FcγRIIIb, which is a GPI-linked Fc-receptor that lacks intrinsic intracellular signaling capacity (4). This receptor is selectively present on neutrophils and on a subset of basophils (6). In spite of the lack for direct signaling through FcγRIIIb evidence from a number of studies show that FcγRIIIb cooperates together with other FcγR in the context of the phagocytosis of opsonized microbes (7). This suggests that the abundantly expressed FcγRIIIb primarily acts to facilitate enhanced recognition and that ITAM signaling via the other FcγR, in particular FcγRIIa, is sufficient, or at least instrumental, to trigger the phagocytic process. The FcγRIIIb-encoding gene, FCGR3B, which only occurs in humans and certain primates (8), is located within the FCGR2/3 locus on human chromosome 1, where it is prone to gene copy number variation (CNV) (9). The CNV of FCGR3B ranges from very rare individuals with no FCGR3B, to individuals with five copies of this gene (10). FCGR3B CNV has been shown to affect various diseases, i.e., a low CNV of FCGR3B was shown to result in an increased susceptibility to autoimmune diseases like systemic lupus erythematosus (SLE) (11, 12), primary Sjogren's syndrome (pSS) (12), Wegener's granulomatosis (WG) (12) and rheumatoid arthritis (RA) (13). A high CNV of FCGR3B has been associated with psoriasis vulgaris in Han Chinese (14). Nevertheless, no enhanced susceptibility to bacterial or fungal infection was observed in very rare individuals lacking FcγRIIIb expression (15), also showing that their neutrophils were able to function normally in regards to phagocytosis and superoxide generation (16). In addition, several polymorphic variants of the FCGR3B gene, known as the NA1, NA2, and SH haplotypes exist (17, 18), which do not result in marked differences in IgG-affinity. On the level of neutrophil-mediated ADCC of cancer cells all polymorphic variants appear similarly effective (3), but

neutrophils from NA1NA1 individuals have been reported to bind and phagocytose IgG-opsonized bacteria and red cells somewhat more effectively than their heterozygous NA1NA2 and homozygous NA2NA2 counterparts (19, 20).

Neutrophils constitute a major first line of host immune defense against fungal and bacterial infection (21). After extravasation from blood circulation they can enter a variety of tissues, including solid tumors (22–25). And even though the role of neutrophils in cancer is complex, with evidence for both positive or negative effects on tumor development (26), it is clear that neutrophils can contribute to the destruction of cancer cells particularly upon treatment with cancer therapeutic antibodies, as demonstrated now in a variety of animal models (27–30). Recently, we have found that neutrophils destroy antibody-opsonized cancer cells by a unique cytotoxic mechanism, termed trogoptosis, where neutrophils take up small pieces of cancer cell membrane, which leads to mechanical injury of the plasma membrane of cancer cells causing necrotic cell death (31). This neutrophil-mediated cytotoxic process can further be enhanced by inhibiting the interaction between the innate inhibitory immunoreceptor signal regulatory protein α (SIRPα) and CD47 (31–33). SIRPα is specifically expressed on myeloid cells and interacts with its ligand CD47, which is expressed ubiquitously, and is often overexpressed on cancer cells, acting as a "don't eat me" signal to prevent phagocytosis by macrophages (33–35). Interference with CD47-SIRPα interactions has also been shown to increase ADCC by monocytes and neutrophils, making this interaction an innate immune checkpoint and an attractive target for enhancing antibody therapy in cancer (32, 33, 36). Obviously, it is of interest to identify other pathways that negatively impact neutrophil ADCC.

Even though FcγRIIIb is a very abundant protein on neutrophils (37), its actual function has remained uncertain. Available evidence in the context of phagocytosis of antibody-opsonized bacteria by human neutrophils suggests that FcγRIIIb cooperates with activating FcγR, like FcγRIIa/c, to promote phagocytosis (7, 38–40), and we have confirmed this in the current study. However, here we show that with respect to neutrophil mediated ADCC, FcγRIIIb rather acts as a decoy receptor for IgG, likewise competing with FcγRIIa for the binding of therapeutic antibodies, thereby resulting in decreased ADCC. Thus, in the context of cancer FcγRIIIb on neutrophils uniquely functions as a limiting factor, thereby identifying it a as potential target for enhancing the therapeutic efficacy of cancer therapeutic antibodies.

MATERIALS AND METHODS

Cells and Culture

The HER2/Neu-positive human breast cancer carcinoma cell line SKBR3 (ATCC) was cultured in IMDM medium (Gibco) supplemented with 20% fetal bovine serum, 2 mM L-glutamine, 100 U/mL penicillin and 100 μg/mL streptomycin at 37°C and 5% CO_2. SKBR3-CD47KD cells were generated by lentiviral transduction of pLKO.1-puro—CD47KD (5′ ccgggcacaattacttgga ctagttctcgagaactagtccaagtaattgtgcttttt 3′), resulting in a CD47 expression of 10–15% of the parental cell line according to

---
Abbreviations: FcγR, Fcγ receptor; ADCC, antibody dependent cellular cytotoxicity; NK cell, natural killer cell; ADCP, antibody dependent cellular phagocytosis; ITAM, immunoreceptor tyrosine-based activation motif; CNV, copy number variation; G-CSF, granulocyte-colony stimulating factor; IFNγ, interferon-γ.

instructions provided by the manufacturer (Sigma), as show previously (32). Transduced cells were selected with $1 \mu g/mL$ of puromycin. As control cell line, empty vector shRNA were used (SKBR3-SCR). The CD47 knockdown cell line was routinely verified by flow cytometry.

The EGFR-positive human epidermoid carcinoma cell line A431 (ATCC) was cultured in RPMI medium (Gibco) supplemented with 10% fetal bovine serum, 2 mM L-glutamine, 100 U/mL penicillin and $100 \mu g/mL$ streptomycin at $37°C$ and 5% CO_2. A431-CD47KO cell lines were generated by lentiviral transduction of pLentiCrispR-v2—CD47KO [pLentiCrispR-v2 was a gift from Feng Zhang (Addgene plasmid #52961)], using $5'$ cagcaacagcgccgctacca $3'$ as the CD47 CrispR target sequence. Transduced cells were selected with $1 \mu g/mL$ of puromycin, followed by limiting dilution. A clone lacking CD47 expression was selected by flow cytometry. An A431-SCR cell line was used as control for the CD47KO generated using CRISPR-Cas9 technology using a scrambled vector.

Neutrophil Isolation

Neutrophils from healthy donors were isolated as previously described (41). In short, granulocytes were isolated from blood by density gradient centrifugation (2,000 rpm, 20 min, 20°C) with isotonic Percoll (1.069 g/mL) and erythrocyte lysis. The pellet fraction was lysed with ice-cold NH4Cl (155 mmol/LNH,CI, 10 mmol/L KHCO, 0.1 mmol/L EDTA, pH 7.4) solution for 5–10 min to destroy erythrocytes. Cells were centrifuged at $4°C$ (1,500 rpm, 5 min), and residual erythrocytes were lysed for another 5 min. After this, granulocytes were washed twice in cold phosphate buffered saline (PBS) containing HSA (0.5% wt/vol).Isolated neutrophils were used at a concentration of 5×10^6 cells/mL. Cells were cultured in HEPES$^+$ medium (containing 132 mM NaCl, 6.0 mM KCl, 1.0 mM $CaCl_2$, 1.0 mM $MgSO_4$, 1.2 mM K_2HPO_4, 20 mM Hepes, 5.5 mM glucose, and 0.5% HSA), in the presence of 10 ng/ml clinical grade G-CSF (Neupogen; Amgen, Breda, The Netherlands) and 50 ng/mL recombinant human interferon-γ (Pepro Tech Inc, USA) at a concentration of 5×10^6 cells/mL for 4 or 16 h. After 16 h, cell viability was determined by the percentage of FITC-Annexin V (BD Pharmingen, San Diego, CA) positive cells on FACS, after which the cell concentration was corrected to 5×10^6 viable cells/mL. Cells were consequently washed and prepared for analysis by ADCC assay. All blood was obtained after informed consent and according to the Declaration of Helsinki principles (version Seoul 2008).

Antibodies and Reagents

FcγR expression was determined on FACS and depicted as MFI (median fluorescent intensity) using the following antibodies: anti-human FcγRI (Clone 10.1, mouse IgG1, BD Pharmingen, San Diego, CA), anti-human FcγRIIa (Clone AT10, mouse IgG1, AbD Serotec, Oxford, U.K.), anti-human FcγRIIIb (Clone 3G8, mouse IgG1, BD Pharmingen, San Diego, CA), all FITC labeled. FcγRs antagonistic antibodies were used in ADCC and trogocytosis assays at a final concentration of $5 \mu g/mL$: monovalent human Fc fragments (Bethyl, USA) for blocking FcγRI as used previously (3), anti-human CD32 F(ab')$_2$ (Clone 7.3, Ancell) to block FcγRIIa/b/c, anti-human

CD16 F(ab')$_2$ (Clone 3G8, Ancell) to block FcγRIIIa/b at a concentration of $10 \mu g/mL$. CD11b expression was determined with the FITC labeled anti-CD11b antibody (Lot 8000236273, Pelicluster), and SIRPα with the FITC labeled mouse IgG$_1$ antibody 12C4, previously described in (32). FITC-labeled mouse IgG1 was used as isotype control (Pelicluster). Afucosylated trastuzumab was generated in our laboratory as described before for afucosylated rituximab (42). Briefly, CHO-KI or Lec13 cells were transfected with antibody LC and HC expression constructs using transfection kit V from the Amaxa Nucleofectior System (Lonza, Cologne, Germany). The medium was exchanged by culture medium after 48 h, which contained $500 \mu g/mL$ hygromycin B. Single-cell subclones were created by limiting dilution. The produced antibodies were purified from the cell culture supernatant using CaptureSelect^{TM} IgG-CH1 Affinity Matrix (Thermo Fisher Scientific). IgA2-HER2 was generated by synthesizing (IDT, Leuven, Belgium) the variable heavy and light chain V gene encoding for trastuzumab (sequence as obtained from https://www.drugbank.ca/) and cloning into pcDNA3.1 expression vectors encoding for the constant regions for IgA2 and kappa, respectively, as described previously (43). The resulting expression vectors were then used to produce the antibodies in HEK Freestyle cells as we described previously (44, 45). Briefly, after transfection, cell supernatant was harvested after 5 days, after which cells were centrifuged ($\geq 4000 g$) and the supernatant was filtered using a 0.45 nm puradisc syringe filter (Whatmann, GE Healthcare, 10462100). Antibody concentration was determined via enzyme-linked immunosorbert assay (ELISA), as described previously (46). To create afucosylated antibodies, the decoy substrates for fucosylation, 2-deoxy-2-fluoro-l-fucose (2FF) (Carbosynth, MD06089) were added 4 h post transfection. Similarly, human anti-pneumococcal serotype 6B Gdob1 antibodies (IgG$_1$) (47, 48), regular and afucosylated were produced in the same system (44, 45). They were used at a concentration of $10 \mu g/mL$ throughout the experiment to opsonize S. pneumoniae. Polyclonal human IgG (IVIG, nanogam, Sanquin) was used to opsonize S. aureus at a concentration of 1 mg/mL for 10 min at $37°C$.

ADCC

Cancer cell lines were labeled with 100 μCi ^{51}Cr (Perkin-Elmer) for 90 min at $37°C$. After 3 washes with PBS, 5×10^3 cells were incubated in RPMI medium supplemented with 10% fetal bovine serum, 2 mM L-glutamine, 100 U/mL penicillin and $100 \mu g/mL$ streptomycin for 4 h at $37°C$ and 5% CO_2 in a 96-wells U-bottom plate together with neutrophils in a E:T ratio of 50:1 in the presence of $5 \mu g/mL$ therapeutic antibody. After the incubation supernatant was harvested and analyzed for radioactivity using a gamma counter (Wallac). The percentage of cytotoxicity was calculated as [(experimental cpm- spontaneous cpm)/ (total cpm–spontaneous cpm)] $\times$ 100%. All conditions were measured in triplicate.

Trogocytosis Assay

To determine the amount of tumor membrane taken up by neutrophils a FACS based assay was used. Cancer cells were labeled with a lipophilic membrane dye (DiO, $5 \mu M$, Invitrogen)

for 30 min at 37°C. After washing the target cells with PBS they were incubated with neutrophils in a U-bottom 96-wells plate at a E:T ratio of 5:1 in the absence or presence of 0.5 μg/mL therapeutic antibody. Samples were fixed with stopbuffer containing 0.5% PFA, 1% BSA and 20 mM NaF and measured by flow cytometry. After gating for neutrophil population, the mean fluorescent intensity (MFI) and the percentage of cells positive for DiO were determined.

Bacterial Phagogytosis

Uptake of FITC labeled *S. aureus* was performed in a 96 wells plate for 15 min at 37°C shaking, with 0.5×10^6 neutrophils and 25×10^6 bacteria in a final volume of 250 μL in HEPES$^+$ medium. Bacteria were opsonized with polyclonal IgG (IVIG) (1 mg/mL) for 10 min at 37°C. Cells were fixed with stopbuffer (0.5% PFA, 1% BSA, 20 mM NaF) for 30 min at 4°C and measured by flow cytometry (BD FACSCanto II). Uptake of Dy488 labeled heat killed *Streptococcus Pneumoniae* was performed in a 96 wells plate for 30 min at 37°C while shaking, with 1.5×10^4 neutrophils and 5×10^6 bacteria in a final volume of 225 μL in HEPES$^+$ medium. When applicable, neutrophils were incubated with FcγR blockers for 15 min at RT. Bacteria were opsonized with GDob1 antibody at a concentration of 10 μg/mL throughout the experiment. Cells were fixed with stopbuffer (0.5% PFA, 1% BSA, 20 mM NaF) for 30 min at 4°C and measured by flow cytometry (BD FACSCanto II).

MLPA

Genotyping of individuals for *FCGR3B* CNV was performed using the *FCGR*-specific Multiplex Ligation-dependent Probe Amplification (MLPA) assay (MRC Holland), using genomic DNA isolated from whole blood with the QIAamp® kit (Qiagen, Hilden, Germany). The MLPA assay was performed as described previously (49). In brief, 5 μL of DNA (20 ng/μL) was denatured at 98°C for 5 min and subsequently cooled to 25°C in a thermal cycler with heated lid; To each sample 1.5 μL buffer and 1.5 μL buffer probe mix were added and incubated for 1 min at 95°C, followed by 16 h at 60°C. After this, 32 μL of ligase-65 mix was added to each sample at 54°C, followed by an incubation of 15 min at 54°C and 5 min at 98°C, followed by a 4 times dilution of the ligation mixture. This was followed by addition of 10 μL of polymerase mix, which contained one single primer pair, after which the polymerase chain reaction (PCR) was started immediately. PCR conditions were 36 cycles of 30 s at 95°C, 30 s at 60°C, and 60 s at 72°C, followed by 20 min at 72°C. After the PCR reaction, 1 μL of the PCR reaction was mixed with 0.5 μL CXR 60–400 (Promega, Madison, WI) internal size standards and 8.5 μL deionized formamide, and the mixture was incubated for 10 min at 90°C. The products were then separated by electrophoresis on an ABI-3130XL (Applied Biosystems, Foster City, CA).Data were analyzed using GeneMarker v1.6 sofware.

IL-8 ELISA

IL-8 production was measured using the Human IL-8 ELISA Ready-SET-Go! (2nd Generation) kit (eBioscience, Thermo Fisher Scientific, Waltham, MA) according to manufacturer's instructions. Wavelengths were measured with an iMark

microplate absorbance reader (Bio-rad Laboratories, Hercules, CA).

Study Approval

The study was performed according to national regulations with respect to the use of human materials from healthy, anonymized volunteers with written informed consent, and the experiments were approved by the Medical Ethical Committee of the Academic Medical Center in Amsterdam according to the Declaration of Helsinki principles (version Seoul 2008).

Data Analysis and Statistics

Statistical differences were determined by either paired or ordinary one way ANOVA, with Sidak or Dunnett's *post-test*, or by paired student's *t*-test, as indicated in the figure legend.

RESULTS

We studied the role of FcγRIIIb during neutrophil ADCC toward solid cancer cells. Although FcγRIIIb is apparently unable to signal by itself, it definitely has the capacity to bind IgG and as such could potentially influence responses via other activating Fcγ-receptors on neutrophils, in either a positive or negative fashion. Such activating FcγRs present on neutrophils include FcγRI, only present after neutrophil activation, and FcγRIIa, which appears to be the main receptor required for ADCC against cancer cells expressing the tumor antigens HER2/Neu or EGFR (**Supplementary Figure 1**) (2, 3). Neutrophil-mediated ADCC toward cancer cells can be enhanced after neutrophil-activation, e.g., by granulocyte-colony stimulating factor (G-CSF) and interferon-γ (IFNγ) (32). This stimulation causes a change in the expression levels of the FcγRs, resulting in expression of FcγRI, a small decrease in expression in FcγRIIa, and, of particular interest, a substantial decrease in FcγRIIIb (**Figure 1A**). The reduction in FcγRIIIb expression could well be due to cleavage of FcγRIIIb by protease release after neutrophil activation (50, 51). As mentioned before FcγRIIIb is subject to considerable gene CNV (9), and the expression levels of FcγRIIIb are directly linked to the number of copies present in the genome (**Figure 1B**). Upon stimulation FcγRIIIb levels on neutrophils are gradually reduced and the variation among individuals with different FcγRIIIb levels are essentially blunted (**Figure 1B**).

FcγRIIIb Functions as a Decoy Receptor During Neutrophil ADCC

We first determined the effect of blocking FcγRIIIb with F(ab')$_2$ fragments of specific anti-FcγRIIIb on both their ability to take up cancer cell fragments (trogocytosis) (**Figure 2A**) as well as their cytotoxic capacity, as measured by ^{51}Cr-release. The use of F(ab')$_2$-fragments is absolutely critical here as intact anti-FcγR antibodies may also exert non-specific blocking by the so called "Kurlander" phenomenon (52). Blocking FcγRIIIb resulted in a prominent increase in both trogocytosis and ADCC, clearly suggesting that FcγRIIIb plays a negative role in neutrophil-mediated antibody-dependent destruction of cancer cells (**Figures 2B–J**). Similar results were obtained

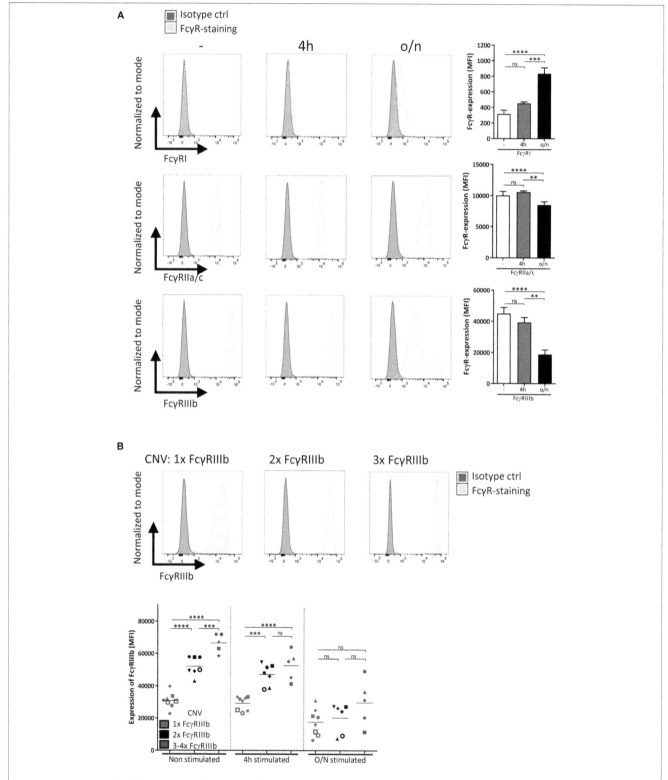

FIGURE 1 | Expression of FcγR on neutrophils depends on activation status and CNV. **(A)** FcγR expression, shown as representative histograms and bar graphs (MFI), was determined for freshly isolated neutrophils and neutrophils stimulated for 4 h or overnight with G-CSF and IFNγ. **(B)** Neutrophils were isolated from donors with different copy numbers of *FCGR3B*, and their FcγRIIIb expression was checked using flow cytometry, before stimulation, after 4 h stimulation and after overnight stimulation with G-CSF and IFNγ. Individuals with only one copy of *FCGR3B* are represented by green dots, donors with two copies by black dots, donors with three or more copies of *FCGR3B* by blue dots. Each symbol represents an individual donor per color. Data shown are mean + SEM **(A)** and mean **(B)** with $N = 20$ **(A)** and $N = 5$–8 **(B)**, statistical analysis was performed by one-way paired ANOVA with Tukey *post-test*. ns, non-significant; **$p < 0.01$, ***$p < 0.001$, and ****$p < 0.0001$.

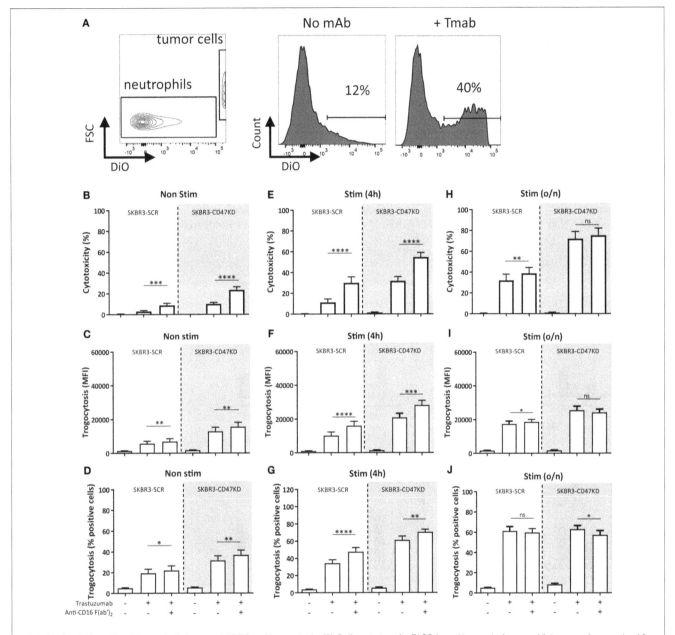

FIGURE 2 | Inhibition of FcγRIIIb results in increased ADCC and trogocytosis. **(A)** Gating strategy for FACS-based trogocytosis assay. Histograms show neutrophil population becoming positive for DiO after incubation with trastuzumab coated SKBR3-scrambled (SKBR3-SCR) cells. **(B–J)** Blocking FcγRIIIb increases ADCC and trogocytosis of trastuzumab coated SKBR3-SCR cells (white background) when using non-stimulated **(B–D)**, 4 h stimulated **(E–G)** and to a lesser extent overnight **(H–J)** stimulated neutrophils (with G-CSF and IFNγ). This effect is also present when inhibiting CD47-SIRPα interactions by CD47 knock-down (SKBR3-CD47KD, gray background). Data shown are means + SEM with **(B)** $N = 26$, **(C)** $N = 20$, **(D)** $N = 20$, **(E)** $N = 17$, **(F)** $N = 18$, **(G)** $N = 18$, **(H)** $N = 14$, **(I)** $N = 8$, **(J)** $N = 8$, statistical analysis was performed by paired t-test. ns, non-significant; $*p < 0.05$, $**p < 0.01$, $***p < 0.001$, and $****p < 0.0001$.

when using other solid cancer cells, such as the EGFR-positive A431 cell line combined with the therapeutic antibody cetuximab (**Supplementary Figures 2A-C**). However, with both tumor targets, this negative role of FcγRIIIb was only visible when using freshly isolated neutrophils or neutrophils that had only been briefly stimulated (i.e., for 4 h; **Figures 2E–G**), when relatively large quantities of FcγRIIIb are still present on the neutrophil cell surface (see **Figure 1**). In contrary,

when evaluated after overnight stimulation with G-CSF and IFNγ both neutrophil trogocytosis and ADCC were higher and the effect of FcγRIIIb blocking eventually disappeared (**Figures 2H–J**), which could be explained, at least in part, by the observed reduction in FcγRIIIb surface expression (**Figure 1**). Of interest, under these conditions the enhancing effect of CD47-SIRPα interference on cytotoxicity was still clearly visible (**Figure 2H**). Whether or not FcγRIIIb is highly expressed on neutrophils, FcγRIIa remains the primary receptor responsible for triggering ADCC (**Supplementary Figure 1**). Thus, the principal FcγR mediating trogocytosis and subsequent ADCC of antibody-opsonized solid cancer cells by human neutrophils is FcγRIIa/c, and FcγRIIIb appears to function as a decoy receptor that apparently competes with FcγRIIa/c for binding to the Fc-portion of the opsonizing cancer therapeutic antibody.

To mimic checkpoint inhibitor blockade, we used SKBR3 cells with shRNA-knock-down for CD47 (reduction by ∼85–90%) (SKBR3-CD47KD) to inhibit the interactions between CD47 and SIRPα (32, 33, 36). The effect of inhibiting both CD47-SIRPα interactions and FcγRIIIb became even more apparent (**Figure 2**, gray background), also indicating that disruption of CD47-SIRPα and

FcγRIIIb blockade were not part of the same inhibitory pathway and that such interferences could generate additive effects.

We hypothesized that blocking of FcγRIIIb could perhaps be resulting in increased production of IL-8 by neutrophils, which was previously described to occur when crosslinking FcαRI on neutrophils (53). The use of IgA therapeutic antibodies enhances neutrophil-mediated ADCC of cancer cells compared to using IgG antibodies (54, 55), which could be in part due to the production of cytokines, such as IL-8, by the neutrophils. We therefore determined the presence of IL-8 in the supernatant after neutrophil-mediated ADCC of SKBR3 cells in the presence or absence of FcγRIIIb blocking antibodies. The IL-8 levels that were produced using an anti-HER2 IgG antibody were significantly lower compared to IgA, as reported before (45),

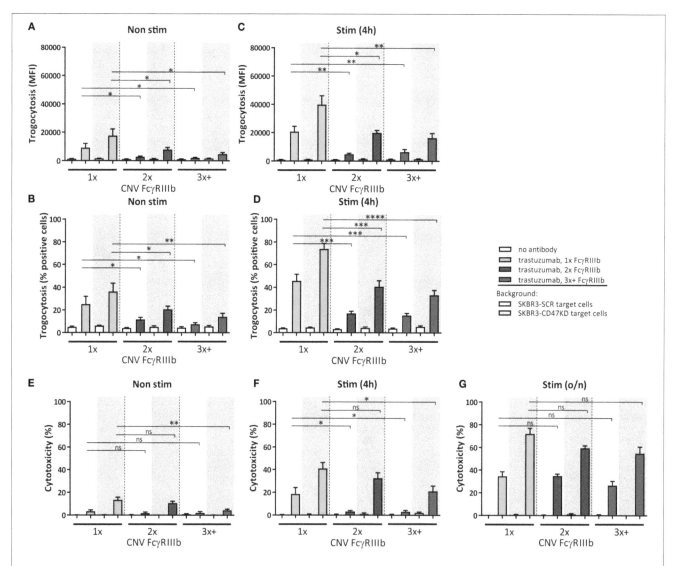

FIGURE 3 | CNV of *FCGR3B* affects ADCC of cancer cells by neutrophils. Trogocytosis **(A–D)** and ADCC **(E–G)** was determined for neutrophils from donors with various copies of *FCGR3B*. Freshly isolated **(A,B,E)**, 4 h stimulated **(C,D,F)** or overnight stimulated **(G)** neutrophils were combined with trastuzumab coated SKBR3-SCR (white background) or SKBR3-CD47KD cells (gray background). Shown are results from individuals with one copy (green), two copies (gray), or three or more copies (blue) of *FCGR3B*. Data shown are means + SEM with results from multiple experiments with donors ranging from $N = 7$–10. Statistical analysis was performed by one-way paired ANOVA with Sidak *post-test*. ns, non-significant; *$p < 0.05$, **$p < 0.01$, ***$p < 0.001$, and ****$p < 0.0001$.

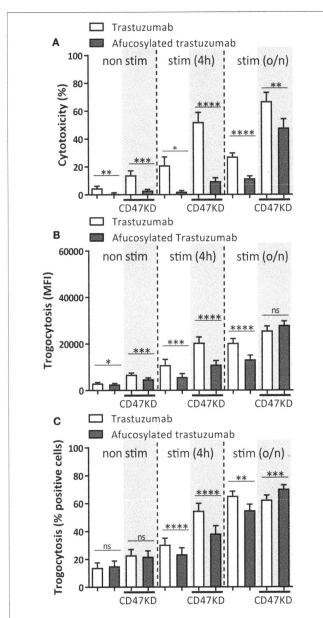

FIGURE 4 | Neutrophil ADCC and trogocytosis are reduced when afucosylated therapeutic antibodies are used. Afucosylated trastuzumab was compared to regularly fucosylated trastuzumab in both trogocytosis **(A,B)**, and ADCC **(C)**. Freshly isolated, 4 h and overnight stimulated (with G-CSF and IFNγ) neutrophils were combined with IgG opsonized SKBR3-SCR (white background) or SKBR3-CD47KD cells (gray background). Data shown are means + SEM with results from multiple experiments with donors ranging from $N = 9$–16. Statistical analysis was performed by paired t-test. ns, non-significant; $*p < 0.05$, $**p < 0.01$, $***p < 0.001$, and $****p < 0.0001$.

and additional inhibition of FcγRIIIb showed no enhanced production of IL-8 (**Supplementary Figure 2D**).

FCGR3B CNV Determines Neutrophil ADCC

As indicated above FcγRIIIb surface expression on neutrophils is subject to considerable variation, and this is largely caused by

gene copy number variation within the *FCGR2/3* locus (15). This enabled us to further study the observed negative contribution of FcγRIIIb to neutrophil ADCC. We therefore evaluated neutrophils from individuals with different copy numbers of *FCGR3B* determined by MPLA-based genotyping (49). Indeed, individuals with one copy of the gene have significantly increased ADCC and trogocytosis capacity compared to individuals with 2 or 3 or more copies, using neutrophils either freshly isolated or after 4 h stimulation with G-CSF and IFNγ (**Figure 3**). However, after overnight stimulation this difference essentially disappeared in all tested individuals and irrespective of *FCGR3* gene copy number (**Figure 1**). When comparing individuals with low (1x) and high FcγRIIIb (2–4x) expression blocking of FcγRIIIb could enhance ADCC to indistinguishable levels (**Supplementary Figure 3**), demonstrating that the difference in ADCC capacity between individuals with different *FCGR3B* CNV can indeed largely be attributed to the difference in FcγRIIIb expression on neutrophils. In these experiments the levels of other surface molecules relevant in the context of neutrophil ADCC (31, 32), including FcγRs, integrins or SIRPα were similar in all donors with different copy numbers of *FCGR3B* (**Supplementary Figure 4**).

When correlating the FcγRIIIb expression to either trogocytosis or ADCC capacity of neutrophils, irrespective of *FCGR3B* genetic status, we also noted a significant inverse correlation, but as expected this occurred only when using either freshly isolated neutrophils (**Supplementary Figures 5A-C**) or 4 h (**Supplementary Figures 5D-F**) stimulated neutrophils, but this correlation disappeared upon overnight neutrophil stimulation (**Supplementary Figures 5G-I**) consistent with the loss of surface FcγRIIIb. By comparison, we did not find any significant correlations when comparing FcγRIIa expression levels and killing (**Supplementary Figure 6**). These findings show that in non-stimulated neutrophils *FCGR3B* CNV is an important determinant of ADCC capacity, with higher levels of CNV and concurrent FcγRIIIb surface expression negatively affecting neutrophil ADCC, thereby providing genetic evidence for a role of FcγRIIIb as a decoy receptor.

Antibody Afucosylation Negatively Impacts Neutrophil ADCC

A number of mutations and posttranslational modifications of therapeutic antibodies have previously been explored for the purpose of improving their clinical potential. One of these alterations is antibody afucosylation, which changes the glycan linked to asparagine at position 297 (N297). Afucosylation of this glycan increases the binding affinity of the antibody to FcγRIIIa (44, 56, 57), and this has been shown to increase ADCC by PBMC, including NK cells and monocytes, that express activating FcγRIIIa (58–61). However, afucosylation also improves binding to FcγRIIIb ~15 fold (44) compared to normal IgG which impacts neutrophil ADCC (2, 62), but to what extend this affects neutrophil trogoptosis toward tumor cells has not been previously investigated. Consistent with the above findings, neutrophil-mediated ADCC of SKBR3 cells using afucosylated trastuzumab resulted in a highly significant and prominent (up to ~80–90%) decrease in ADCC when compared to normally fucosylated trastuzumab (**Figure 4A**). Interestingly, trogocytosis was also substantially affected and showed both a decrease in the net-amount of target membrane uptake on average by neutrophils (**Figure 4B**) and decrease in the number of participating neutrophils (**Figure 4C**), confirming the negative effect of FcγRIIIb under these conditions. As expected from the above the difference in ADCC response between afucosylated and fucosylated trastuzumab became smaller when neutrophils had been activated. Furthermore, by inhibiting FcγRIIIb on neutrophils we were able to completely rescue the ability of afucosylated trastuzumab to perform ADCC and trogocytosis (**Supplementary Figure 7**) showing that the reduced killing of afucosylated trastuzumab by neutrophils can indeed be entirely attributed to its enhanced binding to FcγRIIIb. Clearly, this shows that antibody afucosylation, while enhancing the ADCC capacity of NK cells and monocytes, negatively affects neutrophil ADCC.

FcγRIIIb Contributes to IgG-Mediated Phagocytosis of Bacteria

It has previously been shown that FcγRIIIb does stimulate phagocytosis of bacteria and platelets cooperatively with other activating FcγRs, such as FcγRIIa, which is further stimulated by afucosylation of the opsonizing antibodies (7, 38, 40). To determine whether we could replicate this cooperative role we used S. aureus opsonized with polyclonal human IgG, which is a commercial blood product containing polyclonal IgG isolated and pooled from thousands of donors. We noticed that blocking either FcγRIIa or FcγRIIIb on neutrophils resulted in a decreased phagocytosis of S. aureus, with the most optimal reduction in phagocytosis being achieved by blocking both receptors (**Figure 5A**). No role for FcγRI in bacterial phagocytosis by neutrophils was found. However, since polyclonal IgG contains all IgG isotypes (approx. 65% IgG$_1$) and our ADCC experiments are done using only monoclonal IgG$_1$ antibodies we wanted to be certain that these results were not due to effects of one of the other IgG isotypes. To be able to specifically look at IgG$_1$ mediated effects, we used a

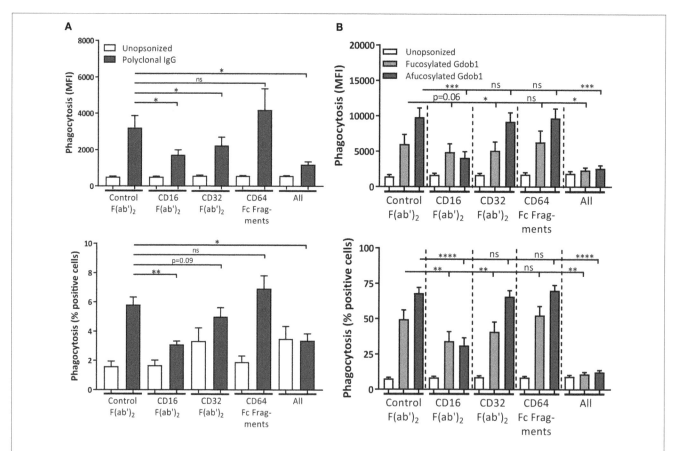

FIGURE 5 | FcγRIIa and FcγRIIIb both contribute to bacterial phagocytosis. FcγRs were blocked on freshly isolated neutrophils during phagocytosis of polyclonal IgG-opsonized S. aureus (gray bars) (A) or heat-killed S. pneumoniae, serogroup 6B, opsonized with GDob1 (IgG$_1$) (dark gray bars) or afucosylated GDob1 (IgG$_1$) (light gray bars) (B). Shown are both percentage of neutrophils phagocytosing (% positive cells) and relative uptake of bacteria (MFI). Data shown are means + SEM with results shown from 3 (A), and 2 (B) experiments with (A) N = 10, (B) N = 7, statistical analysis was performed by one-way paired ANOVA with Dunnett's post-test. ns, non-significant; *p < 0.05, **p < 0.01, ***p < 0.001, and ****p < 0.0001.

heat-killed *Streptococcus pneumoniae* of serogroup 6B, which can be opsonized with a 6B-specific recombinant human IgG1 monoclonal antibody (GDob1) (47). This confirmed a cooperative role of FcγRIIa and FcγRIIIb, with the two receptors functioning in a largely redundant fashion with no additive role for FcγRI (**Figure 5B**; **Supplementary Figure 8**). Of interest, when using an afucosylated variant of GDOb1, with increased affinity for FcγRIIIb, FcγRIIIb clearly became the dominant FcγR mediating phagocytosis (**Figure 5B**). Collectively, this corroborates previous results that FcγRIIIb on human neutrophils plays a facilitating role in microbial phagocytosis, and this strongly contrasts with the negative role of this receptor during ADCC.

DISCUSSION

Here we found that FcγRIIIb on neutrophils acts as a decoy receptor during human neutrophil ADCC toward cancer cells, thereby restricting tumor killing mechanisms exerted via FcγRIIa. This is in line with previous reports showing that signaling through FcγRIIa is apparently entirely essential for active ADCC in neutrophils (2, 3). For phagocytosis, other mechanisms are apparently at play, as we and others found neutrophil FcγRIIIb to actively participate in bacterial ingestion (7, 63). This is possible as FcγRIIIb is a GPI-linked receptor, causing it to preferentially reside in detergent-resistant membranes, or lipid rafts, enriched in signaling

molecules such as myristoylated src-kinases. In addition, it associates through its ectodomains with other receptors, and certainly with other FcγR in *cis* during encounter with IgG-opsonized targets, providing receptor cross-talk (4, 39, 64, 65). The enhanced recognition via FcγRIIIb apparently facilitates phagocytosis, while in contrary it impedes ADCC as we show here. Of interest, this may not only be true for phagocytosis of microbes and/or small particles, but maybe also for relatively small tumor cells such as CLL cells. Here, FcγRIIIb seems to have a beneficial effect (38, 66), although there still seems to be some discussion about whether small tumor cells are phagocytosed or in fact trogocytosed by human neutrophils (67). In general, antibodies of the IgG1 subclass bind to the various Fcγ-receptors expressed on neutrophils with a wide range of affinities. In particular, the binding affinity of FcγRIIIB for IgG1 is approximately 10-fold lower compared to FcγRIIA (68). This might explain the relative high amount of FcγRIIIB molecules on the neutrophil plasma membrane needed to create the "buffering" decoy effect of FcγRIIIB as we describe herein in the context of ADCC specifically (see **Figure 6** for a graphical representation).

In further support that FcγRIIIb negatively affects ADCC, we found a clear gene-dosage effect of *FCGR3B* through the CNV of the gene, with higher numbers gradually decreasing ADCC even further. Potentially *FCGR3B* CNV can be used as a new biomarker for cancer immunotherapy, where patients can be stratified with likelihood of benefitting from therapy when

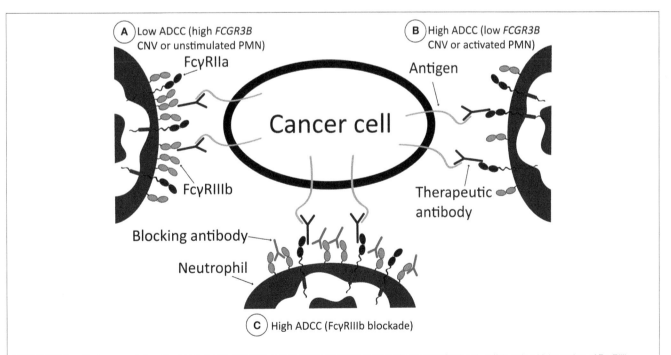

FIGURE 6 | Graphical representation of working model. ADCC by neutrophils is low when neutrophils are not stimulated, or if there is a high number of FcγRIIIb present on the neutrophil cell surface, due to high CNV of *FCGR3B* **(A)**. ADCC is high when neutrophils are stimulated, with G-CSF and IFNγ, or when there is a low number of FcγRIIIb present on the neutrophil cell surface, due to low CNV of *FCGR3B* **(B)**. ADCC by neutrophils can be increased after therapeutic intervention, i.e., by blocking FcγRIIIb with blocking antibodies, which results in high ADCC **(C)**. In all situations, FcγRIIa is required for neutrophil ADCC and is, due to high presence of FcγRIIIb in **(A)**, unable to sufficiently bind the therapeutic antibody opsonizing the cancer cell surface. When there is less FcγRIIIb present on the cell surface **(B)** or after FcγRIIIb blockade **(C)**, neutrophils are more effective in ADCC of solid cancer cells.

patients have a lower *FCGR3B* CNV combined with the right tumor antigens (e.g., HER2/Neu or EGFR).

To date, this FcγRIIIb decoy effect during ADCC has not been possible to study *in vivo* due to the fact that mice do not express a GPI-linked FcγR ortholog or homolog (27–30). However, in the future it might be interesting to study this effect in humanized models [mice expressing human FcγR or mice with human immune system (69)] to see the relative contribution of FcγRIIIb on neutrophils in therapy and if its effect can be circumvented.

Furthermore, our findings raise doubt whether the use of afucosylated monoclonal antibodies for antibody therapy against cancer is beneficial in all situations. Glycoengineering antibodies in this manner is currently being applied to various monoclonal antibodies to increase their capability to enhance ADCC and phagocytosis. This modification is well-documented to increase binding to FcγRIIIa, which is expressed by natural killer cells, monocytes and macrophages, (62, 70, 71). Less consideration has been given to the fact that this type of glycoengineering similarly enhances its affinity to FcγRIIIb, which is only present on granulocytes (44). Here, we confirm that engineered antibodies with enhanced affinity to FcγRIIIb by afucosylation have deleterious effects on ADCC by neutrophils (2, 62). This effect could partially be negated by using a combination of a targeting antibody and preventing the CD47-SIRPα- checkpoint inhibitor axis. Thus, it can be anticipated that the net effect of cancer therapeutic antibody afucosylation is basically a trade-off between the beneficial effects on various immune cells on one hand and the detrimental effects on neutrophils.

One of the obvious implications of our findings is that selective blockade of FcγRIIIb could be a potential way to enhance the effect of cancer therapeutic antibodies and thereby improve clinical outcome for patients and/or reduce their need for other non-specific agents such as chemotherapeutics. However, while interesting to explore further this is not a trivial challenge as the activating FcγRIIIa receptor on other cells has a very similar extracellular region, making it perhaps impossible to achieve the required specificity. Nevertheless, as we show here the effects of blocking FcγRIIIb appear interesting so if the issue of specificity can be solved one way or another this may be an interesting concept to pursue (see also **Figure 6** for a graphical representation).

We have shown in the current study that inhibition of FcγRIIIb also increases ADCC when this is combined with interference of CD47-SIRPα interactions. FcγRIIIb specific

inhibiting agents could thus potentially be combined with antibodies targeting these checkpoint-inhibitor molecules, which are currently in development (www.clinicaltrials.gov identifiers: NCT02216409; NCT02678338, NCT02641002; NCT02367196, NCT02890368; NCT02663518, NCT02953509) (72). In theory, using a monoclonal antibody with an increased affinity to FcγRIIa (2) could also be beneficial to circumvent the decoy effect by FcγRIIIb.

Collectively, we have shown that FcγRIIIb acts as a decoy receptor for IgG during neutrophil-mediated ADCC of solid cancer cells, while it harbors a good potential to stimulate phagocytosis. These results pinpoint FcγRIIIb as a potential target and biomarker for cancer immunotherapy, while underscoring a potential threat using glycoengineered antibodies with enhanced binding to both FcγRIIIa and FcγRIIIb which needs to be further evaluated in patients.

AUTHOR CONTRIBUTIONS

LT, MvH, MH, HM, KF, RvB, TK, MvE, GV, and TvdB designed research. LT, MvH, CB, MH, XZ, JvdH, SN, PV, and JG performed research. SL-T, TV, MP, and GV contributed new reagents analytic tools. LT analyzed data. LT, HM, RvB, and TvdB wrote the paper that was edited and approved by all authors.

FUNDING

LT was supported by a grant (LSBR-1223) from the Landsteiner Foundation for Blood Transfusion Research. HM was supported by a grant (#10300) from the Dutch Cancer Society. TvdB is supported by a research collaboration with Synthon Biopharmaceuticals related to CD47-SIRPalpha targeting in cancer. MH and MvE are supported by the Netherlands Organization for Scientific Research (NWO; VICI 91814650).

ACKNOWLEDGMENTS

We would like to thank Thies Rösner and Steffen Kahle for their contributions to this manuscript.

REFERENCES

1. Guan M, Zhou YP, Sun JL, Chen SC. Adverse events of monoclonal antibodies used for cancer therapy. *Biomed Res Int.* (2015) 2015:428169. doi: 10.1155/2015/428169
2. Derer S, Glorius P, Schlaeth M, Lohse S, Klausz K, Muchhal U, et al. Increasing FcγRIIa affinity of an FcγRIII-optimized anti-EGFR antibody restores neutrophil-mediated cytotoxicity. *MAbs* (2014) 6:409–21. doi: 10.4161/mabs.27457
3. Treffers LW, Zhao XW, van der Heijden J, Nagelkerke SQ, van Rees DJ, Gonzalez P, et al. Genetic variation of human neutrophil Fcγ receptors and SIRPα in antibody-dependent cellular cytotoxicity towards cancer cells. *Eur J Immunol.* (2017) 48:344–54. doi: 10.1002/eji.201747215
4. Vidarsson G, van de Winkel JG. Fc receptor and complement receptor-mediated phagocytosis in host defence. *Curr Opin Infect Dis.* (1998) 11:271–8. doi: 10.1097/00001432-199806000-00002

5. van der Heijden J, Breunis WB, Geissler J, de Boer M, van den Berg TK, Kuijpers TW. Phenotypic variation in IgG receptors by nonclassical FCGR2C alleles. *J Immunol.* (2012) 188:1318–24. doi: 10.4049/jimmunol.1003945

6. Meknache N, Jönsson F, Laurent J, Guinnepain MT, Daëron M. Human basophils express the glycosylphosphatidylinositol-anchored low-affinity IgG receptor FcγRIIIB (CD16B). *J Immunol.* (2009) 182:2542–50. doi: 10.4049/jimmunol.0801665

7. Fossati G, Moots RJ, Bucknall RC, Edwards SW. Differential role of neutrophil Fcγ receptor IIIB (CD16) in phagocytosis, bacterial killing, and responses to immune complexes. *Arthritis Rheum.* (2002) 46:1351–61. doi: 10.1002/art.10230

8. Machado LR, Hardwick RJ, Bowdrey J, Bogle H, Knowles TJ, Sironi M, et al. Evolutionary history of copy-number-variable locus for the low-affinity Fcγ receptor: mutation rate, autoimmune disease, and the legacy of helminth infection. *Am J Hum Genet.* (2012) 90:973–85. doi: 10.1016/j.ajhg.2012.04.018

9. Breunis WB, van Mirre E, Geissler J, Laddach N, Wolbink G, van der Schoot E, et al. Copy number variation at the FCGR locus includes FCGR3A, FCGR2C and FCGR3B but not FCGR2A and FCGR2B. *Hum Mutat.* (2009) 30:E640–50. doi: 10.1002/humu.20997

10. Nagelkerke SQ, Tacke CE, Breunis WB, Geissler J, Sins JW, Appelhof B, et al. Nonallelic homologous recombination of the FCGR2/3 locus results in copy number variation and novel chimeric FCGR2 genes with aberrant functional expression. *Genes Immun.* (2015) 16:422–9. doi: 10.1038/gene.2015.25

11. Tsang-A-Sjoe MW, Nagelkerke SQ, Bultink IE, Geissler J, Tanck MW, Tacke CE, et al. Fc-γ receptor polymorphisms differentially influence susceptibility to systemic lupus erythematosus and lupus nephritis. *Rheumatology* (2016) 55:939–48. doi: 10.1093/rheumatology/kev433

12. Lee YH, Bae SC, Seo YH, Kim JH, Choi SJ, Ji JD, et al. Association between FCGR3B copy number variations and susceptibility to autoimmune diseases: a meta-analysis. *Inflamm Res.* (2015) 64:983–91. doi: 10.1007/s00011-015-0882-1

13. Graf SW, Lester S, Nossent JC, Hill CL, Proudman SM, Lee A, et al. Low copy number of the FCGR3B gene and rheumatoid arthritis: a case-control study and meta-analysis. *Arthritis Res Ther.* (2012) 14:R28. doi: 10.1186/ar3731

14. Wu Y, Zhang Z, Tao L, Chen G, Liu F, Wang T, et al. A high copy number of FCGR3B is associated with psoriasis vulgaris in Han Chinese. *Dermatology* (2014) 229:70–5. doi: 10.1159/000360160

15. de Haas M, Kleijer M, van Zwieten R, Roos D, von dem Borne AE. Neutrophil FcγRIIIb deficiency, nature, and clinical consequences: a study of 21 individuals from 14 families. *Blood* (1995) 86:2403–13.

16. Wagner C, Hänsch GM. Genetic deficiency of CD16, the low-affinity receptor for immunoglobulin G, has no impact on the functional capacity of polymorphonuclear neutrophils. *Eur J Clin Invest.* (2004) 34:149–55. doi: 10.1111/j.1365-2362.2004.01298.x

17. Bux J, Stein EL, Bierling P, Fromont P, Clay M, Stroncek D, et al. Characterization of a new alloantigen (SH) on the human neutrophil Fcγ receptor IIIb. *Blood* (1997) 89:1027–34.

18. Ory PA, Clark MR, Kwoh EE, Clarkson SB, Goldstein IM. Sequences of complementary DNAs that encode the NA1 and NA2 forms of Fc receptor III on human neutrophils. *J Clin Invest.* (1989) 84:1688–91. doi: 10.1172/JCI114350

19. Bredius RG, Fijen CA, De Haas M, Kuijper EJ, Weening RS, Van de Winkel JG, et al. Role of neutrophil FcγRIIa (CD32) and FcγRIIIb (CD16) polymorphic forms in phagocytosis of human IgG1- and IgG3-opsonized bacteria and erythrocytes. *Immunology* (1994) 83:624–30.

20. Salmon JE, Edberg JC, Kimberly RP. Fcγreceptor III on human neutrophils. Allelic variants have functionally distinct capacities. *J Clin Invest.* (1990) 85:1287–95. doi: 10.1172/JCI114566

21. Borregaard N. Neutrophils, from marrow to microbes. *Immunity* (2010) 33:657–70. doi: 10.1016/j.immuni.2010.11.011

22. Heifets L. Centennial of Metchnikoff's discovery. *J Reticuloendothel Soc.* (1982) 31:381–91.

23. Blaisdell A, Crequer A, Columbus D, Daikoku T, Mittal K, Dey SK, et al. Neutrophils oppose uterine epithelial carcinogenesis via debridement of hypoxic tumor cells. *Cancer Cell* (2015) 28:785–99. doi: 10.1016/j.ccell.2015.11.005

24. Trellakis S, Bruderek K, Dumitru CA, Gholaman H, Gu X, Bankfalvi A, et al. Polymorphonuclear granulocytes in human head and neck cancer: enhanced inflammatory activity, modulation by cancer cells and expansion in advanced disease. *Int J Cancer* (2011) 129:2183–93. doi: 10.1002/ijc.25892

25. Fossati G, Ricevuti G, Edwards SW, Walker C, Dalton A, Rossi ML. Neutrophil infiltration into human gliomas. *Acta Neuropathol.* (1999) 98:349–54. doi: 10.1007/s004010051093

26. Treffers LW, Hiemstra IH, Kuijpers TW, van den Berg TK, Matlung HL. Neutrophils in cancer. *Immunol Rev.* (2016) 273:312–28. doi: 10.1111/imr.12444

27. Albanesi M, Mancardi DA, Jönsson F, Iannascoli B, Fiette L, Di Santo JP, et al. Neutrophils mediate antibody-induced antitumor effects in mice. *Blood* (2013) 122:3160–4. doi: 10.1182/blood-2013-04-497446

28. Ring NG, Herndler-Brandstetter D, Weiskopf K, Shan L, Volkmer JP, George BM, et al. Anti-SIRPα antibody immunotherapy enhances neutrophil and macrophage antitumor activity. *Proc Natl Acad Sci USA.* 114:E10578–85. doi: 10.1073/pnas.1710877114

29. Hernandez-Ilizaliturri FJ, Jupudy V, Ostberg J, Oflazoglu E, Huberman A, Repasky E, et al. (2003). Neutrophils contribute to the biological antitumor activity of rituximab in a non-Hodgkin's lymphoma severe combined immunodeficiency mouse model. *Clin Cancer Res.* 9 (16 Pt 1):5866–73.

30. Siders WM, Shields J, Garron C, Hu Y, Boutin P, Shankara S, et al. (2010). Involvement of neutrophils and natural killer cells in the anti-tumor activity of alemtuzumab in xenograft tumor models. *Leuk Lymphoma* (2017) 51:1293–304. doi: 10.3109/10428191003777963

31. Matlung HL, Babes L, Zhao XW, van Houdt M, Treffers LW, van Rees DJ, et al. Neutrophils kill antibody-opsonized cancer cells by trogoptosis. *Cell Rep.* (2018) 23:3946–59.e3946. doi: 10.1016/j.celrep.2018.05.082

32. Zhao XW, van Beek EM, Schornagel K, Van der Maaden H, Van Houdt M, Otten MA, et al. CD47-signal regulatory protein-α (SIRPα) interactions form a barrier for antibody-mediated tumor cell destruction. *Proc Natl Acad Sci USA.* (2011) 108:18342–7. doi: 10.1073/pnas.1106550108

33. Chao MP, Alizadeh AA, Tang C, Myklebust JH, Varghese B, Gill S, et al. Anti-CD47 antibody synergizes with rituximab to promote phagocytosis and eradicate non-Hodgkin lymphoma. *Cell* (2010) 142:699–713. doi: 10.1016/j.cell.2010.07.044

34. Jaiswal S, Jamieson CH, Pang WW, Park CY, Chao MP, Majeti R, et al. CD47 is upregulated on circulating hematopoietic stem cells and leukemia cells to avoid phagocytosis. *Cell* (2009) 138:271–85. doi: 10.1016/j.cell.2009.05.046

35. Kim D, Wang J, Willingham SB, Martin R, Wernig G, Weissman IL. Anti-CD47 antibodies promote phagocytosis and inhibit the growth of human myeloma cells. *Leukemia* (2012) 26:2538–45. doi: 10.1038/leu.2012.141

36. Weiskopf K, Ring AM, Ho CC, Volkmer JP, Levin AM, Volkmer AK, et al. Engineered SIRPα variants as immunotherapeutic adjuvants to anticancer antibodies. *Science* (2013) 341:88–91. doi: 10.1126/science.1238856

37. Fleit HB, Wright SD, Unkeless JC. Human neutrophil Fc γ receptor distribution and structure. *Proc Natl Acad Sci USA.* (1982) 79:3275–9. doi: 10.1073/pnas.79.10.3275

38. Golay J, Da Roit F, Bologna L, Ferrara C, Leusen JH, Rambaldi A, et al. Glycoengineered CD20 antibody obinutuzumab activates neutrophils and mediates phagocytosis through CD16B more efficiently than rituximab. *Blood* (2013) 122:3482–91. doi: 10.1182/blood-2013-05-504043

39. Vossebeld PJ, Homburg CH, Roos D, Verhoeven AJ. The anti-Fcγ RIII mAb 3G8 induces neutrophil activation via a cooperative actin of FcγRIIIb and FcγRIIa. *Int J Biochem Cell Biol.* (1997) 29:465–73. doi: 10.1016/S1357-2725(96)00160-4

40. Kapur R, Kustiawan I, Vestrheim A, Koeleman CA, Visser R, Einarsdottir HK, et al. A prominent lack of IgG1-Fc fucosylation of platelet alloantibodies in pregnancy. *Blood* (2014) 123:471–80. doi: 10.1182/blood-2013-09-527978

41. Kuijpers TW, Tool AT, van der Schoot CE, Ginsel LA, Onderwater JJ, Roos D, et al. Membrane surface antigen expression on neutrophils: a reappraisal of the use of surface markers for neutrophil activation. *Blood* (1991) 78:1105–11.

42. Wirt T, Rosskopf S, Rösner T, Eichholz KM, Kahrs A, Lutz S, et al. An Fc double-engineered CD20 antibody with enhanced ability to trigger complement-dependent cytotoxicity and antibody-dependent

cell-mediated cytotoxicity. *Transfus Med Hemother.* (2017) 44:292–300. doi: 10.1159/000479978

43. Recke A, Trog LM, Pas HH, Vorobyev A, Abadpour A, Jonkman MF, et al. Recombinant human IgA1 and IgA2 autoantibodies to type VII collagen induce subepidermal blistering ex vivo. *J Immunol.* (2014) 193:1600–8. doi: 10.4049/jimmunol.1400160

44. Dekkers G, Treffers L, Plomp R, Bentlage AEH, de Boer M, Koeleman CAM, et al. Decoding the human immunoglobulin G-glycan repertoire reveals a spectrum of Fc-receptor- and complement-mediated-effector activities. *Front Immunol.* (2017) 8:877. doi: 10.3389/fimmu.2017.00877

45. Dekkers G, Plomp R, Koeleman CA, Visser R, von Horsten HH, Sandig V, et al. Multi-level glyco-engineering techniques to generate IgG with defined Fc-glycans. *Sci Rep.* (2016) 6:36964. doi: 10.1038/srep 36964

46. Kapur R, Della Valle L, Verhagen OJ, Hipgrave Ederveen A, Ligthart P, de Haas M, et al. Prophylactic anti-D preparations display variable decreases in Fc-fucosylation of anti-D. *Transfusion* (2015) 55:553–62. doi: 10.1111/trf. 12880

47. Vidarsson G, Stemerding AM, Stapleton NM, Spliethoff SE, Janssen H, Rebers FE, et al. FcRn: an IgG receptor on phagocytes with a novel role in phagocytosis. *Blood* (2006) 108:3573–9. doi: 10.1182/blood-2006-05-024539

48. Saeland E, Vidarsson G, Leusen JH, Van Garderen E, Nahm MH, Vile-Weekhout H, et al. Central role of complement in passive protection by human IgG1 and IgG2 anti-pneumococcal antibodies in mice. *J Immunol.* (2003) 170:6158–64. doi: 10.4049/jimmunol.170.12.6158

49. Breunis WB, van Mirre E, Bruin M, Geissler J, de Boer M, Peters M, et al. Copy number variation of the activating FCGR2C gene predisposes to idiopathic thrombocytopenic purpura. *Blood* (2008) 111:1029–38. doi: 10.1182/blood-2007-03-079913

50. Huizinga TW, van der Schoot CE, Jost C, Klaassen R, Kleijer M, von dem Borne AE, et al. The PI-linked receptor FcRIII is released on stimulation of neutrophils. *Nature* (1988) 333:667–9. doi: 10.1038/333667a0

51. Wang Y, Wu J, Newton R, Bahaie NS, Long C, Walcheck B. ADAM17 cleaves CD16b (FcγRIIIb) in human neutrophils. *Biochim Biophys Acta* (2013) 1833:680–5. doi: 10.1016/j.bbamcr.2012.11.027

52. Kurlander RJ. Reversible and irreversible loss of Fc receptor function of human monocytes as a consequence of interaction with immunoglobulin G. *J Clin Invest.* (1980) 66:773–81. doi: 10.1172/JCI109915

53. van der Steen L, Tuk CW, Bakema JE, Kooij G, Reijerkerk A, Vidarsson G, et al. Immunoglobulin A: Fc(α)RI interactions induce neutrophil migration through release of leukotriene B4. *Gastroenterology* (2009) 137:2018–29.e1-3. doi: 10.1053/j.gastro.2009.06.047

54. Dechant M, Beyer T, Schneider-Merck T, Weisner W, Peipp M, van de Winkel JG, et al. Effector mechanisms of recombinant IgA antibodies against epidermal growth factor receptor. *J Immunol.* (2007) 179:2936–43. doi: 10.4049/jimmunol.179.5.2936

55. Boross P, Lohse S, Nederend M, Jansen JH, van Tetering G, Dechant M, et al. IgA EGFR antibodies mediate tumour killing *in vivo*. *EMBO Mol Med.* (2013) 5:1213–26. doi: 10.1002/emmm.201201929

56. Subedi GP, Hanson QM, Barb AW. Restricted motion of the conserved immunoglobulin G1 N-glycan is essential for efficient FcγRIIIa binding. *Structure* (2014) 22:1478–88. doi: 10.1016/j.str.2014.08.002

57. Ferrara C, Grau S, Jäger C, Sondermann P, Brünker P, Waldhauer I, et al. Unique carbohydrate-carbohydrate interactions are required for high affinity binding between FcγRIII and antibodies lacking core fucose. *Proc Natl Acad Sci USA.* (2011) 108:12669–74. doi: 10.1073/pnas.1108455108

58. Shields RL, Lai J, Keck R, O'Connell LY, Hong K, Meng YG, et al. Lack of fucose on human IgG1 N-linked oligosaccharide improves binding to human Fcγ RIII and antibody-dependent cellular toxicity. *J Biol Chem.* (2002) 277:26733–40. doi: 10.1074/jbc.M202069200

59. Shinkawa T, Nakamura K, Yamane N, Shoji-Hosaka E, Kanda Y, Sakurada M, et al. The absence of fucose but not the presence of galactose or bisecting N-acetylglucosamine of human IgG1 complex-type oligosaccharides shows the critical role of enhancing antibody-dependent cellular cytotoxicity. *J Biol Chem.* (2003) 278:3466–73. doi: 10.1074/jbc.M210665200

60. Niwa R, Hatanaka S, Shoji-Hosaka E, Sakurada M, Kobayashi Y, Uehara A, et al. Enhancement of the antibody-dependent cellular

61. Bruggeman CW, Dekkers G, Bentlage AEH, Treffers LW, Nagelkerke SQ, Lissenberg-Thunnissen S, et al. Enhanced effector functions due to antibody defucosylation depend on the effector cell fcγ receptor profile. *J Immunol.* (2017) 199:204–11. doi: 10.4049/jimmunol.1700116

62. Peipp M, Lammerts van Bueren JJ, Schneider-Merck T, Bleeker WW, Dechant M, Beyer T, et al. Antibody fucosylation differentially impacts cytotoxicity mediated by NK and PMN effector cells. *Blood* (2008) 112:2390–9. doi: 10.1182/blood-2008-03-144600

63. Marois L, Paré G, Vaillancourt M, Rollet-Labelle E, Naccache PH. FcγRIIIb triggers raft-dependent calcium influx in IgG-mediated responses in human neutrophils. *J Biol Chem.* (2011) 286:3509–19. doi: 10.1074/jbc.m110.169516

64. Fernandes MJ, Lachance G, Paré G, Rollet-Labelle E, Naccache PH. Signaling through CD16b in human neutrophils involves the Tec family of tyrosine kinases. *J Leukoc Biol.* (2005) 78:524–32. doi: 10.1189/jlb.0804479

65. Fernandes MJ, Rollet-Labelle E, Paré G, Marois S, Tremblay ML, Teillaud JL, et al. CD16b associates with high-density, detergent-resistant membranes in human neutrophils. *Biochem J.* (2006) 393 (Pt 1):351–9. doi: 10.1042/bj20050129

66. Shibata-Koyama M, Iida S, Misaka H, Mori K, Yano K, Shitara K, et al. Nonfucosylated rituximab potentiates human neutrophil phagocytosis through its high binding for FcγRIIIb and MHC class II expression on the phagocytotic neutrophils. *Exp Hematol.* (2009) 37:309–21. doi: 10.1016/j.exphem.2008.11.006

67. Valgardsdottir R, Cattaneo I, Klein C, Introna M, Figliuzzi M, Golay J. Human neutrophils mediate trogocytosis rather than phagocytosis of CLL B cells opsonized with anti-CD20 antibodies. *Blood* (2017) 129:2636–44. doi: 10.1182/blood-2016-08-735605

68. Bruhns P, Iannascoli B, England P, Mancardi DA, Fernandez N, Jorieux S, et al. Specificity and affinity of human Fcγ receptors and their polymorphic variants for human IgG subclasses. *Blood* (2009) 113:3716–25. doi: 10.1182/blood-2008-09-179754

69. Tsuboi N, Asano K, Lauterbach M, Mayadas TN. Human neutrophil Fcγ receptors initiate and play specialized nonredundant roles in antibody-mediated inflammatory diseases. *Immunity* (2008) 28:833–46. doi: 10.1016/j.immuni.2008.04.013

70. Kol A, Terwissscha van Scheltinga A, Pool M, Gerdes C, de Vries E, de Jong S. ADCC responses and blocking of EGFR-mediated signaling and cell growth by combining the anti-EGFR antibodies imgatuzumab and cetuximab in NSCLC cells. *Oncotarget* (2017) 8:45432–46. doi: 10.18632/oncotarget. 17139

71. Niwa R, Sakurada M, Kobayashi Y, Uehara A, Matsushima K, Ueda R, et al. Enhanced natural killer cell binding and activation by low-fucose IgG1 antibody results in potent antibody-dependent cellular cytotoxicity induction at lower antigen density. *Clin Cancer Res.* (2005) 11:2327–36. doi: 10.1158/1078-0432.CCR-04-2263

72. Weiskopf K. Cancer immunotherapy targeting the CD47/SIRPα axis. *Eur J Cancer* (2017) 76:100–9. doi: 10.1016/j.ejca.2017.02.013

cytotoxicity of low-fucose IgG1 Is independent of FcγRIIIa functional polymorphism. *Clin Cancer Res.* (2004) 10 (18 Pt 1):6248–55. doi: 10.1158/1078-0432.CCR-04-0850

Chronic HIV-1 Infection Alters the Cellular Distribution of FcγRIIIa and the Functional Consequence of the FcγRIIIa-F158V Variant

Ntando G. Phaahla [1,2], Ria Lassaunière [1,3], Bianca Da Costa Dias [1,2], Ziyaad Waja [4,5], Neil A. Martinson [4,5] and Caroline T. Tiemessen [1,2]*

[1] Centre for HIV and STIs, National Institute for Communicable Diseases, Johannesburg, South Africa, [2] Faculty of Health Sciences, University of the Witwatersrand, Johannesburg, South Africa, [3] Department of Virus and Microbiological Special Diagnostics, Statens Serum Institut, Copenhagen, Denmark, [4] Perinatal HIV Research Unit, University of the Witwatersrand, Johannesburg, South Africa, [5] MRC Soweto Matlosana Centre for HIV/AIDS and TB Research, Johannesburg, South Africa

*Correspondence:
Caroline T. Tiemessen
carolinet@nicd.ac.za

Chronic HIV-infection modulates the expression of Fc gamma receptors (FcγRs) on immune cells and their antibody-dependent effector function capability. Given the increasingly recognized importance of antibody-dependent cellular cytotoxicity (ADCC) in HIV-specific immunity, we investigated the cellular distribution of FcγRIIIa on cytotoxic lymphocytes—natural killer cells and CD8$^+$ T cells—and the effect of the FcγRIIIa-F158V variant on ADCC capacity in HIV-infected individuals ($n = 23$) and healthy controls ($n = 23$). Study participants were matched for F158V genotypes, carried two copies of the FCGR3A gene and were negative for FcγRIIb expression on NK cells. The distribution of CD56^{dim}FcγRIIIa^{bright} and CD56^{neg}FcγRIIIa^{bright} NK cell subsets, but not FcγRIIIa surface expression, differed significantly between HIV-1 negative and HIV-1 positive donors. NK cell-mediated ADCC responses negatively correlated with the proportion of the immunoregulatory CD56^{bright}FcγRIIIa$^{dim/neg}$ cells and were lower in the HIV-1 positive group. Intriguingly, the FcγRIIIa-F158V variant differentially affected the NK-mediated ADCC responses for HIV-1 negative and HIV-1 positive donors. Healthy donors bearing at least one 158V allele had higher ADCC responses compared to those homozygous for the 158F allele (48.1 vs. 34.1%), whereas the opposite was observed for the HIV-infected group (26.4 vs. 34.6%), although not statistically significantly different. Furthermore, FcγRIIIa$^+$CD8^{bright} and FcγRIIIa$^+$CD8^{dim} T cell subsets were observed in both HIV-1 negative and HIV-1 positive donors, with median proportions that were significantly higher in HIV-1 positive donors compared to healthy controls (15.7 vs. 8.3%; $P = 0.016$ and 18.2 vs. 14.1%; $P = 0.038$, respectively). Using an HIV-1-specific GranToxiLux assay, we demonstrate that CD8$^+$ T cells mediate ADCC through the delivery of granzyme B, which was overall lower compared to that of autologous NK cells. In conclusion, our findings demonstrate that in the presence of an HIV-1 infection, the cellular distribution of FcγRIIIa is altered and that the functional consequence of FcγRIIIa variant is affected. Importantly, it underscores the need to characterize FcγR expression, cellular distribution and functional consequences of FcγR genetic variants within a specific environment or disease state.

Keywords: NK cells, CD8 T cells, antibody-dependent cellular cytotoxicity, Fc gamma receptor, polymorphism, HIV, infection

INTRODUCTION

Receptors for the Fc domain of immunoglobulin G (IgG), so called Fc gamma receptors (FcγRs), link the specificity of IgG with potent effector functions of the innate immune system. FcγRs comprise a family of activating (FcγRI, FcγRIIa, and FcγRIIIa) and inhibiting (FcγRIIb) receptors that are differentially expressed on innate immune cells such as natural killer (NK) cells, monocytes, dendritic cells, neutrophils, and granulocytes (1–3). During an infection, these receptors play an important role in activating IgG-induced protective inflammatory processes and regulating immune responses (4–7).

Increasing evidence support an important role for FcγR-mediated effector functions, in particular antibody-dependent cellular cytotoxicity (ADCC), in HIV-1-specific immunity (6, 8). In adults, ADCC has been associated with a reduced risk of HIV-1 acquisition in the RV144 vaccine trial, whereas in infants born to HIV-1 infected mothers, passively acquired ADCC activity associated with reduced mortality (9). Similarly, ADCC responses associate with slower disease progression in HIV-1 infected adults (10–14).

In the periphery, CD56^{dim}FcγRIIIa^{bright} NK cells are the primary effectors of ADCC responses (15). During a chronic HIV-1 infection, however, shedding of FcγRIIIa from the surface of cytotoxic CD56^{dim}FcγRIIIa^{bright} NK cells together with an increase in the CD56^{neg}FcγRIIIa^{bright} NK cell subset leads to a significant reduction in NK cell function (16, 17). It is unknown whether this loss in NK cell-mediated ADCC capacity is compensated for by other cytotoxic cells, where FcγR expression is induced upon immune cell activation. For chronic hepatitis C virus or Epstein Barr virus infections, for instance, it has been shown that FcγRIIIa expression is induced on an effector memory CD8$^+$ T cell subset (18, 19). This FcγRIIIa$^+$CD8$^+$ T cell subset acquires NK cell-like functional properties, including ADCC activity accompanied by the release of pore forming perforin and serine protease granzyme B (18, 19). The presence and role of this CD8$^+$ T cell subset in HIV-1 infection is currently undefined.

In addition to the effect of an actively replicating virus on FcγRIIIa expression, host genetics also contribute to variability

of FcγRIIIa expression and/or ADCC responses. *FCGR3A* copy number variation directly correlates with the surface density of FcγRIIIa, with individuals bearing a single *FCGR3A* copy and correspondingly lower FcγRIIIa surface densities, having reduced ADCC responses compared to individuals with two or more gene copies (20). In addition, a phenylalanine (F) to valine (V) substitution at amino acid 158 in the proximal Ig-like domain of FcγRIIIa confers increased binding for IgG1, IgG3, and IgG4, which has been associated with higher NK cell activation and ADCC responses (21–23). Unlike *FCGR3A* copy number and the FcγRIIIa-F158V variant, a deletion of a copy number variable region (CNR) encompassing *FCGR3B* and *FCGR2C*—known as CNR1—does not affect FcγRIIIa directly (24). However, it juxtaposes the 5′-regulatory sequences of *FCGR2C* with the open reading frame of *FCGR2B*, creating a chimeric *FCGR2B'* gene (25). This results in the expression of the inhibitory FcγRIIb on NK cells where it regulates FcγRIIIa-mediated ADCC responses (25, 26).

FCGR variants are rarely adjusted for in studies that compare NK cell-mediated ADCC capacity between HIV-positive and HIV-negative individuals. Moreover, it is unclear if the altered immune milieu accompanying an HIV-1 infection modulates the functional consequences of the aforementioned variants. In this study, we sought to characterize FcγRIIIa expression on cytotoxic lymphocytes—NK cells and CD8$^+$ T cells—and associated ADCC responses in healthy donors and viraemic HIV-1 individuals matched for *FCGR* genetic variants.

MATERIALS AND METHODS
Cohort

All study participants were black South Africans recruited from the city of Johannesburg, Gauteng province, South Africa (**Table 1**). Self-reported HIV-1 uninfected individuals who did not have an acute or chronic illness at the time of sample collection were prospectively recruited from the National Institute for Communicable Diseases as healthy controls. Viraemic, treatment naïve HIV-1 infected individuals were identified from an existing cohort recruited from hospitals in Johannesburg and Soweto. This study was carried out in accordance with the recommendations of the National Health Research Ethics Council (NHREC) of the South African Department of Health. The protocol was approved by the University of the Witwatersrand Ethics Committee (Ethics clearance certificate no. M1511102). All participants provided written informed consent in accordance with the Declaration of Helsinki.

Abbreviations: NK, natural killer cell; IgG, immunoglobulin G; HIV-1, human immunodeficiency virus 1; ADCC, antibody-dependent cellular cytotoxicity; FCGR, Fc gamma receptor gene; FcγR, Fc gamma receptor protein; CNR1, gene copy number variable region 1; EDTA, ethylenediaminetetraacetic acid; HNA, Human neutrophil antigen; MLPA, multiplex ligation-dependent probe amplification; FMO, flurescence minus one; PBMCs, peripheral blood mononuclear cells; KIR2DL2/L3, killer immunoglobulin-like receptor 2 DL2/L3; NKG2A/D, natural killer group 2A or−2D.

TABLE 1 | Clinical and demographic characteristics of study cohort.

	HIV-1 negative	HIV-1 positive	P-value
N	23	23	
Age [mean (SD)]	36.3 [8.5]	40.2 (8.8)	0.143*
Gender [% Females]	69.6	82.6	0.491*
HIV-1 VIRAL LOAD [MEDIAN (IQR)]			
158FF	–	6,931 (3,598–15,090)	0.563[†]
158FV/VV	–	4,732 (1,134–11,430)	
CD4 T CELL COUNT [MEAN (SD)]			
158FF	–	508 (267)	0.629[†]
158FV/VV	–	562 (261)	
OTHER DISEASES OR INFECTIONS			
Mycobacterium tuberculosis	0 (0%)	2 (8.7%)	

*Comparison between HIV-1 negative and HIV-1 positive groups.
[†]Comparison between genotypes.

FCGR Variant Genotyping

Genomic DNA was isolated from ethylenediaminetetraacetic acid (EDTA)-anticoagulated whole blood. Study participants were genotyped for FCGR variants using the FCGR-specific multiplex ligation-dependent probe amplification (MLPA) assay (MRC Holland, Amsterdam, The Netherlands) as previously described (27, 28). This assay detects the genomic copy number of FCGR2A, FCGR2B, FCGR2C, FCGR3A, and FCGR3B and functional allelic variants that include FcγRIIa-H131R (alias H166R, c.497A>G, rs1801274); FcγRIIb-I232T (c.695T>C, rs1050501), FcγRIIIa-F158V (alias F176V, c.634T>G, rs396991), FcγRIIIb-HNA1a/b/c, FCGR2C gene expression variants c.169T>C (X57Q) and c.798+1A>G (rs76277413), and the FCGR2B/C promoter variants c.-386G>C (rs3219018) and c.-120T>A (rs34701572) in two multiplex reactions. Capillary electrophoresis was used to separate the MLPA assay amplicons on an ABI Genetic Analyzer 3500. Data were analyzed with Coffalyser.NET software created by the MLPA assay manufacturer, MRC Holland.

Monoclonal Antibodies and Flow Cytometric Analysis

The following monoclonal antibodies were used: CD3-PerCP (SK7), CD56-AF647 (B159), CD8-APC-H7 (SK1), CD16-PE (3G8), CD16-FITC (NKP15), CD32-FITC (2B6), and CD32-PE (FLI8.26). All antibodies were obtained from BD Biosciences (San Jose, CA). Dead cells were labeled with the BD Horizon™ Fixable Viability Stain 510. Samples were acquired on a BD Fortessa X20 (BD biosciences) and analyzed on FlowJo version 9.8.1 software (Tree Star, San Carlos, CA). Fluorescence-minus-one (FMO) controls were used to set the appropriate gates for analyses.

Isolation of Specific Cell Populations

Peripheral blood mononuclear cells (PBMCs) were isolated from EDTA-anticoagulated whole blood using Ficoll-Paque™ PLUS density gradient centrifugation (GE Healthcare) and stored at −80°C. NK cells and CD8+ T cells were positively selected from overnight rested PBMCs using MACS® magnetic cell separation technology (Miltenyl Biotec). To limit the presence of NK cells in the enriched CD8+ T cell preparation, NK cells were first isolated from PBMCs using CD56+ beads prior to isolation of CD8+ T cells with CD8+ beads. Viability and number of each participant's NK and CD8+ T cells were determined by trypan blue exclusion through direct cell counting on a haemocytometer. The purity of enriched cell fractions was determined by flow cytometric phenotyping assays.

Antibodies

ADCC capacity was evaluated using pooled IgG isolated from the HIV-1 infected individuals included in the study. IgG was isolated from plasma using the Melon Gel IgG Purification kit according to the manufacturer's instructions (Thermo Scientific) and quantitated using the Bicinchoninic acid (BCA) assay. HIV immune globulin (HIVIG; NIH AIDS reagent program) was used as a positive control.

ADCC

NK cells and CD8+ T cells both utilize the pore forming perforin and serine protease granzyme B during cytotoxic responses. It is therefore possible to evaluate ADCC responses of both NK cells and CD8+ T cells with the HIV-specific GranToxiLux assay (15). In brief, CEM.NK^R.CCR5 cells were coated with recombinant HIV-1 ConC gp120, followed by opsonisation with HIV-1-specific antibodies and incubation for 45 min in the presence of NK cells or CD8+ T cells at an effector-to-target (E:T) ratio of 10:1. The optimal concentration of isolated IgG (30 μg/ml) was determined empirically. Samples were acquired on BD Fortessa X20 flow cytometer and data analyzed on FlowJo version 9.8.1 software (Tree Star, San Carlos, CA). Granzyme B activity in the absence of any antibody (background killing) was determined for each subject—NK cells and CD8+ T cells—and subtracted from granzyme B activity in the presence of antibody. The inter assay coefficient of variation, as calculated from a HIVIG-specific ADCC response measured for a single donor included in every run, was <10%.

To assess CD8+ T cell mediated granzyme B responses, HIV-1 positive donors with <5% NK cell contamination in their enriched CD8+ T cell fractions were identified and selected for further analysis. This proportion of NK cells equates to a <0.5:1 NK-to-target ratio in a 10:1 CD8-to-target preparation. In our experience, the NK cell-mediated granzyme B activity at 0.5:1 is on average 14.1% (standard deviation [SD]: 2.8%) of that observed for NK cells at a ratio of 10:1 (**Figure 1**). Using these data, a positivity threshold for CD8+ T cell-mediated granzyme B responses was calculated relative to autologous NK cell-mediated granzyme B responses whereby the mean granzyme B activity for autologous NK cells (E:T = 10:1) was multiplied with 22.4% (14.1% + 3 × SD:2.8%).

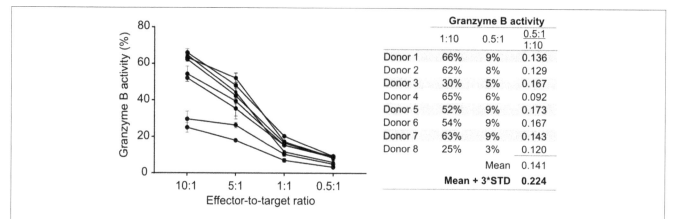

FIGURE 1 | NK cell-mediated ADCC responses at different effector-to-target (E:T) cell ratios. NK cells isolated from eight HIV-1 negative donors were tested at different E:T ratios in an HIV-specific GranToxiLux assay using an ADCC-mediating monoclonal antibody (A32) at 2.5 μg/ml. The mean fraction of Granzyme B activity observed at an E:T of 0.5:1 relative to 10:1 was used to calculate a 99% confidence level cut-off value for NK cell-mediated ADCC responses at an E:T of 0.5:1. Data points represent the mean of triplicate measures and the standard deviation indicated by error bars.

Statistics

All statistical analyses were performed using GraphPad Prism 7 software version 7.04 (GraphPad Software). P-values from 2-tailed tests <0.05 were considered statistically significant. The significance of differences between unpaired data sets were analyzed with the Mann-Whitney U tests and paired data sets with the Wilcoxon matched-pairs signed rank test. The significance of differences between more than two data sets were analyzed using Kruskal-Wallis tests. Correlation analyses of data between two groups were assessed using the non-parametric Spearman rank correlation coefficient. To determine the role of FcγRIIIa-F158V alleles in ADCC responses, the V allele was studied under a dominant model due to the low prevalence of VV homozygotes (29).

RESULTS

Study Population

Thirty-seven chronic HIV-1 infected, viraemic, and antiretroviral naïve individuals with sufficient sample available were identified from an existing cohort of HIV-1 positive individuals (**Figure 2**). Following FCGR genotyping, seven individuals were excluded due to the possession of an FCGR3A gene duplication ($n = 1$), FCGR3A gene deletion ($n = 2$), or CNR1 deletion that results in the expression of the inhibitory FcγRIIb on NK cells ($n = 4$). To ensure that individuals carrying an undetectable CNR1 deletion—possess a duplication of this region on a single chromosome and a deletion on the other—were also excluded, expression of FcγRIIb on NK cells was monitored using flow cytometry. During the eligibility screening of individuals, such an individual was indeed identified and excluded from the study; thus, five HIV-1 positive individuals in total expressed FcγRIIb on their NK cells and were excluded.

Within the HIV-1 positive group, FcγRIIIa-158FF donors were paired with FcγRIIIa-158FV donors according to their HIV-1 RNA plasma viral load. Twenty-three HIV-1 positive

individuals were eligible for further analysis, with the FcγRIIIa-F158V genotype distribution closely resembling that observed in the general black population from the same region in South Africa (29). As a comparative group, thirty-three HIV-1 negative individuals were genotyped for FCGR variants. Six individuals were excluded due to the possession of an FCGR3A duplication ($n = 1$) or CNR1 deletion ($n = 5$). Twenty-three eligible HIV-1 negative individuals were subsequently paired with HIV-1 positive individuals based on the FcγRIIIa-F158V genotype. None of the study participants expressed the activating FcγRIIc on their NK cells, as determined by the FCGR2C c.798+1A>G splice-site variant, or carried the FCGR3A intragenic haplotype previously associated with increased FcγRIIIa surface density (26, 30).

Age and gender did not differ significantly between HIV-1 negative and positive donors (**Table 1**). Two HIV-1 positive individuals had tuberculosis, of which one was an FcγRIIIa-158FF donor and the other an FcγRIIIa-158FV donor. No other infections were noted for these patients. Human cytomegalovirus (HCMV) infection status was not determined for study participants. However, the prevalence is likely 100% for the HIV-1 positive individuals and >85% for HIV-1 negative individuals as observed in other cohorts in rural and urban South Africa [(31) and Tiemessen, unpublished data]. Other sexually transmitted infections were not tested for in the study cohort.

FcγRIIIa Expression on NK Cell Subsets

NK cell subsets were defined based on the relative surface expression of CD56 and FcγRIIIa. Four subsets were identified that include CD56^{bright}FcγRIIIa$^{dim/neg}$, CD56^{dim}FcγRIIIa^{bright}, CD56^{neg}FcγRIIIa^{bright}, and CD56^{dim}FcγRIIIa$^{dim/neg}$ (**Figure 3A**). The distribution of these subsets within the NK cell population differed significantly between HIV-1 positive and HIV-1 negative donors. Compared to the HIV-1 negative group, the HIV-1 positive group had a smaller median proportion of CD56^{dim}FcγRIIIa^{bright} cells (60.2 vs. 77.0%, $P = 0.0002$, **Figure 3B**) that was offset by a larger median

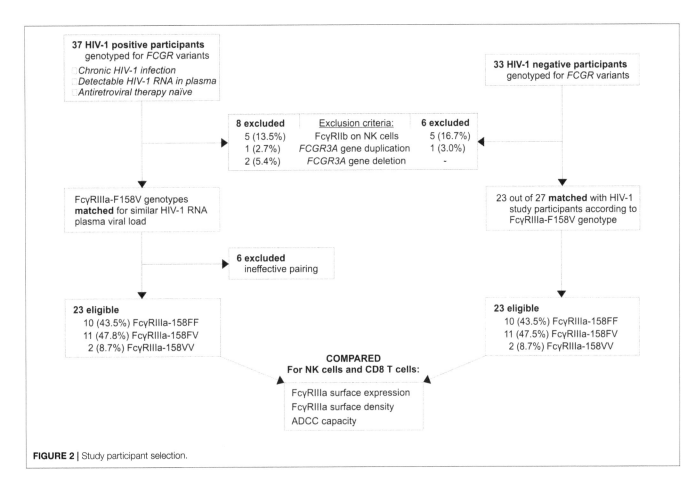

FIGURE 2 | Study participant selection.

proportion of CD56^{neg}FcγRIIIa^{bright} cells (14.9 vs. 2.1%, $P < 0.0001$, **Figure 3B**). The inverse relationship between the NK cell subsets in HIV-1 positive individuals, but not HIV-1 negative individuals, was further observed in a correlation analysis ($R = -0.633$, $P = 0.001$, **Figure 3F**). The relative proportions of CD56^{bright}FcγRIIIa$^{dim/neg}$ and CD56^{dim}FcγRIIIa$^{dim/neg}$ did not differ significantly between HIV-1 positive and HIV-1 negative donors. In contrast to the observed differences in NK cell subsets, FcγRIIIa surface density on neither cytotoxic CD56^{dim}FcγRIIIa^{bright} nor CD56^{neg}FcγRIIIa^{bright} NK cells differed between the two groups ($P = 0.948$ and $P = 0.486$, respectively; **Figure 3C**).

NK Cell-Mediated ADCC Responses

The capacity of CD56$^+$ NK cells to mediate ADCC was tested in an HIV-1-specific granzyme B assay in the presence of pooled IgG isolated from HIV-1-infected South Africans. ADCC responses, measured as granzyme B activity in target cells, were reduced in the HIV-1 positive group compared to the HIV-1 negative group, although not statistically significantly different (31.0 vs. 43.3%, $P = 0.184$, **Figure 3D**). In both groups, the ADCC responses were affected by the FcγRIIIa-F158V variant (**Figure 3E**). Healthy donors bearing at least one V allele had a higher median NK cell-mediated granzyme B activity compared to those homozygous for the F allele (48.1 vs. 34.1%, $P = 0.284$). This trend was, however, not observed in the HIV-1 positive group. In contrast, HIV-1 positive donors bearing at least one V allele had reduced granzyme B activity compared to those homozygous for the F allele (26.4 vs. 34.6%, $P = 0.522$).

ADCC responses of both HIV-1 negative and HIV-1 positive donors negatively correlated with the proportion of immunoregulatory CD56^{bright}FcγRIIIa$^{dim/neg}$ cells ($R = -0.486$, $P = 0.019$; and $R = -0.454$, $P = 0.030$, respectively; **Figure 3F**). Furthermore, ADCC responses of HIV-1 negative donors, but not HIV-1 positive donors, positively correlated with the proportion of CD56^{dim}FcγRIIIa^{bright} cells ($R = 0.665$, $P = 0.0005$; and $R = 0.233$, $P = 0.284$, respectively; **Figure 3F**). FcγRIIIa expression levels on the cytotoxic CD56^{dim}FcγRIIIa^{bright} cell subset did not correlate with ADCC responses in either HIV-1 negative or HIV-1 positive group.

Expression of FcγRIIIa on CD8$^+$ T Cells

During the course of characterizing FcγRIIIa expression on peripheral leukocytes in whole blood obtained from a preliminary cohort of HIV-1 negative and HIV-1 positive donors, we observed a CD8^{bright} T cell subset expressing FcγRIIIa in both groups (**Figure 4**). The proportion of FcγRIIIa$^+$CD8^{bright} T cells within the CD8^{bright} T cell population varied extensively, ranging from 4.4 to 45.9%, with the median proportion significantly higher in the HIV-1 infected group compared to the healthy control group (17.8 vs. 9.8%, $P = 0.002$; **Figure 4**).

In the present validation study, two CD8$^+$ T cell subsets are identified, designated CD8^{bright} and CD8^{dim} (also referred to as

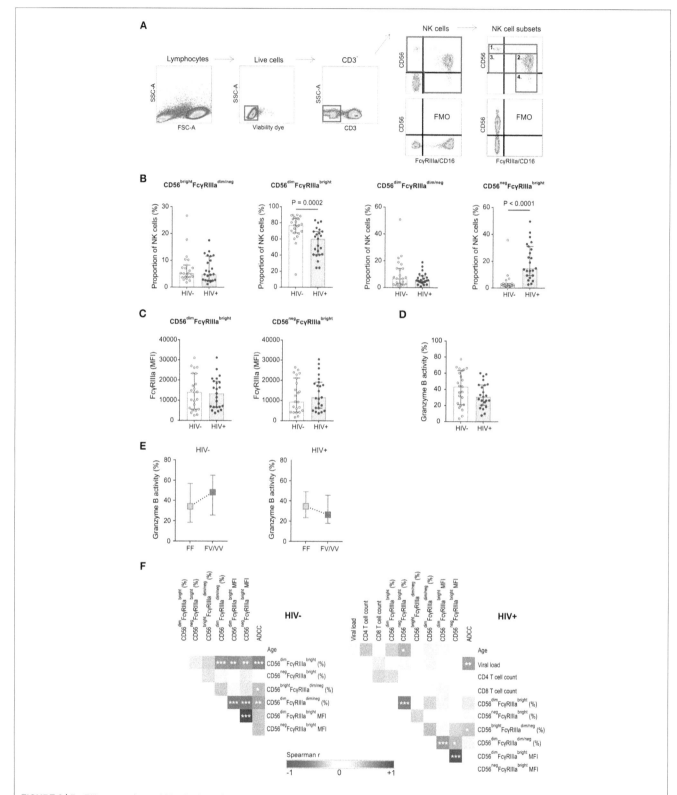

FIGURE 3 | FcγRIIIa expression on NK cell subsets in HIV-1 uninfected and HIV-1 infected individuals matched for *FCGR* genetic variants. **(A)** Gating strategy for defining four NK cell subsets: 1. CD56^{bright}FcγRIIIa$^{dim/neg}$, 2. CD56^{dim}FcγRIIIa^{bright}, 3. CD56^{dim}FcγRIIIa$^{dim/neg}$, and 4. CD56^{neg}FcγRIIIa^{bright}; **(B)** Comparison of NK cell subsets between HIV-1 uninfected and infected individuals; **(C)** FcγRIIIa surface density on FcγRIIIa^{bright} NK cell subsets; **(D)** ADCC activity of NK cells at a target-to-effector cell ratio of 10:1 with isolated IgG pooled from HIV-1 study participants; **(E)** Median ADCC responses for individuals homozygous for the FcγRIIIa-158F allele and individuals bearing at least one FcγRIIIa-158V allele; **(F)** Correlation analysis between demographic, clinical, phenotypic and functional variables in HIV-1 uninfected and HIV-1 infected individuals (***$P < 0.001$; **$P < 0.01$; *$P < 0.05$).

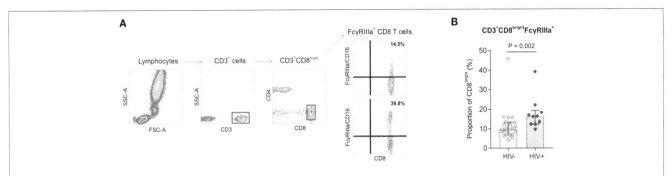

FIGURE 4 | FcγRIIIa expression on CD8 T cells in whole blood obtained from HIV-1 negative and HIV-1 positive donors. **(A)** Gating strategy showing two representative individuals with low and high proportions of FcγRIIIa+CD8bright T cell subsets. **(B)** Frequencies of FcγRIIIa+CD8bright T cells in whole blood isolated from HIV-negative healthy controls (n = 23) and HIV-infected individuals (n = 10).

CD8high and CD8low), according to the relative expression of CD8 on CD3+ T cells (**Figure 5**). The CD8dim subset accounted for 13.9 and 13.4% of the total CD8+ T cell population in HIV-1 negative and HIV-1 positive donors, respectively (P = 0.978). In agreement with our observations in whole blood, 2–44.8% of CD8bright cells and 2–68.4% of CD8dim cells expressed FcγRIIIa. Compared to its FcγRIIIa+CD8bright counterpart, the FcγRIIIa+CD8dim subset expressed significantly higher levels of FcγRIIIa in both the HIV-1 positive and negative group (471 vs. 1610, P < 0.001; and 377 vs. 740, P < 0.001, respectively; data not shown).

Compared to the HIV-1 negative group, the HIV-1 positive group had a significantly higher median proportion of FcγRIIIa+CD8bright and FcγRIIIa+CD8dim T cell subsets (15.7 vs. 8.3%; P = 0.016 and 18.2 vs. 14.1%; P = 0.038, respectively) and correspondingly higher median FcγRIIIa surface densities on both FcγRIIIa+CD8+ T cell subsets (471 vs. 377, P = 0.031; and 1,610 vs. 740, P = 0.021, respectively) (**Figure 5B**). The proportion of FcγRIIIa+CD8bright and FcγRIIIa+CD8dim cells positively correlated in the HIV-1 negative group (R = 0.671, P = 0.001; **Figure 5C**). However, this relationship was not observed for the HIV-1 positive group. In the latter group, neither the presence nor levels of FcγRIIIa correlated with CD4+ T cell count or HIV-1 plasma viral load (**Figure 5C**). However, the proportion of FcγRIIIa on CD8bright T cells negatively correlated with age in both groups, although this correlation was only statistically significant for the HIV-1 positive group (R = −0.510, P = 0.013; **Figure 5C**).

CD8+ T Cells Mediate ADCC

To assess CD8+ T cell-mediated ADCC responses, CD8+ T cells were positively selected from PBMCs after depletion of NK cells. The proportion of potential contaminating NK cells was determined using flow cytometry and six HIV-1 positive donors were identified with <5% NK cells in their enriched CD8+ T cell fractions (mean: 1.3%; range: 0.3–2.9%). A threshold for positive CD8+ T cell-mediated granzyme B responses (5.6%) was calculated based on the corresponding NK cell granzyme B responses at an NK-to-target ratio of 10:1 (described in section Materials and Methods). Five out of six donors had positive CD8+ T cell-mediated granzyme B responses that ranged from

7.5 to 25.6% (mean: 14.5%; **Figure 5E**). Overall, the CD8+ T cell-mediated granzyme B activity was comparatively lower than that observed for their NK cell counterparts (P = 0.031).

DISCUSSION

This study set out to comprehensively characterize FcγRIIIa variability and its effect on ADCC responses in HIV-1 positive and HIV-1 negative South African individuals, the population that bears the largest HIV-1 epidemic. Accurate assessment of FcγRIIIa variability requires careful selection of study participants to exclude confounding genetic variables that modify FcγRIIIa expression and FcγRIIIa-mediated cell activation. Study participants within the comparative groups were further matched for the FcγRIIIa-F158V variant that not only alters ADCC responses, but also affects measurements of FcγRIIIa surface expression with the most commonly used anti-FcγRIIIa antibody, clone 3G8 (32).

In comparing a cohort of Black South African HIV-1 negative and HIV-1 positive donors matched for genotypic variants, we confirmed previously described significant differences in the distribution of NK cell subsets, while differences in FcγRIIIa surface density on cytotoxic NK cells were not observed. NK cell-mediated ADCC responses of HIV-1 positive donors were both reduced and differentially affected by the FcγRIIIa-F158V variant compared to HIV-1 negative donors. In addition, FcγRIIIa expression was identified on a subset of cytotoxic CD8 T cells where it potentially contributes to HIV-1-specific ADCC responses in a granzyme B-dependent manner.

In healthy individuals, NK cells typically comprise a dominant CD56dimFcγRIIIabright population and minor populations that include CD56brightFcγRIIIadim/neg, CD56dimFcγRIIIdim/neg and CD56negFcγRIIIabright. Perturbation of NK cell subsets in the presence of an HIV-1 infection has been extensively described (16, 17, 33). In HIV-1 infected individuals, the cytotoxic CD56dimFcγRIIIabright subset contracts with an associated expansion of the CD56negFcγRIIIabright subset. The latter is characterized by higher levels of inhibitory NK cell receptors, lower levels of natural cytotoxicity receptors, and reduced secretion of cytokines compared to the CD56dimFcγRIIIabright

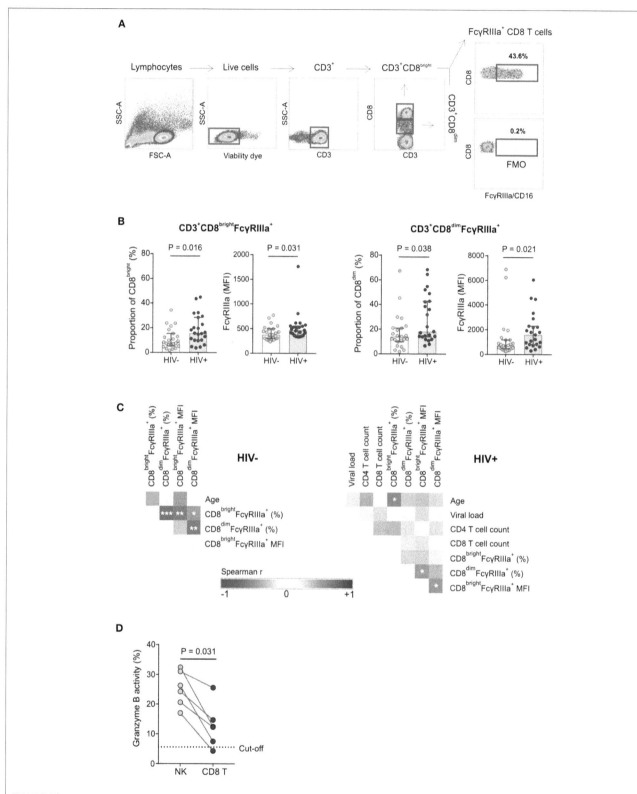

FIGURE 5 | FcγRIIIa expression on CD8 T cells in HIV-1 uninfected and HIV-1 infected individuals matched for *FCGR* genetic variants. **(A)** Gating strategy; **(B)** The proportion of FcγRIIIa+CD8bright and FcγRIIIa+CD8dim T cells and corresponding median fluorescence intensity (MFI) of FcγRIIIa on these FcγRIIIa+CD8+ T cell subsets in a cohort of HIV-1 uninfected and infected individuals; **(C)** Correlation analysis between demographic, clinical, phenotypic, and functional variables in HIV-1 uninfected and HIV-1 infected individuals; **(D)** CD8+ T cell-mediated ADCC responses of HIV-1 positive donors relative to autologous NK cell-mediated ADCC responses at the same effector-to-target cell ratio (***P < 0.001; **P < 0.01; *P < 0.05).

subset (16, 17). This hyporesponsive NK cell subset was similarly increased in the South African HIV-1 positive cohort; however, it did not associate with HIV-1 viral load as observed by Mavilio et al. (16, 34). The lack of an association with HIV-1 viral load may be explained by an ~5- to 6-fold lower median HIV-1 plasma viral load of the South African cohort compared to the other cohorts. Moreover, in the present study, NK cell subsets were studied for overnight rested PBMCs as opposed to freshly isolated negatively-selected NK cells.

The dysregulation of NK cell subsets is typically associated with reduced ADCC responses in HIV-1 infected individuals (16, 17, 35, 36). In the present study, lower ADCC responses were similarly observed for HIV-1 infected individuals. Since ADCC capacity was studied for CD56$^+$ NK cells it precluded an analysis of the association between the CD56^{neg}FcγRIIIa^{bright} subset and ADCC responses, but not for the CD56^{dim}FcγRIIIa^{bright} and CD56^{bright}FcγRIIIa$^{dim/neg}$ subsets. A negative correlation observed between the CD56^{bright}FcγRIIIa$^{dim/neg}$ subset and ADCC responses for both HIV-1 negative and positive donors would suggest that ADCC capacity is similarly affected by the immunoregulatory CD56^{bright}FcγRIIIa$^{dim/neg}$ subset in both groups. However, as demonstrated by a positive correlation between the cytotoxic CD56^{dim}FcγRIIIa^{bright} subset and ADCC responses for HIV-1 negative donors, but not HIV-1 positive donors, not all factors modulating ADCC capacity may be shared between healthy individuals and HIV-1 infected individuals.

Given the association of ADCC-mediating antibody responses with HIV-1 protective immunity, it could be hypothesized that genetic determinants of NK cell-mediated ADCC capacity, in particular the FcγRIIIa-F158V variant, may associate with HIV-1 acquisition risk or disease progression. The FcγRIIIa-158V isoform has greater avidity for complexes comprising IgG1, IgG3, and IgG4 than the FcγRIIIa-158F isoform and confers increased NK cell activation and ADCC responses in healthy individuals (21–23). Despite its potential contribution to ADCC responses, the FcγRIIIa-158V isoform is yet to be positively associated with HIV-1 acquisition and disease progression. On the contrary, the FcγRIIIa-158V isoform has been associated with an increased risk of HIV-1 infection (37), disease progression (37), and HIV-1-associated Kaposi's sarcoma (KS) and Cryptococcal disease (38, 39). Furthermore, homozygosity for the FcγRIIIa-158V allele associated with a higher rate of HIV-1 infection among vaccinated men in the VAX004 trial (40), while homozygosity for the FcγRIIIa-158F allele associated with greater protection from HIV-1 disease progression in male participants in the RV144 vaccine trial (41). Taken together, these findings are more indicative of FcγRIIIa-158V-mediated antibody-dependent enhancement of infection rather than improved ADCC responses to the benefit of the individual. Alternatively, it is possible that the functional consequence of the FcγRIIIa-F158V isoforms may be different in the presence of an HIV-1 infection and that a different mechanism(s) may underlie the aforementioned associations.

FcγRIIa/FcγRIIIb polymorphic variants, for example, show distinct differences in oxidative burst responses of resting neutrophils; however, once neutrophils were pre-activated with IFNγ and G-CSF these differences were no longer observed

(42). Other non-FcγR genetic variants have also been shown to differentially affect gene expression or cytokine production of activated and resting immune cells (43). In the present study, we show a similar trend for the FcγRIIIa-F158V variant, higher ADCC responses for HIV-1 negative donors bearing the FcγRIIIa-158V allele compared to those homozygous for the FcγRIIIa-158F allele, whereas in HIV-1 positive donors this trend was lost or even slightly reversed. The effect of the variant on ADCC responses was, however, not significant in either group. It is possible that the independent effect size of the FcγRIIIa-F158V variant is too small to detect with the current sample size. Larger cohort studies that adjust for other NK cell activation and inhibitory receptors are required to further define the role of this variant in HIV-1 infection. Nonetheless, these findings may partially explain the inconclusive role of FcγRIIIa genetic variants in HIV-1-specific immunity [reviewed by Cocklin and Schmitz (44)].

In addition to modulating the function of an allelic variant, infection can lead to the induction of FcγRIIIa on other cytotoxic cells, including CD8$^+$ T cells. An FcγRIIIa$^+$CD8$^+$ T cell population was first described in the 1980's and has since been characterized in the context of hepatitis C virus and Epstein Barr virus infections (18, 19, 45). These terminally differentiated CD8$^+$ T cells belong to the T effector memory CD45RA$^+$ lymphocyte subset, are perforin positive, directly mediate ADCC *ex vivo*, and increase *in vivo* during hyperlymphocytosis (18, 19). In addition to FcγRIIIa, this cell subset also has increased expression of other NK-like receptors including NKG2A, NKG2D, KIR2DL2/L3 and KIR2DL1/S1 when compared to FcγRIIIa$^-$CD8$^+$ T cells (46). The present study validates the expression of FcγRIIIa on cytotoxic CD8$^+$ T lymphocytes and is in agreement with other studies that have consistently showed an increase in the proportion of FcγRIIIa$^+$CD8$^+$ T cells in the presence of a virus infection (18, 19, 46). Compared to CD8^{bright} cells, the surface density of FcγRIIIa was significantly higher on CD8^{dim} cells, a subset characterized by higher activation levels, increased cytotoxicity and increased cytokine production (47–49). The higher proportions of FcγRIIIa$^+$CD8$^+$ T cells in HIV-1-infected individuals suggests that HIV-1 in its own right is a driver of these cell expansions, whereas increasing age associated with reduced proportions of FcγRIIIa-expressing CD8$^+$ T cells. The increase in FcγRIIIa expression on CD8$^+$ T cells in HIV infection contrasts with decreased proportions of FcγRIIIa expressing NK cells. This suggests the development of an ADCC capacity by CD8$^+$ T cells that could compensate to some extent for the reduction in NK cell ADCC function.

Attributing the otherwise innate cell function of ADCC to CD8$^+$ T cells—mediated through expression of FcγRIIIa and engagement of HIV-1-specific antibodies—is reminiscent of other known examples of innate-like unconventional T cell populations. Among these are invariant NKT cells, mucosal-associated invariant T cells, and γδT cells, that recognize foreign/self-lipid presented by non-classical MHC molecules (50, 51). Another interesting unconventional CD8$^+$ T cell subset is one with a prominent innate/memory phenotype identified by co-expression of eomesodermin (Eomes) and KIR/NKG2A

(52). The current study highlights the addition of another unconventional CD8$^+$ T cell population, capable of ADCC function, that warrants further investigation.

In conclusion, our findings underscore the importance of expanding studies of HIV-specific antibodies to include the influence of different host cell types that share expression of FcγRs (constitutive or induced), the respective functional cellular capabilities, as well as host genotypes, in the context of the presiding immune milieu which is altered as a consequence of chronic HIV infection. Continuing investigations are warranted to further define effector functions, cytokine production and activation status of these different FcγRIIIa$^+$ NK and CD8 T cell subsets in similarly selected individuals.

AUTHOR CONTRIBUTIONS

NP recruited HIV-1 negative donors, performed the majority of the experiments, analyzed the data and wrote the manuscript. RL designed the study, contributed to the data analysis, and writing of the manuscript. BD contributed to the flow cytometry experiments. ZW and NM recruited HIV-1 positive donors, CT in her capacity as head of the laboratory, allocated funds toward the study, supervised the research, and provided the necessary infrastructure to perform the work.

FUNDING

This work is based on the research supported by the Poliomyelitis Research Foundation and the South African Research Chairs Initiative of the Department of Science and Technology and National Research Foundation of South Africa, and the Strategic Health Innovation Partnerships (SHIP) Unit of the South African Medical Research Council (a grantee of the Bill & Melinda Gates Foundation). NP is the recipient of bursaries from the South African National Research Foundation, the Poliomyelitis Research Foundation and a University of the Witwatersrand postgraduate merit award.

ACKNOWLEDGMENTS

The following reagent was obtained through the NIH AIDS Reagent Program, Division of AIDS, NIAID, NIH: Catalog #3957, HIV-IG from NABI and NHLBI. The anti-FcγRIIb/c clone 2B6 was a gift from MacroGenics.

REFERENCES

1. Nimmerjahn F, Ravetch JV. Fcgamma receptors as regulators of immune responses. *Nat Rev Immunol.* (2008) 8:34–47. doi: 10.1038/nri2206
2. Bournazos S, Ravetch JV. Fcγ receptor function and the design of vaccination strategies. *Immunity.* (2017) 47:224–33. doi: 10.1016/j.immuni.2017.07.009
3. Rosales C. Fcγ receptor heterogeneity in leukocyte functional responses. *Front Immunol.* (2017) 8:280. doi: 10.3389/fimmu.2017.00280
4. Ravetch JV, Bolland S. IgG Fc receptors. *Annu Rev Immunol.* (2001) 19:275–90. doi: 10.1146/annurev.immunol.19.1.275
5. Nimmerjahn F, Ravetch JV. Divergent immunoglobulin g subclass activity through selective Fc receptor binding. *Science.* (2005) 310:1510–2. doi: 10.1126/science.1118948
6. Ackerman ME, Dugast A-S, Alter G. Emerging concepts on the role of innate immunity in the prevention and control of HIV infection. *Annu Rev Med.* (2012) 63:113–30. doi: 10.1146/annurev-med-050310-085221
7. Wren LH, Chung AW, Isitman G, Kelleher AD, Parsons MS, Amin J, et al. Specific antibody-dependent cellular cytotoxicity responses associated with slow progression of HIV infection. *Immunology.* (2013) 138:116–23. doi: 10.1111/imm.12016
8. Lewis GK. Role of Fc-mediated antibody function in protective immunity against HIV-1. *Immunology.* (2014) 142:46–57. doi: 10.1111/imm.12232
9. Milligan C, Richardson BA, John-Stewart G, Nduati R, Overbaugh J. Passively acquired antibody-dependent cellular cytotoxicity (ADCC) activity in HIV-infected infants is associated with reduced mortality. *Cell Host Microbe.* (2015) 17:500–6. doi: 10.1016/j.chom.2015.03.002
10. Ahmad R, Sindhu ST, Toma E, Morisset R, Vincelette J, Menezes J, et al. Evidence for a correlation between antibody-dependent cellular cytotoxicity-mediating anti-HIV-1 antibodies and prognostic predictors of HIV infection. *J Clin Immunol.* (2001) 21:227–33. doi: 10.1023/A:1011087132180
11. Banks ND, Kinsey N, Clements J, Hildreth JE. Sustained antibody-dependent cell-mediated cytotoxicity (ADCC) in SIV-infected macaques correlates with delayed progression to AIDS. *AIDS Res Hum Retrovirus.* (2002) 18:1197–205. doi: 10.1089/08892220260387940
12. Gomez-Roman VR, Patterson LJ, Venzon D, Liewehr D, Aldrich K, Florese R, et al. Vaccine-elicited antibodies mediate antibody-dependent cellular cytotoxicity correlated with significantly reduced acute viremia in rhesus macaques challenged with SIVmac251. *J Immunol.* (2005) 174:2185–9. doi: 10.4049/jimmunol.174.4.2185
13. Hessell AJ, Hangartner L, Hunter M, Havenith CE, Beurskens FJ, Bakker JM, et al. Fc receptor but not complement binding is important in antibody protection against HIV. *Nature.* (2007) 449:101–4. doi: 10.1038/nature06106
14. Lambotte O, Ferrari G, Moog C, Yates NL, Liao HX, Parks RJ, et al. Heterogeneous neutralizing antibody and antibody-dependent cell cytotoxicity responses in HIV-1 elite controllers. *AIDS.* (2009) 23:897–906. doi: 10.1097/QAD.0b013e328329f97d
15. Pollara J, Hart L, Brewer F, Pickeral J, Packard BZ, Hoxie JA, et al. High-throughput quantitative analysis of HIV-1 and SIV-specific ADCC-mediating antibody responses. *Cytometry A.* (2011) 79:603–12. doi: 10.1002/cyto.a.21084
16. Mavilio D, Lombardo G, Benjamin J, Kim D, Follman D, Marcenaro E, et al. Characterization of CD56-/CD16+ natural killer (NK) cells: a highly dysfunctional NK subset expanded in HIV-infected viremic individuals. *Proc Natl Acad Sci USA.* (2005) 102:2886–91. doi: 10.1073/pnas.0409872102
17. Brunetta E, Hudspeth KL, Mavilio D. Pathologic natural killer cell subset redistribution in HIV-1 infection: new insights in pathophysiology and clinical outcomes. *J Leukoc Biol.* (2010) 88:1119–30. doi: 10.1189/jlb.0410225
18. Bjorkstrom NK, Gonzalez VD, Malmberg KJ, Falconer K, Alaeus A, Nowak G, et al. Elevated numbers of Fc gamma RIIIA+ (CD16+) effector CD8 T cells with NK cell-like function in chronic hepatitis C virus infection. *J Immunol.* (2008) 181:4219–28. doi: 10.4049/jimmunol.181.6.4219
19. Clemenceau B, Vivien R, Berthome M, Robillard N, Garand R, Gallot G, et al. Effector memory alphabeta T lymphocytes can express FcgammaRIIIa and mediate antibody-dependent cellular cytotoxicity. *J Immunol.* (2008) 180:5327–34. doi: 10.4049/jimmunol.180.8.5327
20. Breunis WB, van Mirre E, Geissler J, Laddach N, Wolbink G, van der Schoot E, et al. Copy number variation at the FCGR locus includes FCGR3A, FCGR2C and FCGR3B but not FCGR2A and FCGR2B. *Hum Mutat.* (2009) 30:E640–650. doi: 10.1002/humu.20997
21. Koene HR, Kleijer M, Algra J, Roos D, von dem Borne AE, de Haas M. Fc gammaRIIIa-158V/F polymorphism influences the binding of IgG by natural killer cell Fc gammaRIIIa, independently of the Fc gammaRIIIa-48L/R/H phenotype. *Blood.* (1997) 90:1109–14.
22. Wu J, Edberg JC, Redecha PB, Bansal V, Guyre PM, Coleman K, et al. A novel polymorphism of FcgammaRIIIa (CD16) alters receptor function

and predisposes to autoimmune disease. *J Clin Invest.* (1997) 100:1059–70. doi: 10.1172/JCI119616

23. Bruhns P, Iannascoli B, England P, Mancardi DA, Fernandez N, Jorieux S, et al. Specificity and affinity of human Fcgamma receptors and their polymorphic variants for human IgG subclasses. *Blood.* (2009) 113:3716–25. doi: 10.1182/blood-2008-09-179754

24. Niederer HA, Willcocks LC, Rayner TF, Yang W, Lau YL, Williams TN, et al. Copy number, linkage disequilibrium and disease association in the FCGR locus. *Hum Mol Genet.* (2010) 19:3282–94. doi: 10.1093/hmg/ddq216

25. Mueller M, Barros P, Witherden AS, Roberts AL, Zhang Z, Schaschl H, et al. Genomic pathology of SLE-associated copy-number variation at the FCGR2C/FCGR3B/FCGR2B locus. *Am J Hum Genet.* (2013) 92:28–40. doi: 10.1016/j.ajhg.2012.11.013

26. van der Heijden J, Breunis WB, Geissler J, de Boer M, van den Berg TK, Kuijpers TW. Phenotypic variation in IgG receptors by nonclassical FCGR2C alleles. *J Immunol.* (2012) 188:1318–24. doi: 10.4049/jimmunol.1003945

27. Schouten JP, McElgunn CJ, Waaijer R, Zwijnenburg D, Diepvens F, Pals G. Relative quantification of 40 nucleic acid sequences by multiplex ligation-dependent probe amplification. *Nucleic Acids Res.* (2002) 30:e57. doi: 10.1093/nar/gnf056

28. Breunis WB, van Mirre E, Bruin M, Geissler J, de Boer M, Peters M, et al. Copy number variation of the activating FCGR2C gene predisposes to idiopathic thrombocytopenic purpura. *Blood.* (2008) 111:1029–38. doi: 10.1182/blood-2007-03-079913

29. Lassaunière R, Tiemessen CT. Variability at the FCGR locus: characterization in Black South Africans and evidence for ethnic variation in and out of Africa. *Genes Immun.* (2015) 17:93. doi: 10.1038/gene.2015.60

30. Lassauniere R, Shalekoff S, Tiemessen CT. A novel FCGR3A intragenic haplotype is associated with increased FcgammaRIIIa/CD16a cell surface density and population differences. *Hum Immunol.* (2013) 74:627–34. doi: 10.1016/j.humimm.2013.01.020

31. Schaftenaar E, Verjans GM, Getu S, McIntyre JA, Struthers HE, Osterhaus AD, et al. High seroprevalence of human herpesviruses in HIV-infected individuals attending primary healthcare facilities in rural South Africa. *PLoS ONE.* (2014) 9:e99243. doi: 10.1371/journal.pone.0099243

32. Congy-Jolivet N, Bolzec A, Ternant D, Ohresser M, Watier H, Thibault G. Fc gamma RIIIa expression is not increased on natural killer cells expressing the Fc gamma RIIIa-158V allotype. *Cancer Res.* (2008) 68:976–80. doi: 10.1158/0008-5472.CAN-07-6523

33. Fauci AS, Mavilio D, Kottilil S. NK cells in HIV infection: paradigm for protection or targets for ambush. *Nat Rev Immunol.* (2005) 5:835–43. doi: 10.1038/nri1711

34. Mavilio D, Benjamin J, Daucher M, Lombardo G, Kottilil S, Planta MA, et al. Natural killer cells in HIV-1 infection: dichotomous effects of viremia on inhibitory and activating receptors and their functional correlates. *Proc Natl Acad Sci USA.* (2003) 100:15011–6. doi: 10.1073/pnas.2336091100

35. Ahmad A, Menezes J. Defective killing activity against gp120/41-expressing human erythroleukaemic K562 cell line by monocytes and natural killer cells from HIV-infected individuals. *AIDS.* (1996) 10:143–9. doi: 10.1097/00002030-199602000-00003

36. Scott-Algara D, Paul P. NK cells and HIV infection: lessons from other viruses. *Curr Mol Med.* (2002) 2:757–68. doi: 10.2174/1566524023361781

37. Poonia B, Kijak GH, Pauza CD. High affinity allele for the gene of FCGR3A is risk factor for HIV infection and progression. *PLoS ONE.* (2010) 5:e15562. doi: 10.1371/journal.pone.0015562

38. Rohatgi S, Gohil S, Kuniholm MH, Schultz H, Dufaud C, Armour KL, et al. Fc Gamma receptor 3A polymorphism and risk for HIV-associated cryptococcal disease. *mBio.* (2013) 4:e00573–13. doi: 10.1128/mBio.00573-13

39. Foster CB, Zhu S, Venzon D, Steinberg SM, Wyvill K, Metcalf JA, et al. Variant genotypes of FcγRIIIA influence the development of Kaposi's sarcoma in HIV-infected men. *Blood.* (2000) 95:2386–90.

40. Forthal DN, Gabriel EE, Wang A, Landucci G, Phan TB. Association of Fcgamma receptor IIIa genotype with the rate of HIV infection after gp120 vaccination. *Blood.* (2012) 120:2836–42. doi: 10.1182/blood-2012-05-431361

41. Kijak, G. (2012). "Modulation of Vaccine Effect by FcGamma Receptor 3a Genetic Polymorphism in RV144", in *19th Conference on Retroviruses and Opportunistic Infections (CROI).* (Seattle, WA).

42. van der Heijden J, Nagelkerke S, Zhao X, Geissler J, Rispens T, van den Berg TK, et al. Haplotypes of FcgammaRIIa and FcgammaRIIIb polymorphic variants influence IgG-mediated responses in neutrophils. *J Immunol.* (2014) 192:2715–21. doi: 10.4049/jimmunol.1203570

43. Jonkers IH, Wijmenga C. Context-specific effects of genetic variants associated with autoimmune disease. *Hum Mol Genet.* (2017) 26:R185–92. doi: 10.1093/hmg/ddx254

44. Cocklin SL, Schmitz JE. The role of Fc receptors in HIV infection and vaccine efficacy. *Curr Opin HIV AIDS.* (2014) 9:257–62. doi: 10.1097/COH.0000000000000051

45. Lanier LL, Kipps TJ, Phillips JH. Functional properties of a unique subset of cytotoxic CD3+ T lymphocytes that express Fc receptors for IgG (CD16/Leu-11 antigen). *J Exp Med.* (1985) 162:2089–106. doi: 10.1084/jem.162.6.2089

46. Clemenceau B, Vivien R, Debeaupuis E, Esbelin J, Biron C, Levy Y, et al. FcγRIIIa (CD16) induction on human T lymphocytes and CD16pos T-lymphocyte amplification. *J Immunother.* (2011) 34:542–9. doi: 10.1097/CJI.0b013e31822801d4

47. Trautmann A, Rückert B, Schmid-Grendelmeier P, Niederer E, Bröcker E-B, Blaser K, et al. Human CD8 T cells of the peripheral blood contain a low CD8 expressing cytotoxic/effector subpopulation. *Immunology.* (2003) 108:305–12. doi: 10.1046/j.1365-2567.2003.01590.x

48. Kienzle N, Baz A, Kelso A. Profiling the CD8low phenotype, an alternative career choice for CD8 T cells during primary differentiation. *Immunol Cell Biol.* (2004) 82:75–83. doi: 10.1111/j.1440-1711.2004.01210.x

49. Falanga YT, Frascoli M, Kaymaz Y, Forconi C, Ong'echa JM, Bailey JA, et al. High pathogen burden in childhood promotes the development of unconventional innate-like CD8+ T cells. *JCI Insight.* (2017) 2:93814. doi: 10.1172/jci.insight.93814

50. Lanier LL. Shades of grey–the blurring view of innate and adaptive immunity. *Nat Rev Immunol.* (2013) 13:73–4. doi: 10.1038/nri3389

51. Godfrey DI, Uldrich AP, McCluskey J, Rossjohn J, Moody DB. The burgeoning family of unconventional T cells. *Nat Immunol.* (2015) 16:1114–23. doi: 10.1038/ni.3298

52. Jacomet F, Cayssials E, Barbarin A, Desmier D, Basbous S, Lefevre L, et al. The hypothesis of the human iNKT/Innate CD8(+) T-cell axis applied to cancer: evidence for a deficiency in chronic myeloid leukemia. *Front Immunol.* (2016) 7:688. doi: 10.3389%2Ffimmu.2016.00688

13

Parameter Identification for a Model of Neonatal Fc Receptor-Mediated Recycling of Endogenous Immunoglobulin G in Humans

Felicity Kendrick[1], Neil D. Evans[1], Oscar Berlanga[2], Stephen J. Harding[2] and Michael J. Chappell[1]*

[1] School of Engineering, University of Warwick, Coventry, United Kingdom, [2] Department of Research and Development, The Binding Site Group Limited, Birmingham, United Kingdom

*Correspondence:
Michael J. Chappell
m.j.chappell@warwick.ac.uk

Salvage of endogenous immunoglobulin G (IgG) by the neonatal Fc receptor (FcRn) is implicated in many clinical areas, including therapeutic monoclonal antibody kinetics, patient monitoring in IgG multiple myeloma, and antibody-mediated transplant rejection. There is a clear clinical need for a fully parameterized model of FcRn-mediated recycling of endogenous IgG to allow for predictive modeling, with the potential for optimizing therapeutic regimens for better patient outcomes. In this paper we study a mechanism-based model incorporating nonlinear FcRn-IgG binding kinetics. The aim of this study is to determine whether parameter values can be estimated using the limited *in vivo* human data, available in the literature, from studies of the kinetics of radiolabeled IgG in humans. We derive mathematical descriptions of the experimental observations—timecourse data and fractional catabolic rate (FCR) data—based on the underlying physiological model. Structural identifiability analyses are performed to determine which, if any, of the parameters are unique with respect to the observations. Structurally identifiable parameters are then estimated from the data. It is found that parameter values estimated from timecourse data are not robust, suggesting that the model complexity is not supported by the available data. Based upon the structural identifiability analyses, a new expression for the FCR is derived. This expression is fitted to the FCR data to estimate unknown parameter values. Using these parameter estimates, the plasma IgG response is simulated under clinical conditions. Finally a suggestion is made for a reduced-order model based upon the newly derived expression for the FCR. The reduced-order model is used to predict the plasma IgG response, which is compared with the original four-compartment model, showing good agreement. This paper shows how techniques for compartmental model analysis—structural identifiability analysis, linearization, and reparameterization—can be used to ensure robust parameter identification.

Keywords: biological systems, lumped-parameter systems, immunoglobulin G, neonatal Fc receptor, parameter estimation, structural identifiability

1. INTRODUCTION

Immunoglobulin G (IgG) is the most abundant immunoglobulin (Ig) isotype in the circulation in humans, with a plasma concentration in healthy adults of 10–16 g l^{-1} (1). Its high concentration is facilitated by the neonatal Fc receptor (FcRn), which binds IgG in intracellular endosomes and transports it to the plasma membrane to be returned to the circulation. A proportion of IgG molecules that are not bound by FcRn are degraded in lysosomes. In this way, FcRn continually protects a proportion of the circulating IgG from degradation. The recycling mechanism is saturable, such that at high plasma IgG concentrations a greater proportion of plasma IgG is degraded. Conversely, at depleted plasma IgG concentrations, a greater proportion is recycled and the half-life is extended beyond the normal 23 days (2).

Recent publications have drawn attention to the importance of FcRn-mediated recycling of endogenous IgG in the bone marrow cancer multiple myeloma. In multiple myeloma, clonal plasma cells secrete an excess of monoclonal Ig into the circulation. Patients undergoing therapy are primarily monitored by quantification of Ig in blood serum samples (3). Mills et al. (4) have suggested that FcRn-mediated recycling of IgG may result in different response rates between patients with IgG-producing multiple myeloma and patients with IgA-producing multiple myeloma. Yan et al. (5) have also suggested that FcRn-mediated recycling of endogenous IgG in patients with multiple myeloma may shorten the half-life of the therapeutic monoclonal antibody daratumumab. These studies highlight the need for a parameterized model of endogenous IgG kinetics for investigating these clinical scenarios.

Numerous mathematical models of IgG kinetics have been presented in the literature, mostly with the aim of describing the pharmacokinetics of therapeutic monoclonal antibodies (mAbs) that are also regulated by FcRn. Many of these models are therefore pharmacokinetic in nature: their parameter values are obtained from animal experiments and they may be physiologically-based, with up to around 10 organs explicitly represented in the model (6–14). Pharmacokinetic models developed for specific mAbs may not be generalizable to endogenous IgG if, for example, they include details such as binding of the mAb to its target. In addition, mAb disposition may be adequately described by linear models in many cases where the plasma concentration of therapeutic mAb is substantially smaller than the plasma concentration of endogenous IgG and the latter is constant (13, 14). However, the assumption of a constant plasma concentration of IgG is not always appropriate; for example, in multiple myeloma the plasma IgG concentration typically shows large changes during the course of therapy. Relative to a less complex model, the more complex model will usually provide a better fit to observed data. However, this alone does not imply that all the parameters in the complex model can be estimated consistently, nor does it imply that the underlying assumptions of the complex model are valid (15).

In this paper we study a mechanism-based model with a single plasma compartment, rather than separate plasma compartments for different organs, which is accessible to measurement in humans. The model, which has been previously shown by Kim et al. (16) and Hattersley (17), has in total four compartments, representing IgG in plasma, IgG in a peripheral compartment (representing less rapidly perfused tissues), unbound IgG in intracellular endosomes and IgG bound to FcRn receptors in intracellular endosomes. The IgG-FcRn interaction is represented by nonlinear receptor-ligand binding kinetics (6, 7, 9). With reliable parameter values for humans, it may be possible to use this model to predict the responses of plasma IgG under various clinical conditions.

The aim of this study is to determine whether the model parameter values can be obtained using the limited *in vivo* human data that are available in the literature. The data are from studies of the kinetics of administered small doses of radiolabeled IgG when the subject's endogenous IgG is in steady state. We consider two measured outputs: the timecourse of the proportion of an administered dose of radiolabeled IgG remaining in plasma and in the body; and the relationship between the fractional catabolic rate and the quantity of endogenous IgG in plasma. Structural identifiability analysis is performed with respect to these outputs and structurally identifiable parameters are estimated from the data.

2. MATHEMATICAL MODELS AND DATA DESCRIPTION

2.1. The Four Compartment Model

The model of IgG metabolism under study (16, 17) has four state variables, nine parameters, and an input function, $I(t)$, representing the synthesis of IgG. The model equations are given by

$$\dot{x}_1(t) = -(k_{21} + k_{31})x_1(t) + k_{12}x_2(t) + k_{14}x_4(t) + I(t)$$
$$\dot{x}_2(t) = k_{21}x_1(t) - k_{12}x_2(t)$$
$$\dot{x}_3(t) = k_{31}x_1(t) - k_{03}x_3(t) - \frac{k_{on}}{v_3}x_3(t)(R_{tot} - x_4(t)) + k_{off}x_4(t)$$
$$\dot{x}_4(t) = \frac{k_{on}}{v_3}x_3(t)(R_{tot} - x_4(t)) - (k_{14} + k_{off})x_4(t),$$

$$(1)$$

where $x_1(t)$, $x_2(t)$, $x_3(t)$, and $x_4(t)$ represent the quantities in μmol of IgG in plasma, IgG in a peripheral compartment, unbound IgG in endosomes and IgG bound to FcRn in endosomes, respectively. $I(t)$ represents the rate of synthesis of IgG in μmol day^{-1}. The rate constants, k_{ij}, represent the rate of material flow from compartment j to compartment i, with the convention that 0 represents the environment outside the system. k_{on} and k_{off} are the receptor-ligand binding constants of IgG and FcRn. We denote the volumes of plasma, the peripheral compartment and the endosomes by v_1, v_2, and v_3, respectively. We assume a constant total (bound and unbound) quantity of FcRn, R_{tot} (6). This means that the quantity of unbound FcRn is represented by $[R_{tot} - x_4(t)]$. The state variables of the model and physiological interpretations of the parameters are summarized in **Table 1**. Note that all states and parameters can only take non-negative values. We refer to **Figure 1** for a schematic of the model.

TABLE 1 | States and parameters of four-compartment model of IgG metabolism, with parameter values sourced in the literature.

Name	Units	Literature value	Physiological interpretation
x_1	μmol	–	Quantity of IgG in the central (plasma) compartment
x_2	μmol	–	Quantity of IgG in the peripheral compartment
x_3	μmol	–	Quantity of unbound IgG in intracellular endosomes
x_4	μmol	–	Quantity of IgG-FcRn complexes in intracellular endosomes
v_1	l	2.9*	Plasma volume
v_2	l	–	Volume of peripheral compartment
v_3	l	0.34†	Total volume of endosomes
k_{21}	day^{-1}	0.51‡	Rate constant of flow of IgG from plasma to peripheral compartment
k_{31}	day^{-1}	0.18§	Rate constant of flow of IgG from plasma into endosomes by pinocytosis
k_{12}	day^{-1}	0.41‡	Rate constant of flow of IgG from peripheral compartment to plasma
k_{14}	day^{-1}	5.0¶	Rate constant of flow of recycled IgG from endosomes back into plasma
k_{03}	day^{-1}	3.0‖	Rate constant of degradation of unbound IgG in endosomes
k_{on}	lμmol day^{-1}	1,000**	Association rate constant of IgG-FcRn binding
R_{tot}	μmol	14¶	Total quantity of FcRn receptors, bound and unbound
k_{off}	day^{-1}	100**	Dissociation rate constant of IgG-FcRn binding

*Solomon et al. (18), †Shah and Betts (19), ‡Hattersley et al. (20), §Waldmann and Strober (21), ¶Ferl et al. (6), ‖ Hansen and Balthasar (22), **Chen and Balthasar (10).

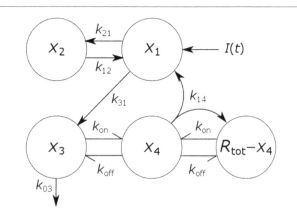

FIGURE 1 | Schematic of four-compartment model of IgG metabolism. Arrows represent material flow between compartments and hooked arrows represent nonlinear receptor-ligand binding. The fifth compartment shown $(R_{tot} - x_4)$ represents unbound FcRn receptors and has been eliminated from the model equations. The arrow, labeled k_{14}, from the IgG-FcRn complex compartment (x_4) to the unbound FcRn receptor compartment $(R_{tot} - x_4)$, represents internalization of FcRn receptors from the plasma membrane to the endosome, after releasing IgG.

When the production rate of IgG is constant, $I(t) = I_0$, the system has a stable equilibrium point given by

$$\hat{x}_1 = \frac{I_0 \left(k_{03}k_{14}v_3 + k_{03}k_{off}v_3 + k_{on}I_0 + k_{14}k_{on}R_{tot}\right)}{k_{31}\left(k_{03}v_3(k_{14} + k_{off}) + k_{on}I_0\right)}$$

$$\hat{x}_2 = \frac{k_{21}}{k_{12}}\hat{x}_1$$

$$\hat{x}_3 = \frac{I_0}{k_{03}}$$

$$\hat{x}_4 = \frac{k_{on}I_0R_{tot}}{k_{03}v_3(k_{14} + k_{off}) + k_{on}I_0}.$$

(2)

A stability analysis for this equilibrium point is provided in the **Supplementary Material**.

2.2. *In vivo* Human Data From the Literature

The data available in the literature were obtained from tracer experiments. These studies entailed intravenous administration of a bolus dose of radiolabeled IgG (the tracer) and monitoring the proportion of the dose remaining in the blood and in the body over time. In this way the administered dose is distinguishable (by the experimenter) from the subject's own endogenous IgG. The quantity of administered tracer is small, so as not to perturb the steady state of the endogenous IgG. The purpose of tracer experiments is to enable observation of processes such as distribution and elimination undergone by the endogenous protein, whilst it is in steady state. The methods are described fully by Waldmann and Strober (21).

The data for an individual subject consist of the timecourse of the proportion of the injected dose of IgG remaining in plasma and the timecourse of the proportion of dose remaining in the body. In this paper we use the data from six such plots available in the literature. We refer to the individuals as subjects A–F. The timecourse data for subjects A–D are from Solomon et al. (18), for subject E from Waldmann and Terry (23), and for subject F from Waldmann and Strober (21). Several of the individuals have health conditions which may result in an increased or decreased plasma IgG concentration. Subjects A and C have IgG multiple myeloma and subject D has macroglobulinemia. Subjects B, E, and F are referred to as "normal" subjects. A spaghetti plot of the data is shown in **Figure 2A**. Subjects A and D show slower dynamics and subject C shows faster dynamics. The dynamics of IgG in these subjects is assumed to be described by the same model, as given by Equations (1), however they may have had altered production rates of IgG due to the diseases.

Also available in the literature is a plot of the fractional catabolic rate (FCR) vs. the subject's plasma concentration of endogenous IgG, obtained from a group of individuals with a

Parameter Identification for a Model of Neonatal Fc Receptor-Mediated Recycling of Endogenous...

167

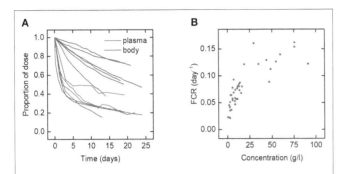

FIGURE 2 | (A) Spaghetti plot of the proportion of administered IgG remaining in plasma (blue) and the body (red) in six subjects; data from Waldmann and Strober (21), Solomon et al. (18), and Waldmann and Terry (23). **(B)** Plasma concentration dependence of the fractional catabolic rate (FCR); redrawn from Waldmann and Strober (21), with permission from S. Karger AG, Basel.

range of plasma IgG concentrations (21). The FCR is defined as the elimination rate of IgG as a fraction of the quantity of IgG in plasma. In practice the FCR is calculated from the rate at which the tracer dose leaves the body at time t divided by the proportion of tracer dose remaining in plasma at time t. The relationship between the FCR and the timecourse data is described further in section 2.6. A plot of the FCR vs. the plasma concentration of endogenous IgG for 41 individuals provided by Waldmann and Strober (21) is shown in **Figure 2B**. Each data point was derived from the timecourse data of an individual subject. All of the data described in this section were extracted from plots in the literature using the Digitizer tool in OriginPro 2016 (24).

2.3. Nonlinear Model of Coupled Tracer and Endogenous IgG Dynamics

The administered tracer and the endogenous IgG are assumed to be indistinguishable by the human body, that is they exhibit identical kinetic (input/output) behavior—a standard assumption in tracer studies (25). We therefore assume that the kinetics of both tracer and endogenous IgG are described by the model given by Equations (1). From Equations (1), letting $x_i(t) = x_{i,T}(t) + x_{i,E}(t)$, where $x_{i,T}(t)$ and $x_{i,E}(t)$ denote the quantities in μmol in compartment i of radiolabeled and endogenous IgG, respectively, gives

$$\dot{x}_{1,T}(t) = -(k_{21} + k_{31})x_{1,T}(t) + k_{12}x_{2,T}(t) + k_{14}x_{4,T}(t)$$

$$\dot{x}_{2,T}(t) = k_{21}x_{1,T}(t) - k_{12}x_{2,T}(t)$$

$$\dot{x}_{3,T}(t) = k_{31}x_{1,T}(t) - k_{03}x_{3,T}(t) - \frac{k_{on}}{v_3}x_{3,T}(t)(R_{tot} - x_{4,E}(t)$$
$$- x_{4,T}(t)) + k_{off}x_{4,T}(t)$$

$$\dot{x}_{4,T}(t) = \frac{k_{on}}{v_3}x_{3,T}(t)(R_{tot} - x_{4,E}(t) - x_{4,T}(t)) - (k_{14} + k_{off})x_{4,T}(t)$$

$$\dot{x}_{1,E}(t) = -(k_{21} + k_{31})x_{1,E}(t) + k_{12}x_{2,E}(t) + k_{14}x_{4,E}(t) + I_E$$

$$\dot{x}_{2,E}(t) = k_{21}x_{1,E}(t) - k_{12}x_{2,E}(t)$$

$$\dot{x}_{3,E}(t) = k_{31}x_{1,E}(t) - k_{03}x_{3,E}(t) - \frac{k_{on}}{v_3}x_{3,E}(t)(R_{tot} - x_{4,E}(t)$$
$$- x_{4,T}(t)) + k_{off}x_{4,E}(t)$$

$$\dot{x}_{4,E}(t) = \frac{k_{on}}{v_3}x_{3,E}(t)(R_{tot} - x_{4,E}(t) - x_{4,T}(t))$$
$$- (k_{14} + k_{off})x_{4,E}(t). \tag{3}$$

I_E (μmol day^{-1}) represents the production rate of endogenous IgG, which is assumed constant. All other parameters are defined in **Table 1**.

The dose of tracer administered at time $t = 0$ days is treated as a non-zero initial condition for $x_{1,T}(t)$. Tracer is administered to the plasma compartment only; therefore the initial conditions of the remaining tracer compartments are zero. The endogenous IgG is assumed to be in steady state throughout the experiment, such that the initial conditions of the endogenous IgG are given by the steady states in Equations (2), with $I_0 = I_E$. In summary, the initial conditions are given by

$$\begin{aligned} x_{1,T}(0) &= D \\ x_{2,T}(0) &= x_{3,T}(0) = x_{4,T}(0) = 0 \\ x_{1,E}(0) &= \hat{x}_1 \\ x_{2,E}(0) &= \hat{x}_2 \\ x_{3,E}(0) &= \hat{x}_3 \\ x_{4,E}(0) &= \hat{x}_4, \end{aligned} \tag{4}$$

where $\hat{x}_i$ is the steady state quantity of endogenous IgG in compartment i, given by Equations (2), and D (μmol) is the administered dose of tracer.

The experimenter observes the proportion of the dose remaining in plasma [denoted by $y_1(t)$] and in the body [denoted by $y_2(t)$] during the experiment. The observation functions are thus given by

$$\begin{aligned} y_1(t) &= \frac{x_{1,T}(t)}{D} \\ y_2(t) &= \frac{x_{1,T}(t) + x_{2,T}(t) + x_{3,T}(t) + x_{4,T}(t)}{D}. \end{aligned} \tag{5}$$

2.4. Linearized Model of Tracer Dynamics

Provided that the administered dose of tracer is sufficiently small, the tracer kinetics can be approximated using the Taylor series expansion of the model state about the equilibrium point. In this way a linear model of the experiment, valid in a neighborhood of the equilibrium point, is derived. Our derivation is provided in the **Supplementary Material**. The derivation of a linearized model for tracer dynamics from a general compartmental model is provided by Anderson (26).

The linear equations describing the tracer kinetics are given by

$$\begin{aligned} \dot{x}_{1,T}(t) &= -(k_{21} + k_{31})x_{1,T}(t) + k_{12}x_{2,T}(t) + k_{14}x_{4,T}(t) \\ \dot{x}_{2,T}(t) &= k_{21}x_{1,T}(t) - k_{12}x_{2,T}(t) \\ \dot{x}_{3,T}(t) &= k_{31}x_{1,T}(t) - k_{03}x_{3,T}(t) - k_{43}x_{3,T}(t) + k_{34}x_{4,T}(t) \\ \dot{x}_{4,T}(t) &= k_{43}x_{3,T}(t) - (k_{14} + k_{34})x_{4,T}(t) \end{aligned} \tag{6}$$

where $x_{1,T}(t)$, $x_{2,T}(t)$, $x_{3,T}(t)$, and $x_{4,T}(t)$ represent the quantities of radiolabeled IgG in the central compartment, in the peripheral compartment, unbound in intracellular endosomes, and bound to FcRn in intracellular endosomes, respectively. The new parameters k_{34} and k_{43} are given by

$$
\begin{aligned}
k_{34} &= k_{\text{off}} \\
k_{43} &= \frac{k_{\text{on}}(R_{\text{tot}} - \hat{x}_4)}{v_3} = \frac{k_{\text{on}} R_{\text{tot}} k_{03}(k_{14} + k_{\text{off}})}{I_E k_{\text{on}} + k_{03} v_3(k_{14} + k_{\text{off}})}.
\end{aligned} \quad (7)
$$

All other parameters are defined in **Table 1**. The initial conditions are given by the first two equations of Equations (4) and the observation functions are given by Equations (5).

2.5. Comparison of Nonlinear Model and Linearized Model for Large Tracer Doses

The linearization of the model of timecourse observations relies on the assumption of a sufficiently small dose of tracer, such that the endogenous IgG can be assumed to remain in steady state. A typical tracer dose is between $3 \cdot 10^{-3}$ and $7 \cdot 10^{-3}$ μmol (18). Simulations of the quantity of tracer in each compartment are shown in **Figure 3**. In **Figure 3A**, a dose of $D = 1$ μmol is assumed and in **Figure 3B**, a dose of $D = 100$ μmol is assumed. The value of 1 μmol was chosen to show that the linear model is a valid approximation of the nonlinear model, even when the dose is more than 100 times typical tracer doses. The extremely large value of 100 μmol was chosen specifically to show the dynamics of the linearized model when it is not a valid approximation of the nonlinear model. The parameter values in **Table 1** are used. A normal IgG synthesis rate of $I_E = 15$ μmol day^{-1} was used; however the linearized model was still valid for $D = 1$ μmol when comparatively very small values of I_E were used. We find that, for a dose of 1 μmol and the particular parameter values used, the linearized model is a valid approximation of the full nonlinear model over a 25-day simulated time course. When the dose is increased to 100 μmol, the assumption that the steady state is not perturbed by the administered dose no longer holds and the two models give different simulation results for the quantities of tracer.

2.6. Fractional Catabolic Rate

We recall that the FCR (μmol day^{-1}) is defined as the elimination rate of IgG as a fraction of the quantity of IgG in plasma and can be defined with respect to the tracer or with respect to the endogenous IgG. The FCR with respect to the tracer is therefore given by

$$
\text{FCR}_T(t) = \frac{k_{03} x_{3,T}(t)}{x_{1,T}(t)}, \quad (8)
$$

where $x_{3,T}(t)$ and $x_{1,T}(t)$ are given by the solution of Equations (6).

Whilst a single value of the FCR is measured for an individual subject (see **Figure 2B**), in actuality $\text{FCR}_T(t)$ is not constant, as shown by the dependence on time in Equation (8). A simulation of $\text{FCR}_T(t)$ during the experiment is shown in **Figure 4**. After around day 5, for the particular parameter values used, $\text{FCR}_T(t)$ approaches a steady state value, which is denoted here by

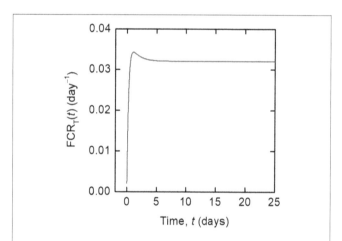

FIGURE 4 | Simulation of $\text{FCR}_T(t)$ given by Equations (12) and (8), for the parameter values in **Table 1** and dose $D = 0.01$ μmol.

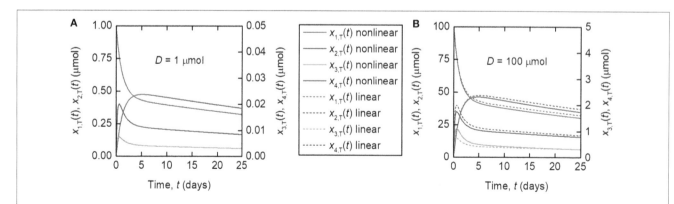

FIGURE 3 | Simulations of the quantities of tracer in each compartment after administration at $t = 0$ days, for a tracer dose of **(A)** 1 μmol and **(B)** 100 μmol. The nonlinear model (Equations 3–4) is represented by solid lines and the linearized model (Equations 6) by dashed lines. The linearized model is valid for the smaller dose but not for the larger dose. Note the different scales for $x_{1,T}(t)$ and $x_{2,T}(t)$, and $x_{3,T}(t)$ and $x_{4,T}(t)$, respectively.

$\text{FCR}_{T,\infty}$:

$$\text{FCR}_{T,\infty} = \lim_{t \to \infty} \frac{k_{03}x_{3,T}(t)}{x_{1,T}(t)}. \quad (9)$$

Solving Equations (6) gives

$$x_{i,T}(t) = A_{i1}\exp(\lambda_1 t) + A_{i2}\exp(\lambda_2 t) + A_{i3}\exp(\lambda_3 t)$$
$$+A_{i4}\exp(\lambda_4 t), i = 1,\ldots,4, \quad (10)$$

where A_{ij} and λ_j $(j = 1,\ldots,4)$ are expressions in terms of the model parameters and $|\lambda_1| > |\lambda_2| > |\lambda_3| > |\lambda_4|$. After sufficient time, $x_{i,T}(t)$ can be approximated by $A_{i4}\exp(\lambda_4 t)$; thus, $\text{FCR}_{T,\infty}$ is given by

$$\text{FCR}_{T,\infty} = k_{03}\frac{A_{34}\exp(\lambda_4 t)}{A_{14}\exp(\lambda_4 t)} = k_{03}\frac{A_{34}}{A_{14}}. \quad (11)$$

The expressions for A_{34} and A_{14} in terms of the model parameters are extremely long. The Mathematica (27) code for generating the expressions for A_{ij} and λ_j is provided in the **Supplementary Material**.

Noting that there is only elimination from the system and no input for $t > 0$, $\text{FCR}_T(t)$ is equal to the rate of change of radiolabeled IgG in all compartments, divided by the quantity of radiolabeled IgG in plasma:

$$\text{FCR}_T(t) = \frac{-\left(\dot{x}_{1,T}(t) + \dot{x}_{2,T}(t) + \dot{x}_{3,T}(t) + \dot{x}_{4,T}(t)\right)}{x_{1,T}(t)} = \frac{-\dot{y}_2(t)}{y_1(t)}. \quad (12)$$

From Equation (12), it can be seen that $\text{FCR}_T(t)$ is equal to the slope of the observation $y_2(t)$ divided by $y_1(t)$, showing how $\text{FCR}_T(t)$ can be obtained from the observations $y_1(t)$ and $y_2(t)$. In practice, the experimenter obtains a value for $\text{FCR}_T(t_N)$, where t_N is a time toward the end of the experiment, such that $\text{FCR}_T(t_N)$ can be assumed a close approximation of $\text{FCR}_{T,\infty}$. Henceforth, the quantity obtained from experiments, $\text{FCR}_T(t_N)$, is referred to simply as FCR_T.

It is also possible to derive an expression for the FCR with respect to the endogenous IgG, FCR_E. If the endogenous IgG is assumed to remain in steady state, then from the definition of the FCR,

$$\text{FCR}_E = \frac{k_{03}\hat{x}_3}{\hat{x}_1}, \quad (13)$$

where $\hat{x}_1$ and $\hat{x}_3$ are the quantities of IgG in compartments 1 and 3 in steady state, given by Equations (2). Substituting the expression for $\hat{x}_3$ from Equations (2) into Equation (13), eliminating I_0 in favor of $\hat{x}_1$ using the first equation of Equations (2), and setting $\hat{x}_1 = x_{1,E}$, gives the following expression for the FCR_E in terms of the quantity of IgG in plasma, $x_{1,E}$:

$$\text{FCR}_E = \frac{1}{2k_{\text{on}}x_{1,E}}\Big(k_{31}k_{\text{on}}x_{1,E} - k_{14}k_{\text{on}}R_{\text{tot}} - k_{03}k_{14}v_3$$
$$- k_{03}k_{\text{off}}v_3 + \big\{4k_{03}k_{31}(k_{14} + k_{\text{off}})k_{\text{on}}x_{1,E}v_3$$
$$+ (-k_{31}k_{\text{on}}x_{1,E} + k_{14}k_{\text{on}}R_{\text{tot}} + k_{03}k_{14}v_3$$
$$+ k_{03}k_{\text{off}}v_3)^2\big\}^{1/2}\Big). \quad (14)$$

3. RESULTS

3.1. Parameter Identification Using Tracer Timecourse Data

In this section we investigate whether it is possible to estimate unknown model parameter values by fitting the linear approximation described in section 2.4 to the timecourse data described in section 2.2. Firstly, a structural identifiability analysis is performed. Parameter values are then estimated from the data by fitting the linearized model described by Equations (6) to the data.

3.1.1. Structural Identifiability Analysis

Structural identifiability addresses the question of whether model parameters can be uniquely identified from the available observations, under the assumption of the availability of ideal (i.e. noise-free) and continuous observational data. Here we determine which of the model parameters are structurally uniquely identifiable from the observations $y_1(t)$ and $y_2(t)$, given by Equations (4–6). The unknown parameter vector is given by $\boldsymbol{\theta} = (k_{21}, k_{31}, k_{12}, k_{14}, k_{03}, k_{43}, k_{34})^T$.

The transfer function method is used (28). To apply this approach the system described by Equations (4–6) is re-written in vector-matrix notation as

$$\dot{\boldsymbol{x}}_T(t, \boldsymbol{\theta}) = \boldsymbol{A}(\boldsymbol{\theta})\boldsymbol{x}_T(t) + \boldsymbol{B}(\boldsymbol{\theta})u(t)$$
$$\boldsymbol{x}_T(0, \boldsymbol{\theta}) = 0 \quad (15)$$
$$\boldsymbol{y}(t, \boldsymbol{\theta}) = \boldsymbol{C}(\boldsymbol{\theta})\boldsymbol{x}_T(t),$$

where $\boldsymbol{x}_T(t, \boldsymbol{\theta}) = \left(x_{1,T}(t), x_{2,T}(t), x_{3,T}(t), x_{4,T}(t)\right)^T$ and $\boldsymbol{y}(t, \boldsymbol{\theta}) = \left(y_1(t), y_2(t)\right)^T$ are column vectors representing the state vector and the observation vector, respectively, and $u(t)$ represents the single input to the system, an impulse at time $t = 0$, given by $u(t) = \delta(t)$. $\boldsymbol{A}(\boldsymbol{\theta})$ is a 4×4 matrix, $\boldsymbol{B}(\boldsymbol{\theta})$ is a column vector and $\boldsymbol{C}(\boldsymbol{\theta})$ is a 2×4 matrix. $\boldsymbol{A}(\boldsymbol{\theta})$, $\boldsymbol{B}(\boldsymbol{\theta})$, and $\boldsymbol{C}(\boldsymbol{\theta})$ are given by

$$\boldsymbol{A}(\boldsymbol{\theta}) = \begin{pmatrix} -(k_{21} + k_{31}) & k_{12} & 0 & k_{14} \\ k_{21} & -k_{12} & 0 & 0 \\ k_{31} & 0 & -(k_{03} + k_{43}) & k_{34} \\ 0 & 0 & k_{43} & -(k_{14} + k_{34}) \end{pmatrix},$$

$$\boldsymbol{B}(\boldsymbol{\theta}) = \begin{pmatrix} D \\ 0 \\ 0 \\ 0 \end{pmatrix},$$

$$\boldsymbol{C}(\boldsymbol{\theta}) = \begin{pmatrix} \frac{1}{D} & 0 & 0 & 0 \\ \frac{1}{D} & \frac{1}{D} & \frac{1}{D} & \frac{1}{D} \end{pmatrix}. \quad (16)$$

Note that the administration of a bolus dose of size D is now represented as an impulse at time $t = 0$, rather than a non-zero initial condition, such that $\boldsymbol{x}_T(0, \boldsymbol{\theta}) = (0, 0, 0, 0)^T$.

Taking Laplace transforms of Equations (15), the input-output relation is given by $\boldsymbol{Y}(s) = \boldsymbol{G}(s)U(s)$, where $\boldsymbol{G}(s)$ is the transfer function matrix, given by $\boldsymbol{G}(s) = \boldsymbol{C}(\boldsymbol{\theta})(s\boldsymbol{I} - \boldsymbol{A}(\boldsymbol{\theta}))^{-1}\boldsymbol{B}(\boldsymbol{\theta})$, where $\boldsymbol{I}$ is the 4×4 identity matrix. $\boldsymbol{G}(s)$ has two elements, corresponding to the two observed outputs, which are given by

$$G_1(s) = \frac{\phi_1 + \phi_2 s + \phi_3 s^2 + s^3}{\phi_4 + \phi_5 s + \phi_6 s^2 + \phi_7 s^3 + s^4}$$
$$G_2(s) = \frac{\phi_8 + \phi_9 s + \phi_{10} s^2 + s^3}{\phi_{11} + \phi_{12} s + \phi_{13} s^2 + \phi_{14} s^3 + s^4},$$
(17)

where the coefficients of s, $\mathbf{\Phi}(\boldsymbol{\theta}) = (\phi_1(\boldsymbol{\theta}), \phi_2(\boldsymbol{\theta}), ..., \phi_{14}(\boldsymbol{\theta}))^T$, are nonlinear expressions in the parameters. The coefficients of s, $\mathbf{\Phi}(\boldsymbol{\theta})$, are given by

$\phi_1(\boldsymbol{\theta}) = k_{12}\left(k_{03}\left(k_{14} + k_{34}\right) + k_{14}k_{43}\right)$

$\phi_2(\boldsymbol{\theta}) = k_{03}\left(k_{12} + k_{14} + k_{34}\right) + k_{14}k_{43} + k_{12}\left(k_{14} + k_{34} + k_{43}\right)$

$\phi_3(\boldsymbol{\theta}) = k_{03} + k_{12} + k_{14} + k_{34} + k_{43}$

$\phi_4(\boldsymbol{\theta}) = \phi_{11}(\boldsymbol{\theta}) = k_{03}k_{12}k_{31}(k_{14} + k_{34})$

$\phi_5(\boldsymbol{\theta}) = \phi_{12}(\boldsymbol{\theta}) = k_{03}((k_{21} + k_{31})(k_{14} + k_{34}) + k_{12}(k_{14} + k_{31}$
$\quad + k_{34})) + k_{14}k_{21}k_{43} + k_{12}(k_{14}(k_{31} + k_{43}) + k_{31}(k_{34} + k_{43}))$

$\phi_6(\boldsymbol{\theta}) = \phi_{13}(\boldsymbol{\theta}) = k_{14}k_{21} + k_{14}k_{31} + k_{21}k_{34} + k_{31}k_{34} + k_{03}(k_{12}$
$\quad + k_{14} + k_{21} + k_{31} + k_{34}) + k_{14}k_{43} + k_{21}k_{43} + k_{31}k_{43} + k_{12}$
$(k_{14} + k_{31} + k_{34} + k_{43})$

$\phi_7(\boldsymbol{\theta}) = \phi_{10}(\boldsymbol{\theta}) = \phi_{14}(\boldsymbol{\theta}) = k_{03} + k_{12} + k_{14} + k_{21} + k_{31}$
$\quad + k_{34} + k_{43}$

$\phi_8(\boldsymbol{\theta}) = k_{03}(k_{12} + k_{21})(k_{14} + k_{34}) + k_{14}k_{21}k_{43}$
$\quad + k_{12}(k_{14}(k_{31} + k_{43}) + k_{31}(k_{34} + k_{43}))$

$\phi_9(\boldsymbol{\theta}) = k_{14}k_{21} + k_{14}k_{31} + k_{21}k_{34} + k_{31}k_{34} + k_{03}(k_{12} + k_{14}$
$+ k_{21} + k_{34}) + k_{14}k_{43} + k_{21}k_{43} + k_{31}k_{43}$
$+ k_{12}(k_{14} + k_{31} + k_{34} + k_{43}).$
(18)

The coefficients $\mathbf{\Phi}(\boldsymbol{\theta})$ are unique with respect to the input-output relationship represented by the transfer function. Introducing an alternative parameter vector, $\bar{\boldsymbol{\theta}} = (\bar{k}_{21}, \bar{k}_{31}, \bar{k}_{12}, \bar{k}_{14}, \bar{k}_{03}, \bar{k}_{43}, \bar{k}_{34})^T$, and equating $\mathbf{\Phi}(\boldsymbol{\theta}) = \mathbf{\Phi}(\bar{\boldsymbol{\theta}})$, the resulting set of simultaneous equations is solved for $\boldsymbol{\theta}$ using the Solve function in Mathematica (27). The only solution is $\boldsymbol{\theta} = \bar{\boldsymbol{\theta}}$; therefore all of the parameters in $\boldsymbol{\theta}$ are structurally uniquely identifiable.

3.1.2. Parameter Estimation

The parameter vector $\boldsymbol{\theta} = (k_{21}, k_{31}, k_{12}, k_{14}, k_{03}, k_{43}, k_{34})^T$ was estimated for each subject using unweighted least squares, by fitting the timecourse data described in section 2.2. The "true" parameter vector for an individual is denoted by $\boldsymbol{\theta}_0$. For an individual subject it is assumed that $y_i(t, \boldsymbol{\theta}_0), i = 1, 2$, is observed with error at measurement times $t_1^{(i)}, \ldots, t_{N_i}^{(i)}, i = 1, 2$, where $t_1^{(1)} = t_1^{(2)} = 0$. The observed (with error) values of $y_i(t, \boldsymbol{\theta}_0), i = 1, 2$, are now denoted by $\tilde{y}_i(t_j^{(i)}, \boldsymbol{\theta}_0)$ for $i = 1, 2$ and $j = 1, \ldots, N_i$. Both outputs y_1 and y_2 were fitted simultaneously, therefore the cost functional for $\boldsymbol{\theta}$ is given by

$$J(\boldsymbol{\theta}_0, \boldsymbol{\theta}) = \sum_{i=1}^{2} J_i(\boldsymbol{\theta}_0, \boldsymbol{\theta}),$$
(19)

TABLE 2 | Settings for differential evolution.

	Subject					
	A	**B**	**C**	**D**	**E**	**F**
Scaling factor (SF)	0.5	0.5	0.7	0.5	0.5	0.7
Crossover probability (CR)	0.9	0.9	0.95	0.9	0.9	0.95

where

$$J_i(\boldsymbol{\theta}_0, \boldsymbol{\theta}) = \sum_{j=1}^{N_i} \left(\tilde{y}_i(t_j^{(i)}, \boldsymbol{\theta}_0) - y_i(t_j^{(i)}, \boldsymbol{\theta})\right)^2.$$
(20)

Differential evolution was implemented using the NonlinearModelFit function in Mathematica (27). The differential evolution algorithm was chosen because there is little information available about the parameters, in particular the parameters k_{14}, k_{03}, k_{43}, and k_{34}. Differential evolution is a stochastic, global minimization algorithm that does not require the user to specify initial guesses for the parameter values (29). All parameters were constrained to be positive. The maximum number of iterations was set to 5,000, which was sufficient for the algorithm to converge in all cases. In differential evolution an initial population of parameter vectors is generated randomly. The algorithm was run for each subject's data with integer seeds for the pseudorandom number generator between 1 and 10; thus 10 estimates for $\boldsymbol{\theta}$ were obtained for each subject.

Differential evolution maintains a population of parameter vectors which evolves iteratively. For each new generation of the algorithm, a mutant and trial vector are produced from the current generation and the trial vector is compared with a target vector from the current generation. Either the target or trial vector is selected to move forward to the new generation based on which has the smallest value of the cost function to be minimized. The scaling factor (SF) is used to produce the mutant vector and generally a larger value of SF means a broader search of the parameter space. The crossover probability (CR) is the probability that each element of the mutant vector is used to produce the trial vector, rather than the corresponding element of the target vector. SF and CR were tuned by trial and error for each subject. The settings $F = 0.5$ and $CR = 0.9$ were tried initially, as recommended by Storn and Price (29) for faster convergence. For subjects C and F the settings were adjusted to $F = 0.7$, for a broader search of the parameter space, and $CR = 0.95$, to speed convergence. The settings for the differential evolution algorithm are given in **Table 2**.

Each run of the algorithm, with a unique seed for the pseudorandom number generator, can produce unique parameter estimates; it is therefore recommended to perform multiple runs with unique, randomly chosen starting populations of parameter vectors (29). The parameter estimates and root mean square error (RMSE) for each run and each subject are tabulated in **Table 3**. The parameter estimates from multiple runs should be close to one another so that they can be averaged (29, 30); however, in some cases, the different runs give very different parameter estimates, implying that the algorithm has

TABLE 3 | Parameter values estimated from timecourse data.

	Run	Parameter (all have units day^{-1})							RMSE
		k_{21}	k_{31}	k_{12}	k_{14}	k_{03}	k_{43}	k_{34}	
Subject A	1	0.391	0.158	1.29	0.0628	0.261	1.88	0.206	0.0124
	2	0.391	0.159	1.29	0.0623	0.294	2.23	0.216	0.0124
	3	0.390	0.159	1.29	0.0616	0.341	2.70	0.225	0.0124
	4	0.390	0.159	1.29	0.0612	0.363	2.91	0.227	0.0124
	5	0.388	0.139	1.11	0.0699	0.0881	0.209	0.0279	0.0123
	6	0.391	0.160	1.30	0.0611	0.395	3.25	0.233	0.0124
	7	0.392	0.160	1.30	0.0616	0.365	2.95	0.229	0.0124
	8	0.386	0.159	1.27	0.0615	0.327	2.54	0.221	0.0124
	9	0.391	0.159	1.29	0.0617	0.336	2.64	0.224	0.0124
	10	0.390	0.159	1.29	0.0619	0.307	2.35	0.218	0.0124
Subject B	1	1.72	0.174	2.96	0.151	1.04	1.23	$1.09 \cdot 10^{-16}$	0.00858
	2	0.101	0.732	0.147	3.18	0.208	1.72	0.00	0.00859
	3	0.0986	1.09	0.146	2.49	0.408	20.2	7.16	0.00865
	4	1.73	0.174	2.98	0.151	1.04	1.23	0.00	0.00858
	5	1.72	0.174	2.96	0.151	1.04	1.23	0.00	0.00858
	6	1.72	0.174	2.96	0.151	1.04	1.23	0.00	0.00858
	7	1.72	0.174	2.96	0.151	1.04	1.23	0.00	0.00858
	8	1.72	0.174	2.96	0.151	1.04	1.23	$3.69 \cdot 10^{-15}$	0.00858
	9	0.101	0.732	0.147	3.18	0.208	1.72	0.00	0.00859
	10	1.72	0.174	2.96	0.151	1.04	1.23	0.00	0.00858
Subject C	1	0.0217	0.438	$6.47 \cdot 10^{-16}$	0.527	0.580	2.10	0.332	0.00682
	2	0.346	0.160	0.537	0.00	1.3126	0.447	0.0880	0.00553
	3	0.0217	0.438	$9.75 \cdot 10^{-15}$	0.527	0.580	2.10	0.332	0.00682
	4	1100	0.349	8590	0.2537	0.765	1.72	0.141	0.00780
	5	0.346	0.160	0.537	$2.81 \cdot 10^{-16}$	1.31	0.447	0.0880	0.00553
	6	203	0.349	1580	0.254	0.764	1.72	0.141	0.00780
	7	0.0217	0.438	$1.51 \cdot 10^{-16}$	0.527	0.580	2.10	0.332	0.00682
	8	0.0217	0.438	$4.65 \cdot 10^{-15}$	0.527	0.580	2.10	0.332	0.00682
	9	284	0.349	2210	0.254	0.765	1.73	0.141	0.00780
	10	0.0217	0.438	$2.75 \cdot 10^{-15}$	0.527	0.580	2.10	0.332	0.00682
Subject D	1	0.346	0.154	0.432	$2.73 \cdot 10^{7}$	20.3	80.2	0.0550	0.0136
	2	0.346	1.50	0.432	$1.45 \cdot 10^{9}$	15.3	725	68.7	0.0136
	3	0.346	0.159	0.432	$4.85 \cdot 10^{16}$	9.08	37.3	94600	0.0137
	4	0.346	0.173	0.432	$1.99 \cdot 10^{7}$	11.5	52.4	1180	0.0137
	5	0.346	0.102	0.432	$2.12 \cdot 10^{17}$	22.2	50.7	0.00	0.0136
	6	0.344	1.95	0.433	$1.16 \cdot 10^{7}$	3.90	240	208	0.0136
	7	0.346	0.0999	0.432	$1.22 \cdot 10^{6}$	15.4	34.1	3.07	0.0137
	8	0.346	0.951	0.432	$2.16 \cdot 10^{11}$	12.8	379	1710	0.0136
	9	0.134	0.242	0.429	0.435	5.49	37.1	0.00	0.0137
	10	0.347	0.142	0.432	$4.14 \cdot 10^{8}$	163	581	0.00	0.0136
Subject E	1	0.412	0.117	0.361	0.273	0.995	1.02	0.326	0.00550
	2	$1.40 \cdot 10^{-6}$	0.445	142	0.452	0.148	0.693	0.00603	0.00379
	3	$2.20 \cdot 10^{-13}$	0.445	8.71	0.452	0.148	0.692	0.00601	0.00379
	4	0.454	0.0795	0.362	$7.12 \cdot 10^{-8}$	4.51	5.30	1.12	0.00550
	5	0.454	0.0795	0.362	$2.97 \cdot 10^{-12}$	5.40	6.76	1.14	0.00550
	6	0.454	0.0795	0.362	0.0000227	3.41	3.52	1.04	0.00550

(Continued)

TABLE 3 | Continued

	Run	Parameter (all have units day^{-1})							RMSE
		k_{21}	k_{31}	k_{12}	k_{14}	k_{03}	k_{43}	k_{34}	
	7	0.00	0.454	$6.91 \cdot 10^7$	0.419	0.175	0.948	0.0586	0.00402
	8	0.454	0.0795	0.362	0.00	4.11	4.66	1.09	0.00550
	9	0.454	0.0795	0.362	0.0000416	3.21	3.20	1.02	0.00550
	10	0.454	0.0795	0.362	$5.41 \cdot 10^{-7}$	51.2	84.0	1.30	0.00550
Subject F	1	0.456	4.22	0.372	19.3	0.956	$1.45 \cdot 10^7$	$5.37 \cdot 10^6$	0.00686
	2	$1.23 \cdot 10^{10}$	0.532	$4.29 \cdot 10^{10}$	0.360	1690	15300	0.214	0.00286
	3	0.456	4.21	0.372	14.6	6.23	$1.21 \cdot 10^8$	$5.22 \cdot 10^6$	0.00686
	4	0.456	4.21	0.372	17.1	1.47	$1.70 \cdot 10^7$	$3.64 \cdot 10^6$	0.00686
	5	0.456	4.21	0.372	15.4	2.87	$1.40 \cdot 10^8$	$1.39 \cdot 10^7$	0.00686
	6	0.456	4.21	0.372	17.6	1.28	$1.54 \cdot 10^7$	$3.88 \cdot 10^6$	0.00686
	7	0.456	4.16	0.372	48.0	0.364	185	407	0.00687
	8	0.456	4.22	0.372	16.1	2.02	$1.42 \cdot 10^7$	$1.42 \cdot 10^7$	0.00686
	9	$4.97 \cdot 10^8$	0.531	$1.73 \cdot 10^9$	0.360	33600	304000	0.214	0.00286
	10	0.456	4.21	0.372	15.7	2.51	$1.44 \cdot 10^8$	$1.65 \cdot 10^7$	0.00686

difficulty finding the global minimum and that there may be many local minima. It is therefore not certain that the global minimum has been found for each subject. It is also possible that certain parameters are highly correlated, such that different parameter vectors produce very similar model outputs. This is reflected in the diversity of parameter vectors obtained within subjects using differential evolution.

In some cases the model parameters are estimated to be zero, or very close to zero, for example k_{34} for subject B, k_{12} and k_{14} for subject C, k_{34} for subject D, and k_{21} and k_{14} for subject E. For each of these subjects the data can be well represented by a reduced model in which either IgG-FcRn binding is irreversible ($k_{34} = 0$), there is no transfer from the peripheral compartment to plasma ($k_{12} = 0$) or vice versa ($k_{21} = 0$), or bound IgG molecules are not recycled into plasma ($k_{14} = 0$). This result suggests that the model complexity is not supported by the available data.

The data and the model outputs using the parameter estimates in **Table 3** are plotted in **Figure 5**. In each panel of **Figure 5**, the model outputs $y_1(t)$ and $y_2(t)$ are plotted for each of the estimated parameter vectors from 10 runs. The model outputs are very similar for all of the estimated parameter vectors for an individual. For some subjects there are small but noticeable differences between the fits, for example: in the first and last 5 days of $y_2(t)$ for subject A; in the first 2 days of $y_1(t)$ for subject B; for all of $y_1(t)$ and the latter part of $y_2(t)$ for subject C; between days 2 and 6 for $y_1(t)$ and the initial 2 days of $y_2(t)$ for subject E; and the first 10 days and final 5 days of $y_2(t)$ for subject F. The similarity between the outputs for the parameter estimates obtained across different runs is shown by the similar values of RMSE within each subject. The model appears to fit the data reasonably well and in some subjects extremely well.

The results of the multiple runs of differential evolution show that in many cases, highly different parameter vectors produce very similar model outputs. The spread of the parameter estimates from multiple runs is conveyed using the coefficient of variation (CV), that is, the standard deviation of the estimates

of a parameter from 10 runs, divided by the mean of those estimates. The CV is tabulated in **Table 4**. For some parameters and subjects, the estimates for the parameters have a small CV, for example the first four parameters for subject A and parameter k_{12} for subject D. In other instances however the CV is much larger, reflecting the highly different estimates obtained for these parameters. The similarly high quality fits produced by diverse parameter vectors implies that, whilst the parameters are structurally identifiable, they are not all *practically* identifiable for the quality of data that are available.

3.2. Parameter Identification Using Fractional Catabolic Rate Data

Authors who have studied a two-compartment model of IgG metabolism have previously estimated parameters from FCR vs. plasma IgG concentration data (16, 21). In this section we investigate whether it is possible to estimate parameters of the four-compartment model from these data, which are described in section 2.2. In section 2.6 two expressions for the FCR were introduced: the FCR of the tracer (Equation 11) and the FCR of the endogenous IgG in steady state (Equation 14). In practice FCR_T is measured; however it is difficult to obtain a closed form expression for FCR_T. In contrast, we can easily obtain an expression for FCR_E in terms of the model parameters and the quantity of endogenous IgG in plasma, $x_{1,E}$, as given by Equation (14). In this section model parameters are estimated by fitting the expression for FCR_E vs. $x_{1,E}$ Equation (14) to the FCR_T vs. $x_{1,E}$ data. It is assumed that FCR_E is a good approximation to FCR_T and the parameter estimates are validated in section 3.2.3 using synthetic data.

3.2.1. Structural Identifiability Analysis

The relationship between FCR_E and $x_{1,E}$ is given by Equation (14). Given that the parameters k_{on} and v_3 only appear in the model (Equations 3) as the ratio k_{on}/v_3, we re-write Equation (14), defining $\phi_1 = k_{on}/v_3$, giving

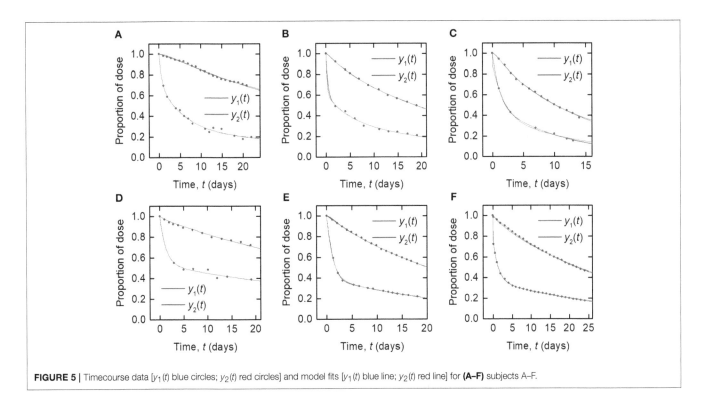

FIGURE 5 | Timecourse data [$y_1(t)$ blue circles; $y_2(t)$ red circles] and model fits [$y_1(t)$ blue line; $y_2(t)$ red line] for **(A–F)** subjects A–F.

$$\mathrm{FCR_E} = \frac{1}{2\phi_1 x_{1,\mathrm{E}}}\left(k_{31}\phi_1 x_{1,\mathrm{E}} - k_{14}\phi_1 R_{\mathrm{tot}} - k_{03}k_{14} - k_{03}k_{\mathrm{off}} \right.$$
$$\left. + \sqrt{4k_{03}k_{31}\left(k_{14}+k_{\mathrm{off}}\right)\phi_1 x_{1,\mathrm{E}} + \left(-k_{31}\phi_1 x_{1,\mathrm{E}} + k_{14}\phi_1 R_{\mathrm{tot}} + k_{03}\left(k_{14}+k_{\mathrm{off}}\right)\right)^2}\right). \tag{21}$$

We wish to know whether the parameter vector $\phi = \left(\phi_1, k_{31}, k_{14}, R_{\mathrm{tot}}, k_{03}, k_{\mathrm{off}}\right)^{\mathrm{T}}$ is structurally identifiable with respect to the relationship in Equation (21). The structural identifiability problem amounts to determining whether there exists an alternative parameter vector $\bar{\phi} = \left(\bar{\phi}_1, \bar{k}_{31}, \bar{k}_{14}, \bar{R}_{\mathrm{tot}}, \bar{k}_{03}, \bar{k}_{\mathrm{off}}\right)^{\mathrm{T}}$ such that $\mathrm{FCR_E}(x_{1,\mathrm{E}}, \phi) = \mathrm{FCR_E}(x_{1,\mathrm{E}}, \bar{\phi})$.

From Equations (13) and (2),

$$\mathrm{FCR_E} = \frac{I_0}{\hat{x}_1}. \tag{22}$$

I_0 is given in terms of $\hat{x}_1$ by the solution of the following quadratic equation, obtained by rearranging the first equation of Equations (2) and setting $\phi_1 = k_{\mathrm{on}}/v_3$:

$$-\phi_1 I_0^2 + \left(-k_{03}\left(k_{14}+k_{\mathrm{off}}\right) + \phi_1\left(k_{31}\hat{x}_1 - k_{14}R_{\mathrm{tot}}\right)\right) I_0$$
$$+k_{03}k_{31}\left(k_{14}+k_{\mathrm{off}}\right)\hat{x}_1 = 0. \tag{23}$$

Substituting $\mathrm{FCR_E}\hat{x}_1$ in place of I_0 and setting $\hat{x}_1 = x_{1,\mathrm{E}}$ gives the following quadratic equation in $\mathrm{FCR_E}$:

$$-\phi_1 x_{1,\mathrm{E}}^2 \mathrm{FCR_E^2} + \left(-k_{03}\left(k_{14}+k_{\mathrm{off}}\right) + \phi_1\left(k_{31}x_{1,\mathrm{E}} - k_{14}R_{\mathrm{tot}}\right)\right)$$
$$x_{1,\mathrm{E}}\mathrm{FCR_E} + k_{03}k_{31}\left(k_{14}+k_{\mathrm{off}}\right)x_{1,\mathrm{E}} = 0. \tag{24}$$

Dividing Equation (24) throughout by the coefficient of $\mathrm{FCR_E^2}$ gives

$$\mathrm{FCR_E^2} + \left(\frac{k_{03}\left(k_{14}+k_{\mathrm{off}}\right) - k_{31}\phi_1 x_{1,\mathrm{E}} + k_{14}\phi_1 R_{\mathrm{tot}}}{\phi_1 x_{1,\mathrm{E}}}\right)\mathrm{FCR_E}$$
$$-\frac{k_{03}k_{31}\left(k_{14}+k_{\mathrm{off}}\right)}{\phi_1 x_{1,\mathrm{E}}} = 0. \tag{25}$$

The expression for $\mathrm{FCR_E}$ given by Equation (21) is one of the two solutions of Equation (25). We therefore wish to know whether there exists an alternative parameter vector $\bar{\phi}$ such that,

$$\mathrm{FCR_E^2} + \left(\frac{k_{03}\left(k_{14}+k_{\mathrm{off}}\right) - k_{31}\phi_1 x_{1,\mathrm{E}} + k_{14}\phi_1 R_{\mathrm{tot}}}{\phi_1 x_{1,\mathrm{E}}}\right)\mathrm{FCR_E}$$
$$-\frac{k_{03}k_{31}\left(k_{14}+k_{\mathrm{off}}\right)}{\phi_1 x_{1,\mathrm{E}}}$$
$$= \mathrm{FCR_E^2} + \left(\frac{\bar{k}_{03}\left(\bar{k}_{14}+\bar{k}_{\mathrm{off}}\right) - \bar{k}_{31}\bar{\phi}_1 x_{1,\mathrm{E}} + \bar{k}_{14}\bar{\phi}_1 \bar{R}_{\mathrm{tot}}}{\bar{\phi}_1 x_{1,\mathrm{E}}}\right)$$
$$\mathrm{FCR_E} - \frac{\bar{k}_{03}\bar{k}_{31}\left(\bar{k}_{14}+\bar{k}_{\mathrm{off}}\right)}{\bar{\phi}_1 x_{1,\mathrm{E}}}. \tag{26}$$

TABLE 4 | Coefficients of variation of parameter estimates obtained from 10 runs of differential evolution, for each of subjects A–F.

Parameter	Coefficient of variation					
	A	**B**	**C**	**D**	**E**	**F**
k_{21}	0.00404	0.634	2.18	0.206	0.691	3.03
k_{31}	0.0405	0.905	0.312	1.24	0.907	0.446
k_{12}	0.0458	0.642	2.18	0.00277	3.16	3.03
k_{14}	0.0417	1.38	0.643	2.58	1.33	0.792
k_{03}	0.280	0.461	0.373	1.71	2.12	3.00
k_{43}	0.360	1.85	0.399	1.15	2.32	1.14
k_{34}	0.305	3.16	0.502	3.05	0.758	1.01

From the uniqueness of interpolating polynomials (31, p. 98), the coefficients of the quadratic in Equation (25) are unique, therefore the problem amounts to solving the simultaneous equations:

$$\frac{k_{03}\left(k_{14}+k_{\text{off}}\right)-k_{31}\phi_1 x_{1,\text{E}}+k_{14}\phi_1 R_{\text{tot}}}{\phi_1 x_{1,\text{E}}}$$
$$=\frac{\bar{k}_{03}\left(\bar{k}_{14}+\bar{k}_{\text{off}}\right)-\bar{k}_{31}\bar{\phi}_1 x_{1,\text{E}}+\bar{k}_{14}\bar{\phi}_1 \bar{R}_{\text{tot}}}{\bar{\phi}_1 x_{1,\text{E}}} \quad (27)$$
$$-\frac{k_{03}k_{31}\left(k_{14}+k_{\text{off}}\right)}{\phi_1 x_{1,\text{E}}}=-\frac{\bar{k}_{03}\bar{k}_{31}\left(\bar{k}_{14}+\bar{k}_{\text{off}}\right)}{\bar{\phi}_1 x_{1,\text{E}}}.$$

The solution was found using the SolveAlways function in Mathematica. The only solution to Equations (27), for all values of $x_{1,\text{E}}$, is given by

$$\bar{k}_{31}=k_{31}$$
$$\bar{k}_{14}\bar{R}_{\text{tot}}=k_{14}R_{\text{tot}}$$
$$\frac{\bar{k}_{03}\left(\bar{k}_{14}+\bar{k}_{\text{off}}\right)}{\bar{\phi}_1}=\frac{k_{03}\left(k_{14}+k_{\text{off}}\right)}{\phi_1}. \quad (28)$$

Therefore, only k_{31} and the expressions $k_{14}R_{\text{tot}}$ and $k_{03}\left(k_{14}+k_{\text{off}}\right)/\phi_1$, containing original parameter combinations, are structurally identifiable with respect to the relationship between FCR_{E} and $x_{1,\text{E}}$.

3.2.2. Parameter Estimation
Having analyzed the structural identifiability of the expression for FCR_{E} vs. $x_{1,\text{E}}$, it becomes clear that we can rewrite the expression in Equation (14) by combining parameters into new structurally identifiable parameters, as follows:

$$\text{FCR}_{\text{E}}(x_{1,\text{E}},\boldsymbol{\psi})=\frac{1}{2x_{1,\text{E}}}\left(k_{31}x_{1,\text{E}}-\psi_1-\psi_2\right. \quad (29)$$
$$\left.+\sqrt{k_{31}^2 x_{1,\text{E}}^2+2k_{31}x_{1,\text{E}}\left(\psi_1-\psi_2\right)+\left(\psi_1+\psi_2\right)^2}\right),$$

TABLE 5 | Parameter estimates from fitting FCR_{E} expression to FCR_{T} vs. $x_{1,\text{E}}$ data.

Parameter	Units	Estimate	Standard error	95% confidence interval
ψ_1	μmol day^{-1}	7.47	2.74	(1.93, 13.0)
ψ_2	μmol day^{-1}	25.7	6.656	(12.3, 39.2)
k_{31}	day^{-1}	0.154	0.00969	(0.135, 0.174)

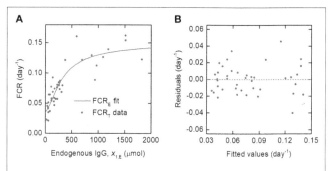

FIGURE 6 | (A) Expression for FCR_{E} vs. $x_{1,\text{E}}$, given by Equation (29), fitted to FCR_{T} vs. $x_{1,\text{E}}$ data from Waldmann and Strober (21). **(B)** Residuals vs. fitted values.

where

$$\psi_1=\frac{k_{03}v_3\left(k_{14}+k_{\text{off}}\right)}{k_{\text{on}}} \quad (30)$$
$$\psi_2=k_{14}R_{\text{tot}}$$

are uniquely identifiable parameters. ψ_1 and ψ_2 have units of μmol day^{-1}. The parameter vector to be estimated is now $\boldsymbol{\psi}=\left(k_{31},\psi_1,\psi_2\right)$.

It is assumed that Equation (29) is a close approximation to the relationship between the measured FCR_{T} and $x_{1,\text{E}}$. Waldmann and Strober (21) provide FCR_{T} vs. plasma IgG concentration data. The plasma concentrations of endogenous IgG were multiplied by the average plasma volume v_1, from **Table 1**, in order to obtain the quantity of endogenous IgG in plasma, $x_{1,\text{E}}$. The data for FCR_{T} vs. $x_{1,\text{E}}$ were then fitted using the interior point algorithm implemented within the NonlinearModelFit function in Mathematica. The starting value for the minimization was set to 1 for each parameter. The parameter estimates were constrained to be positive.

Since the data were obtained from 41 individuals, the estimated parameter values are assumed to represent the average parameter values within the population. The parameter estimates and their standard errors are provided in **Table 5**. The fitted expression given by Equation (29) is plotted alongside the data in **Figure 6A**. The residuals vs. the fitted values are plotted in **Figure 6B**. On inspection, the model appears to fit the data well. The residuals appear reasonably homoscedastic and there is no obvious autocorrelation.

3.2.3. Validation of Parameter Estimates
There are several issues that may cause the estimates of k_{31}, ψ_1, and ψ_2 to be inaccurate. Firstly, the data were obtained from a

sample of 41 individuals, each with their own unique parameter vector; this variability is not accounted for by the estimation procedure. Secondly, the parameters were estimated by fitting the expression for FCR_E vs. $x_{1,E}$; however the data are for the FCR_T, which is not equivalent to the FCR_E. In addition, the FCR_T is in practice calculated from measurements of radioactivity in plasma and urine; the form of the measurement errors is therefore not clear.

Due to the aforementioned issues, the validity of the parameter estimates obtained in section 3.2.2 was investigated by estimating the parameters from synthetic data. It is assumed that the parameter values in **Table 5** are true population parameter values. Data for FCR_T vs. $x_{1,E}$ were simulated according to the experimental methodology, described by Waldmann and Strober (21). The data were simulated for 100 sets of 41 subjects. The parameter values were then estimated from the synthetic data, generating 100 estimates for $\psi = (k_{31}, \psi_1, \psi_2)$.

In order to simulate the FCR_T data, parameter values are required for all model parameters (see Equations 1), not just k_{31}, ψ_1, and ψ_2. Population parameter values are therefore required for all model parameters in order to randomly generate unique parameter vectors for individual subjects. The population parameter values for k_{21}, k_{12}, k_{14}, k_{03}, and k_{off} were fixed to the values from the literature in **Table 1**. The population value of k_{31} was fixed to the estimated value in **Table 5**. The population values of R_{tot} and k_{on}/v_3 were calculated by substituting the previously fixed parameter values into Equations (30) and solving. In this way, a population parameter vector was found, for which k_{31}, ψ_1, and ψ_2 are equal to their estimated values. Unique parameter values for 41 individuals were randomly generated from a lognormal distribution, with the median given by the population parameter values. The variance was tuned by trial and error in order to replicate the size of the errors seen in the real data. This process was repeated to produce 100 sets of 41 individual parameter vectors and thus 100 sets of FCR_T vs. $x_{1,E}$ data. Full details of how the synthetic data were generated are provided in the Mathematica code in the **Supplementary Material**.

The parameter estimates as a proportion of the true parameter values are plotted in **Figure 7**, showing the spread of the parameter estimates. It is clear from this plot that the parameter k_{31} is estimated with higher precision than ψ_1 and ψ_2. The sample mean (μ), sample standard deviation (s.d.), bias (b), and variability (v) of the parameter estimates are given in **Table 6**. The bias is given by

$$b = \mu - p, \tag{31}$$

where p is the true value of the parameter. The variability is given by

$$v = \frac{\sqrt{\text{s.d.}^2 + b^2}}{p}. \tag{32}$$

Variability as defined by Equation (32) has been used by Chen et al. (32) to evaluate the performance of estimation methods when the assumptions relied upon by the methods, in particular relating to noise, are violated. A larger value of v represents a worse performance of an estimation method. The results suggest

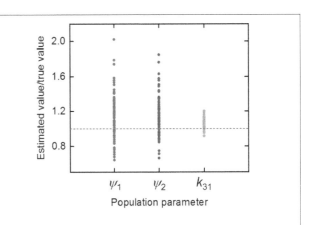

FIGURE 7 | Parameter estimates for k_{31}, ψ_1, and ψ_2 divided by the true parameter value.

TABLE 6 | Mean, standard deviation, bias, and variability of the estimates of k_{31}, ψ_1, and ψ_2.

	Parameter		
	k_{31}	ψ_1	ψ_2
Mean	0.162	8.55	29.0
Standard deviation	0.00758	1.75	5.24
Bias	0.00841	1.08	3.31
Variability	0.0735	0.275	0.241

that k_{31} has been estimated with a good level of accuracy ($v = 0.0735$), but that the parameters ψ_1 and ψ_2 were estimated with a higher level of variability. Based on this result, a future study may look at improving experimental design, for example by increasing the number of subjects, in order to improve upon the variability of the estimates of ψ_1 and ψ_2.

3.3. Simulation of IgG Responses in Multiple Myeloma

It has been shown that parameter estimates obtained using timecourse data are not robust; however, the parameters k_{31}, ψ_1, and ψ_2 may be obtained with reasonably low variability using FCR data. The results from fitting the timecourse data suggest that the model (Equations 1) may be overparameterized with respect to the available data; we therefore ask whether the plasma IgG response can be sufficiently determined using only the parameters k_{21}, k_{12}, k_{31}, ψ_1, and ψ_2.

Firstly we investigate the plasma IgG response given by the full system model (Equations 1), when the parameters k_{31}, ψ_1, and ψ_2 are equal to the values estimated in section 3.2.2. Random values were generated for certain model parameters and the remaining parameter values calculated so that k_{31}, ψ_1, and ψ_2 are equal to their estimated values. Three parameters (not including both R_{tot} and k_{14}) out of k_{03}, R_{tot}, k_{off}, k_{14}, and k_{on}/v_3 were fixed to randomly generated values and substituted into Equations (30), yielding a linear system of two equations in two unknowns. Equations (30) were then solved for the remaining two parameters. There are seven sets of three parameters from

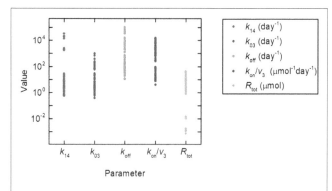

FIGURE 8 | Parameter values used to simulate IgG responses in multiple myeloma, plotted on a logarithmic scale. The method used to generate the parameter values is described in section 3.3. The model predictions generated using these parameter values are shown in **Figure 9A**. Despite the large amount of variation in the parameter values, the model predictions for plasma IgG are extremely similar.

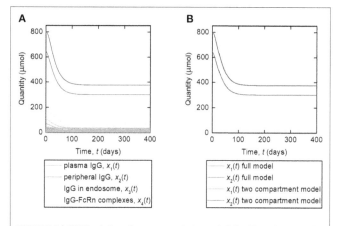

FIGURE 9 | **(A)** Simulation of responses of plasma IgG [$(x_1(t)$], peripheral IgG [$x_2(t)$], IgG in endosomes [$x_3(t)$], and IgG bound to FcRn in endosomes [$x_4(t)$]. The scenario shown represents a decreasing tumor burden during therapy. Each variable is simulated for 70 unique parameter vectors. **(B)** Simulation of responses of plasma IgG [$x_1(t)$], peripheral IgG [$x_2(t)$], compared for the four-compartment model and the proposed two compartment model. The responses are indistinguishable by inspection for the two models.

k_{03}, R_{tot}, k_{off}, k_{14}, and k_{on}/v_3, which can be fixed to give the remaining two parameters. Parameters were generated 10 times, as described, for each of these seven sets, giving 70 parameter vectors in total. The randomly generated parameter values were obtained by assuming a lognormal distribution, in order to ensure positivity, with median set to the parameter value from the literature, given in **Table 1**, and variance 1. The values generated in this way for the parameters k_{03}, R_{tot}, k_{off}, k_{14}, and k_{on}/v_3 are depicted in **Figure 8**, showing the extremely wide range of parameter values used. The parameter k_{31} was set to the estimated value given in **Table 5**. The values for k_{21} and k_{12} were set to the values given in **Table 1**.

In order to simulate the model under realistic clinical conditions, a model for the IgG synthesis rate in multiple myeloma was used, which has been found to predict responses consistent with real patient data (33). The IgG synthesis rate is described by

$$I(t) = (I_0 - I_\infty) \exp(-k_{kill}t) + I_\infty. \tag{33}$$

The following parameter values were used to produce the simulation: $I_0 = 76$ μmol day^{-1}, $I_\infty = 26.5$ μmol day^{-1}, and $k_{kill} = 0.055$ day^{-1} (33).

A simulation of the responses in all four model compartments is shown in **Figure 9A**. Each variable is simulated for 70 unique parameter vectors. The predicted trajectories for plasma IgG and peripheral IgG, respectively, are extremely similar for all 70 parameter vectors; however there is some variation in the responses of IgG in intracellular endosomes, particularly the IgG that is not bound to FcRn receptors. The simulation suggests that, under the investigated conditions, the response in the plasma compartment is relatively insensitive to changes in the individual parameters k_{03}, R_{tot}, k_{off}, k_{14}, and k_{on}/v_3, provided that the parameters k_{31}, ψ_1, and ψ_2 are fixed. The maximal difference between any two trajectories for $x_1(t)$ at any simulated time point is 0.2%.

The lack of variation within the predicted responses for plasma and peripheral IgG, when parameters k_{21}, k_{12}, k_{31}, ψ_1,

and ψ_2 are fixed, suggests that it may be possible to simulate these two variables using a reduced order model based upon the newly derived expression for the FCR (Equation 29). The equations for this model are given by

$$\dot{x}_1(t) = -\left(k_{21} + f(x_1(t))\right)x_1(t) + k_{12}x_2(t) + k_{14}x_4(t) + I(t)$$
$$\dot{x}_2(t) = k_{21}x_1(t) - k_{12}x_2(t), \tag{34}$$

where

$$f(x_1(t)) = \frac{1}{2x_1(t)}\left(k_{31}x_1(t) - \psi_1 - \psi_2 \tag{35}\right.$$
$$\left. + \sqrt{k_{31}^2 x_1(t)^2 + 2k_{31}x_1(t)(\psi_1 - \psi_2) + (\psi_1 + \psi_2)^2}\right).$$

The assumption behind this model is that the fractional rate of IgG catabolism is equal to its fractional rate of catabolism at steady state. A simulation of this model, alongside the original four-compartment model, is shown in **Figure 9B**. The model is simulated with values of k_{21} and k_{12} from **Table 1** and all other parameter values from **Table 5**. The responses for $x_1(t)$ and $x_2(t)$ are very similar for the two models and appear overlayed in **Figure 9B**. The maximal difference between $x_1(t)$ predicted by the two-compartment model and $x_1(t)$ predicted by the four-compartment model, for any of the 70 parameter vectors used and at any simulated time point, is 0.2%. The responses are indistinguishable by inspection for the two models.

The proposed two-compartment model is based upon the assumption that the fractional rate of IgG catabolism is equal to its fractional rate of catabolism in steady state. When the system is in steady state, this assumption is of course true. However, faster dynamics, caused by a rapid change in the IgG synthesis rate, will cause this assumption to progressively weaken. Further study of the proposed model is required to analyse its relationship with the original four-compartment model and to determine under what conditions the proposed model predictions are within an acceptable region of the four-compartment model predictions.

4. DISCUSSION

The motivation behind the research presented in this paper was to investigate a model suitable for predicting IgG responses in patients with IgG multiple myeloma. When producing predictive simulations of a biomedical system, it is important to know the level of confidence in the model parameter values.

There are numerous published models of FcRn-mediated recycling of IgG in the literature, some of which are cited in the Introduction. Most of these models were developed for IgG-based therapeutic monoclonal antibodies and may not be suitable for characterizing endogenous IgG. Those models characterizing endogenous IgG, for example the models of Li et al. (34) and Chen and Balthasar (10), rely upon a mixture of animal and human data for sourcing parameter values.

For example, parameter values provided by Li et al. (34) for endogenous IgG were taken from the literature, apart from the catabolic clearance (corresponding to k_{03} of the present study), the vascular reflection coefficient (not included in our model), and the recycling rate constant (corresponding to k_{14} of the present study). These parameter values were obtained by manually varying the parameters within the model until the results showed a mean half-life of 21 days, a mean IgG synthesis rate of 34 mg kg^{-1} day^{-1} and a realistic fold reduction in IgG concentration when FcRn is not present. The values used for the half-life and synthesis rate are those obtained from normal human data by Waldmann and Strober (21) and Waldmann and Terry (23).

One of the problems with the approach taken in previous papers is that, whilst parameter values have been found that provide a half-life of 21 days for an IgG synthesis rate of 34 mg kg^{-1} day^{-1}, it is not clear what would happen to the half-life when the IgG synthesis rate increases or decreases, under the obtained parameter values. This approach is therefore akin to fitting a model to a curve having only one data point. The nonlinear relationship between synthesis or concentration of IgG and its half-life, which is fundamental to the FcRn-IgG recycling system, may therefore not be captured accurately using this approach.

Another issue with this earlier approach is that it requires the parameter values obtained from the literature to be fixed while the remaining values are varied, therefore implicitly assuming complete confidence in the fixed parameter values that were sourced in the literature. One would question what would happen if one or more of these parameter values were inaccurate by, say, 10% or more, what would be the effect on the corresponding values obtained for k_{14} and k_{03}?

Having considered the models available in the literature and their issues in respect of parameter identifiability, we identified the need for a semi-mechanistic model with parameter values obtained using only *in vivo* human data. This approach necessitated a simpler model than those available in the literature

and previously discussed. The model studied in this paper is therefore missing some of the mechanisms of the more complex models. However, simplified compartmental models can often be derived from complex physiologically-based models by lumping compartments and processes. Lumped models may be adequate for describing processes of interest, for example responses in a central/plasma compartment. Fronton et al. (14) demonstrate the correspondence between a physiologically-based model and several compartmental model structures for IgG. A similar study could be performed using the models presented in this paper in future work.

In this paper, two observed model outputs were considered: the timecourse of the proportion of a dose of IgG remaining in plasma and in the body of an individual subject; and the FCR vs. the quantity of endogenous IgG in plasma, measured in a cohort of subjects with a range of plasma IgG concentrations. We derived mathematical descriptions of these experimental observations based on the underlying model. Structural identifiability analysis was performed with respect to these observations in order to determine which parameters are structurally uniquely identifiable from the available outputs.

In section 3.1 we estimated parameter values using data for the timecourse of an administered dose of radiolabeled IgG in plasma and in the body. We found that all parameters of the linearized model are structurally globally identifiable. Whilst the model is capable of fitting the data well, the results of 10 runs of differential evolution suggest that the parameter estimates are not robust. Highly different parameter vectors, as illustrated by the relative standard deviations of parameter estimates from 10 runs, produce similarly excellent fits to the data. These results suggest that the available data do not support the complexity of the model. A future study may apply a systematic analysis of model sensitivity and parameter correlations, for example using the profile-likelihood method of Raue et al. (35) or generalized sensitivity functions of Thomaseth and Cobelli (36) [extended to multiple output models by Kappel and Munir (37)]. Another potential study for future work could involve estimating model parameters from synthetic timecourse data, to see whether more frequent sampling or a longer observation period provides more stable parameter estimates. However, as highly different parameter values produce similarly excellent fits to the data, the type of data needed for robust parameter estimation is likely to be of a very high quality. As the data are obtained by taking blood samples, there is a practical limitation on the sampling frequency for an individual subject.

The data used were obtained from tracer experiments that were performed between 1963 and 1990. More recent IgG timecourse data are available; however, these data pertain to therapeutic monoclonal antibodies, which can have different kinetics (38). Timecourse data are also available for patients with IgG multiple myeloma, whose serum IgG concentration is monitored during therapy. However, the production rate of IgG in these patients is determined by the status of the disease. Using these data to estimate model parameters would therefore require simultaneous estimation of IgG production parameters. This would require a more complex structural identifiability analysis and may be considered in future work. For these reasons, more recent data were not used in this study.

The structural identifiability of the relationship between FCR$_E$ and the quantity of endogenous IgG in plasma, $x_{1,E}$, was analyzed. We found that the parameter k_{31} and newly defined parameters $\psi_1 = (k_{03}v_3(k_{14}+k_{off}))/k_{on}$ and $\psi_2 = k_{14}R_{tot}$ are structurally globally identifiable. These new parameters were estimated using least squares estimation. Estimation with synthetic data shows that these parameters can be estimated with a reasonable level of variability. The parameters k_{31} and ψ_2 are physiologically meaningful: k_{31} is the rate at which plasma IgG is internalized into intracellular endosomes and ψ_2 is the maximal rate of recycling of IgG from endosomes into plasma. The 95% confidence interval for k_{31} (0.135–0.174 day^{-1}) is similar to other values reported in the literature [0.13 day^{-1} (17); 0.18 day^{-1} (21); 0.16 day^{-1} (33)]. The 95% confidence interval for ψ_2 (12.3–39.2 µmol day^{-1}) is smaller than previously reported values [68.6 µmol day^{-1} (16); 103 µmol day^{-1} (17)]; however it overlaps with the 95% confidence interval (19.1–60.9 µmol day^{-1}) reported by Kendrick et al. (33).

In applications in which the behavior of the variables $x_3(t)$ and $x_4(t)$, representing unbound and bound IgG in intracellular endosomes, respectively, are of great importance, clearly parameter values are required which determine their behavior, including receptor-ligand binding (k_{on}/v_3, k_{off}, and R_{tot}), recycling of bound IgG into plasma (k_{14}) and degradation of unbound IgG (k_{03}). The results presented in this paper suggest that it is not possible to estimate these parameters from the available data that are only based upon measurements in plasma. In section 3.3, it is shown that these parameters can be varied by several orders of magnitude (see **Figure 8**) whilst having a minimal effect on the plasma IgG response (see **Figure 9A**). It is possible that the actions of the parameters determining recycling, degradation, association and dissociation can approximately balance each other out with respect to the dynamics in the plasma compartment, even though the responses of IgG in the endosome are affected by changes in these parameter values. For investigations limited to the behavior of IgG in plasma, model reduction using the parameters k_{31}, ψ_1, and ψ_2 could be investigated in future work. A two-compartment model based upon the newly derived expression for the FCR has been proposed in section 3.3. Further analysis of this model is required to determine whether it is suitable for investigating IgG responses under a range of clinical conditions.

In future work the models studied in this paper could be used to simulate plasma IgG responses in clinical applications, such as the bone marrow cancer multiple myeloma, in which malignant plasma cells secrete large quantities of monoclonal Ig (M-protein). It has been suggested that the FcRn-IgG interaction may play a significant role in the detection of M-protein using a recently-developed mass spectrometry-based method (4). It was found that in patients with IgG-producing disease, the test result was more likely to be positive for M-protein after three months than in patients with IgA-producing disease, whereas after 12 months the patients were equally likely to have a positive test result. Mills et al. (4) have suggested that this effect is due to FcRn-mediated recycling extending the half-life of IgG, emphasizing the importance of assessment times of response. FcRn-mediated

recycling also plays a role in the pharmacokinetics of the novel monoclonal IgG agent for multiple myeloma, daratumumab. Yan et al. (5) found that the isotype of the patient's M-protein has an effect on drug exposure, with IgG patients having significantly lower daratumumab concentrations than patients with other M-protein types. Yan et al. (5) proposed that competition between the IgG M-protein and IgG-based daratumumab for FcRn receptors is the reason for this phenomenon. These recent studies show the importance of FcRn-mediated recycling of IgG in multiple myeloma and the need for mathematical modeling and simulation of this system. The model studied in this paper could be used in future work to investigate such problems.

There is a trade-off in modeling between model accuracy, which is more often represented in complex physiologically-based pharmacokinetic models, and accuracy of parameter values, which is more easily achieved with simplified compartmental models. At present, there are very few studies available on parameter estimation for models of IgG-FcRn kinetics using human data due to issues of parameter identifiability. This paper not only provides useful parameter estimates and suggests a novel model structure, but also exposes some of the difficulties in achieving this aim. Researchers pursuing physiologically-based models of IgG in the future may find it useful to compare the rate of IgG internalization into endosomes and the maximal rate of IgG recycling in their model with the values that we have estimated from human data [considering the approach of Li et al. (34) discussed above]. Furthermore, our paper shows the level of analysis (including structural identifiability analysis, estimation from synthetic data, for example) required in order to have confidence in parameter estimates obtained and an understanding of their meaning to the model.

5. CONCLUSION

It is not possible to estimate all of the model parameters robustly; however certain structurally identifiable parameter combinations have been estimated with a good level of variability. Plasma IgG responses, under typical clinical conditions, are insensitive to large changes in many of the model parameters, provided that certain parameters and parameter combinations are fixed. A reduced-order model, based upon the newly derived expression for the FCR, shows potential for simulating plasma IgG responses under clinical conditions.

AUTHOR CONTRIBUTIONS

FK performed model analyses. FK, MC, and NE wrote the manuscript. SH initiated the work. MC, NE, OB, and SH supervised the work. SH and OB provided discussion on the clinical application of the work. All authors reviewed and approved the final manuscript.

FUNDING

This research was supported by a Biotechnology and Biological Sciences Research Council (BBSRC) studentship, through the Midlands Integrative Biosciences Training Partnership (MIBTP), and an Engineering and Physical Sciences Research Council (EPSRC) Impact Acceleration Account (IAA) award.

REFERENCES

1. Hall A, Yates C, (eds.). *Immunology*. 1st ed. Oxford: Oxford University Press (2010).

2. Junghans RP, Anderson CL. The protection receptor for IgG catabolism is the $\beta 2$-microglobulin-containing neonatal intestinal transport receptor. *Proc Natl Acad Sci USA*. (1996) 93:5512–6.

3. Kumar S, Paiva B, Anderson KC, Durie B, Landgren O, Moreau P, et al. International Myeloma Working Group consensus criteria for response and minimal residual disease assessment in multiple myeloma. *Lancet Oncol*. (2016) 17:328–46. doi: 10.1016/S1470-2045(16)30206-6

4. Mills JR, Barnidge DR, Dispenzieri A, Murray DL. High sensitivity blood-based M-protein detection in sCR patients with multiple myeloma. *Blood Cancer J*. (2017) 7:1–5. doi: 10.1038/bcj.2017.75

5. Yan X, Clemens PL, Puchalski T, Lonial S, Lokhorst H, Voorhees PM, et al. Influence of disease and patient characteristics on daratumumab exposure and clinical outcomes in relapsed or refractory multiple myeloma. *Clin Pharmacokinet*. (2017) 57:529–38. doi: 10.1007/s40262-017-0598-1

6. Ferl GZ, Wu AM, DiStefano JJ. A predictive model of therapeutic monoclonal antibody dynamics and regulation by the neonatal Fc receptor (FcRn). *Ann Biomed Eng*. (2005) 33:1640–52. doi: 10.1007/s10439-005-7410-3

7. Garg A, Balthasar JP. Physiologically-based pharmacokinetic (PBPK) model to predict IgG tissue kinetics in wild-type and FcRn-knockout mice. *J Pharmacokinet Pharmacodyn*. (2007) 34:687–709. doi: 10.1007/s10928-007-9065-1

8. Fang L, Sun D. Predictive physiologically based pharmacokinetic model for antibody-directed enzyme prodrug therapy. *Drug Metab Dispos*. (2008) 36:1153–65. doi: 10.1124/dmd.107.019182

9. Urva S, Yang V, Balthasar J. Physiologically based pharmacokinetic model for T84. 66: a monoclonal anti-CEA antibody. *J Pharm Sci*. (2010) 99:1582–600. doi: 10.1002/jps.21918

10. Chen Y, Balthasar JP. Evaluation of a catenary PBPK model for predicting the *in vivo* disposition of mAbs engineered for high-affinity binding to FcRn. *AAPS J*. (2012) 14:850–9. doi: 10.1208/s12248-012-9395-9

11. Deng R, Meng YG, Hoyte K, Lutman J, Lu Y, Iyer S, et al. Subcutaneous bioavailability of therapeutic antibodies as a function of FcRn binding affinity in mice. *mAbs*. (2012) 4:101–9. doi: 10.4161/mabs.4.1.18543

12. Yan X, Chen Y, Krzyzanski W. Methods of solving rapid binding target-mediated drug disposition model for two drugs competing for the same receptor. *J Pharmacokinet Pharmacodyn*. (2012) 39:543–60. doi: 10.1007/s10928-012-9267-z

13. Ng CM, Loyet KM, Iyer S, Fielder PJ, Deng R. Modeling approach to investigate the effect of neonatal Fc receptor binding affinity and anti-therapeutic antibody on the pharmacokinetic of humanized monoclonal anti-tumor necrosis factor-α IgG antibody in cynomolgus monkey. *Eur J Pharm Sci*. (2014) 51:51–8. doi: 10.1016/j.ejps.2013.08.033

14. Fronton L, Pilari S, Huisinga W. Monoclonal antibody disposition: a simplified PBPK model and its implications for the derivation and interpretation of classical compartment models. *J Pharmacokinet Pharmacodyn*. (2014) 41:87–107. doi: 10.1007/s10928-014-9349-1

15. Xiao JJ. Pharmacokinetic models for FcRn-mediated IgG disposition. *J Biomed Biotechnol*. (2012) 2012:282989. doi: 10.1155/2012/282989

16. Kim J, Hayton WL, Robinson JM, Anderson CL. Kinetics of FcRn-mediated recycling of IgG and albumin in human: pathophysiology and therapeutic implications using a simplified mechanism-based model. *Clin Immunol*. (2007) 122:146–55. doi: 10.1016/j.clim.2006.09.001

17. Hattersley JG. *Mathematical Modelling of Immune Condition Dynamics: A Clinical Perspective*. Ph.D. thesis, University of Warwick (2009).

18. Solomon A, Waldmann T, Fahey J. Metabolism of normal 6.6 s γ-globulin in normal subjects and in patients with macroglobulinemia and multiple myeloma. *J Lab Clin Med*. (1963) 62:1–17.

19. Shah DK, Betts AM. Towards a platform PBPK model to characterize the plasma and tissue disposition of monoclonal antibodies in preclinical species and human. *J Pharmacokinet Pharmacodyn*. (2012) 39:67–86. doi: 10.1007/s10928-011-9232-2

20. Hattersley JG, Chappell MJ, Zehnder D, Higgins RM, Evans ND. Describing the effectiveness of immunosuppression drugs and apheresis in the treatment of transplant patients. *Comput Methods Programs Biomed*. (2013) 109:126–33. doi: 10.1016/j.cmpb.2011.12.013

21. Waldmann TA, Strober W. Metabolism of immunoglobulins. *Progr Allergy* (1969) 13:1–110.

22. Hansen RJ, Balthasar JP. Pharmacokinetic/pharmacodynamic modeling of the effects of intravenous immunoglobulin on the disposition of antiplatelet antibodies in a rat model of immune thrombocytopenia. *J Pharm Sci*. (2003) 92:1206–15. doi: 10.1002/jps.10364

23. Waldmann TA, Terry WD. Familial hypercatabolic hypoproteinemia. A disorder of endogenous catabolism of albumin and immunoglobulin. *J Clin Invest*. (1990) 86:2093–8. doi: 10.1172/JCI114947

24. OriginLab Corporation. *OriginPro 2016*. Northampton (2016).

25. Cobelli C, Foster D, Toffolo G. *Tracer Kinetics in Biomedical Research*. 1st ed. New York, NY: Springer (2002).

26. Anderson DH. *Compartmental Modeling and Tracer Kinetics*. 1st ed. Lecture Notes in Biomathematics. Berlin; Heidelberg: Springer-Verlag (1983).

27. Wolfram Research Inc . *Mathematica Version 11.1*. Champaign, IL (2017).

28. Bellman R, Åström KJ. On structural identifiability. *Math Biosci*. (1970) 7:329–39.

29. Storn R, Price K. Differential evolution– a simple and efficient heuristic for global optimization over continuous spaces. *J Glob Optim.*. (1997) 11:341–59.

30. Ghosh S. A differential evolution based approach for estimating minimal model parameters from IVGTT data. *Comput Biol Med*. (2014) 46:51–60. doi: 10.1016/j.compbiomed.2013.12.014

31. Biswal PC. *Numerical Analysis*. 1st ed. New Delhi: PHI Learning (2008).

32. Chen KW, Huang SC, Yu DC. The effects of measurement errors in the plasma radioactivity curve on parameter estimation in positron emission tomography. *Phys Med Biol*. (1991) 36:1183–200.

33. Kendrick F, Evans ND, Arnulf B, Avet-Loiseau H, Decaux O, Dejoie T, et al. Analysis of a compartmental model of endogenous immunoglobulin G metabolism with application to multiple myeloma. *Front Physiol*. (2017) 8:149. doi: 10.3389/fphys.2017.00149

34. Li L, Gardner I, Dostalek M, Jamei M. Simulation of monoclonal antibody pharmacokinetics in humans using a minimal physiologically based model. *AAPS J*. (2014) 16:1097–109. doi: 10.1208/s12248-014-9640-5

35. Raue A, Kreutz C, Maiwald T, Bachmann J, Schilling M, Klingmüller U, et al. Structural and practical identifiability analysis of partially observed dynamical models by exploiting the profile likelihood. *Bioinformatics.* (2009) 25:1923–9. doi: 10.1093/bioinformatics/btp358

36. Thomaseth K, Cobelli C. Generalized sensitivity functions in physiological system identification. *Ann Biomed Eng.* (1999) 27:607–16.

37. Kappel F, Munir M. Generalized sensitivity functions for multiple output systems. *J Inverse Ill-Posed Problems.* (2017) 25:499–519. doi: 10.1515/jiip-2016-0024

38. Wang W, Wang EQ, Balthasar JP. Monoclonal antibody pharmacokinetics and pharmacodynamics. *Clin Pharmacol Ther.* (2008) 84:548–58. doi: 10.1038/clpt.2008.170

39. Routh EJ. *A Treatise on the Stability of a Given State of Motion: Particularly Steady Motion.* 1st ed. London: Macmillan (1877).

14

Impact of Human FcγR Gene Polymorphisms on IgG-Triggered Cytokine Release: Critical Importance of Cell Assay Format

*Khiyam Hussain [1†], Chantal E. Hargreaves [1,2,3†], Tania F. Rowley [4], Joshua M. Sopp [1],
Kate V. Latham [3], Pallavi Bhatta [4], John Sherington [4], Rona M. Cutler [4],
David P. Humphreys [4], Martin J. Glennie [1], Jonathan C. Strefford [3] and Mark S. Cragg [1**

[1] Antibody and Vaccine Group, Centre for Cancer Immunology, Cancer Sciences, Faculty of Medicine, University of Southampton, Southampton, United Kingdom, [2] Nuffield Department of Medicine, John Radcliffe Hospital, University of Oxford, Oxford, United Kingdom, [3] Cancer Genomics Group, Southampton Experimental Cancer Medicine Centre, Cancer Sciences Unit, Faculty of Medicine, University of Southampton, Southampton, United Kingdom, [4] UCB Pharma, Slough, United Kingdom

***Correspondence:**
Mark S. Cragg
msc@soton.ac.uk

[†] These authors have contributed equally to this work

Monoclonal antibody (mAb) immunotherapy has transformed the treatment of allergy, autoimmunity, and cancer. The interaction of mAb with Fc gamma receptors (FcγR) is often critical for efficacy. The genes encoding the low-affinity FcγR have single nucleotide polymorphisms (SNPs) and copy number variation that can impact IgG Fc:FcγR interactions. Leukocyte-based *in vitro* assays remain one of the industry standards for determining mAb efficacy and predicting adverse responses in patients. Here we addressed the impact of FcγR genetics on immune cell responses in these assays and investigated the importance of assay format. FcγR genotyping of 271 healthy donors was performed using a Multiplex Ligation-Dependent Probe Amplification assay. Freeze-thawed/pre-cultured peripheral blood mononuclear cells (PBMCs) and whole blood samples from donors were stimulated with reagents spanning different mAb functional classes to evaluate the association of FcγR genotypes with T-cell proliferation and cytokine release. Using freeze-thawed/pre-cultured PBMCs, agonistic T-cell-targeting mAb induced T-cell proliferation and the highest levels of cytokine release, with lower but measurable responses from mAb which directly require FcγR-mediated cellular effects for function. Effects were consistent for individual donors over time, however, no significant associations with FcγR genotypes were observed using this assay format. In contrast, significantly elevated IFN-γ release was associated with the *FCGR2A*-131H/H genotype compared to *FCGR2A*-131R/R in whole blood stimulated with Campath ($p \leq 0.01$) and IgG1 Fc hexamer ($p \leq 0.05$). Donors homozygous for both the high affinity *FCGR2A*-131H and *FCGR3A*-158V alleles mounted stronger IFN-γ responses to Campath ($p \leq 0.05$) and IgG1 Fc Hexamer ($p \leq 0.05$) compared to donors homozygous for the low affinity alleles. Analysis revealed significant reductions in the proportion of CD14[hi] monocytes, CD56[dim] NK cells ($p \leq 0.05$) and FcγRIIIa expression ($p \leq 0.05$), in donor-matched freeze-thawed PBMC compared to whole blood samples, likely explaining the difference in association between FcγR genotype and mAb-mediated cytokine release in the different assay formats. These findings highlight the significant impact of *FCGR2A* and *FCGR3A* SNPs on mAb function and the importance of using fresh whole blood assays when evaluating their association with mAb-mediated cytokine release *in vitro*. This knowledge can better inform on the utility of *in vitro* assays for the prediction of mAb therapy outcome in patients.

Keywords: Fc gamma receptors, antibody immunotherapy, Fc gamma receptor polymorphism, cytokine release syndrome, cytokine release assays

INTRODUCTION

The advent of monoclonal antibodies (mAb) has revolutionized the treatment of malignant and autoimmune disease (1, 2). However, there is considerable variability in response to mAb therapy, as some patients may not respond to treatment whilst others experience toxic side effects, of which cytokine release syndrome (CRS) is the most detrimental to patient safety (3). CRS is characterized by rapid immune cell activation and systemic elevations of proinflammatory cytokines, in particular IFN-γ, TNF-α, and IL-6. CRS has been observed with the clinical use of several antibodies, including muromonab (anti-CD3), TGN1412 (anti-CD28), Rituximab (anti-CD20) and alemtuzumab (Campath-1H, anti-CD52) (3–6).

In the first-in-man trial of TGN1412, rapid, life-threatening CRS was observed in healthy volunteers (6). Preclinical *in vitro* testing using soluble TGN1412 to stimulate human whole blood or purified peripheral blood mononuclear cells (PBMCs) failed to predict this toxicity (7). Following these failures, there has been a concerted effort to develop predictive *in vitro* assays that enable a better understanding of mAb *in vivo* action and potential toxicity (8–10). mAb target density, immunoglobulin G (IgG) isotype, tissue microenvironment and Fc gamma receptor (FcγR) expression levels are all key to the outcome of therapy (11). Importantly, several studies have reported that *in vivo* expression levels and distribution of FcγR profoundly influence mAb effector function (12–15). Recapitulating the *in vivo* interaction of the mAb with FcγR *in vitro* is therefore of significant value.

Six FcγR are present in humans, consisting of high and low affinity receptors. The high-affinity FcγRI (CD64) is encoded by *FCGR1A* on chromosome 1q21. The low-affinity receptors, FcγRIIa, FcγRIIb, FcγRIIc, FcγRIIIa, and FcγRIIIb are encoded by genes *FCGR2A*, *FCGR2B*, *FCGR2C*, *FCGR3A*, and *FCGR3B*, respectively, in a 200 kb region on chromosome 1q23-24. These genes are subject to numerous single nucleotide polymorphisms (SNPs) and copy number variation (CNV) (16). There are four reported copy number regions (CNRs) in the low-affinity locus, each encompassing a differing combination of genes (17). Genetic variation can impact upon receptor function and associations have been made between FcγR genetic variants and disease. SNPs in *FCGR2A* (rs1801274; 131H) and *FCGR3A* (rs396991; 158V) increase receptor affinity for IgG (18) while CNV can alter the level of FcγR expressed at the cell surface available for IgG binding. SNPs altering receptor affinity have been associated with superior responses in some cohorts of cancer patients treated with mAb immunotherapy (19–24). *FCGR2A*-131R (25) and *FCGR2B*-232T (26) have been implicated in increased risk of systemic lupus erythematous, while *FCGR3B* HNA 1B and decreased copy number of *FCGR3B* have been associated with reduced immune complex clearance and increased risk of autoimmunity (25, 27).

Given the impact of FcγR SNPs and CNV on receptor function via IgG Fc:FcγR interactions on immune cells (28, 29), studies investigating treatment efficacy and side effect profile in the context of FcγR genotypes and expression levels are warranted. We hypothesized that since the *FCGR2A*-131H and *FCGR3A*-158V alleles in particular, markedly enhance receptor affinity for IgG (18), mAbs and an IgG1 Fc Hexamer construct, have the potential to elicit enhanced cytokine release amongst individuals possessing these gene variants. Furthermore, we aimed to determine the association of several FcγR SNPs with the magnitude of IgG Fc triggered cytokine release in two widely used assay formats: freeze-thawed precultured PBMCs and whole blood. The whole blood assay (but not freeze-thawed PBMC) format recapitulates immune cell subset frequencies, FcγR cellular distribution and expression levels at physiological levels more accurately, revealing associations between FcγR genotype and magnitude of cytokine release in response to mAb treatment. These findings highlight FcγR genotype characterization paired with *vitro* assessment of mAb therapeutics may indeed better predict the magnitude, and variability of responses observed in clinical settings and inform on enhanced therapy design.

MATERIALS AND METHODS

Healthy Donor Cohorts and Ethical Approval

This study comprises two independent cohorts of anonymous healthy donors (total $n = 271$). The Southampton cohort (30), consisted of 178 anonymous healthy donors entering local transfusion services (National Blood Service, Southampton, UK). This study was approved by the University of Southampton Faculty of Medicine Ethics Committee and the National Research Ethics Service Committee South Central, Hampshire, UK. The UCB cohort consisted of 93 anonymous healthy donors based at UCB Celltech, Slough, UK. Blood samples obtained from these donors were taken with informed consent under UCB Celltech UK HTA license number 12504. All donors gave written informed consent in accordance with the Declaration of Helsinki.

PBMC Preparation and Blood Collection

PBMCs were sourced from leukocyte cones (National Blood Service, Southampton, UK) and whole blood was collected from the UCB donor cohort in lithium heparin vacutainers (BD). PBMCs were isolated from these samples immediately by density gradient centrifugation (Lymphoprep, Axis-Shield). Samples were subsequently frozen in 10% DMSO and 90% fetal bovine serum (FBS, Sigma-Aldrich) and stored in liquid nitrogen for 3–24 months.

Genomic DNA Extraction and Multiplex Ligation-Dependent Probe Amplification (MLPA) Assay

Frozen PBMC samples were rapidly thawed and genomic DNA (gDNA) was extracted (DNeasy Blood and Tissue Kit, Qiagen, GmbH, Hilden, Germany). DNA quality was assessed by UV spectrophotometry.

CNV and SNPs in the low-affinity FcγR locus were measured as previously described (30). 100 ng DNA was analyzed in triplicate using the SALSA MLPA P110 and P111 probe mixes (MRC-Holland, Amsterdam, The Netherlands). PCR products were analyzed using the Genetic Analysis System CEQ 8800 capillary electrophoresis machine and GenomeLab software (Beckman Coulter, High Wycombe, UK). CNV across the locus and SNPs in *FCGR2A* 131R/H (rs1801274), *FCGR3A* 158F/V (rs396991), *FCGR2B* 232I/T (rs1050501), *FCGR2C* 57X/Q (rs759550223), *FCGR3B* HNA 1A/B/C isoforms were assessed.

Intra-sample data normalization was performed using the Coffalyser.NET software (MRC-Holland) by comparing the peak heights of PCR products generated by probes detecting regions of interest against the peak heights of PCR products targeting control genes of known normal copy number. Inter-sample normalization was performed by comparing test cases against a reference sample of 96 pooled European Collection of Cell Cultures (ECACC) Human Random Control panel 1 (Porton Down, Public Health England, UK) gDNA samples. Normalized MLPA data was analyzed using Microsoft Excel 2010.

Antibodies and IgG1 Fc Hexamer

Avastin (Bevacizumab) was sourced from Genentech. Hybridoma cells expressing OKT3 (mouse IgG2a) were obtained from the American Type Culture Committee (ATCC) and mAb isolated from tissue culture media by standard procedures in-house. TGN1412 was produced in-house using published sequences (US patent number US7585960). Variable regions were sub-cloned into expression vectors (pEE6.4 heavy chain and pEE12.4 light chain; Lonza) containing constant regions of human IgG4. Heavy- and light-chain vectors were sub-cloned together before transfection into 293F cells for transient production or CHO-K1 cells for stable production. mAb was purified on Protein A-Sepharose, and aggregates were removed by gel filtration. Campath-1H (Campath) human IgG1 was sourced from Professor Geoffrey Hale (University of Cambridge, UK).

To generate a recombinant hexameric Fc construct (IgG1 Fc hexamer), human IgG1 Fc with mature N-termini starting with an IgG1 core hinge (CPPC) were directly fused at their C-terminal lysine residues to the 18 amino-acid C-terminal extension or "tail-piece" (PTLYNVSLVMSDTAGTCY)

of human IgM, which promotes covalent multimerization. IgG1 Fc hexamer was expressed transiently in CHO cells and purified using Protein A and S200 size exclusion chromatography as described previously (28, 29). IgG1 Fc hexamer fraction purity was >98% on analytical HPLC after size exclusion chromatography (SEC). IgG1 Fc hexamer was stored at 4°C in PBS or frozen in aliquots at −80°C.

Endotoxin levels for all antibodies and IgG1 Fc Hexamer used in this study were measured and found to be <1 ng/mg protein (Endosafe-PTS, Charles River Laboratories).

PBMC Assay

Frozen PBMCs were rapidly thawed at 37°C and cultured for 24 h in a flat-bottomed 24-plate at high density (HD), defined as 1.5×10^7 cells/well (total volume 1.5 mL/well), in serum-free medium (CTL-Test Medium, CTL Europe GmbH, Bonn, Germany) supplemented with glutamine (2 mM), pyruvate (1 mM), penicillin, and streptomycin (100 IU/mL), at 37°C in 5% CO_2. PBMCs were washed and cultured in CTL-Test medium at 1×10^5 cells per well, in a round-bottomed 96-well plate. These cultures were then stimulated with soluble Avastin (5 μg/mL), OKT3 (5 μg/mL), TGN1412 (5 μg/mL), Campath (5 μg/mL), or IgG1 Fc Hexamer (100 μg/mL) and incubated at 37°C in 5% CO_2. T-cell proliferation was quantified at 72 h and cytokine release was quantified 24 h post-stimulation.

Whole Blood Assay

Blood from healthy human volunteers was collected into lithium heparin vacutainers (BD) and used within 2 h of the blood draw. Minimally-diluted blood was stimulated with either 100 μg/mL of IgG1 Fc hexamer or 10 μg/mL Campath (Genzyme). Briefly, 12.5 μL of 20x final concentration Avastin (5 μg/mL), OKT3 (5 μg/mL), TGN1412 (5 μg/mL), Campath (5 μg/mL), or IgG1 Fc Hexamer (100 μg/mL) was transferred to a 96-well round bottom tissue culture plate (Costar). 237.5 μL of whole blood was added and mixed gently by pipetting. Plates were incubated at 37°C, 5 % CO_2, 100 % humidity for 24 h, centrifuged at 300 g for 5 min and plasma collected for cytokine analysis. Plasma not analyzed immediately was stored at −80°C until analysis.

Flow Cytometry

1×10^6 PBMCs or 100 μL of whole blood (diluted 1:2 with PBS) were stained with the appropriate fluorochrome-conjugated mAb for 30 min at 4°C and washed once. Samples were stained with anti-CD3 PerCP (clone: SK7), anti-CD56–PE (clone: HCD56), anti-CD19 APC-Cy7 (clone: HIB19), anti-CD14–Pacific Blue (clone: M5E2) and IgG1κ-FITC (clone: MOPC-21) isotype control (all from BioLegend). FcγR staining was carried out using anti-FcγRI FITC (clone: 10.1, F(ab')2), anti-FcγRIIa FITC (clone: E08, F(ab')2), anti-FcγRIIb FITC (clone: 6G11, F(ab')2), anti-hFcγRIIIa FITC (clone: 3G8, F(ab')2), and isotype control human IgG1 FITC (clone: FITC8 F(ab')2), (generated from published sequences in-house or sourced from BioInvent International AB). Results are shown as geometric mean fluorescent intensity (MFI) for FcγR expression on B cells (FSC-A^{lo}SSC-A^{lo}CD19$^+$CD3$^−$), NK cells (FSC-A^{lo}SSC-A^{lo}CD56^{dim}CD3$^−$, CD56^{bright}CD3$^+$ or CD56^{hi}CD3$^+$), classical monocytes (FSC-A^{int}SSC-A^{int}CD14^{hi}), non-classical monocytes (FSC-A^{int}SSC-A^{int}CD14^{lo}) and granulocytes (CD14^{-}SSC^{hi}), (see **Supplementary Figure 1** for FACS gating strategy). FcγR expression levels were corrected by subtracting the geometric MFI of the corresponding isotype control staining.

Intracellular IFN-γ staining of PBMCs was carried out by culturing mAb-treated PBMCs with Golgi plug (BD Biosciences) for 24 h. Cells were stained with anti-CD4 Pacific blue (clone: SK3, BioLegend), anti-CD8 V500 (clone: RPA-T8, BD Biosciences) and anti-CD56 PE (clone: HCD56, BioLegend). PBMCs were fixed with FOXP3 Fix/Perm buffer (BioLegend) and permeabilized with FOXP3 Perm buffer before staining with anti-IFN-γ PE-Cy7 (clone: 4S.B3, eBiosciences). Samples were analyzed on a BD FACSCanto II (BD Biosciences) and data was analyzed using FlowJo Version 9.4.11 (Tree Star).

T-Cell Proliferation Assay

PBMCs were labeled with 2 μM carboxyfluorescein succinimidyl ester (CFSE). Cells were cultured in a 24-well plate at 1×10^7/mL for 24 h prior to the stimulation assays. Cells were transferred into round-bottomed 96-well plates at 1×10^5 per well. On day 3, cells were labeled with anti-CD8-APC (clone: SK1, BioLegend) and anti-CD4-PE (clone C4/120: in-house), and proliferation was assessed by CFSE dilution on a FACSCalibur or FACSCanto flow cytometer (BD Biosciences). CD4^{+} and CD8^{+} T cell division is defined as a percentage of total cells excluding the parent population (first peak).

Cytokine Determination

Supernatants from PBMC and plasma from whole blood assays were taken 24 h post-stimulation. IFN-γ, TNFα, IL-1β, and IL-6 levels were determined using the V-plex Proinflammatory Panel 1 (human) 4-plex Kit (Cat No: K15052D-2, Meso Scale Discovery) as per the manufacturer's protocol.

Statistical Analysis

Chi-squared tests were used to compare cohorts in terms of genotype frequency and to test for Hardy-Weinberg equilibrium. Where appropriate to conform to the assumption of "Normality" and constant variance, continuous data was log-transformed prior to analysis, results back-transformed to give geometric means and cytokine release data plotted with a logarithmic axis. One-way analysis of variance (ANOVA) with *post-hoc* pairwise comparisons was used to compare donor groups with different *FCGR* alleles. Two-way ANOVA with *post-hoc* pairwise comparisons or a paired student's *t*-test were used to compare groups where the same donors were used in each group (e.g., comparing immune cells subset frequencies in donor matched whole blood and freeze-thawed PBMCs). As a large number of statistical tests have been carried out in a range of contexts, there may be an issue with multiplicity of *p*-values. Formal multiplicity adjustments have not been used, so *p*-values should be interpreted with care and within the overall scientific context. Data analysis was carried out using the Graphpad Prism version 8.0.1 software. Statistical significance defined as *$p < 0.05$, **$p < 0.01$ ***$p < 0.001$ and ****$p < 0.0001$ and ns = non-significant.

RESULTS

Low-Affinity FcγR Gene Locus Characterization in Two Independent Cohorts

We assessed the frequency of common SNPs in the low-affinity FcγR locus in two independent cohorts using an FcγR-specific MLPA assay (**Supplementary Table 1**). Genotype frequencies for the combined cohorts are displayed in **Table 1**. Genotyping of the genes not reported to be affected by CNV, *FCGR2A* and *FCGR2B*, showed allele frequencies of 23.99% RR, 52.77% RH and 21.4% HH, and of 77.86% II, 20.66% IT and 0.37% TT, respectively. Genotypes reported for *FCGR3A, FCGR2C,* and *FCGR3B* include those with CNV. Frequencies for *FCGR3A* were 33.58% FF, 49.45% FV, and 8.86% VV; *FCGR2C* were 53.14% XX, 21.03% XQ and 2.21% QQ; and *FCGR3B* were 4.43% AA, 43.54% AB, and 31.37% BB. Reported genotypes were within Hardy-Weinberg equilibrium.

Copy gain (25.8%) across the locus was more prevalent than copy loss (20.2%). We found alterations in CNRs 1 and 2, with CNR2 the most prevalent event (**Table 2**). Frequencies of CNV and CNR events for each cohort are described individually in **Supplementary Tables 2, 3** and for samples with available functional data in **Supplementary Tables 4, 5**.

Immune Cell Subset Frequencies and FcγR Expression on Healthy Donor PBMCs

Using flow cytometry (see **Supplementary Figure 1** for FACS gating strategy), we assessed the cellular constituents and FcγR expression in freeze-thawed PBMC samples from 107 healthy individuals from the Southampton cohort. These donors were selected to generate a cohort with the full range of FcγR SNPs and CNV status with the potential to confer low- and high-affinity IgG binding. As expected, T cells were the most abundant cell type in these samples (median 59.8%, range 38.8–81.8%), followed by monocytes (median 12.3%, range 5.1–30.2%), CD56^{dim} NK cells (median 7.6%, range 1.8–14.3%), CD3^{+} NK cells (median 5.9%, range 1.7–15.1%) and B cells (median 3.9%, range 1.1–10.1%). CD4^{+} T cells (median 47.6%, range 25.2–71.2%) were more abundant than CD8^{+} T cells (median 10.5%, range 3.6–37%) in all donor samples. The frequencies of CD56^{bright} NK cells and dendritic cells (DCs) in these samples were <0.01% of total cells (**Figure 1A**).

Monocytes can be categorized into classical and non-classical subsets on the basis of CD14 high (CD14^{hi}) or low (CD14^{lo}) expression, respectively. FcγR expression levels on each monocyte population were assessed separately. As previously reported (31), CD14^{hi} monocytes abundantly expressed FcγRI and FcγRIIa, but were low or negative for FcγRIIb and FcγRIIIa (**Figure 1B**). In contrast, the less frequent CD14^{lo} non-classical monocytes expressed lower levels of FcγRI and FcγRIIa and higher levels FcγRIIb and FcγRIIIa (**Figure 1C**). B cells expressed high levels of FcγRIIb in comparison to non–classical monocytes but did not express any other FcγR (**Figure 1D**). CD56^{dim} NK cells expressed very variable levels of FcγRIIIa (**Figure 1E**, median MFI 2242, and range 97-8987). Finally, CD3^{+} T and

TABLE 1 | Combined genotype frequencies of common low-affinity FcγR genes in the combined cohorts.

Gene	SNP(s)	Genotype	N	%	p-value	Chi^2 test
FCGR2A	rs1208724	RR	65	23.99	0.42	0.51
		RH	143	52.77		
		HH	58	21.40		
		Failed	5	1.85		
FCGR3A	rs396991	FF	91	33.58	0.42	0.66
		FV	134	49.45		
		VV	24	8.86		
		F	1	0.37		
		V	1	0.37		
		FFF	6	2.21		
		FFV	1	0.37		
		VVV	1	0.37		
		Failed	12	4.43		
FCGR2C	rs759550223	XX	144	53.14	0.48	0.5
		XQ	57	21.03		
		QQ	6	2.21		
		X	17	6.27		
		Q	9	3.32		
		XXX	25	9.23		
		XXQ	4	1.48		
		XQQ	1	0.37		
		QQQ	4	1.48		
		XXXX	1	0.37		
		Failed	3	1.11		
FCGR3B	HNA isoforms (rs200688856 and rs5030738)	AA	12	4.43	0.09	2.86
		AB	118	43.54		
		BB	85	31.37		
		A	8	2.95		
		B	15	5.54		
		AAA	4	1.48		
		AAB	11	4.06		
		ABB	10	3.69		
		BBBB	1	0.00		
		Failed	7	0.37		
FCGR2B	rs1050501	II	211	77.86	0.9	0.02
		IT	56	20.66		
		TT	1	0.37		
		Failed	3	1.11		

HWE was calculated based on diploid genotypes within the population. A p-value >0.05 (Chi^2 >3.84) was considered to be within HWE.

TABLE 2 | Copy number variation event frequencies across low-affinity FcγR genes in the combined cohorts.

Gene	Gene copy	Total (n)	Total (%)
FCGR3A	1	2	0.7
	2	243	90.7
	3	7	2.6
FCGR2C	1	26	9.7
	2	207	77.2
	3	31	11.6
	4	1	0.4
FCGR3B	1	23	8.6
	2	215	80.2
	3	25	9.3
	4	1	0.4

Event	Gain (%)	Loss (%)	Total (%)
CNR1	7 (12.1)	2 (3.4)	9 (15.5)
CNR2	25 (43.1)	23 (39.7)	48 (82.8)
CNR1/2	1 (1.7)	0 (0)	1 (1.8)

In the current study, PBMC samples from healthy donors, were frozen and then re-thawed for use in a PBMC-based cytokine release assay. In these assays, we opted to test the T cell-targeting antibodies, OKT3 (anti-CD3, mouse IgG2a) and TGN1412 (anti-CD28, human IgG4), renowned for inducing CRS in human subjects (5, 6). In order to establish a methodology to predict such CRS *in vitro*, Hunnig et al. developed a modified PBMC-based assay. They showed that PBMCs precultured at high density (HD), but not fresh PBMCs or whole blood, respond to TGN1412 with cytokine release *in vitro*, mimicking the proinflammatory effects observed in the clinic (8). We subsequently reported that the response to TGN1412 was a consequence of a pronounced upregulation of FcγRIIb on monocytes in the HD PBMC culture (10). Given these results and the accepted importance of FcγRs in mediating mAb effector functions, we utilized this PBMC-based HD preculture assay to assess the impact of donor FcγR genotype on T-cell proliferation and cytokine release in response to mAbs of differing functional classes which bind functionally disparate targets.

Consequently, OKT3, TGN1412 and the clinically relevant anti-CD52 (Campath, human IgG1) were used to assess the magnitude and variability of the cytokine release across our donor cohort using this assay platform. We observed a predominant but highly variable, CD8$^+$ T-cell division in response to the anti-CD3 mAb (**Figure 2A**, range 10-92% division of total CD8$^+$ cells). In contrast, TGN1412 predominantly induced CD4$^+$ T-cell division (**Figure 2A**, range 12–74% of total CD4$^+$ cells). T-cell proliferation in response to the control anti-VEGF mAb Avastin was negligible in both T cell subsets (**Figures 2A,B**).

We next assessed cytokine release in response to OKT3, TGN142 and Campath. All 3 mAb induced strong IFN-γ, TNF-α, IL-1β, and IL-6 responses in comparison to Avastin. Cytokine responses to the T-cell specific mAb OKT3 and TGN1412 were

CD3$^+$ NK cells were negative for any cell surface FcγR expression (data not shown).

mAb Mediated T-Cell Proliferation and Cytokine Release Using a PBMC-Based Assay Format

Pre-stored frozen PBMC samples are widely used in academia and industry, to facilitate genotyping and subsequent analysis.

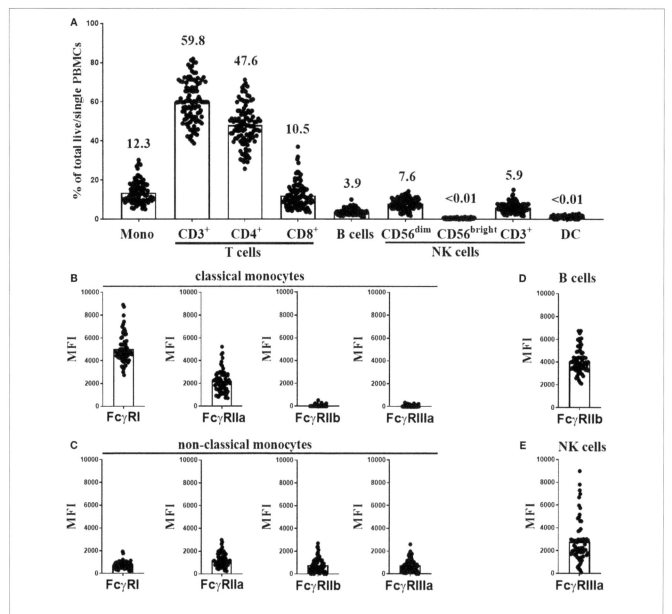

FIGURE 1 | Immune cell subset frequencies and FcγR expression on PBMCs from healthy donors. Immune cell subset frequencies and FcγR expression on freeze-thawed PBMCs using flow cytometry. **(A)** Quantification of monocytes (Mono), CD3+, CD4+, and CD8+ T cells, B cells, CD56dim, CD56bright, and CD3+ NK cells and dendritic cell (DC) frequencies in freeze-thawed PBMCs from healthy human subjects (mean frequency of each cell subset stated above bar). FcγR expression on **(B)** classical, and **(C)** non-classical monocytes, **(D)** FcγRIIb expression on B cells and **(E)** FcγRIIIa expression on CD56dim NK cells ($n = 107$). Each point represents a donor, bars represent group means.

stronger than those observed in Campath-stimulated cultures. However, there was marked variability in the magnitude of donor responses to all three mAb treatments (**Figures 2C–F**). IFN-γ responses to OKT3, TGN1412 and Campath were stable over time, since stimulating PBMCs from the same donor on five separate occasions (over a 6-month period) revealed a similar response on each occasion (**Supplementary Figure 2**). The IFN-γ response to OKT3, TGN1412, and Campath, was significantly correlated with TNF-α, IL-1β, and IL-6 release ($R^2 = 0.27$–0.83, $p \leq 0.002$–0.0001 for IFN-γ vs. the other three cytokines (except

IFN-γ vs. TNF-α for Campath), **Supplementary Figure 3**), and therefore we chose to present IFN-γ release as an exemplar read-out to assess all further cytokine responses in these assays.

To assess the cell populations responsible for this IFN-γ release, we performed intracellular cytokine staining on permeabilized cells stimulated with OKT3, TGN1412, or Campath. Flow cytometry was used to identify and determine the percentage of each cell population secreting IFN-γ. The source of IFN-γ was CD8+ T cells in response to OKT3, both CD4+ and CD8+ T cells in response to TGN1412 and NK cells

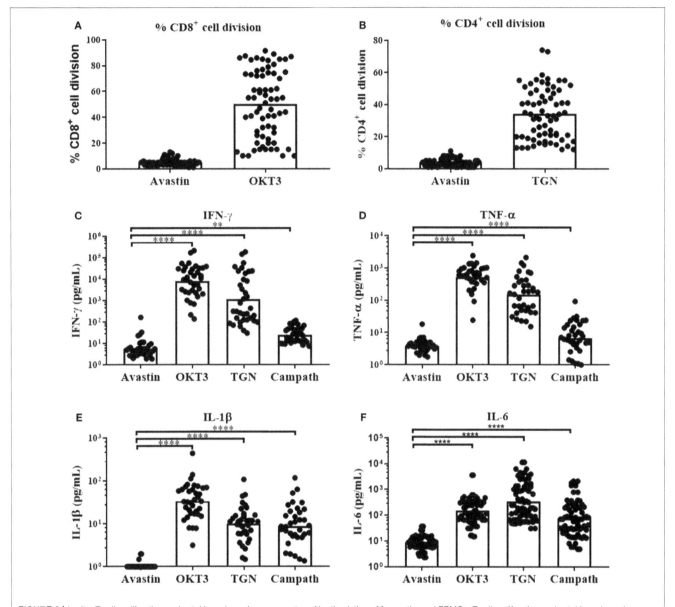

FIGURE 2 | *In vitro* T-cell proliferation and cytokine release in response to mAb stimulation of freeze-thawed PBMCs. T-cell proliferation and cytokine release in response to mAb stimulation. **(A)** % CD8$^+$ cell division in PBMC cultures stimulated with Avastin or OKT3 and **(B)** % CD4$^+$ cell division in PBMC cultures stimulated with Avastin or TGN1412 (TGN), (n = 69, bars represent group means). **(C)** IFN-γ, **(D)** TNF-α, **(E)** IL-1β, and **(F)** IL-6 release by PBMCs stimulated with Avastin, OKT3, TGN1412 or Campath (n = 36, bars represent group geometric means). **p < 0.01 and ****p < 0.0001.

in response to Campath (**Figures 3A,B**). We next assessed the impact of donor FcγR genotype on the magnitude and variability of these responses observed using this HD freeze-thawed PBMC assay format.

FcγR Genotype Does Not Significantly Impact on mAb-Mediated IFN-γ Secretion in a HD PBMC Assay Format

Three key FcγR polymorphisms have been previously associated with mAb effector capacity, defining high or low affinity receptors for FcγRIIa, FcγRIIIa and a stop codon in FcγRIIc (20–24). We

therefore determined the effects of the FcγRIIa 131H/R, FcγRIIIa 158V/F, and FcγRIIc Q/X polymorphisms on IFN-γ release in response to Campath and TGN1412 using the HD PBMC-based cytokine release assay in 36 donors. When stimulating PBMCs with Campath or TGN1412, no significant association of increased IFN-γ release was observed with any of the FcγRIIa, FcγRIIIa, or FcγRIIc alleles (**Figures 4A–F**). Furthermore, no significant associations were observed between FcγR SNPs and magnitude of OKT3 or TGN1412 mediated T-cell proliferation (data not shown). We hypothesized that key properties of the relevant FcγR-expressing immune cell subsets may have been altered during the isolation and storing/thawing/culture

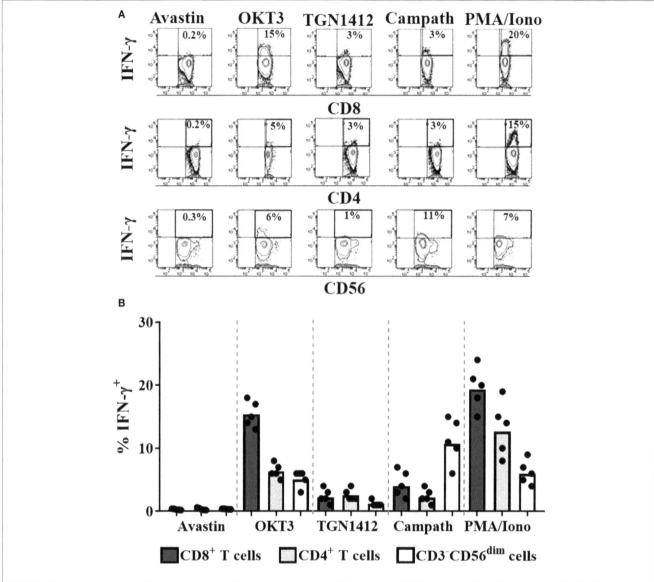

FIGURE 3 | Cellular source of the IFN-γ in response to mAb stimulation. Intracellular IFN-γ staining of PBMCs stimulated for 24 h with Avastin, OKT3, TGN1412, Campath or PMA/Ionomycin (PMA/Iono). **(A)** Representative FACS contour plots of IFN-γ vs. CD8, CD4, or CD56 staining of PBMC cultures stimulated with the aforementioned treatments. **(B)** % CD8[+] T cells, CD4[+] T cells, and CD56[dim] NK cells that are IFN-γ[+] post-stimulation (n = 5, bars represent group means).

of PBMCs, potentially compromising any associations between FcγR genotype and magnitude of mAb mediated IFN-γ response. To address this, we next compared the frequencies of immune cell subsets between donor matched whole blood and freeze-thawed PBMC samples.

Freeze-Thawed PBMCs Display Altered Immune Subset Frequencies and FcγR Expression Profiles Compared to Matched Whole Blood Samples

As expected, whole blood had a significantly higher frequency of granulocytes in comparison to donor matched freeze-thawed (frozen) PBMC samples as a percentage of total live cells

(**Figure 5A**); (Granulocyte median = 54.38% in whole blood compared to 1% for frozen PBMCs, $p < 0.0001$). The proportions of T cells (median = 44.41% for whole blood, 50.04% for frozen PBMCs, $p < 0.05$) were significantly enriched in frozen PBMC samples (**Figure 5B**). In contrast significant reductions in CD14[hi] classical monocytes (median = 7.6% for whole blood and 5.5% for frozen PBMCs, **Figure 5C**), B cells (median = 11.7% for whole blood, 8.9% for frozen PBMCs, **Figure 5E**) and CD56[dim] NK cells (median = 5.9% for whole blood, 5.3% for frozen PBMCs, **Figure 5F**) were observed when comparing whole blood to frozen PBMC samples ($p < 0.05$, $p < 0.001$ and $p < 0.05$, respectively). CD14[lo] non-classical monocyte frequencies were not significantly altered in frozen PBMC when compared to whole blood samples (**Figure 5D**). The proportions of CD56[bright]

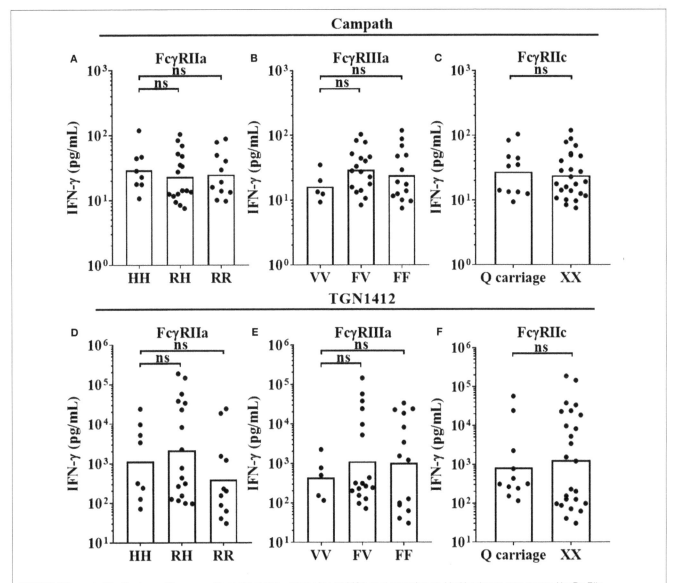

FIGURE 4 | Impact of FcγR polymorphisms on mAb mediated IFN-γ release in a PBMC based assay format. Healthy donors were grouped by FcγRIIa polymorphisms; HH (n = 8), RH (n = 17) and RR (n = 11), FcγRIIIa polymorphisms; VV (n = 5), FV (n = 17) and FF (n = 14), and FcγRIIc polymorphisms; QQ/XQ (n = 11) and XX (n = 25). PBMCs were stimulated with **(A–C)** Campath or **(D–F)** TGN1412 and IFN-γ release was quantified 24 h post-stimulation. Each point represents a donor and bars represent group geometric means. ns = non-significant.

NK cells (median = 0.15% for whole blood, 0.4% for frozen PBMCs, $p < 0.01$) and CD3[+] NK cells (median = 2.4% for whole blood, 4.3% for frozen PBMCs, $p < 0.001$) were significantly enriched in frozen PBMC samples (**Figures 5G,H**).

We also observed significant change in FcγR expression levels when comparing whole blood to frozen PBMCs. Significant reductions in FcγRIIb on B cells (median = 2,904 for whole blood, 2115 for frozen PBMCs, $p < 0.01$ **Figure 6A**) and FcγRIIIa (median = 4,618 for whole blood, 3,144 for frozen PBMCs, $p < 0.05$, **Figure 6B**) on NK cells were observed in frozen PBMCs compared to whole blood. FcγRI expression remained constant whereas FcγRIIa was significantly upregulated on classical monocytes in frozen PBMCs (median = 327 for whole

blood, 1,124 for frozen PBMCs, $p < 0.0001$, **Figure 6C**). FcγRIIa (median = 701 for whole blood, 2,167 for frozen PBMCs, $p < 0.0001$) and FcγRIIb (median = 264 for whole blood, 733 for frozen PBMCs, $p < 0.01$) expression levels were both significantly upregulated on non-classical monocytes (**Figures 6D,E**) in frozen PBMCs, whereas FcγRIIIa expression levels remained unaltered (**Figure 6G**). Granulocytes (present only in whole blood), did not express FcγRI and FcγRIIb, but did express low levels of FcγRIIa and high, but variable levels of FcγRIIIB (**Figure 6H**).

FcγR expression on freeze-thawed PBMCs was also assessed pre- and post-HD culture. As previously reported (10), FcγRI expression on monocytes was not significantly altered (**Supplementary Figure 4A**). In contrast FcγRIIb was markedly

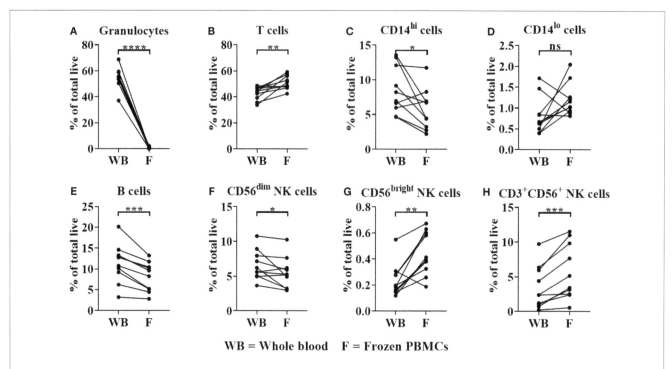

FIGURE 5 | Immune cell subset frequencies in donor matched whole blood (WB) and frozen (F) PBMC samples. Immune cell subset frequencies were quantified in donor matched whole blood, fresh and frozen PBMCs using flow cytometry. Immune cell frequencies were quantified as % of total live/single cells **(A)** % Granulocytes, **(B)** T cells, **(C)** CD14^{hi} monocytes, **(D)** CD14^{lo} monocytes, **(E)** B cells, **(F)** CD3^{-}CD56^{dim}, **(G)** CD3^{-}CD56^{bright}, and **(H)** CD3^{+}CD56^{+} NK cells of total live/single cells. Each point represents a donor, bars represent group means, ($n = 10$). *$p < 0.05$, **$p < 0.01$ ***$p < 0.001$ and ****$p < 0.0001$ and ns = non-significant.

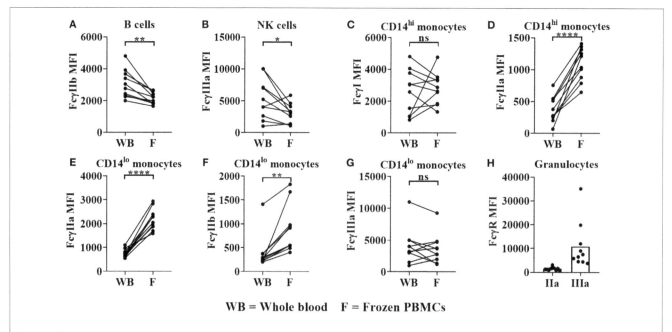

FIGURE 6 | FcγR expression in donor matched whole blood (WB) and frozen (F) PBMCs. Using flow cytometry, FcγR expression was quantified on **(A)** B cells **(B)** NK cells, **(C,D)** classical monocytes, **(E–G)** non-classical monocytes and **(H)** granulocytes in donor matched WB and frozen PBMC samples. FcγRIIa (IIa) and FcγRIIIa (IIIa) expression on granulocytes was quantified in WB only. Each point represents a donor, bars represent group means, ($n = 10$). *$p < 0.05$, **$p < 0.01$, ****$p < 0.0001$ and ns = non-significant.

increased (100-fold increase post-HD culture, $p < 0.01$), whereas increases in FcγRIIa (0.75-fold increase, $p < 0.05$) and FcγRIIIa (3-fold increase, $p < 0.05$) were less pronounced (**Supplementary Figures 4B–D**). FcγRIIb expression on B cells (**Supplementary Figure 4E**) and FcγRIIIa expression on NK cells were also not significantly modified in freeze-thawed PBMCs after HD culture (**Supplementary Figure 4F**).

These effects of freeze-thawing on FcγR expression and NK cell/monocyte frequencies in PBMC samples prompted us to re-assess the IFN-γ response of those therapeutics which induce cytokine release via Fc:FcγR interactions, using a whole blood assay format.

FcγR Polymorphisms Determine the Magnitude of mAb Dependent IFN-γ Secretion in a Whole Blood Assay Format

To determine whether the impact of FcγR polymorphisms on IFN-γ release in response to Campath stimulation (an effect largely mediated by Fc:FcγR interactions) can be assessed *in vitro*, we utilized the whole blood assay format and samples from 88 UCB cohort donors. Furthermore, to restrict ourselves solely to Fc:FcγR effects, without a bias from the target receptor (e.g., CD52) we also stimulated these whole blood samples with an IgG1 Fc hexamer, which is a recombinant human IgG1 Fc construct generated by fusing the human IgG1 Fc domain to the tail-piece domain of human IgM (28). The IgG1 Fc hexamer was designed as a high-avidity FcγR blocking agent, but was demonstrated to induce high levels of pro-inflammatory cytokine release in whole blood *in vitro* assays, but not PBMC assays via a mechanism dependent on the presence of neutrophils and interactions with FcγRIIa and FcγRIIIb (29). We used this IgG1 Fc Hexamer here as a target receptor-independent mimic for ordered immune complexes which may form after mAb infusion and pose a CRS risk.

IFN-γ responses to Campath (median = 4,051 pg/ml) and the IgG1 Fc hexamer (5,588 pg/mL, $p < 0.001$) for both reagents were significantly stronger than PBS-treated controls, (11.72 pg/ml, **Supplementary Figure 5A**). Furthermore, there was a significant correlation ($R^2 = 0.53$, $p < 0.0001$) of IFN-γ release between Campath and IgG1 Fc Hexamer treatment (**Supplementary Figure 5B**). Longitudinal assessment of IFN-γ release over a period of four months using repeat whole blood samples from nine heathy donors, in five separate assays, revealed stable responses from all donors to Campath and IgG1 Fc hexamer stimulation (**Supplementary Figures 6A,B**)—again indicating a stable donor-specific response profile, with potential value as a prognostic test.

This assay format revealed that donors homozygous for the high-affinity *FCGR2A*-131H allele mounted significantly stronger IFN-γ responses to Campath (median = 5,273 pg/mL), than individuals homozygous for the low IgG affinity *FCGR2A*-131R allele (median = 2,788 pg/mL, $p < 0.01$ when comparing HH individuals with RR individuals, **Figure 7A**). Heterozygous individuals (RH) elicited intermediate responses (median = 3,331 pg/mL, $p < 0.05$ when comparing HH individuals with RH individuals, **Figure 7A**). There were no statistically

significant differences in IFN-γ release, between the high affinity homozygous *FCGR3A*-158V allele, heterozygous VF and homozygous *FCGR3A*-158F low IgG affinity donors, in response to Campath stimulation. However, this may have been due to the low numbers of donors homozygous for the high affinity *FCGR3A*-158V allele in our cohort (median; VV = 6,005 pg/mL, VF = 3,847 pg/mL and FF = 2,869 pg/mL, $p = 0.26$ when comparing VV vs. FF donor responses, **Figure 7B**). Significantly greater IFN-γ release was observed in response to Campath stimulation amongst donors homozygous for both high affinity *FCGR2A*-131H and *FCGR3A*-158V SNPs (median = 9204 pg/mL) in comparison to donors homozygous for the low IgG affinity *FCGR2A*-131R and *FCGR3A*-158F alleles (median = 2,684 pg/mL, $p < 0.05$, **Figure 7C**). When comparing *FCGR2C*-57Q SNP-carrying donors, who are predicted to express this additional activatory FcγR on NK cells, with *FCGR2C*-57X homozygous donors who are FcγRIIc negative, no significant associations with IFN-γ release were observed ($p = 0.34$, when comparing QQ/QX with XX donors, **Figure 7D**). Furthermore, no significant associations between the *FCGR3B* and *FCGR2B* SNPs and Campath induced IFN-γ release were revealed using this assay format (**Figures 7E,F**).

For the IgG1 Fc hexamer, *FCGR2A*-131H homozygous high affinity donors mounted significantly stronger IFN-γ responses (median = 7,867 pg/mL) when compared to *FCGR2A*-131R low affinity homozygous donors (median = 3,470 pg/mL, $p < 0.05$). The *FCGR2A*-131RH heterozygous donors mounted an intermediate response (median = 5,066 pg/mL, **Figure 8A**). There were no statistically significant differences in IFN-γ release between the homozygous high affinity *FCGR3A*-158V allele, heterozygous VF and homozygous *FCGR3A*-158F low IgG affinity donors, in response to IgG1 Fc Hexamer stimulation. (median IFN-γ responses (pg/mL); VV = 7441, VF = 5,066 and FF = 5,443.14, **Figure 8B**). IFN-γ release in response to IgG1 Fc hexamer amongst donors homozygous for both the high affinity *FCGR2A*-131H and *FCGR3A*-158V alleles were significantly elevated compared to donors homozygous for the low IgG affinity alleles (median for HH/VV = 9,472 and RR/FF = 4,324 pg/mL, $p < 0.05$, **Figure 8C**). No significant associations between the *FCGR2C*, *FCGR3B* and *FCGR2B* SNPs and IgG1 Fc hexamer induced IFN-γ release were observed using this assay format (**Figures 8D–F**). Assessing the effects of *FCGR3A*, *FCGR2C*, and *FCGR3B* gene CNV with FcγR expression on immune cells or mAb mediated cytokine release was not possible in the current study due to the limited size of donor cohorts and relative rarity of gene CNV >2.

Finally, we stimulated matched whole blood and precultured freeze-thawed PBMC cultures with OKT3, TGN1412, Campath and the IgG1 Fc Hexamer, to directly compare both assay formats and modified IFN-γ release amongst five high IgG affinity *FCGR2A*-131H homozygous donors compared to five low IgG affinity *FCGR2A*-131R homozygous donors. A trend toward increased IFN-γ release was observed in the *FCGR2A*-131H homozygous donors. However, with such small donor numbers a clear statistically significant relationship could not be confirmed using either assay format (data not shown). Altogether, these results demonstrate the importance of donor assay format and

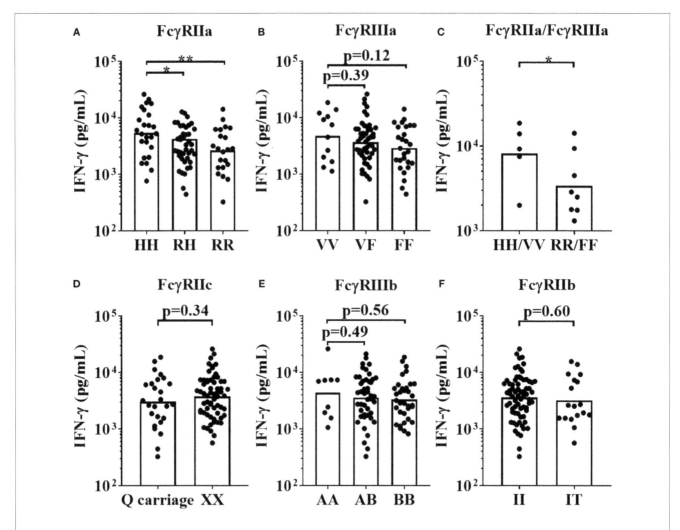

FIGURE 7 | Impact of FcγR polymorphisms on Campath induced IFN-γ release in a whole blood assay format. Healthy donors were grouped by **(A)** FcγRIIa polymorphisms; HH (*n* = 25), RH (*n* = 41) and RR (*n* = 22), **(B)** FcγRIIIa polymorphisms; VV (*n* = 12), FV (*n* = 49) and FF (*n* = 27), **(C)** high affinity FcγR polymorphisms HH/VV (*n* = 5) and low affinity FcγR polymorphisms RR/FF (*n* = 8), **(D)** FcγRIIc polymorphisms; Q carriage (*n* = 26) and XX (*n*= 62), **(E)** FcγRIIIb polymorphisms; AA (*n* = 9), AB (*n* = 45) and BB (*n* = 34) and **(F)** FcγRIIb polymorphisms; II (*n* = 70) and IT (*n* = 18). Whole blood from each donor was stimulated with Campath and IFN-γ release was quantified 24 h post-stimulation. Each point represents a donor, bars represent group geometric means. *$p < 0.05$ and **$p < 0.01$.

sufficient sample numbers when determining the impact of *FCGR2A* and *FCGR3A* polymorphisms on the magnitude of the IFN-γ response elicited by antibodies and IgG constructs with CRS-inducing potential.

DISCUSSION

Beyond their effects resulting from specific binding of cell surface antigens, mAb possess additional biological activity mediated through their Fc:FcγR interactions which are typically critical for efficacious antibody immunotherapy in patients. mAb interactions with FcγRIIa and FcγRIIIa mediate antibody dependent cellular cytotoxicity (ADCC) and antibody dependent cellular phagocytosis (ADCP) by tumor targeting mAb such as Rituximab, Herceptin and Campath. SNPs in *FCGR2A* and

FCGR3A genes influencing mAb affinity for FcγR have previously been shown to modify antibody immunotherapy in cancer patients (32). Here we report that whole blood assays are potentially more sensitive for hazard identification of mAb mediated cytokine release, as well as the assessment of the impact of *FCGR2A* and *FCGR3A* SNPs on the magnitude of this cytokine release *in vitro*.

MLPA remains the current gold standard assay for comprehensive FcγR genotyping. Using PBMC samples from healthy donors, we observed considerable variability across the FcγR locus in the form of SNPs and CNV, with homology between FcγR genes further complicating analysis as a result of the ancestral segmental duplication (33, 34). SNP frequencies described in this study are in line with others (35, 36) and while the reported SNP frequencies are within Hardy-Weinberg equilibrium, it is not optimized for loci with

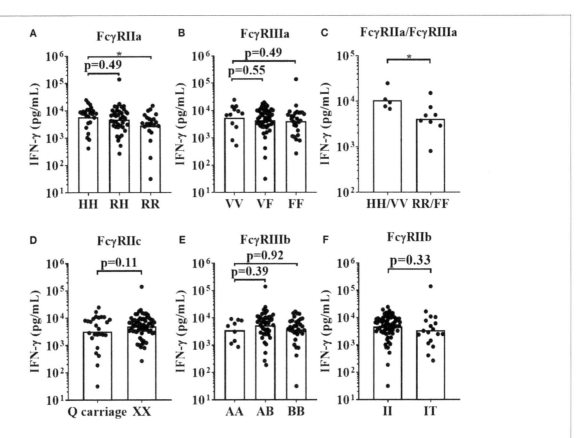

FIGURE 8 | Impact of FcγR polymorphisms on IFN-γ release induced by IgG1 Fc Hexamer stimulation in a whole blood assay format. Healthy donors were grouped by; **(A)** FcγRIIa polymorphisms; HH (n = 25), R/H (n = 41), and RR (n = 22), **(B)** FcγRIIIa polymorphisms; VV (n = 12), FV (n = 49) and FF (n = 27), **(C)** high affinity FcγR polymorphisms HH/VV (n = 5) and low affinity FcγR polymorphisms RR/FF (n = 8), **(D)** FcγRIIc polymorphisms; Q carriage (n = 26) and XX (n= 62), **(E)** FcγRIIIb polymorphisms; AA (n = 9), AB (n = 45) and BB (n = 34) and **(F)** FcγRIIb polymorphisms; II (n = 70) and IT (n = 18). Whole blood from each donor was stimulated with IgG1 Fc Hexamer and IFN-γ release was quantified 24 h post-stimulation. Each point represents a donor, bars represent group geometric means. *p < 0.05.

CNV. CNV represents a significant source of genetic diversity and can affect the function of FcγR gene products. Alterations in copy number of FcγR genes have reported gene dosage effects on protein expression (27, 37). CNV has been described in *FCGR3A*, *FCGR2C*, and *FCGR3B* (30, 35, 37), with rare events reported to affect *FCGR2B* (34). Regions of copy number alteration, CNR1-4, encompassing multiple genes in the locus have been described (17). As previously described (17, 35), CNV of *FCGR3A* is rare (3.6% of individuals), with alterations affecting *FCGR2C* and *FCGR3A* the most common CNV events. To date, these CNV have not been associated with mAb-mediated effects in the clinic, perhaps due to their relative rarity, leading to insufficient statistical power. Similar deficiencies were observed here in our study, with several 100 donors being required to study the impacts of CNV comprehensively. While many studies have reported associations between the high affinity *FCGR2A* and *FCGR3A* alleles and greater mAb efficacy in numerous cancers (20, 23), others have not observed such associations (38, 39), perhaps due to differing and complex biological backgrounds. We postulated that FcγR genotypes may correlate with *in vitro* IFN-γ responses to mAb stimulation and further enable prediction of CRS risk in the clinic.

In recent years, the limited value of rodent models for predicting treatment responses in humans set in motion intensive research to establish *in vitro* assays using human PBMCs; for example to predict the magnitude of cytokine release induced by therapeutic mAb (40). Assessment of mAb function and toxicity *in vitro* often utilizes banked frozen PBMC samples in both commercial pharmaceutical and academic settings. We previously used a PBMC-based assay format in which freeze-thawed PBMCs are first cultured at high density prior to stimulation with mAb. The high density preculture step promotes PBMC sensitivity to TGN1412 which otherwise elicits no immune cell activation in fresh untouched PBMC cultures (8, 10). Thus using this assay format which allows for the assessment of a CRS-inducing mAb (TGN1412), we sought to determine the impact of FcγR SNPs on mAb-induced cytokine release. Although assays were reproducible and stable per donor over time (indicating an inherent factor underpinning the level of response), no significant impact of *FCGR2A*, *FCGR2C*, or *FCGR3A* polymorphisms was observed with any mAb with respect to the magnitude of cytokine release (**Figure 4**). Larger cohorts would be required to accurately study the impact of CNV at the low-affinity locus given the low-frequency of events in *FCGR3A*, for example, whose gene product, FcγRIIIa, is an important mediator of NK cell-mediated ADCC.

This prompted a detailed comparison of immune cell subset frequencies and FcγR expression in whole blood and previously frozen PBMC samples. Significant reductions in monocytes, NK cells (CD3⁻CD56^dim cells) and FcγRIIIa expression on the latter were observed in freeze-thawed PBMCs relative to whole blood (**Figures 5C,F, 6B**). These observations were in concordance with previous studies reporting reduction in FcγRIIIa positive NK cells in freeze-thawed PBMC samples (41). In addition, FcγRIIa expression was significantly increased on monocytes in PBMC samples (**Figures 6D,E**), however, monocyte frequencies were reduced (**Figure 5C**), further impacting the likelihood of observing any *FCGR2A* SNP association with mAb-mediated cytokine release. The absence of FcγR-bearing neutrophils, platelets, donor IgG and complement proteins from serum in PBMC samples further justifies the utility of whole blood assays when determining the effects of FcγR SNPs on mAb-mediated cytokine release.

In the current study minimally diluted whole blood (95% blood / 5% mAb diluent) combined with aqueous mAb presentation was shown to be a useful and promising format, with only minimal sample and mAb manipulation aiming to preserve the natural peripheral blood molecular and cellular composition. We used this system to test Campath which binds CD52, a cell surface membrane antigen abundantly expressed on the surface of B cells, T cells, and monocytes (42). Campath triggering of FcγRIIIa on NK cells directly leads to IFN-γ release (12). We also tested an IgG1 Fc Hexamer construct which interacts with FcγRs, not target antigen. We have previously reported that cytokine release associated with this construct is primarily via interaction with FcγRIIa and FcγRIIIb and dependent on the presence of neutrophils (28, 29). Thus, both Campath and the IgG1 Fc Hexamer were suitable candidates for the assessment of the impact of FcγR SNPs on cytokine release in this assay format.

FcγRIIa is a monomeric receptor possessing an ITAM in its intracellular domain. It is the most broadly distributed FcγR, being expressed on monocytes, macrophages, platelets, and neutrophils and also in a soluble form (FcγRIIa2), (43). Our quantification of FcγRIIa expression in whole blood confirmed expression is restricted to monocytes and neutrophils (**Figure 6**). IgG triggering of FcγRIIa-mediated ITAM signaling results in cellular activation, phagocytosis, oxidative burst and the production of pro-inflammatory cytokines by monocytes and neutrophils (44). In whole blood, we observed a significantly elevated IFN-γ release in response to Campath and IgG1 Fc Hexamer stimulation amongst *FCGR2A*-131H/H donors compared to R/R donors. As Campath primarily stimulates cytokine release by triggering FcγRIIIa on NK cells (12), it was unexpected to observe a significant association with the *FCGR2A*-131H allele (**Figure 7A**). This enhanced IFN-γ release amongst the *FCGR2A*-131H homozygous donors may therefore be an indirect consequence of Campath triggered FcγRIIa activation on monocytes and neutrophils leading to pro-inflammatory cytokine release in these cell types, that then activates NK cells to secrete IFN-γ (45). We have previously demonstrated that the IgG1 Fc hexamer stimulates IFN-γ

production in whole blood in a neutrophil-dependent manner, in contrast to the response to Campath which was not affected by depletion of neutrophils from whole blood (29). Isolated neutrophils have also been shown to be capable of producing pro-inflammatory cytokines (29, 46) and TLR-independent neutrophil-derived IFN-γ is important for host resistance to intracellular pathogens (28), emphasizing the importance of maintaining the presence of these FcγR bearing cells in *in vitro* cytokine release assays, especially when testing reagents with the potential to form immune complexes. Neutrophils express both FcγRIIa and FcγRIIIb and this study, along with our previous data, suggests both receptors are important in this immune-complex induced cytokine response and that polymorphisms in FcγRIIa in particular may modulate this. This is in agreement with earlier studies indicating a complex interplay between FcγRIIa and FcγRIIIb haplotype and sensitivity of neutrophils to IgG-induced respiratory burst (47).

FcγRIIIa is a type I transmembrane receptor and signals via its association with the ITAM-expressing FcRγ chain, encoded by the *FCER1G* gene (48). In whole peripheral blood its expression is largely restricted to CD3⁻CD56^dim NK cells, and non-classical monocytes (**Figures 6B,C**). Additionally, FcγRIIIa is also abundantly expressed on macrophages (not present in whole blood) as well as on tumor-associated macrophages (49). FcγRIIIa has been reported to be the most potent activating receptor on freshly isolated peripheral blood NK cells, able to elicit potent ADCC and cytokine production in response to Campath treatment (50). Although not significant, we observed enhanced IFN-γ responses to Campath and IgG1 Fc hexamer stimulated whole blood cultures sourced *FCGR3A*-158V/V donors relative to *FCGR3A*-158V/F and *FCGR3A*-158F/F donors. Given the lower frequency of the *FCGR3A*-158V/V genotype in Western European populations (<10%), large sample size is essential for these studies to achieve statistically significant associations with mAb mediated cytokine release. In the current study only 12/88 donors (UCB cohort) possessed the *FCGR3A*-158V/V genotype, likely explaining the lack of statistical significance.

In the whole blood assay format, mAb-mediated effector functions are profoundly influenced by simultaneous mAb interactions with FcγRIIa, FcγRIIIa, FcγRIIb, and FcγRIIIb. To partially address the impact of IgG Fc interaction with more than one FcγR species, we analyzed a subset of donors homozygous for high or low affinity *FCGR2A*-131 and *FCGR3A*-158 alleles. The HH/VV donors had a 4-fold higher IFN-γ response to Campath and a 2-fold higher response to IgG1 Fc Hexamer, in comparison to the RR/FF donors. Encouragingly, these significant differences were observed with a relatively low number of donors and were again stable over time (indicating a stable donor-specific response profile), with potential value for development of prognostic tests. However, greater donor numbers are required for sufficient statistical powering for other associations, especially when also taking into account the low frequency of certain SNPs and large variability of cytokine responses to mAb stimulation of whole blood cultures. Based upon power calculations on our data to date, we recommend ≥20 donors for each FcγR SNP for assessing associations of FcγR genotype with mAb-mediated cytokine release hazard identification. This gives more than 80% power to detect a 3-fold difference between groups, using the whole blood IFN-γ release assay (**Supplementary Figure 7**).

Using the whole blood assay format, we did not observe statistically significant associations between *FCGR2C*, *FCGR2B*, or *FCGR3B* SNPs with the magnitude of Campath or IgG1 Fc hexamer-mediated cytokine release. FcγRIIc expression has been reported on NK cells, however, using flow cytometry we observed negligible or no FcγRIIc expression on NK cells, in >100 PBMC or whole blood samples (manuscript in preparation). This may explain the lack of significant association of *FCGR2C* SNPs with the magnitude of cytokine release. In whole blood samples, FcγRIIb expression is almost entirely restricted to B cells, which are unlikely to contribute to Campath or IgG1 Fc Hexamer induced IFN-γ release. Furthermore, it is worth recollecting that FcγRIIb is an ITIM-signaling inhibitory receptor, more likely to restrict cytokine release mediated by ITAM signaling on cell types co-expressing activatory and inhibitory FcγR. In addition, the I232T *FCGR2B* SNP leading to lack of inhibitory signaling, is extremely rare in Caucasian populations and so would require an extremely large cohort to study (26). Although FcγRIIIb has been reported to play a role in IgG1 Fc Hexamer induced cytokine release (29), we observed large variability in the expression levels of this receptor on neutrophils (MFI range 3771-35100) between donor samples. This may have compromised observing significant associations of *FCGR3B* SNPs with the extent of cytokine release in the IgG1 Fc Hexamer treated samples.

In summary, while there is considerable variability in the magnitude of cytokine responses elicited by cytokine storm-inducing IgG1 antibodies and Fc constructs in the whole blood assay format, key cell populations such as NK cells, monocytes and neutrophils remain intact and express FcγR at physiological levels. Our findings suggest that high-throughput genotyping combined with whole blood assays may be a powerful pharmacogenetic approach to predict both mAb therapy outcome and hazard identification but requires sufficient donors of each FcγR genotype if these associations are sought.

AUTHOR CONTRIBUTIONS

KH, CH, TR, KL, and JMS performed experiments. KH, CH, and JS performed statistical analyses. KH, CH, TR, MG, JCS, and MC designed experiments. KH and CH wrote the manuscript with contributions from TR, DH, and MC. All authors contributed to manuscript revision and read and approved the submitted version.

FUNDING

This work was supported by an NC3R CRACKIT grant awarded to MG (Award number: NC3Rs 15402-106217), a CRUK programme grant awarded to MC (Award number: A24721) and a BBSRC iCASE studentship to DH and MC (Award number: BB/N5039927/1).

REFERENCES

1. Glennie MJ, French RR, Cragg MS, Taylor RP. Mechanisms of killing by anti-CD20 monoclonal antibodies. *Mol Immunol.* (2007) 44:3823–37. doi: 10.1016/j.molimm.2007.06.151

2. Lee CS, Cragg M, Glennie M, Johnson P. Novel antibodies targeting immune regulatory checkpoints for cancer therapy. *Br J Clin Pharmacol.* (2013) 76:233–47. doi: 10.1111/bcp.12164

3. Lee DW, Gardner R, Porter DL, Louis CU, Ahmed N, Jensen M, et al. Current concepts in the diagnosis and management of cytokine release syndrome. *Blood.* (2014) 124:188–95. doi: 10.1182/blood-2014-05-552729

4. Coles AJ, Wing MG, Molyneux P, Paolillo A, Davie CM, Hale G, et al. Monoclonal antibody treatment exposes three mechanisms underlying the clinical course of multiple sclerosis. *Ann Neurol.* (1999) 46:296–304. doi: 10. 1002/1531-8249(199909)46:3<296::AID-ANA4>3.0.CO;2-#

5. Norman DJ, Vincenti F, de Mattos AM, Barry JM, Levitt DJ, Wedel NI, et al. Phase I trial of HuM291, a humanized anti-CD3 antibody, in patients receiving renal allografts from living donors. *Transplantation.* (2000) 70:1707–12. doi: 10.1097/00007890-200012270-00008

6. Suntharalingam G, Perry MR, Ward S, Brett SJ, Castello-Cortes A, Brunner MD, et al. Cytokine storm in a phase 1 trial of the anti-CD28 monoclonal antibody TGN1412. *N Engl J Med.* (2006) 355:1018–28. doi: 10.1056/NEJMoa063842

7. Stebbings R, Poole S, Thorpe R. Safety of biologics, lessons learnt from TGN1412. *Curr Opin Biotechnol.* (2009) 20:673–7. doi: 10.1016/j.copbio.2009.10.002

8. Romer PS, Berr S, Avota E, Na SY, Battaglia M, ten Berge I, et al. Preculture of PBMCs at high cell density increases sensitivity of T-cell responses, revealing cytokine release by CD28 superagonist TGN1412. *Blood.* (2011) 118:6772–82. doi: 10.1182/blood-2010-12-319780

9. Bartholomaeus P, Semmler LY, Bukur T, Boisguerin V, Romer PS, Tabares P, et al. Cell contact-dependent priming and Fc interaction with CD32+ immune cells contribute to the TGN1412-triggered cytokine response. *J Immunol.* (2014) 192:2091–8. doi: 10.4049/jimmunol.1302461

10. Hussain K, Hargreaves CE, Roghanian A, Oldham RJ, Chan HT, Mockridge CI, et al. Upregulation of FcgammaRIIb on monocytes is necessary to promote the superagonist activity of TGN1412. *Blood.* (2015) 125:102–10. doi: 10.1182/blood-2014-08-593061

11. Nimmerjahn F. Translating inhibitory fc receptor biology into novel therapeutic approaches. *J Clin Immunol.* (2016) 36 (Suppl. 1):83–7. doi: 10.1007/s10875-016-0249-6

12. Wing MG, Moreau T, Greenwood J, Smith RM, Hale G, Isaacs J, et al. Mechanism of first-dose cytokine-release syndrome by CAMPATH 1-H: involvement of CD16 (FcgammaRIII) and CD11a/CD18 (LFA-1) on NK cells. *J Clin Invest.* (1996) 98:2819–26. doi: 10.1172/JCI119110

13. White AL, Chan HT, Roghanian A, French RR, Mockridge CI, Tutt AL, et al. Interaction with FcgammaRIIB is critical for the agonistic activity of anti-CD40 monoclonal antibody. *J Immunol.* (2011) 187:1754–63. doi: 10.4049/jimmunol.1101135

14. Dahan R, Barnhart BC, Li F, Yamniuk AP, Korman AJ, Ravetch JV. Therapeutic activity of agonistic, human anti-CD40 monoclonal antibodies requires selective fcgammar engagement. *Cancer Cell.* (2016) 29:820–31. doi: 10.1016/j.ccell.2016.05.001

15. Arce Vargas F, Furness JS, Litchfield K, Joshi K, Rosenthal R, Ghorani E, et al. Fc Effector Function Contributes to the Activity of Human Anti-CTLA-4 Antibodies. *Cancer Cell.* (2018) 33:649–63 e4.

16. Hargreaves CE, Rose-Zerilli MJ, Machado LR, Iriyama C, Hollox EJ, Cragg MS, et al. Fcgamma receptors: genetic variation, function, and disease. *Immunol Rev.* (2015) 268:6–24. doi: 10.1111/imr.12341

17. Niederer HA, Willcocks LC, Rayner TF, Yang W, Lau YL, Williams TN, et al. Copy number, linkage disequilibrium and disease association in the FCGR locus. *Hum Mol Genet.* (2010) 19:3282–94. doi: 10.1093/hmg/ddq216

18. Bruhns P, Iannascoli B, England P, Mancardi DA, Fernandez N, Jorieux S, et al. Specificity and affinity of human Fcgamma receptors and their polymorphic variants for human IgG subclasses. *Blood.* (2009) 113:3716–25. doi: 10.1182/blood-2008-09-179754

19. Cartron G, Dacheux L, Salles G, Solal-Celigny P, Bardos P, Colombat P, et al. Therapeutic activity of humanized anti-CD20 monoclonal antibody and polymorphism in IgG Fc receptor FcgammaRIIIa gene. *Blood.* (2002) 99:754–8. doi: 10.1182/blood.V99.3.754

20. Zhang W, Gordon M, Schultheis AM, Yang DY, Nagashima F, Azuma M, et al. FCGR2A and FCGR3A polymorphisms associated with clinical outcome of epidermal growth factor receptor expressing metastatic colorectal cancer patients treated with single-agent cetuximab. *J Clin Oncol.* (2007) 25:3712–8. doi: 10.1200/JCO.2006.08.8021

21. Musolino A, Naldi N, Bortesi B, Pezzuolo D, Capelletti M, Missale G, et al. Immunoglobulin G fragment C receptor polymorphisms and clinical efficacy of trastuzumab-based therapy in patients with HER-2/neu-positive metastatic breast cancer. *J Clin Oncol.* (2008) 26:1789–96. doi: 10.1200/JCO.2007.14.8957

22. Calemma R, Ottaiano A, Trotta AM, Nasti G, Romano C, Napolitano M, et al. Fc gamma receptor IIIa polymorphisms in advanced colorectal cancer patients correlated with response to anti-EGFR antibodies and clinical outcome. *J Transl Med.* (2012) 10:232. doi: 10.1186/1479-5876-10-232

23. Persky DO, Dornan D, Goldman BH, Braziel RM, Fisher RI, Leblanc M, et al. Fc gamma receptor 3a genotype predicts overall survival in follicular lymphoma patients treated on SWOG trials with combined monoclonal antibody plus chemotherapy but not chemotherapy alone. *Haematologica.* (2012) 97:937–42. doi: 10.3324/haematol.2011.050419

24. Lee YH, Bae SC, Song GG. Functional FCGR3A 158 V/F and IL-6−174 C/G polymorphisms predict response to biologic therapy in patients with rheumatoid arthritis: a meta-analysis. *Rheumatol Int.* (2014) 34:1409–15. doi: 10.1007/s00296-014-3015-1

25. Tsang MW, Nagelkerke SQ, Bultink IE, Geissler J, Tanck MW, Tacke CE, et al. Fc-gamma receptor polymorphisms differentially influence susceptibility to systemic lupus erythematosus and lupus nephritis. *Rheumatology (Oxford).* (2016) 55:939–48. doi: 10.1093/rheumatology/kev433

26. Floto RA, Clatworthy MR, Heilbronn KR, Rosner DR, MacAry PA, Rankin A, et al. Loss of function of a lupus-associated FcgammaRIIb polymorphism through exclusion from lipid rafts. *Nat Med.* (2005) 11:1056–8. doi: 10.1038/nm1288

27. Willcocks LC, Lyons PA, Clatworthy MR, Robinson JI, Yang W, Newland SA, et al. Copy number of FCGR3B, which is associated with systemic lupus erythematosus, correlates with protein expression and immune complex uptake. *J Exp Med.* (2008) 205:1573–82. doi: 10.1084/jem.20072413

28. Qureshi OS, Rowley TF, Junker F, Peters SJ, Crilly S, Compson J, et al. Multivalent Fcgamma-receptor engagement by a hexameric Fc-fusion protein triggers Fcgamma-receptor internalisation and modulation of Fcgamma-receptor functions. *Sci Rep.* (2017) 7:17049. doi: 10.1038/s41598-017-17255-8

29. Rowley TF, Peters SJ, Aylott M, Griffin R, Davies NL, Healy LJ, et al. Engineered hexavalent Fc proteins with enhanced Fc-gamma receptor avidity provide insights into immune-complex interactions. *Commun Biol.* (2018) 1:146. doi: 10.1038/s42003-018-0149-9

30. Hargreaves CE, Iriyama C, Rose-Zerilli MJ, Nagelkerke SQ, Hussain K, Ganderton R, et al. Correction: evaluation of high-throughput genomic assays for the Fc gamma receptor locus. *PLoS ONE.* (2016) 11:e0145040. doi: 10.1371/journal.pone.0145040

31. Tutt AL, James S, Laversin SA, Tipton TR, Ashton-Key M, French RR, et al. Development and characterization of monoclonal antibodies specific for mouse and human fcgamma receptors. *J Immunol.* (2015) 195:5503–16. doi: 10.4049/jimmunol.1402988

32. Kim DH, Jung HD, Kim JG, Lee JJ, Yang DH, Park YH, et al. FCGR3A gene polymorphisms may correlate with response to frontline R-CHOP therapy for diffuse large B-cell lymphoma. *Blood.* (2006) 108:2720–5. doi: 10.1182/blood-2006-01-009480

33. Machado LR, Hardwick RJ, Bowdrey J, Bogle H, Knowles TJ, Sironi M, et al. Evolutionary history of copy-number-variable locus for the low-affinity Fcgamma receptor: mutation rate, autoimmune disease, and the legacy of helminth infection. *Am J Hum Genet.* (2012) 90:973–85. doi: 10.1016/j.ajhg.2012.04.018

34. Nagelkerke SQ, Tacke CE, Breunis WB, Geissler J, Sins JW, Appelhof B, et al. Nonallelic homologous recombination of the FCGR2/3 locus results in copy number variation and novel chimeric FCGR2 genes with aberrant functional expression. *Genes Immun.* (2015) 16:422–9. doi: 10.1038/gene.2015.25

35. Breunis WB, van Mirre E, Bruin M, Geissler J, de Boer M, Peters M, et al. Copy number variation of the activating FCGR2C gene predisposes to idiopathic thrombocytopenic purpura. *Blood.* (2008) 111:1029–38. doi: 10.1182/blood-2007-03-079913

36. Lassauniere R, Tiemessen CT. Variability at the FCGR locus: characterization in Black South Africans and evidence for ethnic variation in and out of Africa. *Genes Immun.* (2016) 17:93–104. doi: 10.1038/gene.2015.60

37. Breunis WB, van Mirre E, Geissler J, Laddach N, Wolbink G, van der Schoot E, et al. Copy number variation at the FCGR locus includes FCGR3A, FCGR2C and FCGR3B but not FCGR2A and FCGR2B. *Hum Mutat.* (2009) 30:E640–50. doi: 10.1002/humu.20997

38. Ghesquieres H, Cartron G, Seymour JF, Delfau-Larue MH, Offner F, Soubeyran P, et al. Clinical outcome of patients with follicular lymphoma receiving chemoimmunotherapy in the PRIMA study is not affected by FCGR3A and FCGR2A polymorphisms. *Blood.* (2012) 120:2650–7. doi: 10.1182/blood-2012–05-431825

39. Kenkre VP, Hong F, Cerhan JR, Lewis M, Sullivan L, Williams ME, et al. Fc Gamma Receptor 3A and 2A Polymorphisms Do Not Predict Response to Rituximab in Follicular Lymphoma. *Clin Cancer Res.* (2016) 22:821–6. doi: 10.1158/1078-0432.CCR-15-1848

40. Stebbings R, Findlay L, Edwards C, Eastwood D, Bird C, North D, et al. "Cytokine storm" in the phase I trial of monoclonal antibody TGN1412: better understanding the causes to improve preclinical testing of immunotherapeutics. *J Immunol.* (2007) 179:3325–31. doi: 10.4049/jimmunol.179.5.3325

41. Mata MM, Mahmood F, Sowell RT, Baum LL. Effects of cryopreservation on effector cells for antibody dependent cell-mediated cytotoxicity (ADCC) and natural killer (NK) cell activity in (51)Cr-release and CD107a assays. *J Immunol Methods.* (2014) 406:1–9. doi: 10.1016/j.jim.2014.01.017

42. Coles AJ, Twyman CL, Arnold DL, Cohen JA, Confavreux C, Fox EJ, et al. Alemtuzumab for patients with relapsing multiple sclerosis after disease-modifying therapy: a randomised controlled phase 3 trial. *Lancet.* (2012) 380:1829–39. doi: 10.1016/S0140-6736(12)61768-1

43. Bruhns P, Jonsson F. Mouse and human FcR effector functions. *Immunol Rev.* (2015) 268:25–51. doi: 10.1111/imr.12350

44. Nimmerjahn F, Ravetch JV. Fcgamma receptors as regulators of immune responses. *Nat Rev Immunol.* (2008) 8:34–47. doi: 10.1038/nri2206

45. Sun JC, Madera S, Bezman NA, Beilke JN, Kaplan MH, Lanier LL. Proinflammatory cytokine signaling required for the generation of natural killer cell memory. *J Exp Med.* (2012) 209:947–54. doi: 10.1084/jem.20111760

46. Sturge CR, Benson A, Raetz M, Wilhelm CL, Mirpuri J, Vitetta ES, et al. TLR-independent neutrophil-derived IFN-gamma is important for host resistance to intracellular pathogens. *Proc Natl Acad Sci USA.* (2013) 110:10711–6. doi: 10.1073/pnas.1307868110

47. van der Heijden J, Nagelkerke S, Zhao X, Geissler J, Rispens T, van den Berg TK, et al. Haplotypes of FcgammaRIIa and FcgammaRIIIb polymorphic variants influence IgG-mediated responses in neutrophils. *J Immunol.* (2014) 192:2715–21. doi: 10.4049/jimmunol. 1203570

48. Mandelboim O, Malik P, Davis DM, Jo CH, Boyson JE, Strominger JL. Human CD16 as a lysis receptor mediating direct natural killer cell cytotoxicity. *Proc Natl Acad Sci USA.* (1999) 96:5640–4. doi: 10.1073/pnas.96. 10.5640

49. Grugan KD, McCabe FL, Kinder M, Greenplate AR, Harman BC, Ekert JE, et al. Tumor-associated macrophages promote invasion while retaining Fc-dependent anti-tumor function. *J Immunol.* (2012) 189:5457–66. doi: 10.4049/jimmunol. 1201889

50. Bryceson YT, March ME, Ljunggren HG, Long EO. Synergy among receptors on resting NK cells for the activation of natural cytotoxicity and cytokine secretion. *Blood.* (2006) 107:159–66. doi: 10.1182/blood-2005-04-1351

15

Functional Roles of the IgM Fc Receptor in the Immune System

Hiromi Kubagawa[1]*, Kazuhito Honjo[2], Naganari Ohkura[3], Shimon Sakaguchi[3], Andreas Radbruch[1], Fritz Melchers[1]* and Peter K. Jani[1]*

[1] *Deutsches Rheuma-Forschungszentrum, Berlin, Germany,* [2] *Department of Medicine, School of Medicine, University of Alabama at Birmingham, Birmingham, AL, United States,* [3] *Immunology Frontier Research Center, Osaka University, Osaka, Japan*

*Correspondence:
Fritz Melchers
fritz.melchers@unibas.ch
Peter K. Jani
jani.peter.k@gmail.com
Hiromi Kubagawa
hiromi.kubagawa@drfz.de

It is now evident from studies of mice unable to secrete IgM that both non-immune "natural" and antigen-induced "immune" IgM are important for protection against pathogens and for regulation of immune responses to self-antigens. Since identification of its Fc receptor (FcμR) by a functional cloning strategy in 2009, the roles of FcμR in these IgM effector functions have begun to be explored. Unlike Fc receptors for switched Ig isotypes (e.g., FcγRs, FcεRs, FcαR, Fcα/μR, pIgR, FcRn), FcμR is selectively expressed by lymphocytes: B, T, and NK cells in humans and only B cells in mice. FcμR may have dual signaling ability: one through a potential as yet unidentified adaptor protein non-covalently associating with the FcμR ligand-binding chain via a His in transmembrane segment and the other through its own Tyr and Ser residues in the cytoplasmic tail. FcμR binds pentameric and hexameric IgM with a high avidity of ~ 10 nM in solution, but more efficiently binds IgM when it is attached to a membrane component via its Fab region on the same cell surface (*cis* engagement). Four different laboratories have generated *Fcmr*-ablated mice and eight different groups of investigators have examined the resultant phenotypes. There have been some clear discrepancies reported that appear to be due to factors including differences in the exons of *Fcmr* that were targeted to generate the knockouts. One common feature among these different mutant mice, however, is their propensity to produce autoantibodies of both IgM and IgG isotypes. In this review, we briefly describe recent findings concerning the functions of FcμR in both mice and humans and propose a model for how FcμR plays a regulatory role in B cell tolerance.

Keywords: FcμR, autoantibody, natural IgM, tolerance, Mott cell, epigenetics

INTRODUCTION

Two forms of IgM exist that differ in the carboxyl terminus of the heavy chain (HC). Alternative splicing with a transmembrane exon (μm) generates monomeric membrane-bound IgM as a B cell receptor (BCR) for antigen and with a secretory exon (μs) polymeric IgM secreted by plasma cell as a component of humoral immunity. The secreted form of IgM consists mainly of J chain-containing pentamers. The existence of J chain-deficient hexamers has also been reported albeit at an unknown concentration. To determine the role of secreted IgM in immune responses, two different groups have independently disrupted the exon encoding the μs (μs KO) (1, 2). Such mutant mice normally express IgM and other Ig isotypes on the surface of B cells and secrete all Ig isotypes except for IgM. These mutant mice are unable to control infections, because of inefficient induction of a protective IgG antibody response (3–5). Paradoxically, the autoimmune pathology associated with IgG autoantibody is more severe in μs KO mice than in the control mice, possibly because of impaired clearance of autoantigen-containing apoptotic cells (6, 7). Yet, no studies have directly demonstrated such deficiency in removal of self-antigens. Thus, both natural and immune IgM are important for protection against pathogens as well as in regulation of immune responses to self-antigens (8).

A variety of secreted and cell surface proteins is involved in binding the Fc portion of antibody, thereby participating in its effector function, e.g., complement and various types of Fc receptors (FcRs). Classical FcRs for switched Ig isotypes (i.e., FcγRs, FcεRI, FcαR), the receptor for polymeric IgA and IgM (pIgR), the low affinity FcεRII/CD23, and the FcR for neonatal IgG (FcRn) have thus far extensively been characterized at both genetic and protein levels (9–17) (see also other articles in this issue), and much of the knowledge gained has now been translated to clinical practice (18, 19). On the other hand, the role of the IgM FcR (FcμR) as an effector molecule for IgM antibody, the first Ig isotype appearing during phylogeny, ontogeny and immune responses, has just begun to be explored, since the *FCMR* was identified in 2009 (20). Several FcμR review articles have recently been published elsewhere (21–25). Here we briefly reiterate the biochemical structure of the FcμR and its functional roles in the development of B cell subsets and plasma cells, describe the potential molecular bases for certain discrepancies observed among different *Fcmr* KO mice, and introduce our theoretical model for how FcμR is involved in B cell tolerance.

UNIQUE PROPERTIES OF FcμR

Dual Signaling Ability
FCMR is a single copy gene located on chromosome 1q32.2 adjacent to two other IgM-binding receptors *PIGR* and *FCAMR* (FcR for IgA and IgM) (20). The predicted human FcμR is a type I glycoprotein of 390 amino acids (aa) with a peptide core of $\sim$41 kD, which consists of a signal peptide, a V-set Ig-like domain responsible for Fcμ binding, an additional extracellular region with unknown domain structure (termed the stalk region), a transmembrane (TM) segment containing a charged His residue (H^{253}) and a relatively long cytoplasmic (CY) tail of 118 aa containing conserved, three Tyr and five Ser residues (see **Figure 1A**). Among these Tyr residues, the carboxyl terminal Y^{385} matches the Ig tail Tyr motif (DYxN; x indicates any aa) seen in IgG and IgE (26), but the other two do not correspond to any known Tyr-based signaling motifs, ITAM, ITIM or switch. Two carboxyl terminal Y^{366} and Y^{385} are involved in receptor-mediated endocytosis (27, 28) and the membrane proximal Y^{315} is predominantly involved in the FcμR-mediated protection from IgM anti-Fas monoclonal antibody (mAb)-induced apoptosis (28) (see below). An important role of the H^{253} residue in anchoring the receptor in the plasma membrane became evident when the fate of IgM bound to FcμR in cells stably expressing the wild type (WT) or H253F mutant form of receptor was examined by immunofluorescence microscopy; the mutant showed enhanced cap formation even at 4°C. IgM ligand-binding

activity was found significantly increased in an FcμR mutant with a deletion of most of the CY tail compared to the WT receptor, despite comparable surface levels as determined by receptor-specific mAbs. Based on our preliminary data, this enhancement appears to result from the formation of an oligomeric FcμR as a consequence of its presumably mobile nature within the plasma membrane. This is different from our speculated inside-out regulation of FcμR ligand binding by its CY tail as seen in integrins. Ligation of FcμR with preformed soluble IgM immune complexes induced phosphorylation of both Tyr and Ser residues (20). Intriguingly, the phosphorylated FcμR migrated faster on SDS-PAGE than the unphosphorylated form, unlike most proteins that run slower when phosphorylated. Preliminary data with an epitope-tagged FcμR suggest that there could be cleavage of the CY tail of FcμR, but the precise molecular mechanisms for this cleavage and the functional role of the resultant FcμR stub still need to be elucidated. Collectively, these features of human FcμR suggest a dual signaling ability of FcμR: one via a potential as yet unidentified adaptor protein non-covalently associating with the FcμR via the H^{253} residue and the other from its own Tyr and Ser residues in the CY tail.

While mouse ortholog with 422 aa has relatively low homology ($\sim$54%) with human FcμR, the overall structural characteristics (a single Ig-like domain, a His residue in TM segment, and a long CY tail containing three Tyr and five Ser residues) are conserved. However, the analysis of its biochemical nature including the ligand binding is limited (22, 29).

Lymphocyte-Restricted Distribution
Given the fact that IgM is the first Ig isotype to appear during phylogeny, ontogeny and immune responses, we initially thought that FcμR would have a broad cellular distribution, thereby serving as a first line of defense against pathogens. On the contrary, FcμR was found to be expressed by lymphocytes only: both B and T cells and, to a lesser extent, NK cells in humans, and only B cells in mice (20, 29–32). Unlike the phylogenetically broad distribution of IgM from jawed vertebrates onward (i.e., cartilaginous fish), computational analysis of existing genomic sequence databases unexpectedly reveals that FcμR appears probably in early reptiles and is found in all three major living (extant) groups of mammals (i.e., egg laying, marsupial and placental mammals) (33). FcμR is the only FcR constitutively expressed on human T cells, which are otherwise generally negative for FcRs, and for B cells, FcμR is the only IgM-binding FcR expressed. [In this regard, another IgM-binding receptor, Fcα/μR, was initially reported to be expressed by B cells, but subsequent analyses revealed that the major cell type expressing Fcα/μR in immune system is a follicular dendritic cell in both humans and mice (34).] During B-lineage differentiation, the cell surface expression of FcμR was detectable from pre-B/B transitional stage to plasmablasts, except for a transient down-modulation during germinal center reactions in both humans and mice (20, 29, 30, 32, 35). Collectively, the restriction of FcμR expression to adaptive immune cells is thus remarkable, because FcRs for switched Ig isotypes are expressed by various hematopoietic cells including myeloid cells as central mediators

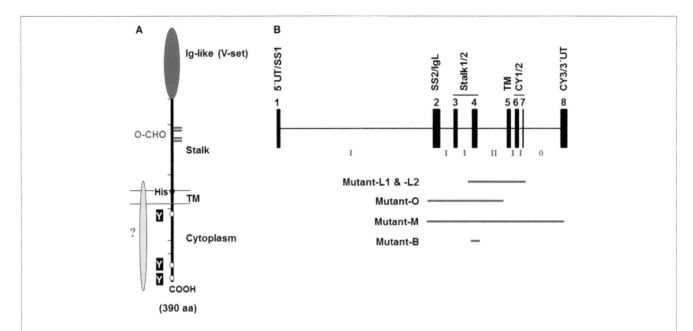

FIGURE 1 | Schematic representation of the FcμR. **(A)** Predicted FcμR protein structure. The human FcμR cDNA encodes a type I transmembrane protein of 390 aa with a peptide core of ~41 kD that consists of a signal peptide (not shown), an Ig-like domain (V-set), remaining extracellular (stalk), transmembrane (TM; between two lines) and cytoplasmic region. Black and brown hatch marks indicate exon boundaries in the *FCMR* gene and O-glycosylation sites, respectively. Small black and yellow circles indicate a TM charged His residue and conserved Tyr residues, respectively. A green fusiform indicates a hypothetical adaptor protein non-covalently associating with the FcμR ligand-binding chain via the His residue. **(B)** Schematic representation of targeted exons in *Fcmr*-ablated mice. The exon (black closed boxes) organization of *Fcmr* is drawn along with intron phases ("phase 0" indicates between the codons; "phase I" between the first and second nucleotide of a codon; "phase II" between the second and third nucleotide). Exons encoding particular regions of the receptor are denoted as follows: the 5′ untranslated (5′UT), the signal peptide (SS1 and 2), the Ig-like domain (IgL), the uncharacterized extracellular (Stalk 1 and 2), the transmembrane (TM), the cytoplasmic (CY1-3), and the 3′ untranslated (3′UT) regions. Red lines indicate the exons targeted in each *Fcmr* knockout mouse strain (see text for details).

coupling innate and adaptive immune responses. Lymphocyte-specific FcμR may thus have a distinct function from myeloid cell FcRs.

Cis Engagement

Cell surface FcμR in humans is a sialoglycoprotein of ~60 kD and one third of the relative molecular mass of the mature FcμR is thus made up of O-linked glycans. It exclusively binds the Fc portion of pentameric and hexameric IgM with strikingly high avidity of ~10 nM as determined by Scatchard plot analysis with the assumption of a 1:1 stoichiometry of FcμR to IgM (20, 25) (**Figure 2A**). Much higher concentrations (>100-fold) are required for binding of monomeric IgM to FcμR-bearing cells, indicating the importance of IgM conformation. This in turn suggests that serum IgM, at its serum concentration of ~1 μM, constitutively binds to FcμR on the surface of lymphocytes. In addition to the high avidity for IgM in solution, a unique ligand-binding property of FcμR was observed when IgM mAbs to lymphocyte surface proteins were used as a ligand. When Fas death receptor is ligated with 10 pM agonistic IgM anti-Fas mAb, apoptosis-prone Jurkat cells undergo robust apoptosis within 1 day, but Jurkat cells stably expressing FcμR do not (**Figures 2B,C**). This finding is thus consistent with previously reported anti-apoptotic activity of Toso (the original name of FcμR) (36). [In this review we will only use "FcμR" as the name of the receptor, based on a recent nomenclature agreement (37).]

However, ligation of Fas with agonistic IgG3 anti-Fas mAb or co-ligation of both Fas and FcμR with the corresponding mouse IgG mAbs plus an appropriate common secondary reagent [e.g., F(ab')$_2$ fragments of anti-mouse γ antibody] had no inhibitory effects on the IgG3 Fas mAb-induced apoptosis (**Figure 2D**). This suggests that FcμR *per se* has no intrinsic activity to inhibit Fas-mediated apoptosis. The anti-apoptotic activity of FcμR depends on usage of the IgM Fas mAb and not on physical proximity of two receptors by artificial co-ligation as observed with ITIM containing receptors such as FcγRIIb and paired Ig-like receptor B (38, 39).

To determine whether the interaction of the Fc portion of IgM Fas mAb with FcμR occurs in *cis* or *trans*, a 10-fold excessive of Fas(−)/FcμR(+) cells as a potential competitive source of FcμR(+) cells was added into the assay but no inhibition of FcμR-mediated protection of Jurkat cells was observed (**Figure 2E**). This suggests that the interaction of the Fc portion of IgM Fas mAb with FcμR occurs in *cis* on the same surface of Jurkat cells (**Figure 2E**), but not in *trans* between neighboring cells (**Figure 2F**). Addition of >10^4 molar excess of IgM or its soluble immune complexes was required for partial, but significant blockade of such a *cis* interaction (**Figure 2E**), suggesting that the soluble IgM immune complexes are not potent competitors in the FcμR-mediated protection from IgM Fas mAb-induced apoptosis. However, when IgM mAb reactive with other surface proteins

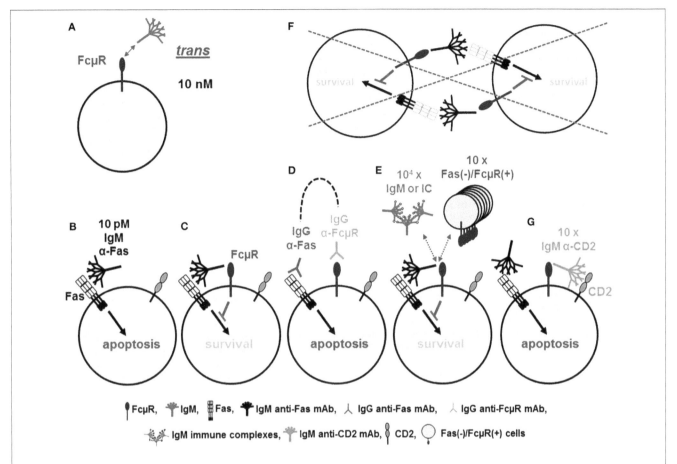

FIGURE 2 | Dominant *cis*, rather than *trans*, interaction of FcμR. **(A)** FcμR positive cells bind IgM pentamers in solution in *trans* with high avidity of ~10 nM. **(B–G)** Ligation of Fas death receptor trimer with agonistic IgM anti-Fas mAb induces apoptosis in WT Jurkat cells **(B)**, but not in FcμR-positive Jurkat cells **(C)**. Co-ligation of Fas and FcμR with the corresponding IgG mAb plus a common secondary reagent (dotted line) has no inhibitory effects on the IgG Fas mAb-induced apoptosis **(D)**. FcμR-mediated protection from IgM Fas mAb-induced apoptosis is not blocked by addition of 10^4 molar excess of IgM or its soluble immune complexes or 10-fold excess of Fas(−)/FcμR(+) cells, suggesting an efficient *cis* interaction of IgM Fas mAb and FcμR on the same cell surface **(E)**, but not a *trans* interaction between neighboring cells **(F)**. Addition of tenfold excess of IgM mAb reactive with CD2 on Jurkat cells can efficiently block the interaction of IgM Fas mAb and FcμR, resulting in apoptosis **(G)**.

expressed on Jurkat cells (e.g., CD2 or TCR) was used as a potential competitor, a 10-fold excess of IgM anti-CD2 or anti-TCR mAb was sufficient to block the *cis* interaction, thereby permitting FcμR(+) cells to undergo apoptosis (**Figure 2G**) (28). Similar results with agonistic IgM vs. IgG3 Fas mAb were observed with Epstein Barr virus-transformed B cell lines simultaneously expressing endogenous FcμR and Fas on the cell surface (20). Furthermore, when BCR and FcμR on blood B cells were co-ligated with a mitogenic IgM anti-κ mAb in the presence of IgG2b anti-FcμR mAbs with blocking or non-blocking activity for IgM-ligand binding, Ca^{2+} mobilization was the same in the absence or presence of FcμR non-blocking mAb. By contrast, the FcμR blocking mAb significantly diminished Ca^{2+} mobilization by blood B cells, suggesting that FcμR provides stimulatory signals upon BCR cross-linkage with IgM mAbs (28). Collectively, these findings of human FcμR indicate that although FcμR binds soluble IgM pentamers and hexamers at a high avidity of ~10 nM, FcμR binds more

efficiently to the Fc portion of IgM when it is attached to a membrane component via its Fab region on the same cell surface. FcμR expressed on lymphocytes may thus have a potential to modulate the function of target antigens or receptors when they are recognized by natural or immune IgM through its *cis* engagement.

In summary, FcμR: (i) is expressed by lymphocytes: B, T and NK cells in humans and only B cells in mice, suggesting that FcμR may have a distinct function compared to other FcRs, which are mainly expressed by myeloid cells, and potential species differences; (ii) may have dual signaling ability: one from a potential adaptor protein that non-covalently associates with FcμR ligand-binding chain via H^{253}, and the other from its own Tyr/Ser residues in the CY tail; and (*iii*) binds more efficiently to the Fc portion of IgM when it is attached to a membrane component via the Fab region on the same cell surface (*cis* engagement), than to the Fc portion of IgM in solution/fluids.

VARIANT RESULTS OBSERVED IN DIFFERENT *Fcmr*-DEFICIENT MICE

Despite the initial prediction of embryonic lethality of *Fcmr* ablation (40), there are now five different *Fcmr* KO mice that have been independently generated by four different groups of investigators [Lee et al. (mutant-L1 and -L2), Ohno et al. (mutant-O), Mak et al. (mutant-M), and Baumgarth et al. (mutant-B)]. Eight different groups of investigators have characterized these mutant mice with clear differences in reported phenotypes (29, 32, 35, 41–50) (see **Table 1**). This is an unusual case in the gene-targeting field. Several discrepancies could be in part due to the following: (i) Investigator's preconception of FcμR or Toso in terms of its cellular distribution (B cells vs. myeloid and T cells) (51, 52) and its function (binding IgM Fc vs. inhibiting Fas- or TNFα-mediated apoptosis) (53, 54). (ii) Differences in embryonic stem cells of C57BL/6 (mutant-L1, -L2, and -B) vs. 129/sv (mutant-O and -M) origin and the extent of the 129 mouse-origin DNA still present around the disrupted *Fcmr* gene after backcrossing onto C57BL/6 background; (iii) Differences in exon targeting strategies [exon 2-4 (mutant-O), 2-8 (mutant-M), 4 (mutant-B) vs. 4-7 (mutant-L1 and -L2) (**Figure 1B**)], global (mutant-O and -M) vs. conditional deletion (mutant-L1, -L2, and -B), and the *Cd19* heterozygosity in the CD19-Cre-mediated deletion vs. the unmanipulated *Cd19* in global deletion, and the presence (mutant-M) vs. absence (other mutants) of the *Neo* gene in the mouse genome; and/or (iv) other factors, e.g., ages of the mice examined, experimental procedures/conditions, environmental factors including intestinal microbiota, or reagents used.

Another factor that could contribute to these discrepancies is the relative difficulty in assessing cell surface FcμR in mice by flow cytometry using receptor-specific mAbs, because of its relative low cell surface density as well as its sensitivity to extracellular IgM concentrations, tissue milieu and cellular activation status (20, 29, 35). This vulnerability could result in the discrepancy in reported cellular distribution of FcμR in mice. In fact, using the same receptor-specific rat mAb (B68 clone), FcμR was expressed by: mouse B cells (55), myeloid cells (43) or CD4 T, CD8 T, and B cells (41). This conflicted cellular distribution data about FcμR is a major reason why some investigators created additional Cre/loxP-mediated, cell type-specific *Fcmr* deletion systems (35, 50). In this regard, EIIa-Cre mediated *Fcmr*-deleted mutant-L1 (equivalent to global deletion) showed more TNFα-induced apoptosis of CD3/CD28-activated CD8 T cells than control mice (41). The abnormality was initially considered as an intrinsic T cell defect since this group originally reported that FcμR was expressed by T cells. However, subsequent results from conditional deletion clearly indicated no phenotypic differences between T cell-specific [or dendritic cell (DC)-specific] *Fcmr* deletion and control counterparts. The only differences were seen with B cell-specific *Fcmr* deletion. The authors thus concluded that FcμR on B cells might indirectly affect certain T cell functions (50), although it remains unclear how this would work. In this review, we will focus on the following aspects of B cell-related findings in *Fcmr* KO mice: (i) alterations in B cell subsets, (ii) IgM homeostasis, and (iii) dysregulated humoral immune responses.

Alteration in B Cell Subsets

The development of B-lineage cells in the bone marrow (BM) was unaffected in most *Fcmr* KO strains (29, 32, 35, 50) except for mutant-M where the numbers of pro-B, pre-B, and immature B cells were significantly diminished as compared to WT controls (42). Since the surface expression of FcμR begins to be detectable at the transitional stage of pre-B to B cells in differentiation, it seems conceivable that FcμR is dispensable in developing B-lineage cells in the BM. However, it is noteworthy that: (i) μs KO mice, which are deficient for secretion of IgM, have significantly altered B cell development from pre-B to the immature B cell transition (42); (ii) this alteration of early B cell development is corrected by administration of natural IgM (56); and (iii) many of the abnormalities observed in *Fcmr* KO mice mirror those seen in μs KO mice. Thus, despite the fact that FcμR is a key sensor of secreted IgM, it remains to be elucidated why, among five *Fcmr* KO mice, only mutant-M has an alteration in development of B cell precursors (42). In this regard, several human pre-B cell lines express FcμR transcripts but not FcμR protein on their cell surface at detectable levels unless stimulated with phorbol myristate acetate (20, 57), suggesting the existence of post-transcriptional controls of FcμR.

Unlike in the BM, in peripheral lymphoid organs there were variable alterations in B cell subsets observed in these mutant mice but, as a general trend, *Fcmr* ablation was found to more profoundly affect innate-like B cells, B-1, and marginal zone (MZ) B cells, rather than the B-2 or follicular (FO) B cell compartment (see **Table 1**). Remarkably, an increase in B-1 B cell numbers, particularly in spleen accompanied by elevated levels of autoantibodies of both IgM and IgG isotypes, has been the sole result consistently observed in all five mutant mice. Thus, FcμR plays an important regulatory role in the homeostasis of B-1 B cell development and autoantibody production (see further discussion below).

For MZ B cells, the mutant-O had age-dependent alterations in their cell numbers, i.e., increase in young (3-wk) and marked decrease in old (>9-wk) mice (49). This age-dependent reduction of MZ B cells might result from their rapid differentiation into plasma cells in the absence of FcμR, as evidenced by the markedly elevated IgM autoantibodies to Smith antigen/ribonuclear protein, which are considered to be derived from MZ B cells (45). Alternatively, FcμR-deficient MZ B cells might undergo cell death due to lack of survival signals through FcμR upon BCR cross-linkage (49), as shown by cross-talk downstream of FcμR and BCR signaling via the non-canonical NFκB pathway (47). Notably, the reduction of MZ B cells was also observed with both Fas- and *Fcmr*-deficient, autoimmune-prone B6.MRL.*Fas^{lpr/lpr}*/*Fcmr* $^{-/-}$ mice (45). In mutant-M, unlike mutant-O, there were no changes in the MZ B cell compartment, whereas in both CD19-Cre-mediated deletion mutant-B and -L2, the number of MZ B cells was not reduced (for mutant-B) or enhanced (for mutant-L2) (35, 50). Since the number of MZ B cells in μs KO mice is increased by 3-fold and this increase can be normalized by passive administration of natural and polyclonal,

TABLE 1 | Phenotypic comparison of five different *Fcmr*-deficient mice.

	Lee et al. (mutant-L1) 4–7; C57BL/6	Ohno et al. (mutant-O) 2–4; 129/Sv					Mak et al. (mutant-M) 2–8; 129/Sv					Baumgarth et al. (mutant-B) 4; C57BL/6	Lee et al. (mutant-L2) 4–7; C57BL/6
Fcmr KO created by / Δ exons; ES cell origin													
Neo cond. KO	Removed Cond. KO (EIIa-Cre)	Removed Global del. (backcrossing with C57BL/6)					Not removed Global del. (backcrossing with C57BL/6)					Removed cond. KO (CD19-Cre)	Removed cond. KO (CD19-, CD4- or CD11c-Cre)
References (year)	(41) (2011)	(29) (2012)	(45) (2014)*	(32) (2012)	(47) (2015)	(49) (2018)	(42) (2013)	(43) (2013)	(44) (2014)	(46) (2015)	(48) (2015)	(35) (2017)	(50) (2018)
Distribution of FcµR+ cells	B68 mAb: CD4 T, CD8 T, NKT, B & Leuko. B in Sp, LN, blood	MM3 mAb: B cells; immat. B to plasma-blast in BM, Sp, LN	NR	4B5 mAb: B cells	4B5 mAb: B cells	MM3 mAb: B cells	mRNA: B, Gr-1+, CD11c+ in Sp	B68 mAb: granulo. & mono. in BM, Sp	NR	NR	NR	4B5 mAb: B cells; TGN in immat. B in BM	B68 mA: B cells
FcµR levels & function in WT mice	α-CD3/CD28 Rx of CD8 T: ↑ > NFB; B1 = B2 PerC: B1a = B2 > B1b	Sp: FOB > MZB > FOB		BM: immat. B > proB/preB Sp: MZB > FOB PP: non-GCB > GCB	α-µ Rx of B: ↑; co-IP of FcµR/IgM BCR; α-µ & α-FcµR Rx: ↑p52,↑BCL-xL		BM: immat. B > pro-B, pre-B; Sp: FOB > MZB > GCB, PC; PerC: B2 > B1a;					BM: mat. B > immat. B > late preB; Sp: MZB > B1 > FOB;	BM: mat. B > immat. B, preB
Lymphocyte populations in BM	NR	Not changed	CD19+ cells↓	Not changed	NR	Not changed	cells↓, proB↓, preB↓, immat. B↓, mat.B→	NR	NR	NR	NR	B1, B1a, B1b→	Not changed
Lymphocyte populations in periphery	Sp, LN and Blood: B↓, CD8 T →, CD4 T →	Sp: B↓, FOB→, MZB↓, B1↑; LN: B→, T→; PerC: T↑	Sp: B↓, B2↓, B1a & 1b →, MZB↓, PC↓	Sp:B→, FOB→, MZB↓, Tr3B↓; IgMhiIgDhi↑	NR	Sp: MZB↑ FOB↑ at 3wk; MZB↓ at 9 wk	Sp: cells↓, FOB↓; PerC: B1a↑, B2↓	NR	NR	NR	NR	Sp: B1↑, B1a↑, FOB↑, MZB→; PerC: B1→, B1a→, B1b→; splenomegaly (8 mo)	Sp: TrB↑, mat. B→, B1↑, B2→, FOB→; MZB↑; PerC: B1a↑, B1b↓;
Effect of Fcmr-ablation	↑Suscept. of act. CD8 T to TNFα-induced apoptosis Resistance to TNF/GalN-induced, iNKT-mediated liver damage	↑Basal serum IgM & IgG3 ↑Nat. autoAb of IgM, IgG3 & IgG2c ↑Ab resp. to TI-2 Ag (subopt. dose) ↓1° IgG1 & ↓2° IgM Ab resp. to TD-Ag	↑Basal serum IgM & IgA at early age ↑Nat. autoAb of IgM & IgG ↑MZB-derived IgM α-Smr/RNP Ab Rapid PC- diff. of MZB cells ↑Mott cell formation	↑Basal serum IgM ↑Nat. autoAb of IgM & IgG ↓Ab resp. to TI & TD Ags ↓Survival after BCR ligation ↓GC formation ↓Memory & PC-diff.	↓Survival of B cells upon α-µ Rx → BCR-mediated endocyto → plkBα & ↓BCL-xL after α-µ Rx	↑Cell death & turnover of MZB cells ↑IgD and MHC II on MZB cells ↓tonic BCR signaling ↓Ab resp. to TI-1 Ag ↑Suscept. to sepsis	Basal serum ↓IgG1 (3 mo), ↓IgG3 & IgA (6 mo) ↑nat. IgG autoAb Ab resp. to: TI-1↑, TI-2→, TD 1° IgG↓ & 2° IgG→ ↓prolif.→ & survival after α-µ Rx	→ Myeloid development ↑ROS after fMLP Rx of granulocytes ↓phagocyte Listeria ↓TNFα, IL-6 after LPS Rx resistance to endotoxin shock in vivo suscept. to Listeria inf.	Resistant to MOG-EAE ↓T & Mφ infiltration in brain → CD4 T function ↓DC act. & maturation ↑Treg diff.	↓Recruit. and act. of iDC in LCMV-liver ↓act. of CD8 T in liver fail to induce autoimmune diabetes	↓IL17A, ↓IL10 & ↑INFγ in Th17- polarizing cells	↑IgM BCR ↑tonic BCR signaling ↑basal serum IgM ↑ASC of IgM & IgG in Sp, BM ↑nat. autoAb of IgM & IgG ↑survival of unstimulated B1 & B2 cells.	↑Susept. to H1N1 infection in CD19-Cre mice only → Ag-specific CD4 & CD8T resp. ↓TNFα & INFγ by CD4 & CD8T ↑B cell survival ↑IL10+ Breg → basal serum IgM & IgG ↑natural autoAb of IgM &IgG

*Mutant-O mice crossed with Fas-deficient autoimmune prone B6/lpr strain.

α-, anti-; Ab, antibody; act., activation; Ag, antigen; ASC, antibody secreting cell; BCR, B cell receptor; BM, bone marrow, cond., conditional; del., deletion; diff., differentiation; FOB, follicular B cells; GCB, germinal center B; iDC, inflammatory dendritic cell; immat., immature; inf., infection; iNKT, invariant NKT; KO, knockout; LN, lymph node; MZB, marginal zone B; nat., natural; NFB, newly formed B; NR, not reported; PC, plasma cell; PerC, peritoneal cavity; PP, Peyer's patch; prolif., proliferation; ROS, reactive oxygen species; Rx, treatment; recruit., recruitment; Sp., spleen; subopt., suboptimal; suscept., susceptibility; Sm/RNP, Smith antigen/ribonuclear protein; TD, T cell dependent; TGN, trans-Golgi network; TI, T cell independent; Tr(3), transitional (3); WT, wildtype; ↑, ↓ & →, increased or enhanced, decreased or diminished, & comparable to WT control mice.

but not monoclonal, IgM, we initially considered that the FcμR and its signals upon IgM-ligand binding might play an important regulatory role in the fate of MZ B cells. This simplistic view, however, may need further consideration based on the above conflicting results.

In addition to the aforementioned changes in cell numbers of B cell subsets, there were some differences in the density of certain cell surface markers (e.g., CD19, CD21, CD23, IgD, IgM) between *Fcmr* KO and WT controls (29, 49, 50). The surface levels of several co-receptors of the BCR complex such as CD21 and CD23 were diminished in certain B cell subsets from mutant-O compared to WT controls (29, 50). This was also the case with CD19 that was also significantly diminished on BM immature B cells, but not on BM recirculating and splenic B cells in mutant-O (our unpublished observation). Notably, the surface IgD levels were higher on splenic MZ B in mutant-O mice than WT controls (49). Indeed, our subsequent analysis of the same mutant mice also revealed higher expression of surface IgD on BM recirculating and splenic MZ B cells, but not on FO B cells, than WT controls (unpublished). The molecular basis for this elevated surface IgD density in mutant-O is unclear, but it has been shown that functionally hypo-responsive anergic B cells are characterized by high levels of IgD BCR and generally turn over rapidly when competing, non-tolerant B cells are present (58, 59).

For surface IgM in mutant-O, IgM staining with fluorochrome-labeled anti-μ mAb, which might include endogenous membrane-bound IgM plus cytophilic IgM bound via FcμR or other potential IgM-binding proteins/receptors, was indistinguishable in these B cell populations including BM immature B cells (29, 49). By contrast, in mutant-B the cell surface expression of IgM BCR was significantly increased as compared to control mice, but this phenotype was only demonstrable 3 days after transferring of *Fcmr*-deficient or control B cells into μs KO mice to avoid the influence of cytophilic IgM (35). The authors implied that this increase in IgM BCR in *Fcmr* KO mutant-B was due to the lack of FcμR-mediated constraints on the IgM BCR (see below), resulting in enhanced tonic BCR signaling, facilitating the spontaneous differentiation of B-1 B cells and the increase in autoantibody production. Stimulated emission-depletion microscopic analysis revealed a strong interaction of FcμR with membrane-bound IgM in the *trans*-Golgi network (TGN) of BM immature B cells, but a weak interaction with the IgM on the plasma membrane in mature B cells, thereby constraining transport of IgM to the plasma membrane. This effect on the exocytotic pathway was proposed to regulate surface expression of IgM and eventually limiting tonic IgM BCR signaling. When we examined the potential interaction of FcμR with IgM BCR on the plasma membrane by fluorescence resonance energy transfer, we also found a very low incidence of such an interaction. By contrast, another group showed the physical interaction of FcμR and IgM BCR on the plasma membrane of mature B cells by confocal microscopy (47) and that tonic BCR signaling was diminished in *Fcmr* KO mutant-O (49). Given the low avidity of FcμR for monomeric IgM in solution, it remains unclear how FcμR could interact with membrane-bound IgM in the TGN of BM immature B cells or on the plasma membrane of mature B cells.

Another remarkable finding related to this issue came from immunofluorescence confocal microscopic analysis: strong staining of intracellular FcμR in a region corresponding to the TGN in murine BM immature B cells (35). The results were in close agreement with the findings of FcμR-mediated endocytosis of IgM by chronic lymphocytic leukemia (CLL) B cells in humans (27). The bulk of the intracellular FcμR protein resided in the TGN and in small vesicles, probably sorting endosomes of CLL cells. While the major function of the TGN is to sort proteins destined for the plasma membrane, endosomal compartment or specialized secretory granules, retrograde transport in the endocytic route to the TGN has been demonstrated for several proteins (60). It is thus worth considering whether DNA- or RNA-containing autoantigens are engulfed into endosomes by IgM BCR on immature B cells in the BM, two thirds of which are known to be autoreactive at least in humans, followed by retrograde transport to the TGN where TLR9 or TLR7 recognizes the respective DNA or RNA/IgM BCR complexes and then FcμR binds the Cμ3/Cμ4 of the resultant oligomerized IgM BCRs in the TGN.

IgM Homeostasis

The pre-immune serum level of IgM or natural IgM was elevated in most *Fcmr* KO mice (29, 32, 35, 50) except for mutant-M (42) and this elevation correlated with the number of *Fcmr* null mutant alleles ($Fcmr^{-/-} > Fcmr^{+/-} > Fcmr^{+/+}$) (32). The frequency of IgM-secreting cells in spleen and BM was significantly higher and the spot sizes in ELISPOT assays were also bigger in mutant-B than their control counterparts (35). FcμR was not expressed by phagocytic cells in spleen and liver including liver sinusoidal endothelial cells, which are thought to be the primary site of IgM catabolism at least in rat, as determined by both immuno-histological and RT-PCR analyses (29). The half-life of injected IgM was comparable between *Fcmr* KO (mutant-O) and WT mice. Thus, the increase in serum IgM levels in naive *Fcmr* KO mice is the consequence of lack of FcμR-mediated regulation of natural IgM production either at the B cell or plasmablast stage in innate-like B cells (29).

Dysregulated Humoral Immune Responses

Antibody responses to T cell-independent (TI) and T cell-dependent (TD) antigens were dysregulated in *Fcmr* KO mice as compared to WT controls, although there were some differences among mutant mice that might result from differences in mouse ages, antigen doses and forms, administration routes, kinetics, etc. Generally, mutant mice exhibited enhanced TI type 2 responses (involving multiple BCR cross-linkage) but impaired TD responses, especially at suboptimal doses. Since similar selective enhancement of TI-2 immune responses are also observed in μs KO mice (2) and mice deficient for components of the BCR complex such as CD19 (61) or CD81 (62), FcμR seems to regulate B cell responses to TI-2 and TD antigens by interacting differently with BCR complexes on the plasma membrane.

In summary, there are clear differences in reported phenotypes in five different *Fcmr* KO mice in terms of development of B cell subsets and plasma cells, IgM homeostasis and humoral immune responses. However, the increase in

B-1 B cell compartment accompanied by elevated levels of autoantibodies of both IgM and IgG isotypes is the sole result consistently observed with all these mutant mice.

EPIGENETIC FINDINGS IN THE *Fcmr-Il10* LOCUS IN Treg CELLS

One of the biggest discrepancies in the field is the cellular distribution of FcμR in mice (B cells vs. non-B cells). While several groups of investigators described the predicted functions of FcμR in non-B cell populations, their actual evidence for the surface expression of FcμR by myeloid, dendritic and T cells was rather weak (41, 43, 51, 52). Most of their functional results came from the comparative analysis in chimeras adoptively transferred by a mixture of *Fcmr* KO and WT BM cells or the direct comparison of cellular function between *Fcmr* KO and WT controls (43, 44, 46, 48). This was the reason why the phrase "functional relevant expression of FcμR" by non-B cells was used (52). Nevertheless, several functional outcomes in non-B cells from some *Fcmr* KO mice could be worthy of consideration because of the clear-cut differences compared to WT controls, even though they might be indirect or bystander effects. For example, mutant-M were resistant to the induction of myelin oligodendrocyte glycoprotein (MOG)-induced autoimmune encephalomyelitis (EAE). The authors initially considered that this resistance was not due to an intrinsic impairment of mutant Th1 and Th17 cell functions (see different observations by another group of investigators below), but rather to the immature and tolerogenic nature of mutant DCs, as characterized by their weak inflammatory responses and increased induction of Treg cells (44). Intriguingly, administration of a recombinant soluble FcμR fusion protein, which consisted of the human FcμR ectodomain and human IgG1 Fc (lacking complement binding activity) (FcμR EC/IgG Fc), into EAE-susceptible WT mice resulted in delaying or ameliorating their disease, depending on the time points of injection. While its mode of action was not discussed, it might be possible that since IgM anti-MOG antibody also participates in the demyelination process in EAE, the soluble FcμR EC/IgG Fc could simply act as a decoy receptor.

By contrast, results from recent single-cell RNA sequencing analysis along with complex algorithmic assessments and its functional annotation indicated that FcμR is one of the four critical regulators of Th17 pathogenicity in MOG-induced EAE (48). [The other three included *Gpr65* (G protein-coupled receptor 65), *Plzp* (promyelocytic leukemia zinc finger transcriptional repressor of the Th2 master regulator *Gata3*) and *Cd5l* (CD5-like antigen, apoptosis inhibitor expressed by macrophages [AIM], or soluble protein α [Spα]). Astonishingly, CD5L/AIM/Spα is a glycoprotein of ~45 kD secreted by macrophages, supports their survival and was originally identified as an IgM binding protein (63–65). Two out of four regulators identified for Th17-mediated EAE were thus capable of binding to IgM, although CD5L/AIM/Spα was annotated as a regulator of lipid biosynthesis (66).] Th17 cells polarized *ex vivo* by differentiation conditions with TGFß+IL-6 or

IL-1ß+IL-23+IL-6 from *Fcmr* KO mutant-M were found to secrete significantly less IL-17A and IL-10 than those from control WT mice (48). Mutant naive CD4 T cells exhibited lower FOXP3 levels during Treg cell differentiation upon TGFß stimulation *in vitro*. The authors considered that FcμR could be a negative regulator in a non-pathologic state but a promoter of pathogenicity (48), although it was difficult to understand its mechanisms. Given our findings that none of the sorted T cells with the phenotype of IL-17$^+$, INFγ$^+$, or IL-17$^+$/IFNγ$^+$ expressed FcμR transcripts, as determined by gene array analysis (25), it is hard to imagine how such a minor population of Th17 cells expresses functional FcμR, possibly at low levels, on their surface and plays a major regulatory role in the pathogenesis of EAE.

To explore the molecular basis for the resistance of *Fcmr* KO mice to EAE as well as for the reduction of IL-10 production by their Th17 cells, a computational epigenetic analysis was performed. Since *Fcmr* and *Il0* genes are ~139 kb apart from each other on chromosome 1, we analyzed the data of the histone post-translational modification by chromatin immunoprecipitation and sequencing and the assay for transposonase-accessible chromatin (ATAC) sequencing available for resting and activated Treg cells at the *Fcmr-Il10* locus (67). These included marks of acetylation of histone H3 at lysine 27 (H3K27ac) as a predictor of enhancer activity (68, 69), albeit not exclusively, and of ATAC as an indication of open chromatin (70). As shown in **Figure 3**, the H3K27ac marks are selectively observed in three loci, i.e., 3′ site of *Fcmr*, 5′ upstream of *Il10* and *Il10*, in activated Treg cells. The ATAC and H3K27ac marks coincided, suggesting that these loci were in an opened chromatin status, hence transcription factors would be highly accessible to these loci. Remarkably, the H3K27ac marks in the *Fcmr* gene of activated Treg cells were restricted to its 3′ region, i.e., exon 5 (TM) to exon 8 (encoding CY tail and 3′ UTR) and were absent in exon 2 (encoding the Ig-like domain responsible for IgM-ligand binding), consistent with the lack of functional FcμR expression by T cells. This 3′ *Fcmr*-restricted H3K27ac mark was not observed with resting Treg cells, suggesting that the potential enhancer activity of 3′ *Fcmr* in Treg cells was dependent on cell activation. By contrast, the H3K27ac marks in the 5′ upstream of *Il10* were observed irrespective of cell activation. Notably, several regions besides exons in the 3′ *Fcmr* were conserved in 40 other placental mammalian *Fcmr* genes as determined by phastCons (not shown). The above H3K27ac marks were not observed in early B-lineage cells, i.e., pro-B cells of either young or old mice. Collectively, these three loci [3′ site of *Fcmr*, 5′ upstream of *Il10*, and *Il10*] could be involved in enhancing IL-10 expression by Treg cells upon cellular activation potentially through a chromatin loop formation.

While the above epigenetic results of the *Fcmr-Il10* locus were derived from Treg cells, it remained to be elucidated whether a similar scenario was applicable for other cell types including Th17 cells. If so, *Fcmr* KO mutant-M, in which exons 2–8 were targeted, do not have this putative 3′ *Fcmr* enhancer element for IL-10 in their genome, and this could account for the reduction of IL-10 production by Th17-polarizing cells (48). For *Il17a*,

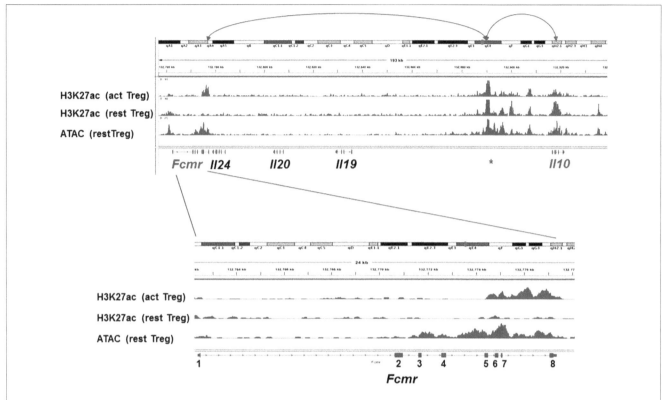

FIGURE 3 | Epigenetic status of the *Fcmr-Il10* locus in Treg cells. Top: Genomic locus (~180 kb) from *Fcmr* to *Il10* is depicted along with the chromosome 1 site designation, distance, marks of the acetylation of histone H3 at lysine 27 (H3K27ac) in activated (act) or resting (rest) Treg cells, marks of the assay for transposonase-accessible chromatin (ATAC) and the exon (square) and intron (line) of indicated genes. Red * indicates the unique region with high H3K27ac marks in both activated and resting Treg cells and of ATAC at 5′ upstream of *Il10* gene. Red arrow lines indicate potential association with the indicated loci by chromatin loop formation. Bottom: Enlarged illustration of *Fcmr* locus with coding exons numbered. 5′ and 3′ UTR regions are indicated by smaller squares.

which is located at ~110 Mb upstream of *Fcmr* on chromosome 1, whether the 3′ *Fcmr* enhancer element is able to form such a long-range interaction with the *Il17a* promoter is an intriguing question. It is also unclear how absence of the 3′ *Fcmr* enhancer element contributes to the resistance to EAE in *Fcmr* KO mutant-M. Nevertheless, given the assumptions that in single-cell RNA sequencing analysis, most identified FcμR transcripts might be derived from its 3′ region and that only the resistance to EAE as the consequence of *Fcmr*-deficiency might be functionally annotated for FcμR, it is thus conceivable and very intriguing that FcμR could be one of the four important regulators of Th17 pathogenicity in EAE, despite the lack of expression of functional FcμR by such T cells (48). Collectively, some of the discrepancies observed in *Fcmr* KO mice could be attributed to differences in the exons disrupted.

In summary, the epigenetic analysis of *Fcmr-Il10* locus reveals that three loci (3′ site of *Fcmr*, 5′ upstream of *Il10*, and *Il10*) may be involved in enhancing IL-10 expression by Treg cells upon cellular activation through chromatin loop formation. The epigenetic alteration selectively at the 3′ site of *Fcmr* may account for the functional abnormalities in non-B cell populations observed in certain *Fcmr* KO mice in conjunction with the exons targeted, even though functional FcμR is not expressed by such non-B cell populations.

FcμR IN CENTRAL DELETION OF AUTOREACTIVE B CELLS DEVELOPING IN BONE MARROW

The common feature among the different *Fcmr* KO mice is the propensity to produce autoantibodies of both IgM and IgG isotypes accompanied by increases in B-1 B cells, indicating an important regulatory role of FcμR in B cell development and central repertoire selection against those B cells expressing autoreactive BCRs. During B cell development in the BM, immature B cells are highly susceptible to deletion by BCR crosslinking. It has been estimated that ~90% of the newly generated BM B cells are deleted before entering the mature B cell compartment (71) and that approximately two thirds of the BM immature B cells in humans are self-reactive (72). During this development, the FcμR expression becomes detectable at the transition from BCR-non-expressing pre-B cells to BCR-expressing immature B cells. In three strains of mutant-O, -B and -L2 (29, 32, 35, 50), however, the sizes of the pro-, pre- and immature B cell compartments showed no alterations, when compared with WT control mice. Only one mutant-M had reduced pro-, pre-, and immature B cell compartments (42). Changes in sizes of BM B-lineage compartment might not become visible in such analyses, because such changes in the number of BCR$^+$ B cells might occur, as the immature B cells exit the BM. Furthermore, the peripheral compartments of immature and mature B cells may fill by homeostasis to unaltered sizes, though with either non-autoreactive or autoreactive B cells.

It is noteworthy that μs KO mice, which are deficient for secreted pentameric IgM, the ligand of FcμR, have significantly altered B cell development at the transition from pre-B to immature B cells (42). This alteration of early B cell development, including the inability to centrally delete autoreactive B cells, can be corrected by administration of natural IgM (56). Therefore, ligation of the FcμR by its ligand, pentameric natural, polyclonal IgM *in vivo* contributes to the negative selection of autoreactive B cells. It remains to be elucidated in this experimental setting whether immature B cells in BM are the prime target of this correction. If so, it suggests that the provision of pentameric, natural, polyclonal IgM binding to FcμR on immature B cells allows *cis*-crosslinking of autoreactive BCRs with autoantigen presented by pentameric IgM ligated to FcμR (**Figure 4**). This crosslinking would be expected to connect signaling from the BCR (e.g., via PI3 kinase) (73) with signaling from FcμR. If FcμR-signaling would downregulate PI3 kinase activity, this could lead to upregulation of FOXO1, which, in turn, could upregulate RAG1/2 expression (74, 75). In this way the immature B cells could continue editing V$_L$-J$_L$-rearranged light chain (LC) gene loci (76, 77) to change the autoreactivity of the BCR. Any loss of autoreactivity would abolish *cis*-crosslinking with autoantigen-bound natural IgM/FcμR, thus terminate RAG expression and allow immature B cells to leave the BM.

FcμR AND MOTT CELL FORMATION IN THE CONTROL OF AUTOIMMUNITY OF B CELLS

Another finding is the marked increase in Mott cells in mutant-O, even though it has only been described by our analysis (45). We propose that the FcμR may control autoantibody production by formation of Mott cells in the scenario described below. Mott cells are a variant form of plasma cells containing Ig inclusion bodies (called Russell bodies) that accumulate in dilated rough endoplasmic reticulum (ER). Mott cells are rarely observed in normal lymphoid tissues, but are found in various pathological conditions, such as Ig-associated neoplasms, chronic inflammatory diseases and autoimmune disorders (78–81). Several mechanisms for formation of Ig inclusions or for the defect in Ig secretion have been suggested, including (i) structural alteration of Ig HCs preventing their appropriate processing, (ii) impairment of Ig LCs in preventing Ig HC aggregation, and (iii) inability to degrade or to export Ig, leading to its aggregation. However, the most relevant mechanism associated with mutant-O seems to be that the Ig becomes stuck in the exocytotic pathway due to its autoreactivity with intracellular membrane components. Several precedents support this idea. (i) Two clonally unrelated IgM Mott cell hybridomas utilize germline Ig variable gene segments and have no obvious structural defects, suggesting their B-1 B cell origin (79). (ii) Ig inclusions are not generated when the Mott Ig μ HC or κ LC is by itself or is

associated with a heterologous κ LC or μ HC, respectively. The inclusion body formation is only reconstituted when Mott V$_H$ and Mott Vκ genes are expressed with an IgM, but not IgG1, constant region, suggesting that both specificity and isotype are critical for Mott cell formation. (iii) LPS or IL-5 stimulation of sorted B-1 B cells from autoimmune mice (NZB/W F$_1$) generates Mott cells *ex vivo* at a frequency of ∼50 times higher than conventional B-2 B cells (81). (iv) In studies of autoantibody transgenic mice, incompletely edited B cells express multi-reactive IgM that accumulates in the Golgi and is released or detached from the membrane as insoluble amyloid-like immune complexes termed spherons reaching up to ∼2 μm in diameter (82, 83).

Given these precedents and the preferential *cis* engagement of FcμR, the following scenario would account for the high incidence of Mott cells in the absence of FcμR. Incompletely edited B cells migrate into peripheral lymphoid tissues and express membrane-bound IgM with self-reactivity to intracellular membrane components (e.g., glycans). The interaction of the monomeric IgM with self-antigens in the ER must be of low affinity. However, when cells receive certain signals such as from TLR4 to facilitate a switch in the usage of μm to μs exon along with J-chain synthesis during transition to the ER-Golgi intermediate compartment (ERGIC) or the Golgi, the resultant pentameric IgM is contained inside the ERGIC/Golgi vesicles and binds a self-antigen on intracellular membranes via its Fab region and simultaneously the FcμR via its Fc portion. This *cis* engagement may prevent further differentiation of such autoreactive B cells, thereby contributing to the peripheral tolerance to self-antigens located on intracellular membranes (**Figure 4**). Based on this hypothesis, Mott cell IgMs in *Fcmr* KO mice are anticipated to have autoantibody activity to intracellular membrane components.

Instead of IgM-opsonized self-antigens, it may be equally possible that DNA and DNA-associated autoantigens or RNA and RNA-associated autoantigens are recognized by the respective IgM on BM immature B cells and delivered to an endosomal or lysosomal compartment where TLR9 or TLR7 binds the corresponding ligand-containing IgM BCR. The resultant oligomerized IgM BCRs are transported via a retrograde route to the TGN where FcμR may bind the Cμ3/Cμ4 domain of the oligomeric IgM BCR. In summary, based on the findings of enhanced autoantibody production in all *Fcmr* KO mice and Mott cell formation in our mutant mice as well as the *cis* engagement of FcμR, we propose a model for how FcμR on B cells plays a regulatory role in central and peripheral tolerance.

FcμR IN DISEASES

The association of FcμR with human CLL has long been suggested, dating back to studies showing that CLL B cells could form rosettes with ox erythrocytes coated with IgM antibody (84, 85). By flow cytometric assays CLL B cells also exhibited specific IgM binding (57, 86). Subsequently, several investigators showed enhanced *TOSO/FCMR* gene expression in CLL and initially considered that this enhancement would

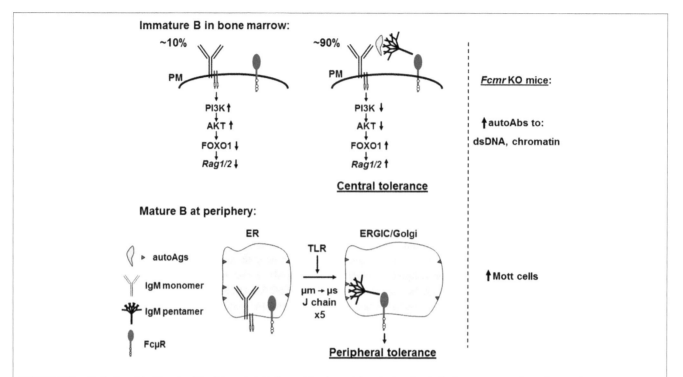

FIGURE 4 | Hypothetical model of the role of FcμR in central deletion and B cell repertoire selection. Top: In the bone marrow, only small populations (~10%) of the newly generated B cells bearing monomeric IgM (Y shape with Igα/Igβ, two purple lines carrying green ITAM) on the plasma membrane (PM) are survived by ligand-independent (or tonic) signals through activation of the PI3K-AKT pathway and suppression of the FOXO1-mediated Rag1/2 activity (left). By contrast, ~90% of the newly generated immature B cells have variable binding affinities for autoantigens (green leaf shape) and are subjected to negative selection by receptor editing or apoptosis (right). Autoantigens opsonized with natural pentameric IgM (broom shape) simultaneously bind the corresponding BCR and FcμR (blue tennis racket shape with three conserved Tyr residues in yellow). The resultant cross-linkage of BCR and FcμR on immature autoreactive B cells may inhibit the BCR-mediated PI3K-AKT pathway, resulting in relief of the AKT-mediated suppression of FOXO1 and leading to activation of Rag1/2 and receptor editing, thereby contributing to negative selection or central tolerance. In the absence of FcμR autoantibodies against dsDNA or chromatin are increased. Bottom: In peripheral lymphoid tissues, incompletely edited B cells express IgM BCR with self-reactivity to membrane components (brown triangles) present on ER membranes, but no interaction of monomeric IgM with the corresponding antigens occurs due to its low affinity. When cells receive signals from TLR, a switch from μm to μs exon usage occurs along with the synthesis of J chain during the translocation from ER to the ER Golgi intermediate compartment (ERGIC) or the Golgi and the resultant pentameric IgM is contained inside the vesicles where it binds membrane components via the Fab regions and its Fc portion binds FcμR. This cis engagement of self-antigen/secreted IgM/FcμR within the vesicles prevents further development of such autoreactive B cells, thereby contributing to peripheral tolerance. In the absence of FcμR, Mott cells containing intracellular Ig inclusion bodies are increased.

contribute to increased resistance of CLL cells to apoptosis (87, 88). We also examined the surface expression of FcμR by B and T cells in CLL using receptor specific mAbs by flow cytometry. CLL B cells (CD19+/CD5+) expressed significantly much higher levels of surface FcμR than B cells from healthy donors. This enhancement was more evident in Ig HC variable region (IGHV)-mutated, better prognostic, CD38− or early Rai-stage CLL than in IGHV-unmutated, poor prognostic, CD38+ or advanced Rai-stage CLL (89). Intriguingly, surface FcμR levels were also significantly elevated in non-CLL B cells (CD19+/CD5−) and T cells (CD19−/CD5+), especially in patients with IGHV-mutated CLL, when compared with the corresponding populations in healthy individuals. This increase in FcμR expression on T cells in CLL was unique, because normal human T cells activated ex vivo with anti-CD3 mAb or PMA down-modulated surface FcμR, whereas normal B cells activated with anti-μ mAb or PMA up-regulated surface FcμR (20). Regarding the enhanced surface expression of FcμR on CLL B cells, CLL-derived BCRs, unlike those from other

B cell malignancies, have been shown to ligate each other via interactions between Ig HC CDR3 of one BCR and the framework region 2 of another BCR irrespective of their IGHV mutation status, thereby providing antigen-independent cell-autonomous signaling (90, 91). This antigen-independent self-ligation of BCR on CLL cells could account for enhanced surface expression of FcμR as well as for the well-known phenomenon of reduced levels of surface IgM and IgD on CLL cells. It remains unclear, however, why surface FcμR levels were also elevated on non-CLL B and T cells in IGHV-mutated CLL patients.

Another remarkable finding was the marked elevation of serum titers of FcμR in CLL patients but not in healthy individuals (89). [One exception was an individual who was found 2 years later to have high serum autoantibody titers against dsDNA.] Detection of the serum FcμR was accomplished by sandwich ELISA using two different receptor-specific mAbs. It was resolved as an ~40 kD protein, distinct from the ~60 kD cell surface FcμR and found by proteomic analysis as a soluble form of the receptor (solFcμR), which was encoded by an alternative spliced FcμR transcript resulting from the direct splicing of exon 4 (stalk 2) to exon 6 (CY1), skipping exon 5 (TM). This splicing event resulted in a reading frame shift in exon 6 and generated a novel 70 aa hydrophilic carboxyl tail, thereby confirming the source of the solFcμR. The functional role of solFcμR in CLL and possibly in autoimmune disorders as observed with aforementioned exceptional control individual remains to be elucidated. In this regard it is noteworthy that administration of another form of solFcμR (FcμR EC/IgG Fc) into EAE-susceptible mice ameliorates the disease (44). Collectively, both membrane-bound and soluble forms of FcμR are elevated in patients with CLL.

Since among leukemia/lymphomas CLL uniquely expresses high levels of FcμR on their surface, two types of immunotherapy targeting for the receptor have thus been developed for CLL cells. One is an immunotoxin-coupled IgM Fc (Cμ2-Cμ4) and the other is chimeric antigen receptor-modified T cells using a single chain fragment-containing the variable region of an anti-FcμR mAb (6B10) (92, 93). In both cases, patient CLL B cells appear to be selectively eliminated *in vitro* without affecting the non-leukemic B and T cells. Apart from FcμR in hematologic malignancy, *FCMR*-deficiency has not yet been identified, but based on the data from *Fcmr* KO mice it may belong to hyper-IgM syndrome. Since FcμR is expressed by B, T, and NK cells in humans, the phenotypic abnormalities of *FCMR* deficiency in affected individuals are predicted to be more complex than those in *Fcmr* KO mice. In patients with selective IgM immunodeficiency, we initially predicted that surface FcμR levels might be high because of lack of ligand-induced down-modulation. Contrary to this assumption, cell surface FcμR levels on a particular circulating B cell subset with a MZ phenotype (IgM$^+$/IgD$^+$/CD27$^+$) in such patients were significantly diminished as compared to age-matched controls, but the molecular basis for this reduction remains to be elucidated (94).

In summary, enhanced levels of both the membrane-bound and secretory forms of FcμR are evident in patients with CLL, possibly as the consequence of antigen-independent autonomous self-ligation of BCR on CLL cells.

EPILOGUE

It has been known for many years that passive administration of IgM antibody enhances the subsequent antibody responses to antigenic challenge, whereas passive administration of IgG antibody suppresses the response. Complement activation, but not its lytic activity, has so far been implicated as a mechanism for this IgM-mediated enhancement, and the inhibitory FcγR is involved in IgG-mediated suppression (95, 96). The existence of FcμR on a variety of cell types has also been suggested for nearly 50 years by many investigators including us, but the FcμR cDNA was identified just 10 years ago by a functional cloning strategy (20). However, since FcμR turned out to be identical to the Toso cDNA, which was also previously cloned by functional strategy as a potent inhibitor of Fas-mediated apoptosis, there have been lively debates regarding the real function of this receptor, IgM Fc binding vs. Fas-apoptosis inhibition. While we have now a general consensus that this is an authentic FcμR, there have been clear discrepancies in the phenotypic abnormalities reported in five different *Fcmr* KO mice. In this article, we have discussed potential molecular mechanisms underlying some of these discrepancies. One of the remarkable outcomes of our analysis is the finding of restricted H3K27ac and ATAC marks to the 3' *Fcmr* in activated, but not resting, Treg cells and could account for some puzzles in T cell function described in certain *Fcmr* KO mice. Given the fact that all *Fcmr* KO mice are prone to produce autoantibodies accompanied by increased B-1 B cells, we introduce our hypothetical model for how FcμR controls autoantibody production. We see that FcμR has a very important role in immature B cell in the BM to control against the development of autoreactivity in B cell repertoire. We hope that this short article may help to resolve many still existing puzzles and will open new avenues of investigation.

AUTHOR CONTRIBUTIONS

PKJ performed the comparative analysis (**Table 1**). KH analyzed the FcμR ligand binding property (**Figure 2**) and the phenotype of mutant-O. NO and SS conducted the epigenetic analysis (**Figure 3**). AR intellectually contributed. HK and FM made the rest of figures (**Figures 1**, **4**) and wrote the paper. All authors listed approved for publication. PKJ was a scholar of the Alexander von Humboldt Foundation.

ACKNOWLEDGMENTS

We thank Dr. Peter Burrows for critical reading and Ms. Beate Löhr for literature support.

REFERENCES

1. Boes M, Esau C, Fischer MB, Schmidt T, Carroll M, Chen J. Enhanced B-1 cell development, but impaired IgG antibody responses in mice deficient in secreted IgM. *J. Immunol.* (1998) 160:4776–87.

2. Ehrenstein MR, O'Keefe TL, Davies SL, Neuberger M S. Targeted gene disruption reveals a role for natural secretory IgM in the maturation of the primary immune response. *Proc. Natl. Acad. Sci. USA.* (1998) 95:10089–93. doi: 10.1073/pnas.95.17.10089

3. Boes M, Prodeus AP, Schmidt T, Carroll MC, Chen J. A critical role of natural immunoglobulin M in immediate defense against systemic bacterial infection. *J. Exp. Med.* (1998) 188:2381–6. doi: 10.1084/jem.188.12.2381

4. Baumgarth N, Herman OC, Jager GC, Brown LE, Herzenberg LA, Chen J. B-1 and B-2 cell-derived immunoglobulin M antibodies are nonredundant components of the protective response to influenza virus infection. *J. Exp. Med.* (2000) 192:271–80. doi: 10.1084/jem.192.2.271

5. Subramaniam KS, Datta K, Quintero E, Manix C, Marks MS, Pirofski LA. The absence of serum IgM enhances the susceptibility of mice to pulmonary

challenge with *Cryptococcus neoformans*. *J. Immunol.* (2010) 184:5755–67. doi: 10.4049/jimmunol.0901638

6. Boes M, Schmidt T, Linkemann K, Beaudette BC, Marshak-Rothstein A, Chen J. Accelerated development of IgG autoantibodies and autoimmune disease in the absence of secreted IgM. *Proc. Natl. Acad. Sci. USA.* (2000) 97:1184–9. doi: 10.1073/pnas.97.3.1184

7. Ehrenstein MR, Cook HT, Neuberger MS. Deficiency in serum immunoglobulin (Ig) M predisposes to development of IgG autoantibodies. *J. Exp. Med.* (2000) 191:1253–8. doi: 10.1084/jem.191.7.1253

8. Ehrenstein MR, Notley CA. The importance of natural IgM: scavenger, protector and regulator. *Nat. Rev. Immunol.* (2010) 10:778–86. doi: 10.1038/nri2849

9. Ravetch JV, Kinet JP. Fc receptors. *Annu. Rev. Immunol.* (1991) 9:457–92. doi: 10.1146/annurev.iy.09.040191.002325

10. Daëron M. Fc receptor biology. *Annu. Rev. Immunol.* (1997) 15:203–34. doi: 10.1146/annurev.immunol.15.1.203

11. Turner H, Kinet JP. Signalling through the high-affinity IgE receptor FcεRI. *Nature.* (1999) 402:B24–30. doi: 10.1038/35037021

12. Ravetch JV, Bolland S. IgG Fc receptors. *Annu. Rev. Immunol.* (2001) 19:275–90. doi: 10.1146/annurev.immunol.19.1.275

13. Conrad DH. FcεRII/CD23: the low affinity receptor for IgE. *Annu. Rev. Immunol.* (1990) 8:623–45. doi: 10.1146/annurev.iy.08.040190.003203

14. Monteiro RC, Van De Winkel JG. IgA Fc receptors. *Annu. Rev. Immunol.* (2003) 21:177–204. doi: 10.1146/annurev.immunol.21.120601.141011

15. Nimmerjahn F, Bruhns P, Horiuchi K, Ravetch JV. FcgRIV: a novel FcR with distinct IgG subclass specificity. *Immunity.* (2005) 23:41–51. doi: 10.1016/j.immuni.2005.05.010

16. Kaetzel CS, Mostov K. Immunoglobulin transport and the polymeric immunoglobulin receptor. In: Mestecky J, Lamm ME, Strober W, Bienenstock J, McGhee JR, Mayer L, editors. *Mucosal Immunology.* Volume 1. San Diego, CA: Elsevier Academic Press (2005). p. 211–250. doi: 10.1016/B978-012491543-5/50016-4

17. Roopenian DC, Akilesh S. FcRn: the neonatal Fc receptor comes of age. *Nat. Rev. Immunol.* (2007) 7:715–25. doi: 10.1038/nri2155

18. Ravetch JV, Nimmerjahn F. Fc receptors and their role in immune regulation and inflammation. In: Paul WE, editor. *Fundamental Immunology.* Philadelphia, PA: Lippincott Williams & Wilkins. (2008) p. 684–705.

19. Schwab I, Nimmerjahn F. Intravenous immunoglobulin therapy: how does IgG modulate the immune system? *Nat. Rev. Immunol.* (2013) 13:176–89. doi: 10.1038/nri3401

20. Kubagawa H, Oka S, Kubagawa Y, Torii I, Takayama E, Kang DW, et al. Identity of the elusive IgM Fc receptor (FcμR) in humans. *J. Exp. Med.* (2009) 206:2779–93. doi: 10.1084/jem.20091107

21. Klimovich VB. IgM and its receptors: structural and functional aspects. *Biochemistry.* (2011) 76:534–49. doi: 10.1134/S0006297911050038

22. Kubagawa H, Oka S, Kubagawa Y, Torii I, Takayama E, Kang DW, et al. The long elusive IgM Fc receptor, FcmR. *J. Clin. Immunol.* (2014) 34(Suppl. 1):S35–45. doi: 10.1007/s10875-014-0022-7

23. Kubagawa H, Kubagawa Y, Jones D, Nasti TH, Walter MR, Honjo K. The old but new IgM Fc receptor (FcmR). *Curr. Top. Microbiol. Immunol.* (2014) 382:3–28. doi: 10.1007/978-3-319-07911-0_1

24. Wang H, Coligan JE, Morse HC III. Emerging functions of natural IgM and its Fc receptor FCMR in immune homeostasis. *Front. Immunol.* (2016) 7:99. doi: 10.3389/fimmu.2016.00099

25. Kubagawa H, Skopnik CM, Zimmermann J, Durek P, Chang HD, Yoo E, et al. Authentic IgM Fc Receptor (FcmR). *Curr. Top. Microbiol. Immunol.* (2017) 408:25–45. doi: 10.1007/82_2017_23

26. Engels N, Wienands J. The signaling tool box for tyrosine-based costimulation of lymphocytes. *Curr. Opin. Immunol.* (2011) 23:324–9. doi: 10.1016/j.coi.2011.01.005

27. Vire B, David A, Wiestner A. TOSO, the Fcμ receptor, is highly expressed on chronic lymphocytic leukemia B cells, internalizes upon IgM binding, shuttles to the lysosome, and is downregulated in response to TLR activation. *J. Immunol.* (2011) 187:4040–50. doi: 10.4049/jimmunol.1100532

28. Honjo K, Kubagawa Y, Kearney JF, Kubagawa H. Unique ligand-binding property of the human IgM Fc receptor. *J. Immunol.* (2015) 194:1975–82. doi: 10.4049/jimmunol.1401866

29. Honjo K, Kubagawa Y, Jones DM, Dizon B, Zhu Z, Ohno H, et al. Altered Ig levels and antibody responses in mice deficient for the Fc receptor for IgM (FcmR). *Proc. Natl. Acad. Sci. USA.* (2012) 109:15882–7. doi: 10.1073/pnas.1206567109

30. Shima H, Takatsu H, Fukuda S, Ohmae M, Hase K, Kubagawa H, et al. Identification of TOSO/FAIM3 as an Fc receptor for IgM. *Int. Immunol.* (2010) 22:149–56. doi: 10.1093/intimm/dxp121

31. Murakami Y, Narayanan S, Su S, Childs R, Krzewski K, Borrego F, et al. Toso, a functional IgM receptor, is regulated by IL-2 in T and NK cells. *J. Immunol.* (2012) 189:587–97. doi: 10.4049/jimmunol.1200840

32. Ouchida R, Mori H, Hase K, Takatsu H, Kurosaki T, Tokuhisa T, et al. Critical role of the IgM Fc receptor in IgM homeostasis, B-cell survival, and humoral immune responses. *Proc. Natl. Acad. Sci. USA.* (2012) E2699–706. doi: 10.1073/pnas.1210706109

33. Akula S, Mohammadamin S, Hellman L. Fc receptors for immunoglobulins and their appearance during vertebrate evolution. *PLoS ONE.* (2014) 9:e96903. doi: 10.1371/journal.pone.0096903

34. Kikuno K, Kang DW, Tahara K, Torii I, Kubagawa HM, Ho KJ, et al. Unusual biochemical features and follicular dendritic cell expression of human Fca/m receptor. *Eur. J. Immunol.* (2007) 37:3540–50. doi: 10.1002/eji.200737655

35. Nguyen TT, Klasener K, Zurn C, Castillo PA, Brust-Mascher I, Imai DM, et al. The IgM receptor FcmR limits tonic BCR signaling by regulating expression of the IgM BCR. *Nat. Immunol.* (2017) 18:321–33. doi: 10.1038/ni.3677

36. Hitoshi Y, Lorens J, Kitada SI, Fisher J, LaBarge M, Ring RZ, et al. Toso, a cell surface, specific regulator of Fas-induced apoptosis in T cells. *Immunity.* (1998) 8:461–71. doi: 10.1016/S1074-7613(00)80551-8

37. Kubagawa H, Carroll MC, Jacob CO, Lang KS, Lee KH, Mak T, et al. Nomenclature of Toso, Fas apoptosis inhibitory molecule 3, and IgM FcR. *J. Immunol.* (2015) 194:4055–7. doi: 10.4049/jimmunol.1500222

38. Ravetch JV, Lanier LL. Immune inhibitory receptors. *Science.* (2000) 290:84–9. doi: 10.1126/science.290.5489.84

39. Bléry M, Kubagawa H, Chen CC, Vely F, Cooper MD, Vivier E. The paired Ig-like receptor PIR-B is an inhibitory receptor that recruits the protein-tyrosine phosphatase SHP-1. *Proc. Natl. Acad. Sci. USA.* (1998) 95:2446–51. doi: 10.1073/pnas.95.5.2446

40. Song Y, Jacob CO. The mouse cell surface protein TOSO regulates Fas/Fas ligand-induced apoptosis through its binding to Fas-associated death domain. *J. Biol. Chem.* (2005) 280:9618–26. doi: 10.1074/jbc.M413609200

41. Nguyen XH, Lang PA, Lang KS, Adam D, Fattakhova G, Foger N, et al. Toso regulates the balance between apoptotic and nonapoptotic death receptor signaling by facilitating RIP1 ubiquitination. *Blood.* (2011) 118:598–608. doi: 10.1182/blood-2010-10-313643

42. Choi SC, Wang H, Tian L, Murakami Y, Shin DM, Borrego F, et al. Mouse IgM Fc receptor, FCMR, promotes B cell development and modulates antigen-driven immune responses. *J. Immunol.* (2013) 190:987–96. doi: 10.4049/jimmunol.1202227

43. Lang KS, Lang PA, Meryk A, Pandyra AA, Boucher LM, Pozdeev VI, et al. Involvement of Toso in activation of monocytes, macrophages, and granulocytes. *Proc. Natl. Acad. Sci. USA.* (2013) 110:2593–8. doi: 10.1073/pnas.1222264110

44. Brenner D, Brustle A, Lin GH, Lang PA, Duncan GS, Knobbe-Thomsen CB, et al. Toso controls encephalitogenic immune responses by dendritic cells and regulatory T cells. *Proc. Natl. Acad. Sci. USA.* (2014) 111:1060–5. doi: 10.1073/pnas.1323166111

45. Honjo K, Kubagawa Y, Suzuki Y, Takagi M, Ohno H, Bucy RP, et al. Enhanced autoantibody and Mott cell formation in FcmR-decient autoimmune mice. *Int. Immunol.* (2014) 26:659–72. doi: 10.1093/intimm/dxu070

46. Lang PA, Meryk A, Pandyra AA, Brenner D, Brustle A, Xu HC, et al. Toso regulates differentiation and activation of inflammatory dendritic cells during persistence-prone virus infection. *Cell Death Differ.* (2015) 22:164–73. doi: 10.1038/cdd.2014.138

47. Ouchida R, Lu Q, Liu J, Li Y, Chu Y, Tsubata T, et al. FcmR interacts and cooperates with the B cell receptor to promote B cell survival. *J. Immunol.* (2015) 194:3096–101. doi: 10.4049/jimmunol.1402352

48. Gaublomme JT, Yosef N, Lee Y, Gertner RS, Yang LV, Wu C, et al. Single-cell genomics unveils critical regulators of Th17 cell pathogenicity. *Cell.* (2015) 163:1400–12. doi: 10.1016/j.cell.2015.11.009

49. Liu J, Zhu H, Qian J, Xiong E, Zhang L, Wang YQ, et al. Fcm receptor promotes the survival and activation of marginal zone B cells and protects mice against bacterial sepsis. *Front. Immunol.* (2018) 9:160. doi: 10.3389/fimmu.2018.00160

50. Yu J, Duong VHH, Westphal K, Westphal A, Suwandi A, Grassl GA, et al. Surface receptor Toso controls B cell-mediated regulation of T cell immunity. *J. Clin. Invest.* (2018) 128:1820–36. doi: 10.1172/JCI97280

51. Honjo K, Kubagawa Y, Kubagawa H. Is Toso/IgM Fc receptor (FcmR) expressed by innate immune cells? *Proc. Natl. Acad. Sci. USA.* (2013) 110:E2540–1. doi: 10.1073/pnas.1304904110

52. Lang KS, Lang PA, Meryk A, Pandyra AA, Merches K, Lee KH, et al. Reply to Honjo et al.: functional relevant expression of Toso on granulocytes. *Proc. Natl. Acad. Sci. U.S.A.* (2013) 110:E2542–3. doi: 10.1073/pnas.1306422110

53. Honjo K, Kubagawa Y, Kubagawa H. Is Toso an antiapoptotic protein or an Fc receptor for IgM? *Blood.* (2012) 119:1789–90. doi: 10.1182/blood-2011-09-380782

54. Nguyen XH, Fattakhova G, Lang PA, Lang KS, Adam D, Foger N, et al. Antiapoptotic function of Toso (Faim3) in death receptor signaling. *Blood.* (2012) 119:1790–1. doi: 10.1182/blood-2011-11-386839

55. Lapke N, Tartz S, Lee KH, Jacobs T. The application of anti-Toso antibody enhances CD8(+) T cell responses in experimental malaria vaccination and disease. *Vaccine.* (2015) 33:6763–70. doi: 10.1016/j.vaccine.2015.10.065

56. Nguyen TT, Elsner RA, Baumgarth N. Natural IgM prevents autoimmunity by enforcing B cell central tolerance induction. *J. Immunol.* (2015) 194:1489–502. doi: 10.4049/jimmunol.1401880

57. Ohno T, Kubagawa H, Sanders SK, Cooper MD. Biochemical nature of an Fcm receptor on human B-lineage cells. *J. Exp. Med.* (1990) 172:1165–75. doi: 10.1084/jem.172.4.1165

58. Goodnow CC, Crosbie J, Adelstein S, Lavoie TB, Smith-Gill SJ, Brink RA, et al. Altered immunoglobulin expression and functional silencing of self-reactive B lymphocytes in transgenic mice. *Nature.* (1988) 334:676–82. doi: 10.1038/334676a0

59. Cyster JG, Hartley SB, Goodnow CC. Competition for follicular niches excludes self-reactive cells from the recirculating B-cell repertoire. *Nature.* (1994) 371:389–95. doi: 10.1038/371389a0

60. Bonifacino JS, Rojas R. Retrograde transport from endosomes to the trans-Golgi network. *Nat. Rev. Mol. Cell Biol.* (2006) 7:568–79. doi: 10.1038/nrm1985

61. Sato S, Steeber DA, Tedder TF. The CD19 signal transduction molecule is a response regulator of B-lymphocyte differentiation. *Proc. Natl. Acad. Sci. USA.* (1995) 92:11558–62. doi: 10.1073/pnas.92.25.11558

62. Tsitsikov EN, Gutierrez-Ramos JC, Geha RS. Impaired CD19 expression and signaling, enhanced antibody response to type II T independent antigen and reduction of B-1 cells in CD81-deficient mice. *Proc. Natl. Acad. Sci. USA.* (1997) 94:10844–9. doi: 10.1073/pnas.94.20.10844

63. Tissot JD, Sanchez JC, Vuadens F, Scherl A, Schifferli JA, Hochstrasser DF, et al. IgM are associated to Spa (CD5 antigen-like). *Electrophoresis.* (2002) 23:1203–6. doi: 10.1002/1522-2683(200204)23:7/8<1203::AID-ELPS1203>3.0.CO;2-1

64. Martinez VG, Moestrup SK, Holmskov U, Mollenhauer J, Lozano F. The conserved scavenger receptor cysteine-rich superfamily in therapy and diagnosis. *Pharmacol.Rev.* (2011) 63:967–1000. doi: 10.1124/pr.111.004523

65. Miyazaki T, Kurokawa J, Arai S. AIMing at metabolic syndrome. -towards the development of novel therapies for metabolic diseases via apoptosis inhibitor of macrophage (AIM). *Circ. J.* (2011) 75:2522–31. doi: 10.1253/circj.CJ-11-0891

66. Wang C, Yosef N, Gaublomme J, Wu C, Lee Y, Clish CB, et al. CD5L/AIM regulates lipid biosynthesis and restrains Th17 cell pathogenicity. *Cell.* (2015) 163:1413–27. doi: 10.1016/j.cell.2015.10.068

67. Kitagawa Y, Ohkura N, Kidani Y, Vandenbon A, Hirota K, Kawakami R, et al. Guidance of regulatory T cell development by Satb1-dependent super-enhancer establishment. *Nat. Immunol.* (2017) 18:173–83. doi: 10.1038/ni.3646

68. Creyghton MP, Cheng AW, Welstead GG, Kooistra T, Carey BW, Steine EJ, et al. Histone H3K27ac separates active from poised enhancers and predicts developmental state. *Proc. Natl. Acad. Sci. USA.* (2010) 107:21931–6. doi: 10.1073/pnas.1016071107

69. Rada-Iglesias A, Bajpai R, Swigut T, Brugmann SA, Flynn RA, Wysocka J. A unique chromatin signature uncovers early developmental enhancers in humans. *Nature.* (2011) 470:279–83. doi: 10.1038/nature09692

70. Lara-Astiaso D, Weiner A, Lorenzo-Vivas E, Zaretsky I, Jaitin DA, David E, et al. Immunogenetics. Chromatin state dynamics during blood formation. *Science.* (2014) 345:943–9. doi: 10.1126/science.1256271

71. Melchers F. Checkpoints that control B cell development. *J. Clin. Invest.* (2015) 125:2203–10. doi: 10.1172/JCI78083

72. Wardemann H, Yurasov S, Schaefer A, Young JW, Meffre E, Nussenzweig MC. Predominant autoantibody production by early human B cell precursors. *Science.* (2003) 301:1374–7. doi: 10.1126/science.1086907

73. Srinivasan L, Sasaki Y, Calado DP, Zhang B, Paik JH, DePinho RA, et al. PI3 kinase signals BCR-dependent mature B cell survival. *Cell.* (2009) 139:573–86. doi: 10.1016/j.cell.2009.08.041

74. Ochodnicka-Mackovicova K, Bahjat M, Maas C, van der Veen A, Bloedjes TA, de Bruin AM, et al. The DNA damage response regulates RAG1/2 expression in Pre-B cells through ATM-FOXO1 signaling. *J. Immunol.* (2016) 197:2918–29. doi: 10.4049/jimmunol.1501989

75. Benhamou D, Labi V, Novak R, Dai I, Shafir-Alon S, Weiss A, et al. A c-Myc/miR17-92/Pten axis controls PI3K-mediated positive and negative selection in B cell development and reconstitutes CD19 deficiency. *Cell Rep.* (2016) 16:419–31. doi: 10.1016/j.celrep.2016.05.084

76. Gay D, Saunders T, Camper S, Weigert M. Receptor editing: an approach by autoreactive B cells to escape tolerance. *J. Exp. Med.* (1993) 177:999–1008. doi: 10.1084/jem.177.4.999

77. Nemazee D. Mechanisms of central tolerance for B cells. *Nat. Rev. Immunol.* (2017) 17:281–94. doi: 10.1038/nri.2017.19

78. Shultz LD, Coman DR, Lyons BL, Sidman CL, Taylor S. Development of plasmacytoid cells with Russell bodies in autoimmune "viable motheaten" mice. *Am. J. Pathol.* (1987) 127:38–50.

79. Tarlinton D, Forster I, Rajewsky K. An explanation for the defect in secretion of IgM Mott cells and their predominant occurrence in the Ly-1 B cell compartment. *Eur. J. Immunol.* (1992) 22:531–9. doi: 10.1002/eji.1830220236

80. Jäck HM, Beck-Engeser G, Sloan B, Wong ML, Wabl M. A different sort of mott cell. *Proc. Natl. Acad. Sci. USA.* (1992) 89:11688–91. doi: 10.1073/pnas.89.24.11688

81. Jiang Y, Hirose S, Hamano Y, Kodera S, Tsurui H, Abe M, et al. Mapping of a gene for the increased susceptibility of B1 cells to Mott cell formation in murine autoimmune disease. *J. Immunol.* (1997) 158:992–7.

82. Khan SN, Cox JV, Nishimoto SK, Chen C, Fritzler MJ, Hendershot LM, et al. Intra-Golgi formation of IgM-glycosaminoglycan complexes promotes Ig deposition. *J. Immunol.* (2011) 187:3198–207. doi: 10.4049/jimmunol.1101336

83. Radic M, Weigert MG, Khan SN, Han J, Kalinina O, Luning Prak ET. Antibodies that bind complex glycosaminoglycans accumulate in the Golgi. *Proc. Natl. Acad. Sci.* (2013) 110:11958–63. doi: 10.1073/pnas.1308620110

84. Pichler WJ, Knapp W. Receptors for IgM-coated erythrocytes on chronic lymphatic leukemia cells. *J. Immunol.* (1977) 118:1010–5.

85. Ferrarini M, Hoffman T, Fu SM, Winchester R, Kunkel HG. Receptors for IgM on certain human B lymphocytes. *J. Immunol.* (1977) 119:1525–9.

86. Sanders SK, Kubagawa H, Suzuki T, Butler JL, Cooper MD. IgM binding protein expressed by activated B cells. *J. Immunol.* (1987) 139:188–93.

87. Proto-Siqueira R, Panepucci RA, Careta FP, Lee A, Clear A, Morris K, et al. SAGE analysis demonstrates increased expression of TOSO contributing to Fas-mediated resistance in CLL. *Blood.* (2008) 112:394–7. doi: 10.1182/blood-2007-11-124065

88. Pallasch CP, Schulz A, Kutsch N, Schwamb J, Hagist S, Kashkar H, et al. Overexpression of TOSO in CLL is triggered by B-cell receptor signaling and associated with progressive disease. *Blood.* (2008) 112:4213–9. doi: 10.1182/blood-2008-05-157255

89. Li FJ, Kubagawa Y, McCollum MK, Wilson L, Motohashi T, Bertoli LF, et al. Enhanced levels of both membrane-bound and soluble forms of IgM Fc receptor (FcmR) in patients with chronic lymphocytic leukemia. *Blood.* (2011) 118:4902–9. doi: 10.1182/blood-2011-04-350793

90. Duhren-von MM, Ubelhart R, Schneider D, Wossning T, Bach MP, Buchner M, et al. Chronic lymphocytic leukaemia is driven by antigen-independent cell-autonomous signalling. *Nature.* (2012) 489:309–12. doi: 10.1038/nature11309

91. Minici C, Gounari M, Ubelhart R, Scarfo L, Duhren-von Minden M, Schneider D, et al. Distinct homotypic B-cell receptor interactions shape the outcome of chronic lymphocytic leukaemia. *Nat. Commun.* (2017) 8:15746. doi: 10.1038/ncomms15746

92. Vire B, Skarzynski M, Thomas JD, Nelson CG, David A, Aue G, et al. Harnessing the Fcm receptor for potent and selective cytotoxic therapy of chronic lymphocytic leukemia. *Cancer Res.* (2014) 74:7510–20. doi: 10.1158/0008-5472.CAN-14-2030

93. Faitschuk E, Hombach AA, Frenzel LP, Wendtner CM, Abken H. Chimeric antigen receptor T cells targeting Fcμ receptor selectively eliminate CLL cells while sparing healthy B cells. *Blood.* (2016) 128:1711–22. doi: 10.1182/blood-2016-01-692046

94. Gupta S, Agrawal S, Gollapudi S, Kubagawa H. FcμR in human B cell subsets in primary selective IgM deficiency, and regulation of FcμR and production of natural IgM antibodies by IGIV. *Hum. Immunol.* (2016) 77:1194–201. doi: 10.1016/j.humimm.2016.10.003

95. Henry C, Jerne NK. Competition of 19S and 7S antigen receptors in the regulation of the primary immune response. *J. Exp. Med.* (1968) 128:133–52. doi: 10.1084/jem.128.1.133

96. Heyman B. Regulation of antibody responses via antibodies, complement, and Fc receptors. *Annu. Rev. Immunol.* (2000) 18:709–37. doi: 10.1146/annurev.immunol.18.1.709

16

Effect of Fc Receptor Genetic Diversity on HIV-1 Disease Pathogenesis

Daniel E. Geraghty[1], Christian W. Thorball[2], Jacques Fellay[2,3] and Rasmi Thomas[4,5]*

[1] Clinical Research Division, Fred Hutchinson Cancer Research Center, Seattle, WA, United States, [2] School of Life Sciences, École Polytechnique Fédérale de Lausanne, Lausanne, Switzerland, [3] Precision Medicine Unit, Lausanne University Hospital and University of Lausanne, Lausanne, Switzerland, [4] U. S. Military HIV Research Program, Walter Reed Army Institute of Research, Silver Spring, MD, United States, [5] Henry M. Jackson Foundation for the Advancement of Military Medicine, Bethesda, MD, United States

*Correspondence:
Rasmi Thomas
rthomas@hivresearch.org

Fc receptor (FcR) genes collectively have copy number and allelic polymorphisms that have been implicated in multiple inflammatory and autoimmune diseases. This variation might also be involved in etiology of infectious diseases. The protective role of Fc-mediated antibody-function in HIV-1 immunity has led to the investigation of specific polymorphisms in FcR genes on acquisition, disease progression, and vaccine efficacy in natural history cohorts. The purpose of this review is not only to explore these known HIV-1 host genetic associations, but also to re-evaluate them in the context of genome-wide data. In the current era of effective anti-retroviral therapy, the potential impact of such variation on post-treatment cohorts cannot go unheeded and is discussed here in the light of current findings. Specific polymorphisms associating with HIV-1 pathogenesis have previously been genotyped by assays that captured only the single-nucleotide polymorphism (SNP) of interest without relative information of neighboring variants. With recent technological advances, variation within these genes can now be characterized using next-generation sequencing, allowing precise annotation of the whole chromosomal region. We herein also discuss updates in the annotation of common FcR variants that have been previously associated with HIV-1 pathogenesis.

Keywords: next-generation sequencing, polymorphism, disease association, Fc receptors, HIV-1

INTRODUCTION

Fc receptors comprise a class of cell surface receptors expressed on various hematopoietic cells that bind to the Fc portion of antibodies to form immune complexes and recruit the complement and/or effector system to defend the body against pathogens. The Fc receptors are classified based on their binding to the Fc domain of immunoglobulin (Ig). The most abundant Ig in serum is IgG which can bind to different classes of FcγR. Other types of FcR including FcεR, Fcα/μR, and FcαR1 are receptors for other Ig classes such as IgE, IgM, and IgA.

More recently vaccine studies in infectious diseases point to a critical role of non-neutralizing antibody functions, which is the ability of an antibody to interact with other immune components and effector cells via their Fc portions to mediate killing or control of the pathogen. These mechanisms include, but are not limited to, antibody dependent cellular cytotoxicity (ADCC), antibody-dependent cell-mediated virus inhibition (ADCVI), antibody dependent cellular phagocytosis (ADCP), and antibody dependent complement deposition (ADCD) (1, 2). These functions are mediated by three distinct classes of FcγRs that are expressed on most human immune cells, with varying levels of expression dependent on cell type such as monocytes, macrophages, natural killer cells, eosinophils, neutrophils, B cells but not on T cells (3). These receptors include FcγRI (CD64), FcγRIIa/b/c (CD32), and FcγRIIIa/b (CD16), which bind the different IgG subclasses with varying proficiency, and can cause either activation or inhibition of the effector cell.

Polymorphisms in the FcγR have been shown to affect binding affinity to the Fc region of IgG and can trigger a range of effector and immunoregulatory functions. Such variation has been shown to play a crucial role in the pathogenesis of a range of chronic inflammatory and autoimmune diseases, as well as susceptibility to infectious pathogens (4, 5). An overview of FcγR biology has been recently summarized and so our focus for this review will be to evaluate the effect of genetic variation in the human Fcγ receptors and their role specifically in HIV-1 disease pathogenesis (6). Although there is evidence that the neonatal Fc receptor (FcRn), an MHC class I-related molecule expressed on many cells, functions in HIV-1 vaccination and infection (7, 8), no significant genetic variation has been identified for this locus, and we have not included it in this review.

FCγ RECEPTOR GENETIC DIVERSITY

The Fcγ receptors are encoded by the FCGR genes located on chromosome 1 in humans, including five FCGRs in a tandem arrangement within ~200 kb of genomic sequence (**Figure 1A**). A sixth gene, FCGR1A, is located ~12 Mb distant from the five gene cluster. Genetic variation at the FCGR gene cluster bears similarity to the Killer Ig-like receptor (KIR) region which is shown in comparison to emphasize both the types and extent of copy number and allelic variation (**Figures 1A,B**) (9). Like KIR, the genes in the FCGR cluster are arranged in haplotypes containing both invariant framework and copy number variant genes. An examination of total nucleotide variation in FCGR from a recent genome build indicates extensive depths of SNP variation, similar in overall extent to KIR and the vast majority of which has not been functionally characterized (**Figures 1B,C**). Both gene families encode receptors for other central components of the immune response (KIR and MHC class I; FCGR and IgG constant domains) placing them in distinct roles but perhaps of equivalent importance in investigations of host genetics and its relationship to immune function. Given the parallels in significance and the similar physical characteristics of both copy number variation and allelic polymorphism, a major difference is that the allelic variations for FCGR genes have been less examined, curated and annotated. This review in part is attempting to address this deficit as an organizing framework of characterized variation possibly guided by established methods for structural and allelic annotation as currently employed for the KIR system (10).

In the FCGR family of six genes, several nonsynonymous single nucleotide polymorphisms (SNP), SNPs encoding altered splice sites, and copy number variants (CNVs) encoding addition, or deletion of one or more gene have been functionally characterized (**Figure 1, Table 1**). Variation in the FCGR1 gene is limited, with the most frequent minor allele characterized at <4%, but there is considerable diversity in the other FCGR genes. The most studied SNPs in the FCGR genes over the past two decades have centered on nonsynonymous substitutions that contribute to differential binding affinity for subclasses of IgG. FCGR2A has two allele variants encoding arginine or histidine at amino acid position 166 (rs1801274), with the latter resulting in a higher affinity for IgG1, and IgG2 (11–13). FCGR3A also has two common allele variants differing by a single SNP, altering codon 176 from phenylalanine to valine (rs396991) resulting in a higher affinity for IgG1, IgG2, IgG3, and IgG4 for the 176V variant (11, 12, 14). This stronger binding affinity is associated with functional capacity of the receptor in different experimental and clinical contexts (15–17). Two adjacent nonsynonymous SNPs in FCGR2A (together altering codon 63 from Q to W; rs201218628) have been studied, although their functional consequence is less clear, and their frequency is rare (18). FCGR2B has an isoleucine to threonine change at position 232 (rs1050501), which alters the transmembrane region, with the 232T allele inhibiting the association of FCGR2B with lipid rafts in a human B cell line measuring downstream function (19). The frequency of this alteration is low at ~1% in Caucasians, and while more prevalent among African Americans and Asians (5–11%) has been less studied.

A major studied polymorphism in the FCGR2C gene is a SNP in exon 3 (rs759550223) that encodes a glutamine or a stop codon resulting in the presence or absence of protein expression (20–22). The frequency of the minor allele varies between populations, and studies have suggested it is expressed on NK cells and is capable of inducing ADCC after receptor cross-linking on purified NK cells as measured by their ability to lyse the target P815 cell line (20, 23). In addition, both alleles have been associated with both null and surface expression on NK cells as measured by anti-FCGR2B/C specific mAb 2B6 (22). However, there may be some confusion regarding this SNP as it is identical to rs10917661, which is assigned to FCGR2B, in a reference SNP identification (rs id) segment where the two genes have identical sequences except at the variant position. Sequence identity between FCGR2B and FCGR2C may lead to incorrect assignment of SNPs to these two loci. Also, rs759550223 has a very low minor allele frequency defined in the SNP database (dbSNP), and the minor allele assigned is identical to the FCGR2B-derived sequence, suggesting the possibility that the SNP has been falsely generated by a combination of variants between two distinct loci. FCGR2C has been previously reported to have arisen from an unequal recombination between the FCGR2A and FCGR2B genes, and encoded a functional molecule that exhibited differential expression in natural killer cells (21, 24, 25). However, FCGR2C is also classified as a gene/pseudogene in the NCBI gene database. These inconsistencies further emphasize the need of validation of the FCGR genes by a combination of methods such as next generation sequencing (NGS) technologies

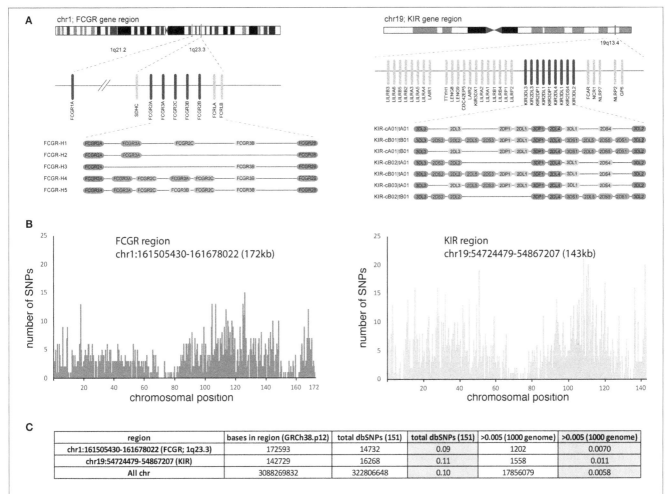

FIGURE 1 | Structure and polymorphism of the FCGR genes. **(A)** Approximate chromosomal locations of the FCGR gene complex containing 5 FCGR genes and the FCGR1A gene located at ~12 Mb centromeric to the FCGR cluster. In comparison, the KIR gene family is illustrated immediately to the right including adjacent genes (FCAR) and gene clusters. For both FCGR and KIR, alternative haplotypes identified in populations are illustrated with the colored bars depicting genes present in a subset of haplotypes and shaded bars depicting genes present in all haplotypes (framework genes). Figure depicting KIR has been reproduced with permission from the Oxford University Press (9). **(B)** The plots show the abundance of SNPs at each position of the indicated regions from chr1 and chr19, using data derived from the UCSC genome browser. **(C)** Approximate number of SNPs in both regions are listed including a summary from all chromosomes for comparison.

as discussed below, in addition to precise curating of allelic variation and flow cytometry phenotyping.

A triallelic nonsynonymous SNP at codon 66 (66R, 66L, 66H; rs10127939) of the FCGR3A gene has also been found to affect affinity for immune complexes (ICs), with the FCGR3A-66R and 66H alleles exhibiting higher affinity (26). Other nonsynonymous SNPs have been identified but none have been characterized functionally or in association analyses. FCRG3B polymorphisms were first described as the human neutrophil antigen (HNA)-1 system (27, 28). The three major HNA-1 variants have differential affinity for IgG1 and IgG3, with the higher affinity HNA-1a and lower affinity HNA-1b differing at 4 nonsynonymous codon positions (rs2290834, rs200688856, rs448740, rs147574249). Consistent with this differential affinity, phagocytosis was lower with HNA-1b through analysis of antibacterial IgG subclass antibodies and with IgG1 and IgG3 anti-Rhesus D (29, 30). A third isoform, termed HNA-1c, of

unknown function is identical to the HNA-1b isoform except at the rs5030738 polymorphic site, where it encodes an asparagine rather than alanine residue (31). Other variants of the HNA-1 antigen system have also been described but to date no functional or association studies interrogating them have been reported (32, 33).

CNV is a hallmark of multicopy gene family genomic regions, including notably among them, those encoding immune response genes (34). In the FCGR region, CNVs include at least five haplotypes with varying combinations of deletions and duplications of the FCGR2C, FCGR3A, and FCGR3B genes, flanked by the invariant framework FCGR2A and FCGR2B genes (**Figure 1A**, *left*) (34–36). FCGR-H1 forms the most common among these haplotypes, containing the five loci, with FCGR-H2 being the most commonly observed CNV [equivalent to CNR1 in Nederer et al. (36)] and FCGR-H3 less prevalent (equivalent to CNR2 or CNR3). Although variants FCGR-H4 and -H5 have not been explicitly described, they form predicted reciprocal structures of the H2 and H3 deletion variants (34). Individuals with FCGR gene copy numbers that may be consistent with those structures have been described (22, 34–38). As discussed above, older genotyping methods focusing on specific regions of the genes may have misassigned SNPs, and the lack of a standard nomenclature of common FGCR coding variants may lead to misinterpretation when comparing different studies. Newer NGS technologies have allowed for updated annotation of the FCGR genes as per the current Human genome database reference hg38. SNPs with a minor allele frequency >0.01 are shown in **Table 1**.

FCGR VARIATION AND HIV-1 DISEASE PATHOGENESIS

The first report of the effect of polymorphisms in the FCGR genes on HIV-1 disease progression was in two natural history HIV-1 cohorts consisting of anti-retroviral therapy (ART) naïve individuals (39). Since then, functional SNPs in the FCGR2A (rs1801274) and FCGR3A (rs396991) genes that affect binding affinity to the Fc domain of IgG have been evaluated in the context of HIV-1 acquisition, disease progression, and vaccine efficacy. Now that most HIV-1 infected individuals are on ART, there is an opportunity to evaluate disease outcomes after ART initiation. With increased high-throughput sequencing, targeted SNP genotyping is being replaced by whole gene and genome sequencing. This gives the opportunity to evaluate previous host genetic findings in the light of genome wide findings and also examine other SNPs in nearby genes. We will discuss the effects of genetic polymorphisms in the FCGR genes and their impact on HIV-1 disease progression, acquisition, post-ART and vaccine outcomes in the next sections.

FCGR Polymorphisms and HIV-1 Disease Progression
Candidate Gene Studies
Forthal et al. identified an association between the FCGR2A low binding RR (rs1801274) genotype and a faster rate of CD4+ T cell decline and progression to AIDS using samples and data from the Multicenter AIDS Cohort Study (MACS) consisting of more than 500 HIV-1 infected males of mostly Western European ancestry (40). Paradoxically, the same RR genotype was also found to associate with a decreased risk of Pneumocystis jiroveci (carinii) pneumonia, an AIDS defining illness, when compared to the HH genotype in the same cohort. At the functional level, cells from RR homozygous carriers demonstrated less efficient phagocytosis of HIV-1/IgG complexes. There was no association of the FCGR2A genotype with viral load setpoint (spVL), defined as the number of HIV-1 RNA copies/ml in a plasma sample collected 18 months after the first seropositive test. The absence of association of FCGR2A variation with spontaneous viral load control was also confirmed in an HIV-1 seroconverting cohort including 253 Kenyan women, in which the associations with disease progression and CD4+ T cell decline were not replicated (41).

No association was observed by Forthal et al. in the MACS cohort between a specific FCGR3A genotype (rs396991) and spontaneous viral control or disease progression (40). Similarly, Weis et al. did not identify any significant genetic associations of FCGR3A variation with disease progression or spVL in the Kenyan's women cohort (41). There is one report of the VV genotype of FCGR3A being overrepresented in 43 untreated controllers compared to 59 HIV positive progressors on ART (42). However, since the HIV positive progressors were on ART, analyses with measures of spVL or CD4+ T cell counts could not be performed and this finding remains inconclusive.

A more consistent finding has been reported by two independent groups showing the association between the FCGR3A FF genotype and decreased risk of Kaposi's sarcoma (KS) (39, 40). In the first study, FCGR3A genotyping was performed in two small cohorts consisting of 119 and 131 HIV-1 infected males of Western European ancestry. A significant association with protection was identified in each cohort independently and in the combined analysis. Forthal et al. replicated this finding in the MACS cohort. KS is the most frequent malignant condition associated with HIV-1 related immunosuppression, and alterations in the cytokine balance have been suggested to play a critical role in its pathogenesis. Differences in genotype have been shown to alter IgG binding that could influence cytokine levels, with the V allele having higher affinity than the F. The authors concluded that FF homozygous individuals might be at lower risk of KS because of a less vigorous proinflammatory response. The VV genotype has been associated with an increased risk of cryptococcal disease in 164 HIV-1 infected men, again in the MACS cohort (43). Of note, this observation extends beyond HIV-1 infection, because the VV genotype was previously associated with cryptococcal disease in non-HIV-infected individuals in a separate study (44).

Genome-Wide Testing
The associations with HIV-1 natural history described above were tested using a candidate gene study design in cohorts with relatively small sample size. The current availability of genome-wide genotyping and sequencing data provides an opportunity to reassess the potential involvement of FCGR variation in HIV-1 disease in larger cohorts, by applying more stringent standards for significance level and including robust population stratification (45). We therefore accessed previously published data generated from cohorts and studies that contributed to the International Collaboration for the Genomics of HIV (ICGH) (46–48) and assessed genetic associations with HIV-1 disease outcomes in the FCGR2A and FCGR3A regions.

The potential associations between FCGR2A or FCGR3A variants and spVL were evaluated using a fixed-effect inverse-variance weighted meta-analysis across cohorts, including a total of 7,266 HIV positive patients of Western European ancestry. We tested all common polymorphisms (minor allele frequency >5%) in a 50 kb window around the gene. In line with previous studies, no significant association with spVL was observed. An additional analysis was performed in a subset of ICGH, consisting of 467 long-term non-progressors (individuals with CD4+ T cell counts consistently above 500 cells/mm (3) for >10 years without treatment) and 517 rapid progressors

TABLE 1 | Characterization of variation in the Fc Receptor genes.

Chr. location (GRCh38.p7)	dbSNP rs#	MAF	Function	RefSeqGene (genomic DNA)	RefSeqGene (mRNA)	SNP variants[a]	RefSeqGene (Protein)	Amino acid change
FCGR2A				NG_012066	NM_021642.3		NP_067674.2	
161506414-161506415	rs201218628	0.006	Missense	6000_6001	184_185	CA>TG	62	Gln>Trp
161509955	rs1801274[d]	0.442	Missense	9641	497	A>G	166	His>Arg
161510070	rs150311303	0.008	Insertion	9657_9658	613_614	insTTC	205	Gln>GlnLeu
161510859	rs11810143	0.055	synonymous	10445	642	A>G	214	Pro>Pro
161510928	rs140474146	0.009	Synonymous	10514	711	G>A	237	Leu>Leu
161518073	rs12029217	0.121	Synonymous	17659	876	C>T	292	Pro>Pro
161518091	rs6694457	0.026	Synonymous	17677	894	T>C	298	Asp>Asp
FCGR2B				NG_023318	NM_004001.4		NP_003992.3	
161671501	rs148030870	0.010	synonymous	13387	243	C>T	81	Ser>Ser
161671594	rs6665610	0.138	Synonymous	13480	336	G>A	112	Thr>Thr
161671618	rs367584808	0.005	Synonymous	13504	360	C>A	120	Leu>Lue
161672984	rs200112434	0.109	Missense	14870	401	T>G	134	Val>Gly
161673192	rs2298022	0.029	Synonymous	15078	609	G>A	203	Thr>Thr
161673195	rs182968886	0.110	Synonymous	15081	612	G>A	204	Leu>Lue
161674008	rs1050501	0.186	Missense	15894	695	T>C	232	Ile>Thr
161675262	rs28651835	0.032	Missense	17148	766	C>T	256	Pro>Ser
FCGR2C				NG_011982	NM_201563.5[b]		NP_963857.3	
161589466	rs114945036	0.245	Intron	13128		C>T		
161589597	rs759550223	0.002	Nonsense	13259	169	C>T	57	Gln>*Ter
161589781	rs138747765	0.194	Missense	13443	353	C>T	118	Thr>Ile
161589930	rs78603008	0.195	Intron	13592		G>A		
161591153	rs370748254	0.134	Missense	14815	401	T>G	134	Val>Gly
161591361	rs74341264	0.199	Synonymous	15023	609	G>A	203	Thr>Thr
161591366	rs76016754	0.034	Missense	15028	614	A>T	205	Tyr>Phe
161599629	rs430178	0.259	Splice acceptor	23291		C>G		
161599779	rs138731942	0.075	Synonymous	23441	948	C>T	316	Asn>Asn
FCGR3A				NG_009066	NM_001127593.1		NP_001121065.1	
161543083	rs115866423	0.006	Missense	12541	694	A>T	232	Asn>Tyr
161544752	rs396991[d]	0.351	Missense	10872	526	T>G	176	Phe>Val
161548509	rs150808747	0.012	Synonymous	7115	231	C>T	77	Asp>Asp
161548524	rs114535887	0.019	Synonymous	7100	216	G>A	72	Ser>Ser
161548543	rs10127939	0.039	Missense	7081	197	T>G/T>A	66	Leu>Arg/Leu>His

(Continued)

TABLE 1 | Continued

Chr. location (GRCh38.p7)	dbSNP rs#	MAF	Function	RefSeqGene (genomic DNA)	RefSeqGene (mRNA)	SNP variants[a]	RefSeqGene (Protein)	Amino acid change
FCGR3B				NG_032926	NM_000570.4		NP_000561.3	
161626224	rs71632957	0.022	Synonymous	10740	498	T>C	166	Asp>Asp
161626242	rs114169903	0.025	Synonymous	10722	480	A>G	160	Pro>Pro
161629781	rs2290834	0.447	Missense	7183	316	A>G	106	Ile>Val
161629800	rs368410676	0.023	Synonymous	7164	297	G>T	99	Pro>Pro
161629853	rs147574249	0.284	Missense	7111	244	A>G	82	Asn>Asp
161629864	rs5030738	0.083	Missense	7100	233	C>A	78	Ala>Asp
161629903	rs448740	0.467	Missense	7061	194	A>G	65	Asn>Ser
161629983	rs527909462	0.135	Synonymous	6981	114	T>C	38	Leu>Leu
161629989	rs200688856	0.128	Missense	6975	108	C>G	36	Ser>Arg
FCGR1A				NG_007578	NM_000566.3		NP_000557.1	
149784005	rs138447715	0.034	Missense	6274	55	A>G	19	Thr>Ala
149784064	rs80039899	0.017	Synonymous	6333	114	C>T	38	Thr>Thr
149784065	rs7531523	0.005	Missense	6334	115	G>A	39	Val>Ile
149784139	rs149926813	0.005	Synonymous	6408	189	T>C	63	Thr>Thr
149784147	rs144081076	0.004	Missense	6416	197	C>T	66	Ser>Leu
149784224	rs74315310	0.004	Nonsense	6493	274	C>T	92	Arg> *Ter
149788436	rs138510822	0.008	Synonymous	10705	378	G>A	126	Ala>Ala
149790290	rs587727639	0.008	Missense	12559	796	G>A	266	Asp>Asn
FCAR				Na[c]	NM_002000.3		NP_001991.1	
54885265	rs61735068	0.006	Missense		101	A>C	34	Lys>Thr
54885488	rs1865096	0.261	Synonymous		324	G>A	108	Arg>Arg
54885501	rs11666735	0.055	Missense		337	G>A	113	Asp>Asn
54888276	rs61735069	0.042	synonymous		631	T>C	211	Leu>Leu
54889758	rs77103719	0.006	Synonymous		759	G>A	253	Thr>Thr
54889796	rs61735070	0.006	Missense		797	C>T	266	Pro>Leu
54889804	rs16986050	0.155	Missense		805	A>G	269	Ser>Gly

[a]Only SNP variants with a MAF of >0.01 are shown.
[b]The status of FCGR2C has been recently changed from gene to pseudogene in genbank.
[c]No unique genome reference sequence has been defined for FCAR in genbank at this point.
[d]rs1801274 and rs396991 have been commonly referenced in the literature as FCGR2A-131R/H and FCGR3A-158F/V, respectively.

(individuals with two or more CD4+ T cell counts below 300 cells/mm (3) within 3 years after the last seronegative test result). We were unable to replicate findings by Forthal et al. and did not observe associations with HIV-1 progression (40). These analyses included the FCGR2A rs1801274 polymorphism; however, the FCGR3A polymorphism rs396991 was not available from the ICGH meta-analysis as it is not directly genotyped on most genotyping arrays and could not be reliably imputed. Thus, in order to evaluate its association with HIV-1 spVL, we reassessed a standard genome-wide association study (GWAS) using exome sequencing data from 395 individuals of European descent in the Swiss HIV Cohort Study (SHCS), following the procedures described in McLaren et al. (48). This analysis did not show any association between rs396991 and HIV-1 spVL ($p = 0.21$). Additionally, the rs1801274 did not show any association with spVL ($p = 0.54$) in the same cohort (**Figure 2**). The inability to replicate previous findings could be attributed to differences in sample size, clinical definition and statistical rigor employed. Globally, these new analyses confirm the previous findings that common human genetic variants in FCGR2A or FCGR3A are not associated with spontaneous control of HIV-1 infection.

Influence of FCGR Diversity on HIV-1 Acquisition

There are no conclusive studies reporting associations of FCGR polymorphisms with HIV-1 acquisition. Two independent

mother-to-child transmission cohorts reported contrasting findings of FCGR2A genotypes associating with increased infection risk in children with the high-affinity HH (rs1801274) genotype (49, 50).

Here again, we evaluated potential associations between FCGR2A and FCGR3A variants and susceptibility to HIV-1 infection by accessing the results of a previous GWAS of HIV-1 acquisition that compared 6,300 HIV-1 infected individuals and 7,200 controls of European ancestry (46). The rs1801274 polymorphism did not show any sign of association with HIV-1 acquisition ($p = 0.81$), and all other tested polymorphisms in a 50 kb window around both FCGR2A and FCGR3A were also non-significant after correction for multiple testing. The FCGR3A SNP (rs396991) was not included on the genotyping chip and could not be reliably imputed and so was not tested directly. This analysis in the largest acquisition cohort published to date adds substantial evidence to the lack of involvement of common FCGR2A and FCGR3A polymorphisms in HIV-1 acquisition.

Role of FCGR Polymorphisms on Outcomes After ART Initiation

Variation in genotype and expression of host genes is well established to impact HIV-1 susceptibility and disease progression in ART-naïve individuals (47). Initiation of ART in acute HIV-1 infection can limit establishment of viral reservoirs and induces post-treatment control in some individuals (51, 52).

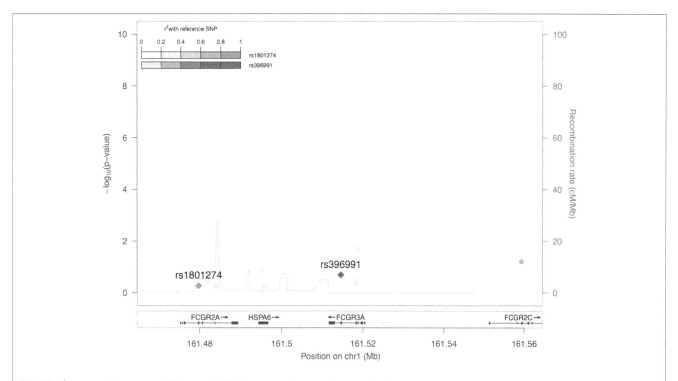

FIGURE 2 | No association between FCGR2A or FCGR3A polymorphisms on HIV-1 set point viral load. Regional association plot highlighting the association between the FCGR2A (rs1801274) and FCGR3A (rs396991) polymorphisms and HIV-1 spVL across 395 exome sequenced patients (48). Color intensities represent the linkage disequilibrium (r^2) of other SNPs in the region with rs1801287 and rs396991, respectively. The blue line indicates the estimated recombination rate in cM/Mb from The International HapMap Consortium (2007).

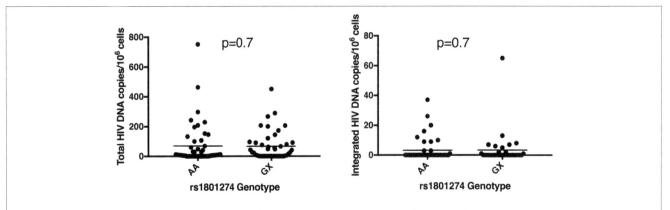

FIGURE 3 | Polymorphism in FCGR2A (CD32a) does not associate with reservoir size. The rs1801274 SNP variant did not associate with levels of total or integrated HIV DNA, determined in $N = 93$ and $N = 78$ of the patients, respectively (55, 56).

Host variation that influences viral reservoir size or reactivation during ART has not been definitively studied and has potential to significantly advance HIV cure research. There is at least one report indicating that broadly neutralizing antibodies (bNAbs) can interfere with establishment of a silent reservoir by Fc-FcR mediated mechanisms in humanized mice when administered early in the infection (53). Recently, Descours et al. identified CD32a (FCGR2A) as a marker of latently infected CD4 T cells (54). Given the previous associations of FCGR2A with HIV-1 disease pathogenesis, we hypothesized that polymorphisms in this gene might affect the size of the viral reservoir in patients that went on ART early in acute infection (55, 56). We examined genetic variation in the FCGR2A gene, characterizing polymorphisms in 436 ART-suppressed patients from the RV254 cohort. We screened for 18 variants in the extracellular domains of FCGR2A including rs1801274 and did not find associations with total or integrated HIV DNA ($p > 0.05$) (**Figure 3**). Surprisingly, recent reports from several independent groups confirm that they were unable to replicate the original findings from the Descours et al. study, showing that associations with post-ART control continue to be elusive (57–60).

Effect of FCGR Variation on HIV-1 Vaccine Efficacy

Variation in host genes can impact vaccine outcomes, and other than HLA, the only other gene to impact HIV-1 vaccine efficacy was in the FCGR locus (61–63). Two studies of HIV-1 vaccine efficacy revealed a remarkable coincidence of FCGR polymorphism associated with opposing directions for efficacy, suggesting that the effect of FCGR genetic variation may be specific to vaccine regimens. The FCGR2C association study of Li et al. (62), used a direct sequencing approach to identify FCGR2C SNPs that associated with vaccine efficacy (VE) against HIV-1 in the RV144 vaccine trial, that showed modest efficacy (64). Individuals with at least one minor allele of three FCGR2C SNPs (rs114945036, rs138747765, and rs78603008) had a vaccine efficacy of 64% against any HIV-1 subtype and 91%

against the CRF01-AE subtype with the protective 169K HIV-1 variant identified previously by sieve analysis (65). Although the functional mechanisms underlying the association were not revealed in this study, a subsequent examination of the FCGR2C SNPs showed rs114945036 correlated with expression levels of FCGR2A/C (66). This effect was found across different populations and was specific to the rs114945036 SNP located in the intron. Further, rs114945036 also associated with the expression of the Fc receptor-like A (FCRLA) gene, an FCGR related gene located within a gene cluster adjacent to FCGR (see **Figure 1A**). These results suggest that the FCGR expression is either influenced by this SNP through an undefined mechanism, or is in linkage with other causal variants that directly affect expression levels.

In the second study, four FCGR2C SNPs significantly modified the hazard ratio in the HVTN505 trial that did not show protection against HIV-1 acquisition (62). Three of the SNPs were common with those previously identified in RV144. In contrast to the RV144 study, in HVTN505 among the recipients carrying the FCGR2C minor alleles, HIV-1 acquisition risk was higher in the vaccine group than in the placebo group, in precisely the opposite direction of that observed in RV144 (efficacy against HIV-1 acquisition hazard ratios (HR) of 9.79 ($p = 0.035$) and 0.36 ($p = 0.04$), respectively). It is not clear how polymorphisms in a pseudogene functions during HIV-1 vaccination and their associations with FCGR expression may provide a novel avenue for further investigation.

Two additional studies of outcomes in Vax004, a trial testing recombinant gp120 vaccination in preventing sexually acquired HIV infection, also implicated FCGR variation in HIV infection and vaccine efficacy. Both studies tested the classical FCGR2A or FCGR3A variants comprised of the FCGR2A-R/H (rs1801274) and FCGR3A-F/V (rs396991) alleles. The first study found that lower affinity receptors (FCG2A-RR or HR and FCGR3A-FF) were associated with higher serum ADCVI activity, which itself predicted the rate of infection (67). A second study by the same group, showed the FCGR3A-VV genotype distinguished the lowest behavioral risk group from the high-risk behavioral group (68). The low risk group had a higher infection rate than low risk vaccinees with one or two F alleles (HR = 3.52; $p = 0.002$) while the high-risk group showed no association. Functional studies may be directed by these findings to interrogate quantitative and qualitative effects on FCGRs and associated antibody production. At a minimum, the intersection of these studies suggests that the impact of FCGR genetic variations on vaccine efficacy should be further investigated.

FCGR AND IGHG—FUTURE DIRECTIONS FOR GENETIC ANALYSIS

It is apparent that the genomic complexity of the FCGR region presents a major challenge for uncovering the underlying causal FCGR variants. Different FCGR have distinct functions and mechanisms of regulation but share highly similar sequences. While FCGR genetic variations are clearly linked to host defense against infectious diseases and other important immune functions as discussed, current approaches measure only a small portion of the existing FCGR variation. The HVTN505 and RV144 studies referenced above were by far the most comprehensive in that regard, measuring ~10 kb of the FCGR region, including functional exons encoding external protein domains and flanking intron sequences from the five FCGR genes. However, the complete FCGR region extends over 200 kb leaving open the likelihood of additional causal variation (**Figure 1A**). Indeed, the lack of phasing of the over 20,000 SNPs documented in the FCGR region significantly limits its direct utility for association analysis and the ultimate goal of identifying causal variants (69). Complete haplotype-resolved FCGR genomic sequences across human populations by approaches such as those used for defining variability in the KIR region may be necessary in order to provide a complete analysis of these loci (70–72).

When considering FCGR host genetics and its relationship to HIV-1 susceptibility and vaccine efficacy—or any association with disease—a natural but not often considered extension to host genetic association studies interrogating FCGR variability lies within the human immunoglobulin constant heavy G chain (IGHG) gene region on chromosomal segment 14q32.3 (73). This region encoding the human IG heavy constant genes (IGHG3, IGHG1, IGHG2, IGHA2, and the IGH locus on chromosome 14) provides access to a system for understanding immunogenicity of the polymorphic IG chains (74, 75). The evident functional relationship between FCGR and IgG constant region variability, which itself is substantial (74), argues strongly for host genetic studies of FCGR to be paired with analysis of IGHG. Although little genomic characterization for the IGHG system is available at present, we anticipate that NGS technologies will rapidly fill that void. Of course, once provided with high quality and high resolution data, significant effort will need to be invested in new sophisticated analytical approaches examining multiple factors simultaneously to find the causal variation revealing operative biological mechanisms.

CONCLUDING REMARKS

Disease pathogenesis of HIV-1 has been shown to be modulated by allelic variants in the FCGR genes. However, such findings have not always been robust, as they were not replicated or in some cases were contradictory. There is however considerable interest in the role of Fc-mediated antiviral functions such as ADCC, ADCP, ADCD, and ADCVI in protective immunity against HIV-1 (76). Host genetics of the Fc receptors that bind to the Fc domain of the IgG antibody might modulate the functional antiviral antibody responses to HIV-1 vaccination. ADCC was previously identified as a correlate of protection in the RV144 human efficacy trial (64). More recently, ADCP has been shown to correlate with protection against acquisition of SIV/SHIV/HIV-1 in multiple preclinical and human efficacy trials (77–80). Given such associations, it would be critical to investigate association of host variation in FCGR genes and such Fc-mediated antiviral functions that are now being generated using technologies such as systems serology (1). Such findings might shed light on the role of Fc gene and receptor genotypes on HIV-1 disease pathogenesis.

AUTHOR CONTRIBUTIONS

RT conceptualized, organized the content of the review and wrote sections Introduction, FCGR polymorphisms and HIV-1 disease progression, Influence of FCGR diversity on HIV-1 acquisition, Role of FCGR polymorphisms on outcomes after ART initiation, and Concluding Remarks. DG contributed to sections Fcγ receptor genetic diversity, Effect of FCGR variation on HIV-1 vaccine efficacy, and FCGR and IGHG–future directions for genetic analysis. JF and CT drafted sections FCGR polymorphisms and HIV-1 disease progression, Influence of FCGR diversity on HIV-1 acquisition. All authors participated in editing and revising the manuscript.

ACKNOWLEDGMENTS

We would like to acknowledge the RV254 study group led by Dr. Jintanat Ananworanich and Dr. Sodsai Tovanabutra, MHRP for providing samples, clinical data, and viral reservoir measurements. We thank Dr. Vicky Polonis, MHRP and Mr. Philip Ehrenberg for thoughtful comments and suggestions. We thank Ms. Aviva Geretz, MHRP for reviewing the compiled FCGR polymorphisms. This work was supported by a cooperative agreement (W81XWH-18-2-0040) between the Henry M. Jackson Foundation for the Advancement of Military Medicine, Inc., and the U. S. Department of Defense (DOD). This research was funded, in part, by the U. S. National Institute of Allergy and Infectious Disease. The views expressed are those of the authors and should not be construed to represent the positions of the U. S. Army or the DOD.

REFERENCES

1. Chung AW, Alter G. Systems serology: profiling vaccine induced humoral immunity against HIV. *Retrovirology.* (2017) 14:57. doi: 10.1186/s12977-017-0380-3

2. Forthal DN, Moog C. Fc receptor-mediated antiviral antibodies. *Curr Opin HIV AIDS.* (2009) 4:388–93. doi: 10.1097/COH.0b013e32832f0a89

3. Cocklin SL, Schmitz JE. The role of Fc receptors in HIV infection and vaccine efficacy. *Curr Opin HIV AIDS.* (2014) 9:257–62. doi: 10.1097/coh.0000000000000051

4. Bournazos S, Woof JM, Hart SP, Dransfield I. Functional and clinical consequences of Fc receptor polymorphic and copy number variants. *Clin Exp Immunol.* (2009) 157:244–54. doi: 10.1111/j.1365-2249.2009.03980.x

5. Li X, Gibson AW, Kimberly RP. Human FcR polymorphism and disease. *Curr Top Microbiol Immunol.* (2014) 382:275–302. doi: 10.1007/978-3-319-07911-0_13.

6. Bournazos S, Ravetch JV. Fcgamma receptor function and the design of vaccination strategies. *Immunity.* (2017) 47:224–33. doi: 10.1016/j.immuni.2017.07.009

7. Kratochvil S, McKay PF, Chung AW, Kent SJ, Gilmour J, Shattock RJ. Immunoglobulin G1 allotype influences antibody subclass distribution in response to HIV gp140 vaccination. *Front Immunol.* 8:1883. (2017) doi: 10.3389/fimmu.2017.01883

8. Gupta S, Gach JS, Becerra JC, Phan TB, Pudney J, Moldoveanu Z, et al. The Neonatal Fc receptor (FcRn) enhances human immunodeficiency virus type 1 (HIV-1) transcytosis across epithelial cells. *PLoS Pathog.* (2013) 9:e1003776. doi: 10.1371/journal.ppat.1003776

9. Shen S, Pyo CW, Vu Q, Wang R, Geraghty DE. The essential detail: the genetics and genomics of the primate immune response. *ILAR J.* (2013) 54:181–95. doi: 10.1093/ilar/ilt043

10. Misra MK, Augusto DG, Martin GM, Nemat-Gorgani N, Sauter J, Hofmann JA, et al. Report from the Killer-cell Immunoglobulin-like Receptors (KIR) component of the 17th International HLA and Immunogenetics Workshop. *Hum Immunol.* (2018) 79:825–33 doi: 10.1016/j.humimm.2018.10.003

11. Bruhns P. Properties of mouse and human IgG receptors and their contribution to disease models. *Blood.* (2012) 119:5640–9. doi: 10.1182/blood-2012-01-380121

12. Bruhns P, Iannascoli B, England P, Mancardi DA, Fernandez N, Jorieux S, et al. Specificity and affinity of human Fcgamma receptors and their polymorphic variants for human IgG subclasses. *Blood.* (2009) 113:3716–25. doi: 10.1182/blood-2008-09-179754

13. Warmerdam PA, van de Winkel JG, Gosselin EJ, Capel PJ. Molecular basis for a polymorphism of human Fc gamma receptor II (CD32). *J Exp Med.* (1990) 172:19–25.

14. Ravetch JV, Perussia B. Alternative membrane forms of Fc gamma RIII(CD16) on human natural killer cells and neutrophils. Cell type-specific expression of two genes that differ in single nucleotide substitutions. *J Exp Med.* (1989) 170:481–97.

15. Seret G, Hanrotel C, Bendaoud B, Le Meur Y, Renaudineau Y. Homozygous FCGR3A-158F mutation is associated with delayed B-cell depletion following rituximab but with preserved efficacy in a patient with refractory lupus nephritis. *Clini Kidney J.* (2013) 6:74–6. doi: 10.1093/ckj/sfs162

16. Shimizu, Tanaka Y, Tazawa H, Verma S, Onoe T, Ishiyama K, et al. Fc-gamma receptor polymorphisms predispose patients to infectious complications after liver transplantation. *Am J Transplant.* (2016) 16:625–33. doi: 10.1111/ajt.13492

17. Taylor RJ, Saloura V, Jain A, Goloubeva O, Wong S, Kronsberg S, et al. *Ex vivo* antibody-dependent cellular cytotoxicity inducibility predicts efficacy of cetuximab. *Cancer Immunol Res.* (2015) 3:567–74. doi: 10.1158/2326-6066.cir-14-0188

18. Flinsenberg TW, Janssen WJ, Herczenik E, Boross P, Nederend M, Jongeneel LH, et al. A novel FcgammaRIIa Q27W gene variant is associated with common variable immune deficiency through defective FcgammaRIIa downstream signaling. *Clin Immunol.* (2014) 155:108–17. doi: 10.1016/j.clim.2014.09.006

19. Kono H, Kyogoku C, Suzuki T, Tsuchiya N, Honda H, Yamamoto K, et al. FcgammaRIIB Ile232Thr transmembrane polymorphism associated with human systemic lupus erythematosus decreases affinity to lipid rafts and attenuates inhibitory effects on B cell receptor signaling. *Hum Mol Genet.* (2005) 14:2881–92. doi: 10.1093/hmg/ddi320

20. Ernst LK, Metes D, Herberman RB, Morel PA. Allelic polymorphisms in the FcgammaRIIC gene can influence its function on normal human natural killer cells. *J Mol Med.* (2002) 80:248–57. doi: 10.1007/s00109-001-0294-2

21. Metes D, Ernst LK, Chambers WH, Sulica A, Herberman RB, Morel PA. Expression of functional CD32 molecules on human NK cells is determined by an allelic polymorphism of the FcgammaRIIC gene. *Blood.* (1998) 91:2369–80.

22. Nagelkerke SQ, Tacke CE, Breunis WB, Geissler J, Sins JW, Appelhof B, et al. Nonallelic homologous recombination of the FCGR2/3 locus results in copy number variation and novel chimeric FCGR2 genes with aberrant functional expression. *Genes Immun.* (2015) 16:422–9. doi: 10.1038/gene.2015.25

23. van der Heijden J, Breunis WB, Geissler J, de Boer M, van den Berg TK, Kuijpers TW. Phenotypic variation in IgG receptors by nonclassical FCGR2C alleles. *J Immunol.* (2012) 188:1318–24. doi: 10.4049/jimmunol.1003945

24. Metes D, Galatiuc C, Moldovan I, Morel PA, Chambers WH, DeLeo AB, et al. Expression and function of Fc gamma RII on human natural killer cells. *Nat Immun.* (1994) 13:289–300.

25. Qiu WQ, de Bruin D, Brownstein BH, Pearse R, Ravetch JV. Organization of the human and mouse low-affinity Fc gamma R genes: duplication and recombination. *Science.* (1990) 248:732–5.

26. de Haas M, Koene HR, Kleijer M, de Vries E, Simsek S, van Tol MJ, et al. A triallelic Fc gamma receptor type IIIA polymorphism influences the binding of human IgG by NK cell Fc gamma RIIIa. *J Immunol.* (1996) 156:2948–55.

27. Ory PA, Clark MR, Kwoh EE, Clarkson SB, Goldstein IM. Sequences of complementary DNAs that encode the NA1 and NA2 forms of Fc receptor III on human neutrophils. *J Clin Invest.* (1989) 84:1688–91. doi: 10.1172/jci114350

28. Ory PA, Goldstein IM, Kwoh EE, Clarkson SB. Characterization of polymorphic forms of Fc receptor III on human neutrophils. *J Clin Invest.* (1989) 83:1676–81. doi: 10.1172/jci114067

29. Bredius RG, Fijen CA, De Haas M, Kuijper EJ, Weening RS, Van de Winkel JG, et al. Role of neutrophil Fc gamma RIIa (CD32) and Fc gamma RIIIb (CD16) polymorphic forms in phagocytosis of human IgG1- and IgG3-opsonized bacteria and erythrocytes. *Immunology.* (1994) 83:624–30.

30. Salmon JE, Edberg JC, Kimberly RP. Fc gamma receptor III on human neutrophils. Allelic variants have functionally distinct capacities. *J Clin Invest.* (1990) 85:1287–95. doi: 10.1172/jci114566

31. Bux J, Stein EL, Bierling P, Fromont P, Clay M, Stroncek D, et al. Characterization of a new alloantigen (SH) on the human neutrophil Fc gamma receptor IIIb. *Blood.* (1997) 89:1027–34.

32. Flesch BK, Doose S, Siebert R, Ntambi E, Neppert J. FCGR3 variants and expression of human neutrophil antigen-1a,−1b, and−1c in the populations of northern Germany and Uganda. *Transfusion.* (2002) 42:469–75. doi: 10.1046/j.1525-1438.2002.00087.x

33. Reil A, Sachs UJ, Siahanidou T, Flesch BK, Bux J. HNA-1d: a new human neutrophil antigen located on Fcgamma receptor IIIb associated with neonatal immune neutropenia. *Transfusion.* (2013) 53:2145–51. doi: 10.1111/trf.12086

34. Hollox EJ, Hoh BP. Human gene copy number variation and infectious disease. *Human Genet.* (2014) 133:1217–33. doi: 10.1007/s00439-014-1457-x

35. Breunis WB, van Mirre E, Geissler J, Laddach N, Wolbink G, van der Schoot E, et al. Copy number variation at the FCGR locus includes FCGR3A, FCGR2C, and FCGR3B but not FCGR2A and FCGR2B. *Human Mutat.* (2009) 30:E640–50. doi: 10.1002/humu.20997

36. Niederer HA, Willcocks LC, Rayner TF, Yang W, Lau YL, Williams TN, et al. Copy number, linkage disequilibrium and disease association in the FCGR locus. *Hum Mol Genet.* (2010) 19:3282–94. doi: 10.1093/hmg/ddq216

37. Hargreaves CE, Rose-Zerilli MJ, Machado LR, Iriyama C, Hollox EJ, Cragg MS, et al. Fcgamma receptors: genetic variation, function, and disease. *Immunol Rev.* (2015) 268:6–24. doi: 10.1111/imr.12341

38. Machado LR, Hardwick RJ, Bowdrey J, Bogle H, Knowles TJ, Sironi M, et al. Evolutionary history of copy-number-variable locus for the

low-affinity Fcgamma receptor: mutation rate, autoimmune disease, and the legacy of helminth infection. *Am J Hum Genet*. (2012) 90:973–85. doi: 10.1016/j.ajhg.2012.04.018

39. Lehrnbecher TL, Foster CB, Zhu S, Venzon D, Steinberg SM, Wyvill K, et al. Variant genotypes of FcgammaRIIIA influence the development of Kaposi's sarcoma in HIV-infected men. *Blood*. (2000) 95:2386–90.

40. Forthal DN, Landucci G, Bream J, Jacobson LP, Phan TB, Montoya B. FcgammaRIIa genotype predicts progression of HIV infection. *J Immunol*. (2007) 179:7916–23. doi: 10.4049/jimmunol.179.11.7916

41. Weis JF, McClelland RS, Jaoko W, Mandaliya KN, Overbaugh J, Graham SM, et al. Short communication: Fc gamma receptors IIa and IIIa genetic polymorphisms do not predict HIV-1 disease progression in Kenyan women. *AIDS Res Hum Retroviruses*. (2015) 31:288–92. doi: 10.1089/AID.2014.0209

42. Poonia B, Kijak GH, Pauza CD. High affinity allele for the gene of FCGR3A is risk factor for HIV infection and progression. *PLoS ONE*. (2010) 5:e15562. doi: 10.1371/journal.pone.0015562

43. Rohatgi S, Gohil S, Kuniholm MH, Schultz H, Dufaud C, Armour KL, et al. Fc gamma receptor 3A polymorphism and risk for HIV-associated cryptococcal disease. *MBio*. (2013) 4:e00573–13. doi: 10.1128/mBio.00573-13

44. Meletiadis J, Walsh TJ, Choi EH, Pappas PG, Ennis D, Douglas J, et al. Study of common functional genetic polymorphisms of FCGR2A, 3A and 3B genes and the risk for cryptococcosis in HIV-uninfected patients. *Med Mycol*. (2007) 45:513–8. doi: 10.1080/13693780701390140

45. Little J, Higgins JP, Ioannidis JP, Moher D, Gagnon F, von Elm E, et al. STrengthening the REporting of Genetic Association Studies (STREGA): an extension of the STROBE statement. *PLoS Med*. (2009) 6:e22. doi: 10.1371/journal.pmed.1000022

46. McLaren PJ, Coulonges C, Ripke S, van den Berg L, Buchbinder S, Carrington M, et al. Association study of common genetic variants and HIV-1 acquisition in 6,300 infected cases and 7,200 controls. *PLoS Pathog*. (2013) 9:e1003515. doi: 10.1371/journal.ppat.1003515

47. McLaren PJ, Carrington M. The impact of host genetic variation on infection with HIV-1. *Nat Immunol*. (2015) 16:577–83. doi: 10.1038/ni.3147

48. McLaren PJ, Pulit SL, Gurdasani D, Bartha I, Shea PR, Pomilla C, et al. Evaluating the impact of functional genetic variation on HIV-1 control. *J Infect Dis*. (2017) 216:1063–9. doi: 10.1093/infdis/jix470

49. Brouwer KC, Lal RB, Mirel LB, Yang C, van Eijk AM, Ayisi J, et al. Polymorphism of Fc receptor IIa for IgG in infants is associated with susceptibility to perinatal HIV-1 infection. *AIDS*. (2004) 18:1187–94. doi: 10.1097/00002030-200405210-00012

50. Milligan C, Richardson BA, John-Stewart G, Nduati R, Overbaugh J. FCGR2A and FCGR3A genotypes in human immunodeficiency virus mother-to-child transmission. *Open Forum Infect Dis*. (2015) 2:ofv149. doi: 10.1093/ofid/ofv149

51. Ananworanich J, Chomont N, Eller LA, Kroon E, Tovanabutra S, Bose M, et al. HIV DNA set point is rapidly established in acute HIV infection and dramatically reduced by early ART. *EBioMedicine*. (2016) 11:68–72. doi: 10.1016/j.ebiom.2016.07.024

52. Saez-Cirion A, Bacchus C, Hocqueloux L, Avettand-Fenoel V, Girault I, Lecuroux C, et al. Post-treatment HIV-1 controllers with a long-term virological remission after the interruption of early initiated antiretroviral therapy ANRS VISCONTI Study. *PLoS Pathog*. (2013) 9:e1003211. doi: 10.1371/journal.ppat.1003211

53. Halper-Stromberg A, Lu CL, Klein F, Horwitz JA, Bournazos S, Nogueira L, et al. Broadly neutralizing antibodies and viral inducers decrease rebound from HIV-1 latent reservoirs in humanized mice. *Cell*. (2014) 158:989–99. doi: 10.1016/j.cell.2014.07.043

54. Descours B, Petitjean G, López-Zaragoza JL, Bruel T, Raffel R, Psomas C, et al. CD32a is a marker of a CD4 T-cell HIV reservoir harbouring replication-competent proviruses. *Nature*. (2017) 543:564–7. doi: 10.1038/nature21710

55. De Souza MS, Phanuphak N, Pinyakorn S, Trichavaroj R, Pattanachaiwit S, Chomchey N, et al. Impact of nucleic acid testing relative to antigen/antibody combination immunoassay on the detection of acute HIV infection. *AIDS*. (2015) 29:793–800. doi: 10.1097/QAD.0000000000000616

56. Ananworanich J, Fletcher JL, Pinyakorn S, van Griensven F, Vandergeeten C, Schuetz A, et al. A novel acute HIV infection staging system based on 4th generation immunoassay. *Retrovirology*. (2013) 10:56. doi: 10.1186/1742-4690-10-56

57. Abdel-Mohsen M, Kuri-Cervantes L, Grau-Exposito J, Spivak AM, Nell RA, Tomescu C, et al. CD32 is expressed on cells with transcriptionally active HIV but does not enrich for HIV DNA in resting T cells. *Sci Transl Med*. (2018) 10:eaar6759. doi: 10.1126/scitranslmed.aar6759

58. Osuna CE, Lim SY, Kublin JL, Apps R, Chen E, Mota TM, et al. Evidence that CD32a does not mark the HIV-1 latent reservoir. *Nature*. (2018) 561:E20–8. doi: 10.1038/s41586-018-0495-2

59. Bertagnolli LN, White JA, Simonetti FR, Beg SA, Lai J, Tomescu C, et al. The role of CD32 during HIV-1 infection. *Nature*. (2018) 561:E17–9. doi: 10.1038/s41586-018-0494-3

60. Perez L, Anderson J, Chipman J, Thorkelson A, Chun TW, Moir S, et al. Conflicting evidence for HIV enrichment in CD32(+) CD4 T cells. *Nature*. (2018) 561, E9–16. doi: 10.1038/s41586-018-0493-4

61. Prentice HA, Tomaras GD, Geraghty DE, Apps R, Fong Y, Ehrenberg PK, et al. HLA class II genes modulate vaccine-induced antibody responses to affect HIV-1 acquisition. *Sci Transl Med*. (2015) 7:296ra112. doi: 10.1126/scitranslmed.aab4005

62. Li SS, Gilbert PB, Tomaras GD, Kijak G, Ferrari G, Thomas R, et al. FCGR2C polymorphisms associate with HIV-1 vaccine protection in RV144 trial. *J Clin Invest*. (2014) 124:3879–90. doi: 10.1172/JCI75539

63. Gartland AJ, Li S, McNevin J, Tomaras GD, Gottardo R, Janes H, et al. Analysis of HLA A*02 association with vaccine efficacy in the RV144 HIV-1 vaccine trial. *J Virol*. (2014) 88:8242–55. doi: 10.1128/JVI.01164-14

64. Rerks-Ngarm S, Pitisuttithum P, Nitayaphan S, Kaewkungwal J, Chiu J, Paris R, et al. Vaccination with ALVAC and AIDSVAX to prevent HIV-1 infection in Thailand. *N Engl J Med*. (2009) 361:2209–20. doi: 10.1056/NEJMoa0908492

65. Rolland M, Edlefsen PT, Larsen BB, Tovanabutra S, Sanders-Buell E, Hertz T, et al. Increased HIV-1 vaccine efficacy against viruses with genetic signatures in Env V2. *Nature*. (2012) 490:417–20. doi: 10.1038/nature11519

66. Peng X, Li SS, Gilbert PB, Geraghty DE, Katze MG. FCGR2C polymorphisms associated with HIV-1 vaccine protection are linked to altered gene expression of Fc-gamma receptors in human B cells. *PLoS ONE*. (2016) 11:e0152425. doi: 10.1371/journal.pone.0152425

67. Forthal DN, Gilbert PB, Landucci G, Phan T. Recombinant gp120 vaccine-induced antibodies inhibit clinical strains of HIV-1 in the presence of Fc receptor-bearing effector cells and correlate inversely with HIV infection rate. *J Immunol*. (2007) 178:6596–603.

68. Forthal DN, Gabriel EE, Wang A, Landucci G, Phan TB. Association of Fcgamma receptor IIIa genotype with the rate of HIV infection after gp120 vaccination. *Blood*. (2012) 120:2836–42. doi: 10.1182/blood-2012-05-431361

69. EMBL-EBI. *Ensembl Variation Database*. (2018). Avaliable online at: https://www.ensembl.org/info/genome/variation/index.html

70. Pyo CW, Guethlein LA, Vu Q, Wang R, Abi-Rached L, Norman PJ, et al. Different patterns of evolution in the centromeric and telomeric regions of group A and B haplotypes of the human killer cell Ig-like receptor locus. *PLoS ONE*. (2010) 5:e15115. doi: 10.1371/journal.pone.0015115

71. Pyo CW, Wang R, Vu Q, Cereb N, Yang SY, Duh FM, et al. Recombinant structures expand and contract inter and intragenic diversification at the KIR locus. *BMC Genomics*. (2013) 14:89. doi: 10.1186/1471-2164-14-89

72. Roe D, Vierra-Green C, Pyo CW, Eng K, Hall R, Kuang R, et al. Revealing complete complex KIR haplotypes phased by long-read sequencing technology. *Genes Immun*. (2017) 18:127–34. doi: 10.1038/gene.2017.10

73. Oxelius VA, Pandey JP. Human immunoglobulin constant heavy G chain (IGHG) (Fcgamma) (GM) genes, defining innate variants of IgG molecules and B cells, have impact on disease and therapy. *Clin Immunol*. (2013) 149:475–86. doi: 10.1016/j.clim.2013.10.003

74. Lefranc MP, Lefranc G. Human Gm, Km, and Am allotypes and their molecular characterization: a remarkable demonstration of polymorphism. *Methods Mol Biol*. (2012) 882:635–80. doi: 10.1007/978-1-61779-842-9_34

75. Pandey JP, Li Z. The forgotten tale of immunoglobulin allotypes in cancer risk and treatment. *Exper Hematol Oncol*. (2013) 2:6. doi: 10.1186/2162-3619-2-6

76. Lewis GK. Role of Fc-mediated antibody function in protective immunity against HIV-1. *Immunology*. (2014) 142:46–57. doi: 10.1111/imm.12232

77. Barouch DH, Alter G, Broge T, Linde C, Ackerman ME, Brown EP, et al. Protective efficacy of adenovirus/protein vaccines against SIV challenges in rhesus monkeys. *Science*. (2015) 349:320–4. doi: 10.1126/science.aab3886

78. Barouch DH, Tomaka FL, Wegmann F, Stieh DJ, Alter G, Robb ML, et al. Evaluation of a mosaic HIV-1 vaccine in a multicentre, randomised, double-blind, placebo-controlled, phase 1/2a clinical trial (APPROACH) and in rhesus monkeys (NHP 13-19). *Lancet*. (2018) 392:232–43. doi: 10.1016/S0140-6736(18)31364-3

79. Barouch DH, Stephenson KE, Borducchi EN, Smith K, Stanley K, McNally AG, et al. Protective efficacy of a global HIV-1 mosaic vaccine against heterologous SHIV challenges in rhesus monkeys. *Cell*. (2013) 155:531–9. doi: 10.1016/j.cell.2013.09.061

80. Issac B, Ehrenberg PK, Eller M, Alter G, Sekaly RP, Robb ML, et al. Vaccine-induced gene signature correlates with protection against acquisition in three independent vaccine efficacy trials including RV144. In: *Conference Abstract. HIV Research for Prevention HIVR4P*. Madrid (2018).

17

The Roles of Host and Viral Antibody Fc Receptors in Herpes Simplex Virus (HSV) and Human Cytomegalovirus (HCMV) Infections and Immunity

Jennifer A. Jenks[1]*, Matthew L. Goodwin[1] and Sallie R. Permar[1,2]

[1] *Duke Human Vaccine Institute, Duke University Medical Center, Durham, NC, United States,* [2] *Department of Pediatrics, Children's Health and Discovery Institute, Durham, NC, United States*

*Correspondence:
Jennifer A. Jenks
jennifer.jenks@duke.edu

Herpesvirus infections are a leading cause of neurodevelopmental delay in newborns and end-organ disease in immunocompromised patients. One leading strategy to reduce the disease burden of herpesvirus infections such as herpes simplex virus (HSV) and human cytomegalovirus (HCMV) is to prevent primary acquisition by vaccination, yet vaccine development remains hampered by limited understanding of immune correlates of protection against infection. Traditionally, vaccine development has aimed to increase antibody titers with neutralizing function, which involves the direct binding of antibodies to viral particles. However, recent research has explored the numerous other responses that can be mediated by engagement of the antibody constant region (Fc) with Fc receptors (FcR) present on immune cells or with complement molecules. These functions include antiviral responses such as antibody-dependent cell-mediated cytotoxicity (ADCC) and antibody-dependent cellular phagocytosis (ADCP). Uniquely, herpesviruses encode FcR that can act as distractor receptors for host antiviral IgG, thus enabling viral evasion of host defenses. This review focuses on the relative roles of neutralizing and non-neutralizing functions antibodies that target herpesvirus antigens for HSV and HCMV, as well as the roles of Fc-FcR interactions for both host defenses and viral escape.

Keywords: HSV, HCMV, herpes simplex virus, cytomegalovirus, FcR, Fc receptor, non-neutralizing antibodies, neutralizing antibodies

Herpesvirus infections are the leading cause of infectious brain damage in infants and a leading source of morbidity and mortality in immunosuppressed individuals. Neonatal herpes simplex virus (HSV) has 50% mortality in neonates who develop disseminated disease, even among those who receive appropriate antiviral therapy (1), and congenital human cytomegalovirus (HCMV) is the most common infectious cause of sensorineural hearing loss worldwide (2). In immunocompromised patients, HSV and HCMV infection can both cause severe end-organ disease. HSV-2 causes severe, sometimes refractory disease including orofacial and genital lesions in patients with HIV/AIDS and other immunocompromising conditions (3), and HCMV is a major infectious cause of morbidity and mortality in immunocompromised patients, such as recipients of allogeneic hematopoietic stem cell transplants (4). One strategy to reduce disease burden is to prevent primary acquisition or viral reactivation by vaccination. In fact, a vaccine to prevent HCMV has been designated a "Tier I priority" by the Institute of Medicine since 2000 (5). Yet despite major advancements in research and multiple clinical trials of HSV and HCMV vaccines over the last 20 years, development of efficacious vaccines remains elusive. These challenges may be due in part to a limited understanding of the immune correlates of protection against viral infection, as well as complex mechanisms of herpesvirus evasion of these immune responses.

Traditionally, vaccine developments for HSV and HCMV have predominantly focused on the generation of neutralizing responses to prevent primary acquisition. Neutralization occurs upon direct binding of antibodies to viral antigens by their antibody binding (Fab) regions and can often be mediated in the absence of the antibody constant (Fc) region, as in the case of isolated F(ab) or F(ab)'2 fragments which are enzyme-cleaved immunoglobulin G (IgG) that lack the Fc portions. Thus, neutralization is generally achieved by antibody masking of target cell receptor binding sites or inhibition of conformational change in viral spike proteins required for fusion between the viral lipid envelope and cellular plasma membrane (6). However, the results of animal vaccine studies and recent clinical trials of HSV and HCMV vaccines have suggested that neutralization may be only one of several antibody functions that protect against HSV and HCMV infections, respectively. A previous trial of an HSV-2 subunit vaccine targeting glycoprotein D (gD), which is required for HSV entry into cells (7), elicited robust neutralization but did not confer protection against genital HSV-2 infection (8).

Similarly, a subunit vaccine against HCMV glycoprotein B (gB), which is required for viral entry (9), conferred ∼50% protection in multiple phase II studies of HCMV but elicited negligible neutralizing responses against heterologous HCMV strains (10, 11).

Thus, recent vaccine efforts have aimed to measure both neutralizing and non-neutralizing antibody responses. These responses include antibody-dependent cellular cytotoxicity (ADCC), antibody-dependent cellular phagocytosis (ADCP), antibody-dependent complement deposition (ADCD), and antibody-dependent respiratory burst (ADRB), of which ADCC and ADCP occur upon engagement of Fc and Fc receptors (FcR) (**Figure 1**). ADCC is an adaptive immune response wherein IgG Fc-FcR engagement triggers lysis of target cells. Although ADCC activity is largely mediated by NK cells, it can also be mediated by non-NK cell populations in peripheral blood and mucosal compartments including monocytes, macrophages, and granulocytes. In ADCP, phagocytic cells such as monocytes, macrophages, neutrophils, and dendritic cells (DCs) express FcRs that enable them to efficiently uptake antibody-opsonized particles, enabling both clearance and presentation of viral antigens. The FcR most involved in the non-neutralizing antibody functions ADCC and ADCP are of the FcγR family.

FcγR is which is one of the five main FcR classes, which includes FcγR, FcεRI, FcμR, FcαRI, and FcRn, so named for the IgG that they recognize. The FcγR family is broadly categorized into three groups: FcγRI (CD64), FcγRII (CD32), and FcγRIII

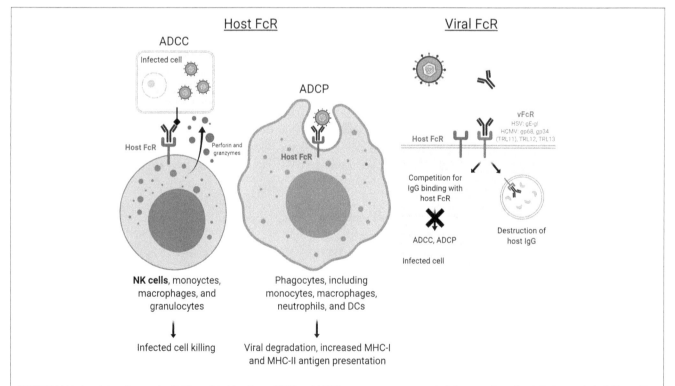

FIGURE 1 | Host and virus Fc receptor (FcR)-mediated functions. ADCC and ADCP occur upon engagement of virus-specific antibody Fc fragments to FcR, resulting in cytotoxic killing of infected cells and whole virion degradation, respectively. Herpesviruses also encode their own viral FcRs (FcRs), which recognize the Fc regions of host immunoglobulins. Mimicking host FcRs, vFcRs enable herpesviruses to reduce and evade antiviral immune responses. Figure created with BioRender.

(CD16), each of which coordinate different functions and are expressed on different cell types. The FcγRI family are high affinity (10^9/M) receptors, which can bind monomeric IgG, and are constitutively expressed on monocytes and macrophages (12). By contrast, FcγRII and FcγRIII are low-affinity (10^6/M) receptors, which bind only immune-complexed IgG, and are expressed on many hematopoietic cells. The FcγRII family is categorized into FcγRIIa, FcγRIIb, and FcγRIIc. FcγRIIa is the most widely distributed FcγR, found on neutrophils, eosinophils, B lymphocytes, platelets, mast cells, Langerhans cells, placental endothelial cells, and dendritic cells (12). In contrast to all other FcγRs which are activating, FcγRIIb is the only inhibitory FcγR, due to its unique inhibitory cytoplasmic signaling motif (13). The FcγRIII family includes two receptors: FcγRIIIa, which is expressed on monocytes, DCs, and macrophages; and FcγRIIIb, which is expressed on neutrophils, mast cells, and eosinophils. The various combinations of FcγRs play a significant role in determining an antiviral cellular response in the context of virus-specific IgG.

In humans, non-neutralizing antibody responses rely on engagement of IgG with particular FcγRs. ADCC is predominantly mediated by FcγRIIIα, FcγRI, FcγRII, FcγRIIIb, and FcαRI (CD89) (14–16). ADCP regulation is multilayered and can involve a myriad of factors, including FcR genetics, phagocyte cell type, and receptor expression pattern, tissue environment, and antibody immune complex, including specificity, isotype, subclass, and glycoforms (17). Notably, antibodies that mediate non-neutralizing functions may also mediate neutralization, and there may be not only complementary but potentially synergistic humoral effector functions for antiviral antibodies. Thus, the relative contributions of neutralizing and non-neutralizing antibody functions against HSV and HCMV for both protection and viral clearance are likely very complex.

Uniquely, herpesviruses also encode their own viral FcRs (FcRs), which recognize the Fc regions of host immunoglobulins. These vFcRs mimic host FcRs, enabling herpesviruses to reduce and evade antiviral immune responses. The elucidation of the mechanisms by which vFcRs evade host antiviral immune responses has exposed their potential as targets for novel vaccine development.

This review will discuss non-neutralizing antibody functions in HSV and HCMV, with a particular focus on functions mediated by Fc-FcR binding, as well as the role of vFcRs to mimic host FcR and to evade immune responses. An improved understanding of the distinct humoral immune correlates of protection will ultimately aid development of efficacious vaccines against herpesvirus pathogens.

FCR-MEDIATED IMMUNITY AGAINST HSV

The hallmark of HSV is its ability to establish lifelong persistent infection in sensory neurons and reactivate to cause recurrent disease or viral shedding. In HSV-infected individuals, control and clearance of the virus has been attributed to the generation of cellular immunity (18), but HSV antibodies are known to play a major role in prevention of HSV infection (19–23). In

congenital HSV, maternal antibodies against HSV are known to reduce disease severity in infants (24). Women who are infected with sufficient time to transmit HSV antibodies to their infants are less likely to have infants with neonatal HSV-2 disease than women with acute HSV-2 infection at the time of childbirth (24). Thus, antibody-mediated immunity has been a central focus for HSV vaccines.

Of particular interest for HSV vaccine development are the HSV glycoproteins gD, gB, and gH/gL, which are essential for cell entry and which have been targets for multiple vaccine trials in humans (25–27). A vaccine trial of HSV-2 gD2 induced both cellular and humoral immune responses in HSV-2-seronegative patients, and despite inducing high-titer gD2-specific antibodies at levels exceeding those induced by natural infection and neutralizing antibodies, the vaccine failed to prevent HSV genital infection after 1 year of follow-up. As compared to the control group, the vaccinated demonstrated only 20% protection against genital disease (27). Surprisingly, protection against viral acquisition (with or without disease) against HSV-1 was 35% whereas there was no vaccine efficacy against HSV-2 (27). Cross-protection was expected in this trial given the high sequence homology between gD1 and gD2, yet it remained unclear what properties of the vaccine-elicited antibodies were partially protective against HSV-1 infection. In a subsequent study of the HSV-2 gD2-vaccinated women, antibody titers to HSV-2 gD2 correlated with protection against HSV-1 infection, with higher antibody concentration associated with higher efficacy, but there was no correlation between HSV-2-specific antibody titers in serum with HSV-2 protection (21). Of note, follow-up studies revealed that in sera drawn 1 month after the final dose of the HSV-2 gD2 vaccine, mean neutralizing titers to HSV-1 were 3.5 times than to HSV-2, and the mean neutralization titer against HSV-2 was 1:29, well-below that seen in natural infection (28). The results of this follow-up study may partially explain the lack of protection observed against HSV-2. Thus, although the vaccine elicited high antibody and mixed neutralizing titers to HSV but had poor efficacy against genital disease, it remains unclear if neutralization is sufficient for protection.

In addition to neutralization, recent studies have aimed to measure non-neutralizing functions of HSV-specific antibodies (**Table 1**). Mouse studies have revealed that passively infused intact HSV-specific IgG can protect against viral challenges by footpad injection, whereas F(ab')2 fragments, which can only mediate neutralization, confer only moderate protection, indicating the importance of Fc-mediated antibody functions against HSV (30). In mice, passive transfer of non-neutralizing monoclonal antibodies with in vitro ADCC activity protected complement-deficient mice against lethal HSV-2 challenge (29). Furthermore, in a murine challenge model of HSV-1 and HSV-2, a single-cycle HSV deleted of glycoprotein D (ΔgD-2), which is a major target of neutralizing antibodies, provided complete protection against lethal intravaginal or skin challenge, as well as rapid clearance and elimination of latent virus (39). Yet, interestingly, the vaccine-elicited antibodies had limited neutralization function and had enhanced FcR-mediated functions, namely ADCP and ADCC, as measured by activation of murine FcγRIII or FcγRIV, which of note is not expressed

TABLE 1 | Studies implicating host FcR-mediated functions in protection against HSV and HCMV infections.

Virus	Model	Functions implicated	Relevant observations	References
HSV-2	Mice	ADCC	Passively transferred non-neutralizing monoclonal antibodies with known ADCC function, measured by ^{51}Cr release, protected complement-deficient mice from HSV-2 challenge	(29)
HSV-1	Mice	FcR-mediated functions	Passive immunization with IgG, as compared to F(ab')2 treatment, reduced viral titer, and viral spread in HSV-1 challenged mice	(30)
HSV-2	Humans	ADCC	High maternal or neonatal anti-HSV ADCC antibody levels, measured by infected cell release of ^{51}Cr label, or high neonatal antiviral neutralizing levels were independently associated with an absence of disseminated HSV infection	(31)
HSV-1	Mice	ADCC	Antibodies against HSV gB or gD given with human mononuclear cells protected against lethal challenge in neonatal mice with HSV-1, and protection was associated with monoclonal ADCC activity	(32)
HSV-1	Mice	ADCC	Both neutralization and ADCC activity were independently associated with *in vivo* protection against HSV-1 challenge	(33)
HSV-2	Humans	ADCC	Among HSV-2 gB-2 and gD-2-vaccinated subjects, low ADCC responses were implicated in poor vaccine efficacy against HSV-2	(34)
HSV-2	Mice	ADCC	Antibody dependent protection against genital HSV-2 infection occurs in an Fcγ-receptor dependent mechanism	(35)
HSV-1	Mice	ADCC	HSV-1 FcγR protected the virus by blocking IgG Fc-mediated complement activation and NK cell-mediated ADCC *in vivo*.	(36)
HSV-2	Mice and guinea pigs	Not specified	Neutralization and IFNγ T cell responses did not correlate with vaccine efficacy for HSV-2 subunit vaccines containing gD or gB alone or in combination, together with CpG adjuvant	(37)
HSV-2	Mice	ADCC	The majority of sera collected from mice immunized with mature gG-2 plus CpG adjuvant showed complement-mediated cytolysis and macrophage-mediated ADCC, measured by infected cell release of ^{51}Cr label, but not neutralization	(38)
HSV-1 and HSV-2	Mice	ADCC	Single-cycle HSV ΔgD-2 vaccine conferred protection against skin challenge with clinical isolates, as well as rapid clearance and elimination of latent virus. Protection was associated with target cell killing	(39)
HSV-1 and HSV-2	Mice	ADCC, ADCP	Single-cycle HSV ΔgD-2 vaccine conferred protection against skin challenge with clinical isolates, and protection was associated with activation of HSV-specific murine FcγRIII and FcγRIV	(40)
HSV-1	Human mAbs	ADCC	mAbs derived from humans vaccinated with the HVEM binding domain of HSV-1 gD mediated neutralization and ADCC, measured by NK cell activation, and reduced ocular disease in infected mice	(41)
HSV-1 and HSV-2	Mice	ADCC, ADCP	Single-cycle HSV ΔgD-2 vaccine conferred protection against skin challenge with clinical isolates, and protection was associated with activation of HSV-specific murine FcγRIV	(42)
HCMV	Mice	Not specified	Prophylactic treatment with HCMV gB-specific neutralizing and non-neutralizing antibodies protected equally against CMV challenge. In the setting of established infection, neutralizing and non-neutralizing antibodies provided protection, with neutralizing antibodies being superior	(43)
HCMV	Humans	ADCP	An HCMV gB vaccine that afforded 50% protection in a clinical trial in post-partum women elicited limited neutralization of autologous virus and negligible neutralization of heterologous strains but robust ADCP	(10)
HCMV	Humans	ADCP	An HCMV gB vaccine that afforded partial protection in a clinical trial in transplant recipients elicited limited neutralization of autologous virus and negligible neutralization of heterologous strains but robust ADCP	(11)

gB, glycoprotein B; gD, glycoprotein D; IFNγ, interferon-gamma; gG, glycoprotein G; HSV ΔgD-2, HSV deleted of glycoprotein D.

in humans but in mice is expressed on macrophages and neutrophils (39, 40, 44). Thus, both neutralizing antibodies and ADCC appear to contribute to protection against HSV in animal models.

In human studies, non-neutralizing antibody functions are correlated with protection against infection. In follow-up studies of the HSV-2 gB2 and gD2 combination vaccine, which failed to confer protection against HSV-2 in HSV-2-seronegative women, found that the vaccine induced neutralization but had limited ADCC, as measured by target cells activation (34). A neonatal herpes study evaluated both neutralizing antibodies and ADCC titers in newborns and noted that each independently correlated with protection against neonatal HSV infection (31). These results were also recapitulated in mice (32). Previous vaccine studies also trialed a recombinant HIV glycoprotein 120 (gp120) construct fused to the HSV-1 gD herpesvirus entry mediator binding domain (HVEM) (41), which is a cellular receptor for HSV and is expressed on lymphocytes, fibroblasts, and epithelial cells (45). Monoclonal antibodies isolated from HVEM-vaccinated individuals had both neutralization and ADCC function (45). In an *in vivo* challenge model, these human monoclonal antibodies from HVEM-vaccinated subjects protected mice from lethal infection and resulted in reduced disease burden, namely reduced ocular disease and modestly reduced virus shedding and latency after corneal inoculation with HSV-1 (45). These studies indicate the importance of Fc-mediated functions, namely ADCC, in protection against HSV in both humans and murine models and are under current investigation in HSV vaccine development.

Immunoglobulin G (IgG) genetic variations and FcγR polymorphisms are known to exert effects on ADCC functions, although this has not yet been explored extensively in the context of HSV. Previous studies have demonstrated that homozygosity for the higher-affinity allele CD16A-158V (which encodes FcγR3α) protects against symptomatic HSV-1 infection, whereas the CD32A-131H/R (which encodes FcγR2α-C) dimorphism does not (46). In a follow-up study, NK cell degranulation was consistently enhanced against opsonized HSV-1-infected targets in specifically CD16A-158V/V carriers as compared with CD16A-158F/F carriers (47). Other genetic polymorphisms for IgG and FcγR in the context of non-neutralizing antibody functions such as ADCC warrant future study.

FCR-MEDIATED IMMUNITY AGAINST HCMV

Many current vaccine strategies against HCMV infection have been designed to induce neutralizing antibody responses (48–53). However, it remains unclear whether HCMV transmission will be impacted by plasma neutralization, as reinfection occurs routinely in individuals with pre-existing immunity. *In vivo* HCMV is known to be largely cell-associated, spreading intracellularly and via cell-to-cell without diffusing into extracellular spaces as a cell-free virion (54), and clinical strains *in vitro* recapitulate this feature (54, 55). Yet, *in vitro* studies of HCMV have largely relied on laboratory strains that produce high titers of cell-free virus (56), which may be more vulnerable to neutralizing antibodies, IFN, and cellular restriction factors, as compared with virus transmitted by cell-free entry. A reconstructed wild-type HCMV strain that spread via direct cell-cell contact demonstrated that high expression of the pentameric gH/gL/gpUL128-131A complex enabled resistance to neutralizing antibodies, providing insight into potential mechanisms that facilitate the *in vivo* persistence of HCMV (57).

Although early studies had suggested that neutralizing antibodies may be protective against congenital HCMV transmission, recent randomized controlled trials in humans have indicated that neutralizing antibodies are insufficient to protect against congenital transmission, implicating a potentially important role for FcR-mediated non-neutralizing antibody responses. In a 2005, non-controlled study of HCMV congenital

transmission, administration of HCMV-specific hyperimmune globulin to pregnant women with primary infection decreased the rate of mother-to-fetus transmission from 40 to 16% ($p = 0.04$), and the risk of congenital disease decreased from 50 to 3% ($p < 0.001$) (58). Subsequent non-randomized studies showed a decrease in the number of congenitally infected infants born to mothers who had been treated with hyperimmune globulin or improved outcomes in HCMV-infected infants (59–62). However, in a randomized clinical trial, the administration of polyclonal human IgG containing high titers of neutralizing antibodies failed to prevent congenital infection (63). Regarding primary infection, the most efficacious HCMV vaccine to-date was a protein subunit vaccine targeting HCMV glycoprotein B (gB), which is essential for viral entry into all cell types (9), with an MF59 adjuvant (gB/MF59), and although it achieved 50% protection against primary acquisition in multiple phase two clinical trials (64–66), sera from gB/MF59 vaccinees exhibited poor neutralization of heterologous HCMV strains (10, 11). Furthermore, a correlation between anti-gB antibody titers and protection in vaccinated transplant recipients was found to be independent of neutralization activity (11). These results suggested that the partial protection conferred by the gB/MF59 vaccine was not due to neutralizing antibodies but perhaps due to non-neutralizing antibody responses.

Follow-up studies have aimed to better characterize FcR-mediated non-neutralizing responses protective against HCMV (**Table 1**). Although the HCMV gB/MF59 vaccine did not elicit neutralizing antibodies against heterologous HCMV strains in populations of post-partum women and transplant recipients, sera from post-partum vaccinees mediated robust ADCP of both gB protein-coated beads and fluorescently-labeled whole HCMV virions by human monocytes (10, 11). Interestingly, the gB/MF59 vaccine preferentially induced high binding magnitude gB-specific responses of the IgG3 isotype (10), which is known to demonstrate high avidity for FcR on monocytes and macrophages and which has been shown to coordinated multiple antibody effector functions including ADCC and ADCP (67, 68). Vaccine-elicited antibody enhancement of phagocytosis is thought to have contributed to the partial efficacy of the HCMV gB subunit vaccine, though it remains unclear if ADCP is necessary or sufficient for protection against disease and warrants further study.

In HCMV, ADCC appears to play a role in antiviral immunity for naturally infected individuals, but its importance in protection for vaccine-elicited responses remains to be determined. Studies of pooled human IgG from naturally seropositive individuals (Cytogam) can promote antibody-mediated NK cell lysis (69), and ADCC is measurable in naturally seropositive subjects (10). However, postnatal and transplant subjects vaccinated with gB/MF59 demonstrated no substantial ADCC-promoting antibody response in *in vitro* assays with human NK cells (10, 11). In a murine model of CMV infection, prophylactic administration of HCMV gB-specific monoclonal antibodies before infection was also protective, and both neutralizing and non-neutralizing mAbs were equally effective in preventing lethal infection of immunodeficient mice (43). Thus, FcR-mediated non-neutralizing antibody functions such as ADCP and ADCC against HCMV appear to be involved in the antiviral immune response, but their separate and overlapping contributions with neutralizing responses remain to be determined.

HSV AND HCMV VIRAL FCR IN IMMUNE EVASION

Uniquely, members of the α- and β-subfamily of *herpesviridae* establish permanent, lifelong infections in their hosts. They achieve this in part by encoding surface glycoproteins that bind to the Fc region of host IgG and facilitate evasion from the host immune response (70). HSV and HCMV encode a number of immunomodulating proteins such as decoy receptors and chemokines, which are theorized to protect against both innate and adaptive immune responses (71).

HSV-1 encodes surface glycoproteins gE and gI, which can form a complex on infected cells or on the virion surface that binds to the Fc domain of host IgG (72, 73). This complex acts as a vFcR and is associated with cell-to-cell spread of infection (72, 73). The HSV gE-gI complex is required for the binding of monomeric non-immune IgG, but HSV gE alone is sufficient for binding polymeric IgG (74). The HSV gE-gI complex is thought to facilitate degradation of antiviral host antibodies through pH-specific binding. In this process, host anti-HSV IgG antibodies participate in antibody bipolar bridging, whereby an HSV-specific host antibody simultaneously binds to the HSV gE-gI complex with its Fc region and to a specific HSV-antigen (e.g., gC or gD) with its Fab arms (75–78). At the basic pH of the cell surface, anti-HSV antibody can bind to both HSV gE-gI complex and HSV antigen, but once this antibody is endocytosed and trafficked into the late endosomes, the HSV gE-gI complex dissociates from the antibody Fc region. The host antibody bound to HSV antigen is then localized to the lysosome, where both are degraded, whereas the HSV gE-gI complex can be recycled back to the cell surface. This process of antibody bipolar bridging protects virally infected cells from antibody- and complement-dependent neutralization (78), ADCC (36), and granulocyte attachment (79), and is thus an important mechanism of host immune evasion from antibody-mediated clearance.

One novel strategy for vaccine development against HSV infection aims to prevent these viral immune evasion activities (**Figure 1**). In fact, a trivalent HSV vaccine composed of the vFcγR HSV-2 glycoproteins C, D, and E has been tested in animal challenge studies, in which the vaccine protected seronegative rhesus macaques against intravaginal challenge and seronegative guinea pigs against severe genital disease (80). These glycoproteins were selected due to the involvement of HSV-2 gC in complement cascade inhibition, thus contributing to immune evasion (81); gD in virus entry (26); and gE in blocking host IgG Fc thus also contributing to immune evasion (82). Immunogenicity data revealed that the vaccine induced plasma and mucosa neutralizing antibodies, antibodies that block gC2 and gE2 immune evasion activities, and stimulated CD4 T cell responses (80). In guinea pigs previously infected intravaginally with HSV-2, the vaccine reduced the frequency of recurrent genital lesions and the frequency and duration of vaginal shedding. These studies demonstrate the potential for

vaccine candidates aimed at preventing HSV evasion from host defenses in the context of both primary infection and reactivation and require further studies in humans.

Human HCMV encodes four glycoproteins that act as vFcγR and interfere with IgG-mediated immunity against HCMV: gp68, gp34 (toll-like receptor 11/TLR11), TLR12, and TLR13 (83–85), each with a unique binding pattern to host IgG. Distinct from host FcγR, HCMV vFcγR demonstrate glycan independent binding (86), and all HCMV FcγR genes are transcribed with relatively delayed kinetics during the protracted viral replication cycle, reaching abundant protein amounts during the late phase of infection (83). HCMV gp68 and gp34 are specific for binding human IgG but do not discriminate among the IgG subclasses (87). Recent studies reported formation of antibody bipolar bridging complexes with gp68 and with gp34, and that HCMV lacking gp34 or/and gp68 elicited much stronger activation of host FcγRI, FcγRIIA, and FcγRIIIA by polyclonal HCMV-immune IgG as compared to wildtype HCMV (71). These results implicate HCMV gp34 and gp68 in evading the host FcR-mediated immune response. Unlike the HSV-1 gE-gI complexes, the gp68-Fc interaction is broadly stable across acidic and basic pHs (86), resulting in degradation of the HCMV vFcγR gp68 with the host antibody and HCMV antigen. It is clear that vFcRs are a unique viral immune evasion factor, and further investigation will be required to understand the role of these receptors in both viral pathogeneses, and as potential novel targets for vaccine development.

CONCLUSION

Herpes simplex virus (HSV) and HCMV infections are a serious cause of morbidity and mortality among infants and immunocompromised patients worldwide. There is an urgent need for efficacious vaccines against these pathogens, both to prevent primary acquisition as well as reactivation of latent virus. Historically, vaccine development has aimed to increase the titer of neutralizing antibodies against HSV or HCMV to confer protection, but recent clinical trial data and follow-up immunogenicity studies have investigated the roles of antibody Fc-mediated functions, namely ADCC and ADCP. Furthermore, herpesviruses uniquely encode vFcRs that promote destruction of antiviral host IgG and may enable immune evasion. An improved understanding of non-neutralizing antiviral immune responses and herpesvirus vFcRs may illuminate new pathways for the development of more efficacious vaccines against HSV and HCMV infections.

AUTHOR CONTRIBUTIONS

JJ wrote the majority of the manuscript. MG wrote and edited the manuscript. SP is the PI of JJ and MG. She oversaw the writing and made significant editing contributions.

FUNDING

This work was supported by a National Institutes of Health R21 grant (5R21-AI136556).

REFERENCES

1. Gnann JW, Sköldenberg B, Hart J, Aurelius E, Schliamser S, Studahl M, et al. Herpes simplex encephalitis: lack of clinical benefit of long-term valacyclovir therapy. *Clin Infect Dis.* (2015) 61:683–91. doi: 10.1093/cid/civ369

2. Dollard SC, Grosse SD, Ross DS. New estimates of the prevalence of neurological and sensory sequelae and mortality associated with congenital cytomegalovirus infection. *Rev Med Virol.* (2007) 17:355–63. doi: 10.1002/rmv.544

3. Siegal FP, Lopez C, Hammer GS, Brown AE, Kornfeld SJ, Gold J, et al. Severe acquired immunodeficiency in male homosexuals, manifested by chronic perianal ulcerative herpes simplex lesions. *N Engl J Med.* (1981) 305:1439–44. doi: 10.1056/NEJM198112103052403

4. Takenaka K, Nishida T, Asano-Mori Y, Oshima K, Ohashi K, Mori T, et al. Cytomegalovirus reactivation after allogeneic hematopoietic stem cell transplantation is associated with a reduced risk of relapse in patients with acute myeloid leukemia who survived to day 100 after transplantation: the Japan Society for hematopoietic cell transplantation transplantation-related complication working group. *Biol Blood Marrow Transplant.* (2015) 21:2008–16. doi: 10.1016/j.bbmt.2015.07.019

5. Stratton KR, Durch JS, Lawrence RS. (editors). *Vaccines for the 21st Century: A Tool for Decisionmaking.* Washington, DC: National Academies Press (US) (2000).

6. Reading SA, Dimmock NJ. Neutralization of animal virus infectivity by antibody. *Arch Virol.* (2007) 152:1047–59. doi: 10.1007/s00705-006-0923-8

7. Whitbeck JC, Peng C, Lou H, Xu R, Willis SH, Ponce de Leon M, et al. Glycoprotein D of herpes simplex virus (HSV) binds directly to HVEM, a member of the tumor necrosis factor receptor superfamily and a mediator of HSV entry. *J Virol.* (1997) 71:6083–93.

8. Belshe RB, Leone PA, Bernstein DI, Wald A, Levin MJ, Stapleton JT, et al. Efficacy results of a trial of a herpes simplex vaccine. *N Engl J Med.* (2012) 366:34–43. doi: 10.1056/NEJMoa1103151

9. Vanarsdall AL, Johnson DC. Human cytomegalovirus entry into cells. *Curr Opin Virol.* (2012) 2:37–42. doi: 10.1016/j.coviro.2012.01.001

10. Nelson CS, Huffman T, Jenks JA, Cisneros de la Rosa E, Xie G, Vandergrift N, et al. HCMV glycoprotein B subunit vaccine efficacy mediated by nonneutralizing antibody effector functions. *Proc Natl Acad Sci USA.* (2018) 115:6267–72. doi: 10.1073/pnas.1800177115

11. Baraniak I, Kropff B, Ambrose L, McIntosh M, McLean GR, Pichon S, et al. Protection from cytomegalovirus viremia following glycoprotein B vaccination is not dependent on neutralizing antibodies. *Proc Natl Acad Sci USA.* (2018) 115:6273–8. doi: 10.1073/pnas.1800224115

12. Hayes JM, Cosgrave EF, Struwe WB, Wormald M, Davey GP, Jefferis R, et al. Glycosylation and Fc receptors. *Curr Top Microbiol Immunol.* (2014) 382:165–99. doi: 10.1007/978-3-319-07911-0_8

13. Smith KG, Clatworthy MR. FcgammaRIIB in autoimmunity and infection: evolutionary and therapeutic implications. *Nat Rev Immunol.* (2010) 10:328–43. doi: 10.1038/nri2762

14. Wallace PK, Howell AL, Fanger MW. Role of Fc gamma receptors in cancer and infectious disease. *J Leukoc Biol.* (1994) 55:816–26. doi: 10.1002/jlb.55.6.816

15. Tudor G, Alley M, Nelson CM, Huang R, Covell DG, Gutierrez P, et al. Cytotoxicity of RH1: NAD(P)H:quinone acceptor oxidoreductase (NQO1)-independent oxidative stress and apoptosis induction. *Anticancer Drugs.* (2005) 16:381–91. doi: 10.1097/00001813-200504000-00004

16. Horner H, Frank C, Dechant C, Repp R, Glennie M, Herrmann M, et al. Intimate cell conjugate formation and exchange of membrane lipids precede apoptosis induction in target cells during antibody-dependent, granulocyte-mediated cytotoxicity. *J Immunol.* (2007) 179:337–45. doi: 10.4049/jimmunol.179.1.337

17. Tay MZ, Wiehe K, Pollara J. Antibody-dependent cellular phagocytosis in antiviral immune responses. *Front Immunol.* (2019) 10:332. doi: 10.3389/fimmu.2019.00332

18. Kinchington PR, Leger AJ, Guedon JM, Hendricks RL. Herpes simplex virus and varicella zoster virus, the house guests who never leave. *Herpesviridae.* (2012) 3:5. doi: 10.1186/2042-4280-3-5

19. Awasthi S, Balliet JW, Flynn JA, Lubinski JM, Shaw CE, DiStefano DJ, et al. Protection provided by a herpes simplex virus 2 (HSV-2) glycoprotein C and D subunit antigen vaccine against genital HSV-2 infection in HSV-1-seropositive guinea pigs. *J Virol.* (2014) 88:2000–10. doi: 10.1128/JVI.03163-13

20. Awasthi S, Friedman HM. A paradigm shift: vaccine-induced antibodies as an immune correlate of protection against herpes simplex virus type 1 genital herpes. *J Infect Dis.* (2014) 209:813–5. doi: 10.1093/infdis/jit658

21. Belshe RB, Heineman TC, Bernstein DI, Bellamy AR, Ewell M, van der Most R, et al. Correlate of immune protection against HSV-1 genital disease in vaccinated women. *J Infect Dis.* (2014) 209:828–36. doi: 10.1093/infdis/jit651

22. Peng T, Ponce-de-Leon M, Jiang H, Dubin G, Lubinski JM, Eisenberg RJ, et al. The gH-gL complex of herpes simplex virus (HSV) stimulates neutralizing antibody and protects mice against HSV type 1 challenge. *J Virol.* (1998) 72:65–72.

23. Nicola AV, Ponce de Leon M, Xu R, Hou W, Whitbeck JC, Krummenacher C, et al. Monoclonal antibodies to distinct sites on herpes simplex virus (HSV) glycoprotein D block HSV binding to HVEM. *J Virol.* (1998) 72:3595–601.

24. Sullender WM, Miller JL, Yasukawa LL, Bradley JS, Black SB, Yeager AS, et al. Humoral and cell-mediated immunity in neonates with herpes simplex virus infection. *J Infect Dis.* (1987) 155:28–37. doi: 10.1093/infdis/155.1.28

25. Browne H, Bruun B, Minson T. Plasma membrane requirements for cell fusion induced by herpes simplex virus type 1 glycoproteins gB, gD, gH and gL. *J Gen Virol.* (2001) 82(Pt 6):1419–22. doi: 10.1099/0022-1317-82-6-1419

26. Eisenberg RJ, Atanasiu D, Cairns TM, Gallagher JR, Krummenacher C, Cohen GH. Herpes virus fusion and entry: a story with many characters. *Viruses.* (2012) 4:800–32. doi: 10.3390/v4050800

27. Langenberg AG, Burke RL, Adair SF, Sekulovich R, Tigges M, Dekker CL, et al. A recombinant glycoprotein vaccine for herpes simplex virus type 2: safety and immunogenicity. *Ann Intern Med.* (1995) 122:889–98. doi: 10.7326/0003-4819-122-12-199506150-00001

28. Awasthi S, Belshe RB, Friedman HM. Better neutralization of herpes simplex virus type 1 (HSV-1) than HSV-2 by antibody from recipients of GlaxoSmithKline HSV-2 glycoprotein D2 subunit vaccine. *J Infect Dis.* (2014) 210:571–5. doi: 10.1093/infdis/jiu177

29. Balachandran N, Bacchetti S, Rawls WE. Protection against lethal challenge of BALB/c mice by passive transfer of monoclonal antibodies to five glycoproteins of herpes simplex virus type 2. *Infect Immun.* (1982) 37:1132–7.

30. McKendall RR. IgG-mediated viral clearance in experimental infection with herpes simplex virus type 1: role for neutralization and Fc-dependent functions but not C' cytolysis and C5 chemotaxis. *J Infect Dis.* (1985) 151:464–70. doi: 10.1093/infdis/151.3.464

31. Kohl S, West MS, Prober CG, Sullender WM, Loo LS, Arvin AM. Neonatal antibody-dependent cellular cytotoxic antibody levels are associated with the clinical presentation of neonatal herpes simplex virus infection. *J Infect Dis.* (1989) 160:770–6. doi: 10.1093/infdis/160.5.770

32. Kohl S, Strynadka NC, Hodges RS, Pereira L. Analysis of the role of antibody-dependent cellular cytotoxic antibody activity in murine neonatal herpes simplex virus infection with antibodies to synthetic peptides of glycoprotein D and monoclonal antibodies to glycoprotein B. *J Clin Invest.* (1990) 86:273–8. doi: 10.1172/JCI114695

33. Mester JC, Glorioso JC, Rouse BT. Protection against zosteriform spread of herpes simplex virus by monoclonal antibodies. *J Infect Dis.* (1991) 163:263–9. doi: 10.1093/infdis/163.2.263

34. Kohl S, Charlebois ED, Sigouroudinia M, Goldbeck C, Hartog K, Sekulovich RE, et al. Limited antibody-dependent cellular cytotoxicity antibody response induced by a herpes simplex virus type 2 subunit vaccine. *J Infect Dis.* (2000) 181:335–9. doi: 10.1086/315208

35. Chu CF, Meador MG, Young CG, Strasser JE, Bourne N, Milligan GN. Antibody-mediated protection against genital herpes simplex virus type 2 disease in mice by Fc gamma receptor-dependent and -independent mechanisms. *J Reprod Immunol.* (2008) 78:58–67. doi: 10.1016/j.jri.2007.08.004

36. Lubinski JM, Lazear HM, Awasthi S, Wang F, Friedman HM. The herpes simplex virus 1 IgG fc receptor blocks antibody-mediated complement activation and antibody-dependent cellular cytotoxicity *in vivo. J Virol.* (2011) 85:3239–49. doi: 10.1128/JVI.02509-10

37. Gregg KA, Harberts E, Gardner FM, Pelletier MR, Cayatte C, Yu L, et al. Single and combination herpes simplex virus type 2 glycoprotein vaccines adjuvanted with CpG oligodeoxynucleotides or monophosphoryl lipid A

exhibit differential immunity that is not correlated to protection in animal models. *Clin Vaccine Immunol.* (2011) 18:1702–9. doi: 10.1128/CVI.05071-11

38. Görander S, Harandi AM, Lindqvist M, Bergström T, Liljeqvist JÅ. Glycoprotein G of herpes simplex virus 2 as a novel vaccine antigen for immunity to genital and neurological disease. *J Virol.* (2012) 86:7544–53. doi: 10.1128/JVI.00186-12

39. Petro C, González PA, Cheshenko N, Jandl T, Khajoueinejad N, Bénard A, et al. Herpes simplex type 2 virus deleted in glycoprotein D protects against vaginal, skin and neural disease. *Elife.* (2015) 4:e06054. doi: 10.7554/eLife.06054

40. Petro CD, Weinrick B, Khajoueinejad N, Burn C, Sellers R, Jacobs WR, et al. HSV-2 DeltagD elicits FcgammaR-effector antibodies that protect against clinical isolates. *JCI Insight.* (2016) 1:e88529. doi: 10.1172/jci.insight.88529

41. Wang K, Tomaras GD, Jegaskanda S, Moody MA, Liao HX, Goodman KN, et al. Monoclonal antibodies, derived from humans vaccinated with the RV144 HIV vaccine containing the HVEM binding domain of herpes simplex virus (HSV) glycoprotein D, neutralize HSV infection, mediate antibody-dependent cellular cytotoxicity, and protect mice from ocular challenge with HSV-1. *J Virol.* (2017) 91:e00411–17. doi: 10.1128/JVI.00411-17

42. Burn C, Ramsey N, Garforth SJ, Almo S, Jacobs WR, Herold BC. A herpes simplex virus (HSV)-2 single-cycle candidate vaccine deleted in glycoprotein D protects male mice from lethal skin challenge with clinical isolates of HSV-1 and HSV-2. *J Infect Dis.* (2018) 217:754–8. doi: 10.1093/infdis/jix628

43. Bootz A, Karbach A, Spindler J, Kropff B, Reuter N, Sticht H, et al. Protective capacity of neutralizing and non-neutralizing antibodies against glycoprotein B of cytomegalovirus. *PLoS Pathog.* (2017) 13:e1006601. doi: 10.1371/journal.ppat.1006601

44. Nimmerjahn F, Bruhns P, Horiuchi K, Ravetch JV. FcgammaRIV: a novel FcR with distinct IgG subclass specificity. *Immunity.* (2005) 23:41–51. doi: 10.1016/j.immuni.2005.05.010

45. Spear PG. Herpes simplex virus: receptors and ligands for cell entry. *Cell Microbiol.* (2004) 6:401–10. doi: 10.1111/j.1462-5822.2004.00389.x

46. Moraru M, Cisneros E, Gómez-Lozano N, de Pablo R, Portero F, Cañizares M, et al. Host genetic factors in susceptibility to herpes simplex type 1 virus infection: contribution of polymorphic genes at the interface of innate and adaptive immunity. *J Immunol.* (2012) 188:4412–20. doi: 10.4049/jimmunol.1103434

47. Moraru M, Black LE, Muntasell A, Portero F, López-Botet M, Reyburn HT, et al. NK cell and Ig interplay in defense against herpes simplex virus type 1: epistatic interaction of CD16A and IgG1 allotypes of variable affinities modulates antibody-dependent cellular cytotoxicity and susceptibility to clinical reactivation. *J Immunol.* (2015) 195:1676–84. doi: 10.4049/jimmunol.1500872

48. Macagno A, Bernasconi NL, Vanzetta F, Dander E, Sarasini A, Revello MG, et al. Isolation of human monoclonal antibodies that potently neutralize human cytomegalovirus infection by targeting different epitopes on the gH/gL/UL128-131A complex. *J Virol.* (2010) 84:1005–13. doi: 10.1128/JVI.01809-09

49. Freed DC, Tang Q, Tang A, Li F, He X, Huang Z, et al. Pentameric complex of viral glycoprotein H is the primary target for potent neutralization by a human cytomegalovirus vaccine. *Proc Natl Acad Sci USA.* (2013) 110:E4997–5005. doi: 10.1073/pnas.1316517110

50. Wen Y, Monroe J, Linton C, Archer J, Beard CW, Barnett SW, et al. Human cytomegalovirus gH/gL/UL128/UL130/UL131A complex elicits potently neutralizing antibodies in mice. *Vaccine.* (2014) 32:3796–804. doi: 10.1016/j.vaccine.2014.05.004

51. Wussow F, Chiuppesi F, Martinez J, Campo J, Johnson E, Flechsig C, et al. Human cytomegalovirus vaccine based on the envelope gH/gL pentamer complex. *PLoS Pathog.* (2014) 10:e1004524. doi: 10.1371/journal.ppat.1004524

52. Wussow F, Yue Y, Martinez J, Deere JD, Longmate J, Herrmann A, et al. A vaccine based on the rhesus cytomegalovirus UL128 complex induces broadly neutralizing antibodies in rhesus macaques. *J Virol.* (2013) 87:1322–32. doi: 10.1128/JVI.01669-12

53. Kabanova A, Perez L, Lilleri D, Marcandalli J, Agatic G, Becattini S, et al. Antibody-driven design of a human cytomegalovirus gHgLpUL128L subunit vaccine that selectively elicits potent neutralizing antibodies. *Proc Natl Acad Sci USA.* (2014) 111:17965–70. doi: 10.1073/pnas.1415310111

54. Ziemann M, Hennig H. Prevention of transfusion-transmitted cytomegalovirus infections: which is the optimal strategy? *Transfus Med Hemother.* (2014) 41:40–4. doi: 10.1159/000357102

55. Waldman WJ, Sneddon JM, Stephens RE, Roberts WH. Enhanced endothelial cytopathogenicity induced by a cytomegalovirus strain propagated in endothelial cells. *J Med Virol.* (1989) 28:223–30. doi: 10.1002/jmv.1890280405

56. Murrell I, Tomasec P, Wilkie GS, Dargan DJ, Davison AJ, Stanton RJ. Impact of sequence variation in the UL128 locus on production of human cytomegalovirus in fibroblast and epithelial cells. *J Virol.* (2013) 87:10489–500. doi: 10.1128/JVI.01546-13

57. Murrell I, Bedford C, Ladell K, Miners KL, Price DA, Tomasec P, et al. The pentameric complex drives immunologically covert cell-cell transmission of wild-type human cytomegalovirus. *Proc Natl Acad Sci USA.* (2017) 114:6104–9. doi: 10.1073/pnas.1704809114

58. Nigro G, Adler SP, La Torre R, Best AM. Passive immunization during pregnancy for congenital cytomegalovirus infection. *N Engl J Med.* (2005) 353:1350–62. doi: 10.1056/NEJMoa043337

59. Buxmann H, Stackelberg OM, Schlößer RL, Enders G, Gonser M, Meyer-Wittkopf M, et al. Use of cytomegalovirus hyperimmunoglobulin for prevention of congenital cytomegalovirus disease: a retrospective analysis. *J Perinat Med.* (2012) 40:439–46. doi: 10.1515/jpm-2011-0257

60. Nigro G, Adler SP, Parruti G, Anceschi MM, Coclite E, Pezone I, et al. Immunoglobulin therapy of fetal cytomegalovirus infection occurring in the first half of pregnancy–a case-control study of the outcome in children. *J Infect Dis.* (2012) 205:215–27. doi: 10.1093/infdis/jir718

61. Visentin S, Manara R, Milanese L, Da Roit A, Forner G, Salviato E, et al. Early primary cytomegalovirus infection in pregnancy: maternal hyperimmunoglobulin therapy improves outcomes among infants at 1 year of age. *Clin Infect Dis.* (2012) 55:497–503. doi: 10.1093/cid/cis423

62. Japanese Congenital Cytomegalovirus Infection Immunoglobulin Fetal Therapy Study G. A trial of immunoglobulin fetal therapy for symptomatic congenital cytomegalovirus infection. *J Reprod Immunol.* (2012) 95:73–9. doi: 10.1016/j.jri.2012.05.002

63. Revello MG, Lazzarotto T, Guerra B, Spinillo A, Ferrazzi E, Kustermann A, et al. A randomized trial of hyperimmune globulin to prevent congenital cytomegalovirus. *N Engl J Med.* (2014) 370:1316–26. doi: 10.1056/NEJMoa1310214

64. Pass RF, Zhang C, Evans A, Simpson T, Andrews W, Huang ML, et al. Vaccine prevention of maternal cytomegalovirus infection. *N Engl J Med.* (2009) 360:1191–9. doi: 10.1056/NEJMoa0804749

65. Griffiths PD, Stanton A, McCarrell E, Smith C, Osman M, Harber M, et al. Cytomegalovirus glycoprotein-B vaccine with MF59 adjuvant in transplant recipients: a phase 2 randomised placebo-controlled trial. *Lancet.* (2011) 377:1256–63. doi: 10.1016/S0140-6736(11)60136-0

66. Bernstein DI, Munoz FM, Callahan ST, Rupp R, Wootton SH, Edwards KM, et al. Safety and efficacy of a cytomegalovirus glycoprotein B (gB) vaccine in adolescent girls: a randomized clinical trial. *Vaccine.* (2016) 34:313–9. doi: 10.1016/j.vaccine.2015.11.056

67. Tay MZ, Liu P, Williams LD, McRaven MD, Sawant S, Gurley TC, et al. Antibody-mediated internalization of infectious HIV-1 virions differs among antibody isotypes and subclasses. *PLoS Pathog.* (2016) 12:e1005817. doi: 10.1371/journal.ppat.1005817

68. Vidarsson G, Dekkers G, Rispens T. IgG subclasses and allotypes: from structure to effector functions. *Front Immunol.* (2014) 5:520. doi: 10.3389/fimmu.2014.00520

69. Forthal DN, Phan T, Landucci G. Antibody inhibition of cytomegalovirus the role of natural killer and macrophage effector cells. *Transpl Infect Dis.* (2001) 3:31–4. doi: 10.1034/j.1399-3062.2001.00006.x

70. Budt M, Reinhard H, Bigl A, Hengel H. Herpesviral Fcgamma receptors: culprits attenuating antiviral IgG? *Int Immunopharmacol.* (2004) 4:1135–48. doi: 10.1016/j.intimp.2004.05.020

71. Corrales-Aguilar E, Hoffmann K, Hengel H. CMV-encoded Fcgamma receptors: modulators at the interface of innate and adaptive immunity. *Semin Immunopathol.* (2014) 36:627–40. doi: 10.1007/s00281-014-0448-2

72. Baucke RB, Spear PG. Membrane proteins specified by herpes simplex viruses. V. Identification of an Fc-binding glycoprotein. *J Virol.* (1979) 32:779–89.

73. Watkins JF. Inhibition of spreading of hela cells after infection with herpes simplex virus. *Virology.* (1964) 23:436–8. doi: 10.1016/0042-6822(64)90270-3

74. Dubin G, Frank I, Friedman HM. Herpes simplex virus type 1 encodes two Fc receptors which have different binding characteristics for monomeric immunoglobulin G (IgG) and IgG complexes. *J Virol.* (1990) 64:2725–31.

75. Dubin G, Socolof E, Frank I, Friedman HM. Herpes simplex virus type 1 Fc receptor protects infected cells from antibody-dependent cellular cytotoxicity. *J Virol.* (1991) 65:7046–50.

76. Ndjamen B, Farley AH, Lee T, Fraser SE, Bjorkman PJ. The herpes virus Fc receptor gE-gI mediates antibody bipolar bridging to clear viral antigens from the cell surface. *PLoS Pathog.* (2014) 10:e1003961. doi: 10.1371/journal.ppat.1003961

77. Sprague ER, Wang C, Baker D, Bjorkman PJ. Crystal structure of the HSV-1 Fc receptor bound to Fc reveals a mechanism for antibody bipolar bridging. *PLoS Biol.* (2006) 4:e148. doi: 10.1371/journal.pbio.0040148

78. Frank I, Friedman HM. A novel function of the herpes simplex virus type 1 Fc receptor: participation in bipolar bridging of antiviral immunoglobulin G. *J Virol.* (1989) 63:4479–88.

79. Van Vliet KE, De Graaf-Miltenburg LA, Verhoef J, Van Strijp JA. Direct evidence for antibody bipolar bridging on herpes simplex virus-infected cells. *Immunology.* (1992) 77:109–15.

80. Awasthi S, Hook LM, Shaw CE, Pahar B, Stagray JA, Liu D, et al. An HSV-2 trivalent vaccine is immunogenic in rhesus macaques and highly efficacious in guinea pigs. *PLoS Pathog.* (2017) 13:e1006141. doi: 10.1371/journal.ppat.1006141

81. Awasthi S, Lubinski JM, Shaw CE, Barrett SM, Cai M, Wang F, et al. Immunization with a vaccine combining herpes simplex virus 2 (HSV-2) glycoprotein C (gC) and gD subunits improves the protection of dorsal root ganglia in mice and reduces the frequency of recurrent vaginal shedding of HSV-2 DNA in guinea pigs compared to immunization with gD alone. *J Virol.* (2011) 85:10472–86. doi: 10.1128/JVI.00849-11

82. Awasthi S, Huang J, Shaw C, Friedman HM. Blocking herpes simplex virus 2 glycoprotein E immune evasion as an approach to enhance efficacy of a trivalent subunit antigen vaccine for genital herpes. *J Virol.* (2014) 88:8421–32. doi: 10.1128/JVI.01130-14

83. Atalay R, Zimmermann A, Wagner M, Borst E, Benz C, Messerle M, et al. Identification and expression of human cytomegalovirus transcription units coding for two distinct Fcgamma receptor homologs. *J Virol.* (2002) 76:8596–608. doi: 10.1128/JVI.76.17.8596-8608.2002

84. Lilley BN, Ploegh HL, Tirabassi RS. Human cytomegalovirus open reading frame TRL11/IRL11 encodes an immunoglobulin G Fc-binding protein. *J Virol.* (2001) 75:11218–21. doi: 10.1128/JVI.75.22.11218-11221.2001

85. Cortese M, Calò S, D'Aurizio R, Lilja A, Pacchiani N, Merola M. Recombinant human cytomegalovirus (HCMV) RL13 binds human immunoglobulin G Fc. *PLoS ONE.* (2012) 7:e50166. doi: 10.1371/journal.pone.0050166

86. Sprague ER, Reinhard H, Cheung EJ, Farley AH, Trujillo RD, Hengel H, et al. The human cytomegalovirus Fc receptor gp68 binds the Fc CH2-CH3 interface of immunoglobulin G. *J Virol.* (2008) 82:3490–9. doi: 10.1128/JVI.01476-07

87. Corrales-Aguilar E, Trilling M, Hunold K, Fiedler M, Le VT, Reinhard H, et al. Human cytomegalovirus Fcgamma binding proteins gp34 and gp68 antagonize Fcgamma receptors I, II and III. *PLoS Pathog.* (2014) 10:e1004131. doi: 10.1371/journal.ppat.1004131

18

Monkeying Around: Using Non-Human Primate Models to Study NK Cell Biology in HIV Infections

Cordelia Manickam[1†], Spandan V. Shah[1†], Junsuke Nohara[2], Guido Ferrari[2] and R. Keith Reeves[1,3*]

[1] Center for Virology and Vaccine Research, Beth Israel Deaconess Medical Center, Harvard Medical School, Boston, MA, United States, [2] Department of Surgery, Duke University School of Medicine, Durham, NC, United States, [3] Ragon Institute of Massachusetts General Hospital, MIT, and Harvard, Cambridge, MA, United States

*Correspondence:
R. Keith Reeves
rreeves@bidmc.harvard.edu

[†] These authors have contributed equally to this work

Natural killer (NK) cells are the major innate effectors primed to eliminate virus-infected and tumor or neoplastic cells. Recent studies also suggest nuances in phenotypic and functional characteristics among NK cell subsets may further permit execution of regulatory and adaptive roles. Animal models, particularly non-human primate (NHP) models, are critical for characterizing NK cell biology in disease and under homeostatic conditions. In HIV infection, NK cells mediate multiple antiviral functions via upregulation of activating receptors, inflammatory cytokine secretion, and antibody dependent cell cytotoxicity through antibody Fc-FcR interaction and others. However, HIV infection can also reciprocally modulate NK cells directly or indirectly, leading to impaired/ineffective NK cell responses. In this review, we will describe multiple aspects of NK cell biology in HIV/SIV infections and their association with viral control and disease progression, and how NHP models were critical in detailing each finding. Further, we will discuss the effect of NK cell depletion in SIV-infected NHP and the characteristics of newly described memory NK cells in NHP models and different mouse strains. Overall, we propose that the role of NK cells in controlling viral infections remains incompletely understood and that NHP models are indispensable in order to efficiently address these deficits.

Keywords: HIV, SIV, non-human primates, innate immunity, natural killer cells, animal models

INTRODUCTION

Natural killer (NK) cells have previously been thought simplistically and aptly named, but recent characterizations suggest their roles in both innate and adaptive immunity are in fact quite diverse and complex. In humans, traditional phenotyping identifies NK cells as large non-B, non-T cells expressing CD56 and CD16, and in peripheral blood they are broadly classified into two subpopulations—CD56^{bright} cytokine-secreting and CD56^{dim}CD16$^+$ cytotoxic cells. The major function of NK cells in viral infections and cancer is lysis of target cells by rapidly releasing cytolytic mediators such as perforin and granzyme B and/or secretion of inflammatory cytokines which include but are not limited to interferon (IFN)-γ, tumor growth factor (TGF), tumor necrosis factor (TNF), interleukin (IL)-6, IL-10, granulocyte macrophage-colony stimulation factor (GM-CSF), and G-CSF. NK cell functions are controlled by a balance of activating receptors such as natural cytotoxicity receptors (1) (NKp30, NKp44, and NKp46), activating killer immunoglobulin receptors (KIRs) and C-type lectin receptors (NKG2D and NKG2C), and inhibitory receptors including inhibitory KIRs and NKG2A (2, 3). Recent studies in humans and mouse models have uncovered the existence of an array of NK cell subsets of diverse phenotypes and differential functions. Indeed, NK cell diversity in a single individual could range from 6,000 to 30,000 distinct phenotypes (4) and their functional repertoire now includes long lived memory-like responses, antigen specific memory responses and immunoregulatory roles in addition to their previously known innate functions (5–13). Given their unique nuances in phenotype, maturation, and function in blood and different tissue compartments, it is imperative to understand the role of NK cells in infections, specifically mucosal infections such as human immunodeficiency virus (HIV) and others. To this end, animal models, both mice and non-human primates (NHP), have proved useful in deepening our knowledge on NK cell biology, subsets, and tissue specific responses in health and disease. In the context of animal models to recapitulate the role of NK against HIV-1 infection, this review will primarily focus on these aspects of NK cells in human responses and its analogous modeling in non-human primates (NHP), which has been summarized in **Figure 1**.

CAVEATS OF MODELING HUMAN NK CELL BIOLOGY IN MICE

Mouse models have played significant and historic roles in understanding the interplay of the immune system and infections, with basic NK cell biology as a particularly notable example. However, critical differences between human and murine NK cells can sometimes complicate direct comparisons. Murine NK cells do not express CD56 but have

approximate functional homologs—$CD11b^{low}CD27^{high}$ and $CD11b^{high}CD27^{low}$ NK cells have been correlated to the human $CD56^{bright}$ and $CD56^{dim}$ subsets respectively (14). However, the $CD27^{low}$ subset is not capable of antibody dependent cell cytotoxicity functions (ADCC). Murine NK cells lack NKp44 and NKp30 expression altogether, and indeed NKp46 is the only NCR that is expressed on both murine and human NK cells (15). Further, while both murine and human NK cells express NKG2D, the ligands differ between the species. Murine NKG2D binds to 3 members of the minor histocompatibility family, 5 members of the retinoic acid early inducible gene 1 (Rae-1) family of proteins and murine UL-16-binding protein-like transcript (MULT1). Human NKG2D ligands include MHC I-like (MIC) molecules, MHC-I chain-related A, MHC-I chain-related B and UL16 binding (ULBP) protein family (16). The MIC family proteins are highly polymorphic with more than 70 alleles, and the NKG2D ligands of both species diversified independently, and thus are not orthologous (17). The trafficking markers, and hence the tissue distribution, also vary between the two species. For example, human NK cells are generally present homeostatically in lymph nodes (LN), albeit at low levels, whereas NK cells are observed in murine LN only after stimulation (18). A major difference, as well as an evolutionary disparity, is the recognition of their cognate MHC class I molecules. Murine NK cells use the Ly49 family of proteins which have C-type lectin domains, for cognition of MHC I molecules (19). Human NK cells lack Ly49 proteins and rather express the highly divergent Ig superfamily receptors called KIR that recognize MHC-I (20). Both Ly49 and KIRs act as functional analogs, but they vary to a large extent in their genetic and structural properties and exhibit qualitative differences in their MHC-I interaction. While mouse studies have significantly expanded our current knowledge of NK cell subsets and their functionality, some of these significant differences complicate the modeling of NK cell biology for some

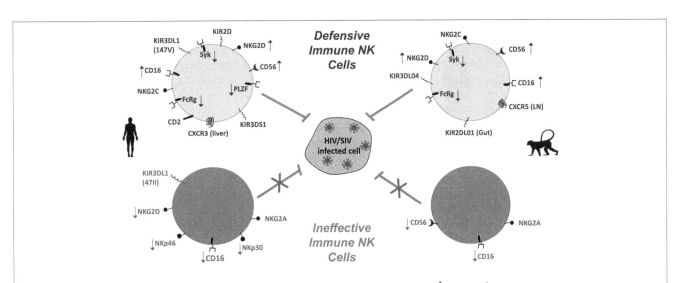

FIGURE 1 | NK cells in HIV/SIV infections of humans **(Left)** and macaques **(Right)**. Differential expression (↑ increase, ↓ decrease) of NK cell markers indicative of defensive and effective anti-HIV/SIV functions (blue) are compared to virus-induced impaired (pink) functions. Overall, the balance of activating and inhibitory receptors is indicative of NK cell functionality and contribution to pathogenic outcomes.

human diseases. Indeed, the limited lifespan, differences in antibody repertoires, and most critically for HIV-1 infection, the lack of lentiviral tropism in mice, has restricted their use as an animal model to understand the role of NK cells against HIV-1.

MODELING NK CELL BIOLOGY IN NHP

NHP NK cells are generally much more similar to human NK cells than murine NK cells and the possibility of *in-vivo* manipulations, such as depleting NK cell numbers, offer opportunities to specifically address NK cell biology. The peripheral NK cell frequency in Old World monkeys, which includes rhesus, cynomolgus and pig-tailed macaques, sooty mangabeys and African green monkeys (AGM), averages ~10% of blood lymphocytes similar to humans. Whereas, in neotropical primates such as common marmosets and cotton-top tamarins, the NK frequency is typically < 5% (21–26). Phylogenetic studies comparing multiple mammalian species have identified KIR3DL as the first ancestral gene originating from simian primates (27). Similar to human NK cells, great apes and Old World monkeys have a rich diversity of KIR3DL1, whereas the New World monkey KIRs diverged from the Old World monkeys, apes and humans, and their KIR3DL1 is more specific to their species. NHP NK cells also have a few dissimilarities such as the low expression of CD56, universal expression of CD8α and NKG2A/C by all subsets of NK cells compared to human NK cells (21, 25, 26, 28, 29). Due to this, the major delineating markers commonly used to identify NK cells in Old World and New World monkeys are CD8α/NKG2A/C and NKp46 respectively.

NHP NK cells, particularly those in rhesus macaques (MAC), have been studied in detail over the last two decades. Gating for CD56 and CD16 expression on circulating NKG2A/C$^+$ MAC NK cells, defines three distinct populations: CD56$^+$CD16$^-$ cells which are functionally equivalent to human CD56^{bright} NK cells; CD56$^-$CD16$^+$ cells corresponding to the human CD56^{dim} NK cells and the CD56$^-$CD16$^-$ (DN) cells for which an analogous phenotype in humans is not yet clearly defined (30, 31). Although NK cell differentiation is dynamic, the CD56 expression pattern can denote the functional maturation of human NK cells, whereby downregulation of CD56 expression indicates a mature differentiated cytotoxic profile (32–34). Hong et al. (35) identified expression patterns in MAC NK cell subsets similar to human NK cells by transcriptional analysis. Expression pattern of transcripts in MAC CD56$^+$ cells were consistent with primitively differentiated cytokine producing cells evidenced as IL-7R, TNF receptor super family member 1B, GATA-3, TCF-7, CD53, amphiregulin, and Granzyme K among others. Conversely, transcripts of effector proteins, such as CCL3, CCL4, and CCL5, were highly expressed in CD16$^+$ cells. Interestingly, Hong et al. (35) found the DN subset to be an intermediary stage between the CD56$^+$ and CD16$^+$ subsets based on the transcriptional profile. While CD57 has also been proposed as a marker of mature, functionally distinct population of NK cells in humans (36), a simian analog has not been identified yet. Overall, the phenotypic, functional and transcriptional profiling has

shown that NHP NK cells are well-suited to model their human counterparts as it will be discussed in the following sections.

NK CELL MODULATION OF HIV AND SIV INFECTIONS VIA KIR/HLA

Epidemiological studies of long-term non-progressors and elite controllers of HIV infection have indicated that the co-expression of KIR3DS1 and a specific HLA-B haplotype known as the HLA-Bw480I correlates with lower viral load, a slower decline of CD4$^+$ T-cell counts and delayed progression to AIDS (37–39). In fact, the NK cell subsets upregulate KIRs and KIR-like molecules in their effort to control virus replication as demonstrated by the protective role of HLA-Bw480I that can potentially bind KIR3DL1 on the membrane of NK cells, contribute to their expansion (40) and increase their cytolytic function (41). In addition to the polymorphism in the HLA-Bw4 variants associated with protection from disease progression, it has been recently reported that a single isoleucine-to-valine substitution in position 47 (I47V) of the KIR3DL1 was responsible for a less protective role in controlling HIV-1 infection compared to the 47VV (not reaching significance) and a significantly more protective role than the 47II genotype (42); the protective role was confined to its interaction with the HLA-B*57:01 and not with the HLA-B*57:03. These data suggest that the KIR-HLA interaction is specifically tuned to impact control of HIV-1 replication. These observations are also supported by the findings that both KIRDL2 and KIRDL3 expressing NK cells can mediate control of HIV-1 via interaction with HLA-C molecules (43, 44). In addition to the polymorphism of the KIR receptor, higher copy numbers of KIR3DS1 and KIR3DL1 in the presence of their ligands were associated with lower viral set point. NK cells from individuals with multiple copies of KIR3DL1 in the presence of KIR3DS1 and their ligands were able to inhibit *in vitro* replication more robustly (37).

Similar observations on the importance of the interaction between KIR and class I HLA molecules have been reported in MAC models and linked with their ability to control SIV infection. The polymorphisms of MAC KIR differs from human (45), but several activating KIR, defined as KIR3DL or KIR3DH, have been associated with lower virus load and longer survival alone or in association with the class I Mamu-A1*001 allele (46) [see also review by Walter and Ansari FI 2015 (47)]. Enhanced copies of KIR3DL04 (or KIR3DH04) were also reported to associate with decreased loss of CD4$^+$ T cells and increased CD56/16 DN NK production of IFN-γ (48). Lastly, a unique profile of circulation and tissue accumulation of the KIR3DL01$^+$ NK subset during acute SIV infection was reported to indicate that this subset (and not the KIR3DL05$^+$) accumulate in gut tissues. These cells also displayed higher proliferation, activation, and antiviral function during chronic infection (49). The study did not correlate the findings with the outcome on control of viremia or disease progression, but raises the important issue of the dynamic changes that take place within the NK subsets during infection, with regard to their frequencies and tissue distribution. An important outcome for the recognition of infected cells by NK cells through the KIR/HLA interaction is related to the ability of NK cells to exert immune pressure on HIV-1 sequence (50, 51), similar to what was described for the CD8$^+$ T cell responses (52, 53).

As discussed above, KIRs play important roles in controlling both HIV and SIV infections. However, one must be judicious when using NHP models to study the impact of KIRs on retroviral infection, due to the disparities between the KIR repertoires of human and that of NHP (54). For instance, the KIR subtype with only one extracellular domain, KIR1D, has been identified in MAC, which seems to be unique to NHP and there is no corresponding counterpart in human (55). Even though the nucleic acid sequence contains two Ig-like domains, the expressed protein is truncated at the second domain due to a frame shift mutation (55). Consequently, the KIR1D subtype lacks the cytoplasmic domain as well, and although it's *in vivo* function is still currently unknown, it is speculated to be secreted extracellularly (56). Another major feature that differentiates the human and NHP KIR is their complexity of KIR2D and KIR3D subtypes. Based on the structure and MHC molecule specificity, the KIR genes can be divided into 4 main lineages, I, II, III, and V (54, 57). While only 3 distinct lineage II KIR3D genes have been characterized in human, MAC has been reported to have a highly diverse lineage II repertoire, consisting of 10 KIR3DL genes and 9 KIR3DS genes (56, 58, 59). This may have evolved to complement the expanded HLA-A and B genes that are observed in NHP, and indeed, some of the KIR3DL/S has been shown to bind to HLA-A/B molecules (27, 58, 60). Conversely, humans have more diverse lineage III KIR genes that are absent in Old-World monkeys, such as MAC (55, 61), which is consistent with the higher variability of HLA-C molecules in human (62). Thus, the KIR gene repertoire for NHP seems to be much more complex than that of humans. The latest studies identified a total of 22 different KIR genes for MAC (59, 63), as compared to 15 KIR genes and 2 pseudogenes in humans (64). In general, the complexity of KIR genotype and expression in relation to the class I HLA molecules should be carefully considered when expression of KIR on human and NHP NK subsets are evaluated for their correlation with the outcome of retroviral infections. Furthermore, it is clear that, in both humans and NHP, KIR, and HLA class I polymorphism can influence the outcome of infection, but the evolutionary advantage of these molecules has not been elucidated yet.

FC-RECEPTOR (FCR) MEDIATED NK CELL FUNCTIONS IN HIV/SIV INFECTIONS

Among the immunomodulatory and effector functions mediated by NK cells, their role as effector cells in Fc-dependent antibody functions represented by ADCC is very important in HIV-1 and SIV infections. This is best highlighted by the correlation between vaccine-induced ADCC responses and control of virus replication (65–68) and protection (69), and in pre-clinical studies conducted in MAC and recent observations in mother-to-child transmission (70, 71). Moreover, the only human

vaccine clinical trial that provided limited success, the RV144 study conducted in Thailand, suggested a crucial role for non-neutralizing Ab responses capable of mediating ADCC as correlates with lower risk of infection (72, 73). The NK cells provide the effector cell component to these type of responses, upon engagement of their FcγR III (CD16) by the Fc region of an antibody that can recognize antigens expressed on the membrane of infected cells (74). In humans as well as in NHP, the canonical ADCC-mediating effector NK cell subset has been described as those that are lineage negative (lacking expression of markers defining major T and B cell subsets) and CD16$^+$, which are the peripheral CD56^{dim}CD16^{bright} cells in humans and CD3$^-$CD20$^-$CD8$^+$NKG2A/C$^+$CD16$^+$in MAC. The effector function of these cellular subsets is in general regulated by the fine interaction between the Ab subclasses and the polymorphisms of the FcRs that present substantial differences between the human and NHP (75–77). In addition to the classical Fc-FcR engagement of ADCC effector cell subsets, it has also been reported that recognition of the infected target cells requires engagement of NKG2D-receptor, suggesting that the NKG2D may serve as a co-receptor for ADCC-mediated NK cell functions (78). In addition to the CD8α$^+$CD16$^+$ NK subset, it has been reported that the CD8α$^-$ NK cells can also be potent ADCC effector cells in MAC and co-express the CD56, CD16, NKG2D, and KIR2D receptors. These cells represent approximately 35% of the macaque CD8α$^-$ cells and are responsive to stimulation by IL-15 to upregulate the CD69 receptor and produce IFN-γ and TNF- cytokines, providing additional functions to the cytotoxicity (79).

IMPACT OF HIV AND SIV INFECTION ON NK DISTRIBUTION AND FUNCTION

In healthy humans, tissue NK cells are more heterogeneous, complex and less studied than their peripheral blood counterparts due to limited access to human tissues. Tissue-resident NK cells differ by their pattern of chemokine and adhesion receptors, which are specialized based on their homing properties and/or *in-situ* maturation (80, 81). CD56^{bright} NK cells in human blood express trafficking markers CD62L, CCR7, CXCR3, and CXCR4 that allow their migration into secondary lymphoid organs, inflamed tissues, and tumors, whereas tissue resident CD56^{bright} NK cells do not express CD62L but other adhesion markers such as CD49a and CD103 (18, 82–84). The CD56^{dim} subset expresses receptors that are necessary for migration into inflamed sites including CXCR4, CX3CR1, CXCR2, and CXCR3 and low levels of CD62L and no CCR7. On the other hand, CD56^{bright} NK cells express high levels of CCR7 and CD62L and constitute a large proportion of NK cells in the lymph node because of their affinity to high endothelial venules (HEV) (18, 85). In fact, LNs have been proposed as a site of maturation for some NK cells (86). CD56^{bright} NK cells are also the predominant population in the gut and participate in the gut homeostasis (87). However, multiple pathogens including

HIV-1, can disrupt the overall homeostatic NK cell distribution in tissues.

It has been previously reported that NK cells undergo redistribution amongst different tissue compartments during the acute phase of HIV infection, as indicated by the increased frequency of circulating $CD3^{neg}CD56^{neg}CD16^{pos}$ NK cells with perturbed functional profiles and reduced presence of $CD3^{neg}CD56^{pos}$ NK cells (88). Despite this body of evidence that suggests an important role for NK cells in the control of HIV-1 replication, they are not able to clear the infection. This may be attributed, at least in part, to the overall subversion of the immune system caused by HIV-1, where NK cells are not only altered functionally but may be impaired in trafficking and tissue infiltration. In fact, it was described very early that NK cells were dysfunctional in HIV-1 infected subjects (89) and this effect could be detected at the level of their ability to perform FcR-mediated functions (90), as well as expression of KIR, activation markers, and cytokine production (91, 92). The impairment of NK cells could be due to the direct effect of HIV-1 or, due to the effect of cytokine milieu on NKp30 and NKG2D expression (93) and/or CD4 dysfunction. The latter has been recently demonstrated to be the case because blockade of PD-1 and IL-10 pathways can restore the HIV-1 specific CD4 T cells *in vitro* and enhance cytokine expression and cytolytic function of the NK subsets (94). The presence of impaired NK subsets is not solely observed during HIV-1 infection as reported by Meier et al. (95). In fact, they described a similar alteration of the NK subsets in HIV-1 and Hepatitis C virus (HCV) infections with a clear decline in the frequency of the $CD56^{dim}$ NK that resulted in reduction of IFN-γ production and cytotoxic function (95). Similar observations on the impairment of NK cell function has been described in SIV-infected MAC related to differentiation, cytokine secretion, and expression of activation/homing markers (96, 97). The importance of these dysfunctions in the context of hampering the ability of NK subsets to fully control retroviral infection is indicated by the demonstration that in chronically SIV-infected MAC, the frequency of CD56/16 DN NK cells in the spleen and liver of infected animals with high virus load was significantly lower than in animals with lower virus load (98). Moreover, frequency of the liver-resident $CXCR3^{+}$ NK cells and circulating $NKG2D^{+}$ cells were inversely correlated with plasma viremia (98). These data suggest that differences in the location and function of the NK subsets have a relevant impact on the outcome of virus replication in the SIV model and the same may occur in HIV-1 infection. To support the complexity of this reality, data was collected from the animals that can naturally survive the SIV infection. In fact, the analysis of the distribution of NK cells within the LN in the pathogenic and non-pathogenic SIV-infection models represented by the MAC and AGM, respectively, revealed unique differential aspects (99). In the pathogenic model, the NK cells were found in a random distribution and did not accumulate in the follicles, whereas a significantly higher frequency of NK cells was observed in the AGM LN mostly around or within the follicles. The AGM NK cells also expressed CXCR5 and the frequency of $CXCR5^{+}$ NK cells in the AGM LN was significantly higher.

This distribution persisted throughout the time of observation of the infected animals and was associated with a significantly higher frequency of cells with membrane-bound IL-15 in the AGM. Anti-IL-15 treatment of AGM depleted NK cells from LN, spleen, and gut, and it induced a significantly increased plasma viral load as well as the amount of cell-associated viral RNA and DNA in the LN, compared to the untreated animals. Collectively, these data indicated that the unique control of virus in non-pathogenic AGM is at least partially mediated by NK cells.

IMPACT OF *IN VIVO* NK DEPLETION IN SIV-INFECTED ANIMALS

A major argument for the importance of $CD8^{+}$ T cell responses in control of retroviral infection was initially provided by seminal studies conducted by Letvin and collaborators, who reported the immediate rebound in SIV replication in MAC upon depletion of $CD8^{+}$ T cells by infusion of targeted monoclonal antibodies (100). Similar experiments have now been conducted in MAC models to address the role of NK cells in virus control, but thus far have provided contrasting results. Initially, $CD16^{+}$ NK depletion performed using the 3G8 mAb 24 h before infection with SIV did not impact the level of viremia observed in the infused animals during the first 11 days of infection compared to those receiving a control mAb. These data suggested that $CD16^{+}$ NK cells did not contribute to initial control of SIV replication (101), although the assay had several caveats, such as the emergence of idiotypic antibodies (102) and the lack of $CD16^{-}$NK cells depletion from lymph nodes that are largely responsible for controlling virus replication (85, 103). More recently, depletion of NK cells in the periphery and in intestinal mucosal tissues following administration of JAK3 inhibitors induced a modest but significant increase of plasma viral load in all six animals tested and in tissue viral load in 5 out of 6 animals. The latter was not related to an increase in frequency of $CD4^{+}$ T cells, suggesting an increased production of the virus on a per cell basis. (104). A follow-up study investigated prolonged administration of the JAK3 inhibitor during the acute phase of infection and recapitulated the finding of significant higher virus replication during the chronic phase (>12 weeks) of infection in JAK3-treated MAC, but not during the acute phase of infection. One caveat to the latter study was related to the concomitantly observed partial depletion of $CD8^{+}$ T cell subsets, among other immune cells, and the unresolved contribution that this could have had on the outcome of the study, mainly implicating depletion of NK subsets in the gastrointestinal tissue (105). The different outcomes of these studies could either be related to the stage of infection, acute vs. chronic infection, or to the depletion procedure, that could impact different NK cell subsets. Overall, the data do not provide a definitive determination of the impact that NK cells could have on the control of SIV infection in MAC. The anti-IL-15 neutralization approach to deplete NK cells has been shown to be effective in AGM and MAC (99, 106), but full evaluation has not been performed during acute and chronic infection of a pathogenic species.

MEMORY NK CELLS AND HIV/SIV

The possibility of NK cells with adaptive features perhaps emerged from an unexpected observation by Boehncke et al. (107) wherein wild-type (WT) and T-cell deficient mice responded similarly to 4-dinitro-1-fluorobenzene (DNFB)-induced contact hypersensitivity (CHS). NK cell memory, as an emerging field of study, was further solidified by O' Leary et al. (108) in a CHS mouse model with the observation of T- and B-cell independent adaptive immunity that was mediated by NK cells. These responses were elicited by haptens and persisted for at least 4 weeks following sensitization. The same group later demonstrated (109) that liver-resident NK cells in mice were not only capable of generating a memory pool against haptens but also against influenza, vesicular stomatitis virus (VSV) and HIV; and that the chemokine receptor CXCR6 plays a critical role in this process. Subsequently, the phenomenon has since been observed in other mouse models, non-human primates, as well as in humans (reviewed in (12, 110, 111)).

As our understanding of the memory NK cell response expands, multiple subpopulations that may mediate antigen recall through differing mechanisms have emerged. These different subtypes are, however, somewhat fluid. For practical purposes, we will comment on four categorizations of these cells:

1) True *antigen-specific memory NK* cells respond to an antigen presented analogously to classical adaptive cells. Antigens include haptens (112), cytomegalovirus (CMV) (13, 113–115), HIV (13, 109), and others (109, 116, 117).

2) *Cytokine-induced memory* NK cells seem to respond to specific cytokines (IL-12, IL-15, and IL-18) with a brief pre-activation period followed by enhanced activity in response to cytokine receptor stimulation (118). Cytokine-induced memory NK cells have been reported against influenza virus (119), leukemia (120) and melanoma (121). A recent article also reports the generation of "tumor-induced memory-like" (TIML-) NK cells (122).

3) *Memory-like* (adaptive) NK cells comprise a unique subset of NK cells that have reduced expression of the CD16 adaptor molecules, FcR γ-chain, and Syk, specifically induced in responses to CMV infection (123–127). Memory-like NK cell numbers have also been shown to expand in HIV (128, 129), HCV (130) and Epstein Bar Virus (EBV) (131–133) infections.

4) *Evolved memory* (adaptive) NK cells overlap with antigen-specific and memory-like NK cells with a response induced by CMV infection. A critical difference is the expression of a specific receptor, Ly49H, by NK cells that interact with MCMV glycoprotein m157 (134, 135) in mouse models, and more recently, Ly49I and Ly49C were also shown to interact with specific MCMV peptides (136). An analogous NKG2C$^+$ cell type has also been described in humans although the mechanisms are less well-defined (137). Collectively, an evolved memory NK cell can be considered as one that expresses a receptor (or perhaps a precise combination of known and unknown receptors) that is induced to control a specific pathogen.

Paust et al. (109) demonstrated that murine NK cells can develop memory against HIV antigens, a virus which cannot infect mice, and thus there is no evolutionary component. Primed hepatic NK cells (but not splenic NK cells) mounted a vigorous recall response in recipient mice, and the chemokine receptor CXCR6 was deemed critical for this function. Later, our group showed that NK cells in MAC were capable of mounting a recall response against SIV/SHIV and HIV vaccine antigens (13), and NKG2C was indicated to play a critical role in this process.

To our knowledge, memory-like FcR γ-chain deficient NK cells have not been reported in mice. One possibility is the exclusive association of CD16 to FcR γ-chain homodimers in mice, compared to the association with homodimers and heterodimers of FcR γ-chain and CD3ζ in humans (138). Thus, murine NK cells might not be able to respond to CMV infection in a manner similar to human NK cells. Nonetheless, the prevalence of other subtypes of NK cells (cytokine-induced and antigen-specific) suggests murine NK cells have likely devised alternate strategies to control viral infections. Other such subtle variations of these cells almost certainly exist, but the exact interplay between the pathogen and NK cells that induces each population still needs significant assessment.

The defining characteristics of "memory-like" NK cells are the lack of the FcR γ signaling chain and Syk adaptor proteins, likely resulting from epigenetic reprogramming of these subsets of NK cells by CMV (126, 139). The initial observation made by Leeansyah et al. suggested persistent lack of FcR γ-chain expression in NK cells from HIV-1 positive subjects receiving cART (140); however, CMV infection status of these patients was not reported in this study. A follow-up study by the same group suggested that these cells had significantly reduced NCR (NKp46 and NKp30) expression and showed greater ADCC against opsonized targets (128), but the role of HIV *per se* in the induction of these cells is not clear. CMV is likely the primary source of induction of these cells (124, 125), but how HIV can also modulate these phenotypes in NK cells is unclear. Our own assessment in MAC suggests SIV infection does not have a significant impact on total numbers of γ-chain$^-$ Syk$^-$ NK cells, which is modulated by rhesus CMV (rhCMV), but the migration into tissues was heavily influenced by SIV infection (127). In blood, rhCMV titers were correlated to adaptive NK cell numbers in both rhCMV-infected, as well as rhCMV/SIV co-infected animals (127). This observation was similar to observations made by Zhou et al. (128), where adaptive NK cell prevalence generally correlated with CMV antibody titers, but was further modulated by HIV infection. This discrepancy could simply be explained by host species-specific differences, or perhaps by HIV specific responses exerted by NK cells in humans. Furthermore, SIV was able to subvert the enhanced responses of adaptive NK cells by suppressing the alternate signaling mechanism induced by rhCMV (127). The data explaining the effect of HIV/SIV infection on adaptive NK cells, in the absence of prior CMV infection, are sorely lacking. It is imperative to address the skewed observations in SIV infection, which could have arisen due to the confounding effects of co-infection with CMV. Most importantly, we need to address the question of protective features of CMV induced NK cells against other viral infections such as HIV-1.

Similar questions have been posited for other memory NK cell subsets as well, particularly NKG2C$^+$ evolved NK cells induced by CMV infection (141). Similar to the expansion of γ-chain$^-$Syk$^-$ NK cell populations in SIV/HIV$^+$ subjects, the expansion of the NKG2C$^+$ population in HIV-1$^+$ subjects is attributed to concurrent HCMV infection (142). A recent study suggests that adaptive NK cells induced by CMV in HIV-1 infected individuals are further modulated and marked by reduced expression of the transcription factor promyelocytic leukemia zinc finger (PLZF) (129, 129) and that these cells are distinguished from other adaptive NK cells expressing NKG2C or CD57. Intriguingly, HIV might be directly affecting NKG2C$^+$ NK cell numbers, since p24 has been reported to stabilize HLA-E expression on lymphocytes of HIV$^+$ patients (143). Overall, the questions regarding the protective ability of memory/adaptive/cytokine-induced NK cell subsets against HIV remain unanswered. Information on the unadulterated effect of HIV on the NK cell receptor repertoire, functional abilities, epigenetic reprogramming and specific subset expansion *in vivo* needs significant in-depth investigation and may direct specific preventative and curative strategies against HIV infections.

CONCLUDING REMARKS

Many studies have highlighted the crucial role of NK cells in mediating control of HIV transmission, dissemination, disease, and reciprocally virus-mediated subversion of NK cells. Unlike many other pathogens, mouse models have contributed in a more limited way to this body of knowledge, due to the lack of tropism of lentiviruses and caveats of humanized mouse models. These circumstances have created one of the best examples of the significant utility of studying immunology in NHP, specifically SIV infection of various MAC species. Overall, these studies have revealed multiple layers of NK cell-virus interplay in lentivirus infection including: (1) KIR-HLA; (2) induction of CD2 and NKG2-related molecules; (3) interaction of Fc-receptor bearing NK cells and Ab-opsonized virus infected cells; and (4) development of HIV/SIV-specific NK cell memory-like responses. Although many unanswered questions remain regarding NK cell correlates of virus control, the significant contribution of NHP models cannot be overstated and rapidly evolving *in vivo* and *ex vivo* manipulations will undoubtedly continue to advance studies of HIV vaccine and other therapeutic modality development.

AUTHOR CONTRIBUTIONS

CM, SS, JN, and GF contributed to writing of specific sections. RR and GF oversaw overall preparation of the manuscript, contributed to writing. RR edited the final version of the manuscript.

FUNDING

This work was supported by National Institutes of Health (NIH) grants P01 AI120756, R01 DE026014, and R01 AI120828. The funders had no role in study design, data collection and analysis, decision to publish, or preparation of the manuscript.

REFERENCES

1. Treml LS, Carlesso G, Hoek KL, Stadanlick JE, Kambayashi T, Bram RJ, et al. TLR stimulation modifies BLyS receptor expression in follicular and marginal zone B cells. *J Immunol.* (2007) 178:7531–9. doi: 10.4049/jimmunol.178.12.7531
2. Moretta A, Biassoni R, Bottino C, Mingari MC, Moretta L. Natural cytotoxicity receptors that trigger human NK-cell-mediated cytolysis. *Immunol Today.* (2000) 21:228–34. doi: 10.1016/S0167-5699(00)01596-6
3. Long EO, Kim HS, Liu D, Peterson ME, Rajagopalan S. Controlling natural killer cell responses: integration of signals for activation and inhibition. *Annu Rev Immunol.* (2013) 31:227–58. doi: 10.1146/annurev-immunol-020711-075005
4. Horowitz A, Strauss-Albee DM, Leipold M, Kubo J, Nemat-Gorgani N, Dogan OC, et al. Genetic and environmental determinants of human NK cell diversity revealed by mass cytometry. *Sci Transl Med.* (2013) 5:208ra145. doi: 10.1126/scitranslmed.3006702
5. Holder KA, Comeau EM, Grant MD. Origins of natural killer cell memory: special creation or adaptive evolution. *Immunology.* (2018) 154:38–49. doi: 10.1111/imm.12898
6. Sun JC, Lanier LL. Is there natural killer cell memory and can it be harnessed by vaccination? NK cell memory and immunization strategies against infectious diseases and cancer. *Cold Spring Harb Perspect Biol.* (2017)10:a029538. doi: 10.1101/cshperspect.a029538
7. Peng H, Tian Z. Natural killer cell memory: progress and implications. *Front Immunol.* (2017) 8:1143. doi: 10.3389/fimmu.2017.01143
8. Holmes TD, Bryceson YT. Natural killer cell memory in context. *Semin Immunol.* (2016) 28:368–76. doi: 10.1016/j.smim.2016.05.008
9. O'Sullivan TE, Sun JC, Lanier LL. Natural killer cell memory. *Immunity.* (2015) 43:634–45. doi: 10.1016/j.immuni.2015.09.013
10. O'Sullivan TE, Sun JC. Generation of natural killer cell memory during viral infection. *J Innate Immun.* (2015) 7:557–62. doi: 10.1159/000375494
11. Marcus A, Raulet DH. Evidence for natural killer cell memory. *Curr Biol.* (2013) 23:R817–20. doi: 10.1016/j.cub.2013.07.015
12. Paust S, von Andrian UH. Natural killer cell memory. *Nat Immunol.* (2011) 12:500–8. doi: 10.1038/ni.2032
13. Reeves RK, Li H, Jost S, Blass E, Li H, Schafer JL, et al. Antigen-specific NK cell memory in rhesus macaques. *Nat Immunol.* (2015) 16:927–32. doi: 10.1038/ni.3227
14. Hayakawa Y, Huntington ND, Nutt SL, Smyth MJ. Functional subsets of mouse natural killer cells. *Immunol Rev.* (2006) 214:47–55. doi: 10.1111/j.1600-065X.2006.00454.x
15. Montaldo E, Del Zotto G, Della Chiesa M, Mingari MC, Moretta A, De Maria A, et al. Human NK cell receptors/markers: a tool to analyze NK cell development, subsets and function. *Cytometry A.* (2013) 83:702–13. doi: 10.1002/cyto.a.22302
16. Mestas J, Hughes CC. Of mice and not men: differences between mouse and human immunology. *J Immunol.* (2004) 172:2731–8. doi: 10.4049/jimmunol.172.5.2731
17. Raulet DH. Roles of the NKG2D immunoreceptor and its ligands. *Nat Rev Immunol.* (2003) 3:781–90. doi: 10.1038/nri1199
18. Fehniger TA, Cooper MA, Nuovo GJ, Cella M, Facchetti F, Colonna M, et al. CD56bright natural killer cells are present in human lymph nodes and are activated by T cell-derived IL-2: a potential new link between adaptive and innate immunity. *Blood.* (2003) 101:3052–7. doi: 10.1182/blood-2002-09-2876

19. Webb JR, Lee SH, Vidal SM. Genetic control of innate immune responses against cytomegalovirus: MCMV meets its match. *Genes Immun.* (2002) 3:250–62. doi: 10.1038/sj.gene.6363876

20. Lanier LL. NK cell receptors. *Annu Rev Immunol.* (1998) 16:359–93. doi: 10.1146/annurev.immunol.16.1.359

21. Carville A, Evans TI, Reeves RK. Characterization of circulating natural killer cells in neotropical primates. *PLoS ONE.* (2013) 8:e78793. doi: 10.1371/journal.pone.0078793

22. Pereira LE, Johnson RP, Ansari AA. Sooty mangabeys and rhesus macaques exhibit significant divergent natural killer cell responses during both acute and chronic phases of SIV infection. *Cell Immunol.* (2008) 254:10–9. doi: 10.1016/j.cellimm.2008.06.006

23. Ibegbu C, Brodie-Hill A, Kourtis AP, Carter A, McClure H, Chen ZW, et al. Use of human CD3 monoclonal antibody for accurate CD4+ and CD8+ lymphocyte determinations in macaques: phenotypic characterization of the CD3- CD8+ cell subset. *J Med Primatol.* (2001) 30:291–8. doi: 10.1034/j.1600-0684.2001.300601.x

24. Wei Q, Stallworth JW, Vance PJ, Hoxie JA, Fultz PN. Simian immunodeficiency virus (SIV)/immunoglobulin G immune complexes in SIV-infected macaques block detection of CD16 but not cytolytic activity of natural killer cells. *Clin Vaccine Immunol.* (2006) 13:768–78. doi: 10.1128/CVI.00042-06

25. Jacquelin B, Petitjean G, Kunkel D, Liovat AS, Jochems SP, Rogers KA, et al. Innate immune responses and rapid control of inflammation in African green monkeys treated or not with interferon-alpha during primary SIVagm infection. *PLoS Pathog.* (2014) 10:e1004241. doi: 10.1371/journal.ppat.1004241

26. Rutjens E, Mazza S, Biassoni R, Koopman G, Ugolotti E, Fogli M, et al. CD8+ NK cells are predominant in chimpanzees, characterized by high NCR expression and cytokine production, and preserved in chronic HIV-1 infection. *Eur J Immunol.* (2010) 40:1440–50. doi: 10.1002/eji.200940062

27. Parham P, Abi-Rached L, Matevosyan L, Moesta AK, Norman PJ, Older Aguilar AM, et al. Primate-specific regulation of natural killer cells. *J Med Primatol.* (2010) 39:194–212. doi: 10.1111/j.1600-0684.2010.00432.x

28. Carter DL, Shieh TM, Blosser RL, Chadwick KR, Margolick JB, Hildreth JE, et al. CD56 identifies monocytes and not natural killer cells in rhesus macaques. *Cytometry.* (1999) 37:41–50. doi: 10.1002/(SICI)1097-0320(19990901)37:1<41::AID-CYTO5>3.0.CO;2-4

29. Mavilio D, Benjamin J, Kim D, Lombardo G, Daucher M, Kinter A, et al. Identification of NKG2A and NKp80 as specific natural killer cell markers in rhesus and pigtailed monkeys. *Blood.* (2005) 106:1718–25. doi: 10.1182/blood-2004-12-4762

30. Webster RL, Johnson RP. Delineation of multiple subpopulations of natural killer cells in rhesus macaques. *Immunology.* (2005) 115:206–14. doi: 10.1111/j.1365-2567.2005.02147.x

31. Reeves RK, Gillis J, Wong FE, Yu Y, Connole M, Johnson RP. CD16- natural killer cells: enrichment in mucosal and secondary lymphoid tissues and altered function during chronic SIV infection. *Blood.* (2010) 115:4439–46. doi: 10.1182/blood-2010-01-265595

32. Yu J, Mao HC, Wei M, Hughes T, Zhang J, Park IK, et al. CD94 surface density identifies a functional intermediary between the CD56bright and CD56dim human NK-cell subsets. *Blood.* (2010) 115:274–81. doi: 10.1182/blood-2009-04-215491

33. Beziat V, Duffy D, Quoc SN, Le Garff-Tavernier M, Decocq J, Combadiere B, et al. CD56brightCD16+ NK cells: a functional intermediate stage of NK cell differentiation. *J Immunol.* (2011) 186:6753–61. doi: 10.4049/jimmunol.1100330

34. Romagnani C, Juelke K, Falco M, Morandi B, D'Agostino A, Costa R, et al. CD56brightCD16- killer Ig-like receptor- NK cells display longer telomeres and acquire features of CD56dim NK cells upon activation. *J Immunol.* (2007) 178:4947–55. doi: 10.4049/jimmunol.178.8.4947

35. Hong HS, Rajakumar PA, Billingsley JM, Reeves RK, Johnson RP. No monkey business: why studying NK cells in non-human primates pays off. *Front Immunol.* (2013) 4:32. doi: 10.3389/fimmu.2013.00032

36. Lopez-Verges S, Milush JM, Pandey S, York VA, Arakawa-Hoyt J, Pircher H, et al. CD57 defines a functionally distinct population of mature NK cells in the human CD56dimCD16+ NK-cell subset. *Blood.* (2010) 116:3865–74. doi: 10.1182/blood-2010-04-282301

37. Pelak K, Need AC, Fellay J, Shianna KV, Feng S, Urban TJ, et al. Copy number variation of KIR genes influences HIV-1 control. *PLoS Biol.* (2011) 9:e1001208. doi: 10.1371/annotation/7e17b146-a69c-4e83-9230-7340486d9dc8

38. Long BR, Ndhlovu LC, Oksenberg JR, Lanier LL, Hecht FM, Nixon DF, et al. Conferral of enhanced natural killer cell function by KIR3DS1 in early human immunodeficiency virus type 1 infection. *J. Virol.* (2008) 82:4785–92. doi: 10.1128/JVI.02449-07

39. Alter G, Martin MP, Teigen N, Carr WH, Suscovich TJ, Schneidewind A, et al. Differential natural killer cell–mediated inhibition of HIV-1 replication based on distinct KIR/HLA subtypes. *J Exp Med.* (2007) 204:3027–36. doi: 10.1084/jem.20070695

40. Alter G, Rihn S, Walter K, Nolting A, Martin M, Rosenberg ES, et al. HLA class I subtype-dependent expansion of KIR3DS1+ and KIR3DL1+ NK cells during acute human immunodeficiency virus type 1 infection. *J Virol.* (2009) 83:6798–805. doi: 10.1128/JVI.00256-09

41. Kiepiela P, Leslie AJ, Honeyborne I, Ramduth D, Thobakgale C, Chetty S, et al. Dominant influence of HLA-B in mediating the potential co-evolution of HIV and HLA. *Nature.* (2004) 432:769–75. doi: 10.1038/nature03113

42. Martin MP, Naranbhai V, Shea PR, Qi Y, Ramsuran V, Vince N, et al. Killer cell immunoglobulin-like receptor 3DL1 variation modifies HLA-B*57 protection against HIV-1. *J Clin Invest.* (2018) 128:1903–12. doi: 10.1172/JCI98463

43. Lin Z, Kuroki K, Kuse N, Sun X, Akahoshi T, Qi Y, et al. HIV-1 control by NK Cells via reduced interaction between KIR2DL2 and HLA-C*12:02/C*14:03. *Cell Rep.* (2016) 17:2210–20. doi: 10.1016/j.celrep.2016.10.075

44. Mori M, Leitman E, Walker B, Ndung'u T, Carrington M, Goulder P. Impact of HLA Allele-KIR Pairs on HIV Clinical Outcome in South Africa. *J Infect. Dis.* (2018) 219:1456–63. doi: 10.1093/infdis/jiy692

45. Sambrook JG, Bashirova A, Palmer S, Sims S, Trowsdale J, Abi-Rached L, et al. Single haplotype analysis demonstrates rapid evolution of the killer immunoglobulin-like receptor (KIR) loci in primates. *Genome Res.* (2005) 15:25–35. doi: 10.1101/gr.2381205

46. Albrecht C, Malzahn D, Brameier M, Hermes M, Ansari AA, Walter L. Progression to AIDS in SIV-infected rhesus macaques is associated with distinct KIR and MHC class I polymorphisms and NK cell dysfunction. *Front. Immunol.* (2014) 5:600. doi: 10.3389/fimmu.2014.00600

47. Walter L, Ansari AA. MHC and KIR polymorphisms in rhesus macaque SIV infection. *Front Immunol.* (2015) 6:163–7. doi: 10.3389/fimmu.2015.00540

48. Hellmann I, Letvin NL, Schmitz JE. KIR2DL4 copy number variation is associated with CD4+ T-cell depletion and function of cytokine-producing NK cell subsets in SIV-infected Mamu-A*01-negative rhesus macaques. *J Virol.* (2013) 87:5305–10. doi: 10.1128/JVI.02949-12

49. Ries M, Reynolds MR, Bashkueva K, Crosno K, Capuano S, Prall TM, et al. KIR3DL01 upregulation on gut natural killer cells in response to SIV infection of KIR- and MHC class I-defined rhesus macaques. *PLoS Pathog.* (2017) 13:e1006506. doi: 10.1371/journal.ppat.1006506

50. Alter G, Heckerman D, Schneidewind A, Fadda L, Kadie CM, Carlson JM, et al. HIV-1 adaptation to NK-cell-mediated immune pressure. *Nature.* (2011) 476:96–100. doi: 10.1038/nature10237

51. Hölzemer A, Thobakgale CF, Cruz CAJ, Garcia-Beltran WF, Carlson JM, van Teijlingen NH, et al. Selection of an HLA-C*03:04-Restricted HIV-1 p24 gag sequence variant is associated with viral escape from KIR2DL3+ natural killer cells: data from an observational cohort in South Africa. *PLoS Med.* (2015) 12:e1001900. doi: 10.1371/journal.pmed.1001900

52. Goonetilleke N, Liu MK, Salazar-Gonzalez JF, Ferrari G, Giorgi E, Ganusov VV, et al. The first T cell response to transmitted/founder virus contributes to the control of acute viremia in HIV-1 infection. *J Exp Med.* (2009) 206:1253–72. doi: 10.1084/jem.20090365

53. Ferrari G, Korber B, Goonetilleke N, Liu MK, Turnbull EL, Salazar-Gonzalez JF, et al. Relationship between functional profile of HIV-1 specific CD8 T cells and epitope variability with the selection of escape mutants in acute HIV-1 infection. *PLoS Pathog.* (2011) 7:e1001273. doi: 10.1371/journal.ppat.1001273

54. Bimber BN, Evans DT. The killer-cell immunoglobulin-like receptors of macaques. *Immunol Rev.* (2015) 267:246–58. doi: 10.1111/imr.12329

55. Hershberger KL, Shyam R, Miura A, Letvin NL. Diversity of the killer cell Ig-like receptors of rhesus monkeys. *J Immunol.* (2001) 166:4380–90. doi: 10.4049/jimmunol.166.7.4380

56. LaBonte ML, Hershberger KL, Korber B, Letvin NL. The KIR and CD94/NKG2 families of molecules in the rhesus monkey. *Immunol Rev.* (2001) 183:25–40. doi: 10.1034/j.1600-065x.2001.1830103.x

57. Bruijnesteijn J, van der Wiel MKH, Swelsen WTN, Otting N, de Vos-Rouweler AJM, Elferink D, et al. Human and rhesus macaque KIR haplotypes defined by their transcriptomes. *J Immunol.* (2018) 200:1692–1701. doi: 10.4049/jimmunol.1701480

58. Moreland AJ, Guethlein LA, Reeves RK, Broman KW, Johnson RP, Parham P, et al. Characterization of killer immunoglobulin-like receptor genetics and comprehensive genotyping by pyrosequencing in rhesus macaques. *BMC Genomics.* (2011) 12:295. doi: 10.1186/1471-2164-12-295

59. Blokhuis JH, van der Wiel MK, Doxiadis GGM, Bontrop RE. The mosaic of KIR haplotypes in rhesus macaques. *Immunogenetics.* 62:295–306. doi: 10.1007/s00251-010-0434-3

60. Maloveste SM, Chen D, Gostick E, Vivian JP, Plishka RJ, Iyengar R, et al. Degenerate recognition of MHC class I molecules with Bw4 and Bw6 motifs by a killer cell Ig-like receptor 3DL expressed by macaque NK cells. *J Immunol.* (2012) 189:4338–48. doi: 10.4049/jimmunol.1201360

61. Boyson JE, Shufflebotham C, Cadavid LF, Urvater JA, Knapp LA, Hughes AL, et al. The MHC class I genes of the rhesus monkey. different evolutionary histories of MHC class I and II genes in primates. *J Immunol.* (1996) 156:4656–65.

62. Kaur G, Gras S, Mobbs JI, Vivian JP, Cortes A, Barber T, et al. Structural and regulatory diversity shape HLA-C protein expression levels. *Nat Commun.* (2017) 8:15924. doi: 10.1038/ncomms15924

63. Blokhuis JH, van der Wiel MK, Doxiadis GGM, Bontrop RE. The extreme plasticity of killer cell Ig-like receptor (KIR) haplotypes differentiates rhesus macaques from humans. *Eur J Immunol.* (2011) 41:2719–28. doi: 10.1002/eji.201141621

64. Robinson J, Mistry K, McWilliam H, Lopez R, Marsh SGE. IPD—the immuno polymorphism database. *Nucleic Acids Res.* (2010) 38(suppl 1):D863–9. doi: 10.1093/nar/gkp879

65. Gomez-Roman VR, Patterson LJ, Venzon D, Liewehr D, Aldrich K, Florese R, et al. Vaccine-elicited antibodies mediate antibody-dependent cellular cytotoxicity correlated with significantly reduced acute viremia in rhesus macaques challenged with SIVmac251. *J Immunol.* (2005) 174:2185–9. doi: 10.4049/jimmunol.174.4.2185

66. Patterson LJ, Beal J, Demberg T, Florese RH, Malkevich N, Venzon D, et al. Replicating adenovirus HIV/SIV recombinant priming alone or in combination with a gp140 protein boost results in significant control of viremia following a SHIV89.6P challenge in Mamu-A*01 negative rhesus macaques. *Virology.* (2008) 374:322–37. doi: 10.1016/j.virol.2007.12.037

67. Alpert MD, Harvey JD, Lauer WA, Reeves RK, Piatak M Jr, Carville A, et al. ADCC develops over time during persistent infection with live-attenuated SIV and is associated with complete protection against SIV(mac)251 challenge. *PLoS Pathog.* (2012) 8:e1002890. doi: 10.1371/journal.ppat.1002890

68. Lambotte O, Pollara J, Boufassa F, Moog C, Venet A, Haynes BF, et al. High antibody-dependent cellular cytotoxicity responses are correlated with strong CD8 T cell viral suppressive activity but not with B57 status in HIV-1 elite controllers. *PLoS ONE.* (2013) 8:e74855. doi: 10.1371/journal.pone.0074855

69. Bradley T, Pollara J, Santra S, Vandergrift N, Pittala S, Bailey-Kellogg C, et al. Pentavalent HIV-1 vaccine protects against simian-human immunodeficiency virus challenge. *Nat Commun.* (2017) 8:15711. doi: 10.1038/ncomms15711

70. Mabuka J, Nduati R, Odem-Davis K, Peterson D, Overbaugh J. HIV-specific antibodies capable of ADCC are common in breastmilk and are associated with reduced risk of transmission in women with high viral loads. *PLoS Pathog.* (2012) 8:e1002739. doi: 10.1371/journal.ppat.1002739

71. Ronen K, Dingens AS, Graham SM, Jaoko W, Mandaliya K, McClelland RS, et al. Comprehensive characterization of humoral correlates of human immunodeficiency virus 1 superinfection acquisition in high-risk kenyan women. *EBioMed.* (2017) 18:216–24. doi: 10.1016/j.ebiom.2017.04.005

72. Haynes BF, Gilbert PB, McElrath MJ, Zolla-Pazner S, Tomaras GD, Alam SM, et al. Immune-correlates analysis of an HIV-1 vaccine efficacy trial. *N Engl J Med.* (2012) 366:1275–86. doi: 10.1056/NEJMoa1113425

73. Tomaras GD, Ferrari G, Shen X, Alam SM, Liao HX, Pollara J, et al. Vaccine-induced plasma IgA specific for the C1 region of the HIV-1 envelope blocks binding and effector function of IgG. *Proc Natl Acad Sci USA.* (2013) 110:9019–24. doi: 10.1073/pnas.1301456110

74. Pollara J, Bonsignori M, Moody MA, Pazgier M, Haynes BF, Ferrari G. Epitope specificity of human immunodeficiency virus-1 antibody dependent cellular cytotoxicity [ADCC] responses. *Curr HIV Res.* (2013) 11:378–87. doi: 10.2174/1570162X113116660059

75. Ramesh A, Darko S, Hua A, Overman G, Ransier A, Francica JR, et al. Structure and diversity of the rhesus macaque immunoglobulin loci through multiple de novo genome assemblies. *Front Immunol.* (2017) 8:1407. doi: 10.3389/fimmu.2017.01407

76. Cocklin SL, Schmitz JE. The role of Fc receptors in HIV infection and vaccine efficacy. *Curr Opin HIV AIDS.* (2014) 9:257–62. doi: 10.1097/COH.0000000000000051

77. Boesch AW, Osei-Owusu NY, Crowley AR, Chu TH, Chan YN, Weiner JA, et al. Biophysical and functional characterization of rhesus macaque IgG subclasses. *Front Immunol.* (2016) 7:589. doi: 10.3389/fimmu.2016.00589

78. Parsons MS, Richard J, Lee WS, Vanderven H, Grant MD, Finzi A, et al. NKG2D Acts as a co-receptor for natural killer cell-mediated anti-HIV-1 antibody-dependent cellular cytotoxicity. *AIDS Res Hum Retroviruses.* (2016) 32:1089–96. doi: 10.1089/aid.2016.0099

79. Vargas-Inchaustegui DA, Demberg T, Robert-Guroff M. A CD8alpha subpopulation of macaque circulatory natural killer cells can mediate both antibody-dependent and antibody-independent cytotoxic activities. *Immunology.* (2011) 134:326–40. doi: 10.1111/j.1365-2567.2011.03493.x

80. Lugthart G, Melsen JE, Vervat C, van Ostaijen-Ten Dam MM, Corver WE, Roelen DL, et al. Human lymphoid tissues harbor a distinct CD69+CXCR6+ NK cell population. *J Immunol.* (2016) 197:78–84. doi: 10.4049/jimmunol.1502603

81. Bernardini G, Sciume G, Santoni A. Differential chemotactic receptor requirements for NK cell subset trafficking into bone marrow. *Front Immunol.* (2013) 4:12. doi: 10.3389/fimmu.2013.00012

82. Carrega P, Bonaccorsi I, Di Carlo E, Morandi B, Paul P, Rizzello V, et al. CD56(bright)perforin(low) noncytotoxic human NK cells are abundant in both healthy and neoplastic solid tissues and recirculate to secondary lymphoid organs via afferent lymph. *J Immunol.* (2014) 192:3805–15. doi: 10.4049/jimmunol.1301889

83. Hudspeth K, Donadon M, Cimino M, Pontarini E, Tentorio P, Preti M, et al. Human liver-resident CD56(bright)/CD16(neg) NK cells are retained within hepatic sinusoids via the engagement of CCR5 and CXCR6 pathways. *J Autoimmun.* (2016) 66:40–50. doi: 10.1016/j.jaut.2015.08.011

84. Cichocki F, Sitnicka E, Bryceson YT. NK cell development and function-plasticity and redundancy unleashed. *Semin Immunol.* (2014) 26:114–26. doi: 10.1016/j.smim.2014.02.003

85. Ferlazzo G, Thomas D, Lin SL, Goodman K, Morandi B, Muller WA, et al. The abundant NK cells in human secondary lymphoid tissues require activation to express killer cell Ig-like receptors and become cytolytic. *J Immunol.* (2004) 172:1455–62. doi: 10.4049/jimmunol.172.3.1455

86. Freud AG, Becknell B, Roychowdhury S, Mao HC, Ferketich AK, Nuovo GJ, et al. A human CD34(+) subset resides in lymph nodes and differentiates into CD56bright natural killer cells. *Immunity.* (2005) 22:295–304. doi: 10.1016/j.immuni.2005.01.013

87. Chinen H, Matsuoka K, Sato T, Kamada N, Okamoto S, Hisamatsu T, et al. Lamina propria c-kit+ immune precursors reside in human adult intestine and differentiate into natural killer cells. *Gastroenterology.* (2007) 133:559–73. doi: 10.1053/j.gastro.2007.05.017

88. Alter G, Teigen N, Davis BT, Addo MM, Suscovich TJ, Waring MT, et al. Sequential deregulation of NK cell subset distribution and function starting in acute HIV-1 infection. *Blood.* (2005) 106:3366–9. doi: 10.1182/blood-2005-03-1100

89. Sirianni MC, Tagliaferri F, Aiuti F. Pathogenesis of the natural killer cell deficiency in AIDS. *Immunol Today.* (1990) 11:81–2. doi: 10.1016/0167-5699(90)90032-5

90. Tyler DS, Stanley SD, Nastala CA, Austin AA, Bartlett JA, Stine KC, et al. Alterations in antibody-dependent cellular cytotoxicity during the course of HIV-1 infection. humoral and cellular defects. *J Immunol.* (1990) 144:3375–84.

91. Eger KA, Unutmaz D. Perturbation of natural killer cell function and receptors during HIV infection. *Trends Microbiol.* (2004) 12:301–3. doi: 10.1016/j.tim.2004.05.006

92. Zulu MZ, Naidoo KK, Mncube Z, Jaggernath M, Goulder PJR, Ndung'u T, et al. Reduced expression of siglec-7, NKG2A, and CD57 on terminally differentiated CD56-CD16+ natural killer cell subset is associated with natural killer cell dysfunction in chronic HIV-1 clade C infection. *AIDS Res Hum Retroviruses.* (2017) 33:1205–13. doi: 10.1089/aid.2017.0095

93. Castriconi R, Cantoni C, Della Chiesa M, Vitale M, Marcenaro E, Conte R, et al. Transforming growth factor beta 1 inhibits expression of NKp30 and NKG2D receptors: consequences for the NK-mediated killing of dendritic cells. *Proc Natl Acad Sci USA.* (2003) 100:4120–5. doi: 10.1073/pnas.0730640100

94. Porichis F, Hart MG, Massa A, Everett HL, Morou A, Richard J, et al. Immune checkpoint blockade restores HIV-specific CD4 T cell help for NK cells. *J Immunol.* (2018) 201:971–81. doi: 10.4049/jimmunol.1701551

95. Meier UC, Owen RE, Taylor E, Worth A, Naoumov N, Willberg C, et al. Shared alterations in NK cell frequency, phenotype, and function in chronic human immunodeficiency virus and hepatitis C virus infections. *J Virol.* (2005) 79:12365–74. doi: 10.1128/JVI.79.19.12365-12374.2005

96. LaBonte ML, McKay PF, Letvin NL. Evidence of NK cell dysfunction in SIV-infected rhesus monkeys: impairment of cytokine secretion and NKG2C/C2 expression. *Eur J Immunol.* (2006) 36:2424–33. doi: 10.1002/eji.200635901

97. Li H, Evans TI, Reeves RK. Loss of bone marrow NK cells during SIV infection is associated with increased turnover rates and cytotoxicity but not changes in trafficking. *J Med Primatol.* (2013) 42:230–6. doi: 10.1111/jmp.12063

98. Vargas-Inchaustegui DA, Helmold Hait S, Chung HK, Narola J, Hoang T, Robert-Guroff M. Phenotypic and functional characterization of circulatory, splenic, and hepatic NK cells in simian immunodeficiency virus-controlling macaques. *J Immunol.* (2017) 199:3202–11. doi: 10.4049/jimmunol.1700586

99. Huot N, Jacquelin B, Garcia-Tellez T, Rascle P, Ploquin MJ, Madec Y, et al. Natural killer cells migrate into and control simian immunodeficiency virus replication in lymph node follicles in African green monkeys. *Nat Med.* (2017) 23:1277–86. doi: 10.1038/nm.4421

100. Schmitz JE, Kuroda MJ, Santra S, Sasseville VG, Simon MA, Lifton MA, et al. Control of viremia in simian immunodeficiency virus infection by CD8+ lymphocytes. *Science.* (1999) 283:857–60. doi: 10.1126/science.283.5403.857

101. Choi EI, Reimann KA, Letvin NL. In Vivo natural killer cell depletion during primary simian immunodeficiency virus infection in rhesus monkeys. *J Virol.* (2008) 82:6758–61. doi: 10.1128/JVI.02277-07

102. Choi EI, Wang R, Peterson L, Letvin NL, Reimann KA. Use of an anti-CD16 antibody for *in vivo* depletion of natural killer cells in rhesus macaques. *Immunology.* (2008) 124:215–22. doi: 10.1111/j.1365-2567.2007.02757.x

103. Fehniger TA, Herbein G, Yu H, Para MI, Bernstein ZP, O'Brien WA, et al. Natural killer cells from HIV-1+ patients produce C-C chemokines and inhibit HIV-1 infection. *J Immunol.* (1998) 161:6433–8.

104. Takahashi Y, Mayne AE, Khowawisetsut L, Pattanapanyasat K, Little D, Villinger F, et al. In Vivo administration of a JAK3 inhibitor to chronically SIV infected rhesus macaques leads to NK cell depletion associated with transient modest increase in viral loads. *PLoS ONE.* (2013) 8:e70992–10. doi: 10.1371/journal.pone.0070992

105. Takahashi Y, Byrareddy SN, Albrecht C, Brameier M, Walter L, Mayne AE, et al. In vivo administration of a JAK3 inhibitor during acute SIV infection leads to significant increases in viral load during chronic infection. *PLoS Pathog.* (2014) 10:e1003929. doi: 10.1371/journal.ppat.1003929

106. DeGottardi MQ, Okoye AA, Vaidya M, Talla A, Konfe AL, Reyes MD, et al. Effect of Anti-IL-15 administration on T Cell and NK cell homeostasis in rhesus macaques. *J Immunol.* (2016) 197:1183–98. doi: 10.4049/jimmunol.1600065

107. Boehncke WH, Schon MP, Girolomoni G, Griffiths C, Bos JD, Thestrup-Pedersen K, et al. Leukocyte extravasation as a target for anti-inflammatory therapy - which molecule to choose? *Exp Dermatol.* (2005) 14:70–80. doi: 10.1111/j.0906-6705.2005.290a.x

108. O'Leary JG, Goodarzi M, Drayton DL, von Andrian UH. T cell- and B cell-independent adaptive immunity mediated by natural killer cells. *Nat Immunol.* (2006) 7:507–16. doi: 10.1038/ni1332

109. Paust S, Gill HS, Wang BZ, Flynn MP, Moseman EA, Senman B, et al. Critical role for the chemokine receptor CXCR6 in NK cell-mediated antigen-specific memory of haptens and viruses. *Nat Immunol.* (2010) 11:1127–35. doi: 10.1038/ni.1953

110. Rapp M, Wiedemann GM, Sun JC. Memory responses of innate lymphocytes and parallels with T cells. *Sem Immunopathol.* (2018) 40:343–55. doi: 10.1007/s00281-018-0686-9

111. Paust S, Blish CA, Reeves RK. Redefining memory: building the case for adaptive NK cells. *J Virol.* (2017) 91:e00169–17. doi: 10.1128/JVI.00169-17

112. Peng H, Jiang X, Chen Y, Sojka DK, Wei H, Gao X, et al. Liver-resident NK cells confer adaptive immunity in skin-contact inflammation. *J Clin Invest.* (2013) 123:1444–56. doi: 10.1172/JCI66381

113. Kielczewska A, Pyzik M, Sun T, Krmpotic A, Lodoen MB, Munks MW, et al. Ly49P recognition of cytomegalovirus-infected cells expressing H2-Dk and CMV-encoded m04 correlates with the NK cell antiviral response. *J Exp Med.* (2009) 206:515–23. doi: 10.1084/jem.20080954

114. Scalzo AA, Manzur M, Forbes CA, Brown MG, Shellam GR. NK gene complex haplotype variability and host resistance alleles to murine cytomegalovirus in wild mouse populations. *Immunol Cell Biol.* (2005) 83:144–9. doi: 10.1111/j.1440-1711.2005.01311.x

115. Rolle A, Meyer M, Calderazzo S, Jager D, Momburg F. Distinct HLA-E peptide complexes modify antibody-driven effector functions of adaptive NK cells. *Cell Rep.* (2018) 24:1967–76 e4. doi: 10.1016/j.celrep.2018.07.069

116. Venkatasubramanian S, Cheekatla S, Paidipally P, Tripathi D, Welch E, Tvinnereim AR, et al. IL-21-dependent expansion of memory-like NK cells enhances protective immune responses against *Mycobacterium tuberculosis.* *Mucosal Immunol.* (2017) 10:1031–42. doi: 10.1038/mi.2016.105

117. Gillard GO, Bivas-Benita M, Hovav AH, Grandpre LE, Panas MW, Seaman MS, et al. Thy1+ NK [corrected] cells from vaccinia virus-primed mice confer protection against vaccinia virus challenge in the absence of adaptive lymphocytes. *PLoS Pathog.* (2011) 7:e1002141. doi: 10.1371/annotation/b29086ef-e08d-444c-8113-18a6dd429a7c

118. Cooper MA, Yokoyama WM. Memory-like responses of natural killer cells. *Immunol Rev.* (2010) 235:297–305. doi: 10.1111/j.0105-2896.2010.00891.x

119. Goodier MR, Rodriguez-Galan A, Lusa C, Nielsen CM, Darboe A, Moldoveanu AL, et al. Influenza vaccination generates cytokine-induced memory-like NK cells: impact of human cytomegalovirus infection. *J Immunol.* (2016) 197:313–25. doi: 10.4049/jimmunol.1502049

120. Romee R, Rosario M, Berrien-Elliott MM, Wagner JA, Jewell BA, Schappe T, et al. Cytokine-induced memory-like natural killer cells exhibit enhanced responses against myeloid leukemia. *Sci Transl Med.* (2016) 8:357ra123. doi: 10.1126/scitranslmed.aaf2341

121. Ni J, Holsken O, Miller M, Hammer Q, Luetke-Eversloh M, Romagnani C, et al. Adoptively transferred natural killer cells maintain long-term antitumor activity by epigenetic imprinting and CD4(+) T cell help. *Oncoimmunology.* (2016) 5:e1219009. doi: 10.1080/2162402X.2016.1219009

122. Pal M, Schwab L, Yermakova A, Mace EM, Claus R, Krahl AC, et al. Tumor-priming converts NK cells to memory-like NK cells. *Oncoimmunology.* (2017) 6:e1317411. doi: 10.1080/2162402X.2017.1317411

123. Hwang I, Zhang T, Scott JM, Kim AR, Lee T, Kakarla T, et al. Identification of human NK cells that are deficient for signaling adaptor FcRgamma and specialized for antibody-dependent immune functions. *Int Immunol.* (2012) 24:793–802. doi: 10.1093/intimm/dxs080

124. Zhang T, Scott JM, Hwang I, Kim S. Cutting edge: antibody-dependent memory-like NK cells distinguished by FcRgamma deficiency. *J Immunol.* (2013) 190:1402–6. doi: 10.4049/jimmunol.1203034

125. Lee J, Zhang T, Hwang I, Kim A, Nitschke L, Kim M, et al. Epigenetic modification and antibody-dependent expansion of memory-like NK cells in human cytomegalovirus-infected individuals. *Immunity.* (2015) 42:431–42. doi: 10.1016/j.immuni.2015.02.013

126. Schlums H, Cichocki F, Tesi B, Theorell J, Beziat V, Holmes TD, et al. Cytomegalovirus infection drives adaptive epigenetic diversification of NK cells with altered signaling and effector function. *Immunity.* (2015) 42:443–56. doi: 10.1016/j.immuni.2015.02.008

127. Shah SV, Manickam C, Ram DR, Kroll K, Itell H, Permar SR, et al. CMV primes functional alternative signaling in adaptive deltag NK cells but is subverted by lentivirus infection in rhesus macaques. *Cell Rep.* (2018) 25:2766–74 e3. doi: 10.1016/j.celrep.2018.11.020

128. Zhou J, Amran FS, Kramski M, Angelovich TA, Elliott J, Hearps AC, et al. An NK cell population lacking FcRgamma is expanded in chronically infected HIV patients. *J Immunol.* (2015) 194:4688–97. doi: 10.4049/jimmunol.1402448

129. Peppa D, Pedroza-Pacheco I, Pellegrino P, Williams I, Maini MK, Borrow P. Adaptive reconfiguration of natural killer cells in HIV-1 infection. *Front Immunol.* (2018) 9:474. doi: 10.3389/fimmu.2018.00474

130. Oh JS, Ali AK, Kim S, Corsi DJ, Cooper CL, Lee SH. NK cells lacking FcepsilonRIgamma are associated with reduced liver damage in chronic hepatitis C virus infection. *Eur J Immunol.* (2016) 46:1020–9. doi: 10.1002/eji.201546009

131. Lunemann A, Vanoaica LD, Azzi T, Nadal D, Munz C. A distinct subpopulation of human NK cells restricts B cell transformation by EBV. *J Immunol.* (2013) 191:4989–95. doi: 10.4049/jimmunol.1301046

132. Hatton O, Strauss-Albee DM, Zhao NQ, Haggadone MD, Pelpola JS, Krams SM, et al. NKG2A-expressing natural killer cells dominate the response to autologous lymphoblastoid cells infected with Epstein-Barr virus. *Front Immunol.* (2016) 7:607. doi: 10.3389/fimmu.2016.00607

133. Jud A, Kotur M, Berger C, Gysin C, Nadal D, Lunemann A. Tonsillar CD56brightNKG2A+ NK cells restrict primary Epstein-Barr virus infection in B cells via IFN-gamma. *Oncotarget.* (2017) 8:6130–41. doi: 10.18632/oncotarget.14045

134. Brown MG, Dokun AO, Heusel JW, Smith HR, Beckman DL, Blattenberger EA, et al. Vital involvement of a natural killer cell activation receptor in resistance to viral infection. *Science.* (2001) 292:934–7. doi: 10.1126/science.1060042

135. Smith HR, Heusel JW, Mehta IK, Kim S, Dorner BG, Naidenko OV, et al. Recognition of a virus-encoded ligand by a natural killer cell activation receptor. *Proc Natl Acad Sci USA.* (2002) 99:8826–31. doi: 10.1073/pnas.092258599

136. Wight A, Mahmoud AB, Scur M, Tu MM, Rahim MMA, Sad S, et al. Critical role for the Ly49 family of class I MHC receptors in adaptive natural killer cell responses. *Proc Natl Acad Sci USA.* (2018) 115:11579–84. doi: 10.1073/pnas.1722374115

137. Hammer Q, Ruckert T, Borst EM, Dunst J, Haubner A, Durek P, et al. Peptide-specific recognition of human cytomegalovirus strains controls adaptive natural killer cells. *Nat Immunol.* (2018) 19:453–63. doi: 10.1038/s41590-018-0082-6

138. Colucci F, Di Santo JP, Leibson PJ. Natural killer cell activation in mice and men: different triggers for similar weapons? *Nat Immunol.* (2002) 3:807–13. doi: 10.1038/ni0902-807

139. Hammer Q, Romagnani C. About training and memory: NK-cell adaptation to viral infections. *Adv Immunol.* (2017) 133:171–207. doi: 10.1016/bs.ai.2016.10.001

140. Leeansyah E, Zhou J, Paukovics G, Lewin SR, Crowe SM, Jaworowski A. Decreased NK Cell FcRgamma in HIV-1 infected individuals receiving combination antiretroviral therapy: a cross sectional study. *PLoS ONE.* (2010) 5:e9643. doi: 10.1371/journal.pone.0009643

141. Peppa D. Natural killer cells in human immunodeficiency virus-1 infection: spotlight on the impact of human cytomegalovirus. *Front Immunol.* (2017) 8:1322. doi: 10.3389/fimmu.2017.01322

142. Guma M, Cabrera C, Erkizia I, Bofill M, Clotet B, Ruiz L, et al. Human cytomegalovirus infection is associated with increased proportions of NK cells that express the CD94/NKG2C receptor in aviremic HIV-1-positive patients. *J Infect Dis.* (2006) 194:38–41. doi: 10.1086/504719

143. Nattermann J, Nischalke HD, Hofmeister V, Kupfer B, Ahlenstiel G, Feldmann G, et al. HIV-1 infection leads to increased HLA-E expression resulting in impaired function of natural killer cells. *Antivir Ther.* (2005) 10:95–107.

Permissions

All chapters in this book were first published by Frontiers; hereby published with permission under the Creative Commons Attribution License or equivalent. Every chapter published in this book has been scrutinized by our experts. Their significance has been extensively debated. The topics covered herein carry significant findings which will fuel the growth of the discipline. They may even be implemented as practical applications or may be referred to as a beginning point for another development.

The contributors of this book come from diverse backgrounds, making this book a truly international effort. This book will bring forth new frontiers with its revolutionizing research information and detailed analysis of the nascent developments around the world.

We would like to thank all the contributing authors for lending their expertise to make the book truly unique. They have played a crucial role in the development of this book. Without their invaluable contributions this book wouldn't have been possible. They have made vital efforts to compile up to date information on the varied aspects of this subject to make this book a valuable addition to the collection of many professionals and students.

This book was conceptualized with the vision of imparting up-to-date information and advanced data in this field. To ensure the same, a matchless editorial board was set up. Every individual on the board went through rigorous rounds of assessment to prove their worth. After which they invested a large part of their time researching and compiling the most relevant data for our readers.

The editorial board has been involved in producing this book since its inception. They have spent rigorous hours researching and exploring the diverse topics which have resulted in the successful publishing of this book. They have passed on their knowledge of decades through this book. To expedite this challenging task, the publisher supported the team at every step. A small team of assistant editors was also appointed to further simplify the editing procedure and attain best results for the readers.

Apart from the editorial board, the designing team has also invested a significant amount of their time in understanding the subject and creating the most relevant covers. They scrutinized every image to scout for the most suitable representation of the subject and create an appropriate cover for the book.

The publishing team has been an ardent support to the editorial, designing and production team. Their endless efforts to recruit the best for this project, has resulted in the accomplishment of this book. They are a veteran in the field of academics and their pool of knowledge is as vast as their experience in printing. Their expertise and guidance has proved useful at every step. Their uncompromising quality standards have made this book an exceptional effort. Their encouragement from time to time has been an inspiration for everyone.

The publisher and the editorial board hope that this book will prove to be a valuable piece of knowledge for researchers, students, practitioners and scholars across the globe.

List of Contributors

Maria L. Visciano, Neelakshi Gohain, Rebekah Sherburn, Robin Flinko, Amir Dashti, William D. Tolbert and Marzena Pazgier
Division of Vaccine Research of Institute of Human Virology, University of Maryland School of Medicine, Baltimore, MD, United States

J. Sjef Verbeek, Sachiko Hirose and Hiroyuki Nishimura
Department of Biomedical Engineering, Toin University of Yokohama, Yokohama, Japan

Luc Lyonnet
Department of Hematology, Hopital de la Conception, INSERM CIC-1409, Assistance Publique-Hôpitaux Marseille (AP-HM), Marseille, France

Pascale Paul and Françoise Dignat-George
Department of Hematology, Hopital de la Conception, INSERM CIC-1409, Assistance Publique-Hôpitaux Marseille (AP-HM), Marseille, France
INSERM 1263, INRA, C2VN, Aix-Marseille Université (AMU), INSERM, Marseille, France

Pascal Pedini, Mathieu Pelardy and Agnes Basire
Établissement Français du Sang PACA-Corse 13005, Marseille, France

Jacques Chiaroni and Christophe Picard
Établissement Français du Sang PACA-Corse 13005, Marseille, France
"Biologie des Groupes Sanguins", UMR 7268 ADÉS Aix-Marseille Université/EFS/CNRS, Marseille, France

Julie Di Cristofaro
"Biologie des Groupes Sanguins", UMR 7268 ADÉS Aix-Marseille Université/EFS/CNRS, Marseille, France

Anderson Loundou
Département de santé Publique - EA 3279, Assistance Publique-Hôpitaux Marseille (AP-HM), Aix-Marseille Université, Marseille, France

Pascal Thomas
Service de Chirurgie Thoracique et Transplantation Pulmonaire, CHU Nord Assistance Publique-Hôpitaux Marseille (AP-HM), Aix-Marseille Université, Marseille, France

Leo Koenderman
Department of Respiratory Medicine and Laboratory of Translational Immunology, University Medical Center Utrecht, Utrecht Netherlands

Martine Reynaud-Gaubert
Service de Pneumologie et Transplantation Pulmonaire, CHU Nord Assistance Publique-Hôpitaux Marseille (AP-HM) - IHU Méditerranée Infection Aix-Marseille-Université, Marseille, France

Sanae Ben Mkaddem and Marc Benhamou
INSERM U1149, Centre de Recherche sur l'Inflammation, Paris, France
CNRS ERL8252, Paris, France
Faculté de Médecine, Université Paris Diderot, Sorbonne Paris Cité, Site Xavier Bichat, Paris, France, Inflamex Laboratory of Excellence, Paris, France

Renato C. Monteiro
INSERM U1149, Centre de Recherche sur l'Inflammation, Paris, France
CNRS ERL8252, Paris, France
Faculté de Médecine, Université Paris Diderot, Sorbonne Paris Cité, Site Xavier Bichat, Paris, France, Inflamex Laboratory of Excellence, Paris, France
Service d'Immunologie, DHU Fire, Hôpital Bichat-Claude Bernard, Assistance Publique de Paris, Paris, France

Krishanu Ray and Marzena Pazgier
Institute of Human Virology, University of Maryland School of Medicine, Baltimore, MD, United States
Department of Biochemistry and Molecular Biology, University of Maryland School of Medicine, Baltimore, MD, United States

Meron Mengistu and Anthony L. DeVico
Institute of Human Virology, University of Maryland School of Medicine, Baltimore, MD, United States
Department of Medicine, University of Maryland School of Medicine, Baltimore, MD, United States

George K. Lewis
Institute of Human Virology, University of Maryland School of Medicine, Baltimore, MD, United States
Department of Microbiology and Immunology, University of Maryland School of Medicine, Baltimore, MD, United States
Division of Vaccine Research of Institute of Human Virology, University of Maryland School of Medicine, Baltimore, MD, United States

Alicia M. Chenoweth
Centre for Biomedical Research, Burnet Institute, Melbourne, VIC, Australia
Department of Immunology and Pathology, Central Clinical School, Monash University, Melbourne, VIC, Australia

Bruce D. Wines and P. Mark Hogarth
Centre for Biomedical Research, Burnet Institute, Melbourne, VIC, Australia
Department of Immunology and Pathology, Central Clinical School, Monash University, Melbourne, VIC, Australia
Department of Pathology, The University of Melbourne, Melbourne, VIC, Australia

Tatjana Srdic-Rajic
Department of Experimental Pharmacology, National Cancer Research Center, Belgrade, Serbia

Heinz Kohler
Department of Microbiology and Immunology, University of Kentucky, Lexington, KY, United States

Vladimir Jurisic
Faculties of Medicinal Science, University of Kragujevac, Kragujevac, Serbia

Radmila Metlas
Vinča Institute of Nuclear Science, University of Belgrade Serbia

Kashyap R. Patel, Jacob T. Roberts and Adam W. Barb
Roy J. Carver Department of Biochemistry, Biophysics, and Molecular Biology, Iowa State University, Ames, IA, United States

Ingrid Teige, Linda Mårtensson and Björn L. Frendéus
BioInvent, Lund, Sweden

Louise W. Treffers , Michel van Houdt, Christine W. Bruggeman, Xi Wen Zhao, Joris van der Heijden, Paul J. J. H. Verkuijlen, Judy Geissler, Suzanne Lissenberg-Thunnissen, Katka Franke, Robin van Bruggen, Gestur Vidarsson and Hanke L. Matlung
Sanquin Research, and Landsteiner Laboratory, Amsterdam UMC, University of Amsterdam, Amsterdam, Netherlands

Timo K. van den Berg
Sanquin Research, and Landsteiner Laboratory, Amsterdam UMC, University of Amsterdam, Amsterdam, Netherlands
Department of Molecular Cell Biology and Immunology, Amsterdam UMC, Amsterdam Infection and Immunity Institute, Vrije Universiteit Amsterdam, Amsterdam, Netherlands

Marieke H. Heineke and Marjolein van Egmond
Department of Molecular Cell Biology and Immunology, Amsterdam UMC, Amsterdam Infection and Immunity Institute, Vrije Universiteit Amsterdam, Amsterdam, Netherlands

Sietse Q. Nagelkerke and Taco W. Kuijpers
Sanquin Research, and Landsteiner Laboratory, Amsterdam UMC, University of Amsterdam, Amsterdam, Netherlands
Emma Children's Hospital, Amsterdam UMC, University of Amsterdam, Amsterdam, Netherlands

Thomas Valerius and Matthias Peipp
Division of Stem Cell Transplantation and Immunotherapy, Department of Internal Medicine II, Kiel University, Kiel, Germany

Ntando G. Phaahla, Bianca Da Costa Dias and Caroline T. Tiemessen
Centre for HIV and STIs, National Institute for Communicable Diseases, Johannesburg, South Africa
Faculty of Health Sciences, University of the Witwatersrand, Johannesburg, South Africa

Ria Lassaunière
Centre for HIV and STIs, National Institute for Communicable Diseases, Johannesburg, South Africa
Department of Virus and Microbiological Special Diagnostics, Statens Serum Institut, Copenhagen, Denmark

Ziyaad Waja and Neil A. Martinson
Perinatal HIV Research Unit, University of the Witwatersrand, Johannesburg, South Africa, MRC Soweto Matlosana Centre for HIV/AIDS and TB Research, Johannesburg, South Africa

Felicity Kendrick, Neil D. Evans and Michael J. Chappell
School of Engineering, University of Warwick, Coventry, United Kingdom

Oscar Berlanga and Stephen J. Harding
Department of Research and Development, The Binding Site Group Limited, Birmingham, United Kingdom

Khiyam Hussain, Joshua M. Sopp, Martin J. Glennie and Mark S. Cragg
Antibody and Vaccine Group, Centre for Cancer Immunology, Cancer Sciences, Faculty of Medicine, University of Southampton, Southampton, United Kingdom

Kate V. Latham and Jonathan C. Strefford
Cancer Genomics Group, Southampton Experimental Cancer Medicine Centre, Cancer Sciences Unit, Faculty of Medicine, University of Southampton, Southampton, United Kingdom

Tania F. Rowley, Pallavi Bhatta, John Sherington, Rona M. Cutler and David P. Humphreys
UCB Pharma, Slough, United Kingdom

Chiara Orlandi
Division of Vaccine Research of Institute of Human Virology, University of Maryland School of Medicine, Baltimore, MD, United States
Institute of Human Virology, University of Maryland School of Medicine, Baltimore, MD, United States
Department of Medicine, University of Maryland School of Medicine, Baltimore, MD, United States

Chantal E. Hargreaves
Antibody and Vaccine Group, Centre for Cancer Immunology, Cancer Sciences, Faculty of Medicine, University of Southampton, Southampton, United Kingdom
Nuffield Department of Medicine, John Radcliffe Hospital, University of Oxford, Oxford, United Kingdom
Cancer Genomics Group, Southampton Experimental Cancer Medicine Centre, Cancer Sciences Unit, Faculty of Medicine, University of Southampton, Southampton, United Kingdom

Hiromi Kubagawa, Andreas Radbruch, Fritz Melchers and Peter K. Jani
Deutsches Rheuma - Forschungszentrum, Berlin, Germany

Kazuhito Honjo
Department of Medicine, School of Medicine, University of Alabama at Birmingham, Birmingham, AL, United States

Naganari Ohkura and Shimon Sakaguchi
Immunology Frontier Research Center, Osaka University, Osaka, Japan

Jacques Fellay
Precision Medicine Unit, Lausanne University Hospital and University of Lausanne, Lausanne, Switzerland
U. S. Military HIV Research Program, Walter Reed Army Institute of Research, Silver Spring, MD, United States

Daniel E. Geraghty
Clinical Research Division, Fred Hutchinson Cancer Research Center, Seattle, WA, United States

Christian W. Thorball
School of Life Sciences, École Polytechnique Fédérale de Lausanne, Lausanne, Switzerland

Rasmi Thomas
U. S. Military HIV Research Program, Walter Reed Army Institute of Research, Silver Spring, MD, United States
Henry M. Jackson Foundation for the Advancement of Military Medicine, Bethesda, MD, United States

Matthew L. Goodwin
Duke Human Vaccine Institute, Duke University Medical Center, Durham, NC, United States

Sallie R. Permar
Duke Human Vaccine Institute, Duke University Medical Center, Durham, NC, United States
Department of Pediatrics, Children's Health and Discovery Institute, Durham, NC, United States Herpesvirus

Cordelia Manickam and Spandan V. Shah
Center for Virology and Vaccine Research, Beth Israel Deaconess Medical Center, Harvard Medical School, Boston, MA, United States

Junsuke Nohara and Guido Ferrari
Department of Surgery, Duke University School of Medicine, Durham, NC, United States

R. Keith Reeves
Center for Virology and Vaccine Research, Beth Israel Deaconess Medical Center, Harvard Medical School, Boston, MA, United States
Ragon Institute of Massachusetts General Hospital, MIT, and Harvard, Cambridge, MA, United States

Index

Printed in the USA
CPSIA information can be obtained
at www.ICGtesting.com
JSHW051413091023
49903JS00006B/398